The Cognitive and Neural Bases of Spatial Neglect

Oxford Medical Publications

The Cognitive and Neural Bases of Spatial Neglect

Edited by

Hans-Otto Karnath

Department of Cognitive Neurology
University of Tübingen
Germany

A. David Milner

Department of Psychology
University of Durham
UK

and

Giuseppe Vallar

Department of Psychology
University of Milan-Bicocca
Italy

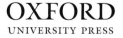

OXFORD
UNIVERSITY PRESS

OXFORD
UNIVERSITY PRESS

Great Clarendon Street, Oxford OX2 6DP

Oxford University Press is a department of the University of Oxford.
It furthers the University's objective of excellence in research, scholarship,
and education by publishing worldwide in

Oxford New York

Auckland Bangkok Buenos Aires Cape Town Chennai
Dar es Salaam Delhi Hong Kong Istanbul Karachi Kolkata
Kuala Lumpur Madrid Melbourne Mexico City Mumbai Nairobi
São Paulo Shanghai Taipei Tokyo Toronto

Oxford is a registered trade mark of Oxford University Press
in the UK and in certain other countries

Published in the United States
by Oxford University Press Inc., New York

A catalogue record for this title is available from the British Library

Library of Congress Cataloging in Publication Data
(Data available)

ISBN 0 19 850833 6 (Hbk)

10 9 8 7 6 5 4 3 2 1

Typeset by Newgen Imaging Systems (P) Ltd., Chennai, India
Printed in Great Britain on acid-free paper by
T.J. International Ltd, Padstow, Cornwall

Preface

Research on unilateral spatial neglect and related disorders has developed rapidly over the past 30 years. What is so interesting about this neurological disorder that has motivated so many studies, not only by investigators within clinical neurology, but also by scientists in many other disciplines including cognitive psychology, neurophysiology, and even philosophy? First, spatial neglect is a very intriguing and amazing clinical phenomenon in its own right, and one that immediately arouses fascination when observed for the first time on a neurological ward. It seems unbelievable that patients, although not blind to the side opposite to the damaged hemisphere, do not react or respond to persons or objects located in that side of space. But over and above studies devoted to a more in-depth understanding of unilateral neglect and to the development of diagnostic and rehabilitation procedures, the attention of an increasing number of researchers has been drawn to spatial neglect for more general reasons. The phenomena of neglect may greatly help our understanding of the normal mechanisms of directing and maintaining spatial attention, and of the anatomo-functional characteristics of representations of space. Furthermore, research in this field is highly relevant to the contemporary search for the cerebral correlates of conscious experience and voluntary action, and may ultimately offer a fuller understanding of the very nature of the integrated self and of personal identity.

This book presents many of the main facts and theories that guide contemporary research on spatial neglect and related disorders. While much of the work has been done in neuropsychological studies of patients with brain damage, major contributions have also been made in behavioral studies of animal models of the condition. In addition, relevant data have accrued from functional neurophysiology in animals and, increasingly, from functional neuroimaging in humans. An overview of this wide field of scientific endeavor is given, bringing together previous findings within an up-to-date synthesis of the most recent observations and results.

The text is divided into seven main sections. Section 1 provides a historical and clinical introduction to spatial neglect. Section 2 deals with the anatomical and neurophysiological bases of the disorder. Most neglect patients have large lesions which disable different brain systems, both cortical and subcortical. Attempts have been made to explore animal models, where more precisely localized lesions and single-cell responses can be studied.

Section 3 is devoted to the important issue of the different frameworks involved in spatial neglect. While neglect, by definition, affects the contralesional side of perceptual space, 'space' is itself an elusive concept. There is evidence, for example, that neglect is delineated differently in near and far peripersonal space, and that neglect patients not only misperceive objects in leftward parts of their egocentric space, but also misperceive the leftward parts of individual objects in any part of their visual space.

Section 4 gives prominence to perceptual and motor factors in neglect, and their interactions. Proposals have been made that neglect patients may experience subjective distortions in their visual perception of the world. The section discusses the various forms of such distortions, and the distinction, drawn by several authors, between 'perceptual' and 'premotor' aspects of unilateral neglect. The section also considers the role of defective visual processing in shaping some manifestations of neglect, as well as the use of visual illusions to tease apart preserved versus defective perceptual processes and to simulate some putative mechanisms underlying the disorder. Finally, the ability of neglect patients to navigate in three-dimensional space is reviewed.

Section 5 concerns the time-honored view that has conceptualized neglect as an attentional disorder, considering first the anatomo-functional basis of spatial attention. Indeed, selective attention to individual items within a visual or haptic array is a *sine qua non* for the efficient search of that array, and search deficits are arguably a central component of neglect. Extinction to double simultaneous stimulation is also observed in many patients with unilateral neglect, and this too is thought to be an attentional deficit.

Section 6 highlights the contribution of neglect and extinction to our understanding of the correspondence between stimulus processing and its conscious experience, of binding effects in vision, and of the impact of disturbed spatial working memory on neglect behavior. Furthermore, the relationships between putative primary sensory disorders and neglect are discussed.

Finally, Section 7 considers possible strategies which may be used to ameliorate spatial neglect in a more or less specific manner in order to shorten the period of necessary treatment, possibly enabling earlier discharge. On the basis of recently discovered mechanisms of visual, vestibular, and proprioceptive contributions to space perception, exciting new approaches to the rehabilitation of neglect patients have been developed.

We are grateful to all the contributors to this volume, whose combined expertise has allowed us to put together a comprehensive state-of-the-art overview of current knowledge about unilateral spatial neglect and related disorders. We are particularly delighted that the two greatest pioneering researchers in the field, Edoardo Bisiach (Lurago Marinone, Italy) and Kenneth H. Heilman (Gainesville, USA), whose work has provided the inspiration for much of the material to be found in these pages, have contributed chapters to the book. We respectfully dedicate the volume to them. We hope that readers will be as excited as we are by the fascinating clinical and experimental phenomena that are described here, and will themselves be stimulated to develop new ideas in their daily clinical work and in their own research in the future.

Hans-Otto Karnath

David Milner

Giuseppe Vallar

Tübingen, Durham, Milan, 2002

Acknowledgements

Most chapters in this book are based on papers presented at a conference, organized to take stock of the achievements made in the past 30 years in the field of unilateral neglect, held in the Villa Olmo of the Centro di Cultura Scientifica A. Volta, Como, Italy, in September 2000. The conference was funded by the European Commission (Research DG, Human Potential Programme, High-Level Scientific Conferences, HPCF-CT-1999-00029) and the European Brain and Behaviour Society. We are grateful to the staff of the Centro di Cultura Scientifica A. Volta, particularly Chiara Stefanetti, for their assistance in the organization of the meeting. Also, the conference would not have been possible without the tireless efforts of Dagmar Heller-Schmerold, Department of Cognitive Neurology, University of Tübingen, Germany, who was involved in many aspects of its organization and the administration of the European Commission grant. Finally, we would like to thank Richard Marley and Carol Maxwell, Oxford University Press, who have been extremely supportive and helpful throughout the whole period of editing this book.

Contents

List of Contributors

Britt Anderson Brain Science Program, Brown University, Providence RI, USA
Marlene Behrmann Department of Psychology, Carnegie Mellon University, Pittsburgh PA, USA
Anna Berti Department of Psychology, University of Turin, Turin, Italy
Alain Berthoz LPPA College de France, Paris, France
Edoardo Bisiach Lurago Marinone (Como), Italy
Verity J Brown School of Psychology, University of St Andrews, St Andrews, UK
Subhojit Chakraborty Department of Neurology, University of Pennsylvania, Philadelphia PA, USA
Anjan Chatterjee Department of Neurology, University of Pennsylvania, Philadelphia PA, USA
Maurizio Corbetta Department of Neurology, Washington University School of Medicine, St Louis MO, USA
Roberta Daini Department of Psychology, University of Milano-Bicocca, Milan, Italy
Fabrizio Doricchi Department of Psychology, University of Rome 'La Sapienzia', Rome, Italy
Jon Driver Institute of Cognitive Neuroscience, University College London, London, UK
Jean-Rene Duhamel Institut de Sciences Cognitives, CNRS, Bron, France
Patrizia Fattori Department of Human Physiology, University of Bologna, Bologna, Italy
Gaspare Galati Department of Psychology, University of Rome 'La Sapienza', Rome, Italy
Claudio Galletti Department of Human Physiology, University of Bologna, Bologna, Italy
Joy J Geng Department of Psychology, Carnegie Mellon University, Pittsburgh PA, USA
Barry Giesbrecht Center for Cognitive Neuroscience, Duke University, Durham NC, USA
Cecilia Guariglia Department of Psychology, University of Rome 'La Sapienza', Rome, Italy
Peter Halligan School of Psychology, Cardiff University, Cardiff, UK
Thomas Haarmeier Department of Neurology, University of Tübingen, Tübingen, Germany
Kenneth M Heilman Department of Neurology, University of Florida College of Medicine, Gainesville FL, USA
Glyn W Humphreys Behavioural Brain Sciences, School of Psychology, University of Birmingham, Birmingham, UK
Masud Husain Division of Neuroscience & Psychological Medicine, Charing Cross Hospital, London, UK
Giuseppe Iaria Department of Psychology, University of Rome 'La Sapienza', Rome, Italy
Sumio Ishiai Department of Rehabilitation, Tokyo Metropolitan Institute for Neuroscience, Tokyo, Japan
Hans-Otto Karnath Department of Cognitive Neurology, University of Tübingen, Tübingen, Germany
Michelle J Kincade Department of Psychology, Washington University School of Medicine, St Louis MO, USA
Elisabetta Làdavas CNC, Centro di Neuroscienze Cognitive, Cesena, University of Bologna, Bologna, Italy
Axel Lindner Department of Cognitive Neurology, University of Tübingen, Tübingen, Germany

Rob D McIntosh   Department of Psychology, University of Durham, Durham, UK

George R Mangun   Center for Mind Sciences, University of California, Davis CA, USA

Tom Manly   MRC, Cognitive and Brain Sciences Unit, Cambridge, UK

John C Marshall   University Department of Clinical Neurology, Radcliffe Infirmary, Oxford, UK

Carlo A Marzi   Dipartimento di Scienze Neurologiche e della Visione, University of Verona, Verona, Italy

Jason B Mattingley   Department of Psychology, School of Behavioural Science, University of Melbourne, Parkville, Victoria, Australia

M-Marsel Mesulam   Cognitive Neurology & Alzheimer's Disease Center, Northwestern University Medical School, Chicago IL, USA

A David Milner   Department of Psychology, University of Durham, Durham, UK

Elena Natale   Dipartimento di Scienze Neurologiche e della Visione, University of Verona, Verona, Italy

Marco Neppi-Modona   Department of Psychology, University of Turin, Turin, Italy

Matthias Niemeier   Department of Cognitive Neurology, University of Tübingen, Tübingen, Germany (now at Department of Physiology, University of Toronto, Canada)

Etienne Olivier   Institut de Sciences Cognitives, CNRS, Bron, France

Luigi Pizzamiglio   Department of Psychology, University of Rome 'La Sapienza', Rome, Italy

Raffaella Ricci   Department of Psychology, University of Turin, Turin, Italy

M Jane Riddoch   Behavioural Brain Sciences, School of Psychology, University of Birmingham, Edgbaston, UK

Giacomo Rizzolatti   Istituto di Fisiologia Umana, University of Parma, Parma, Italy

Ian H Robertson   Department of Psychology, Trinity College, University of Dublin, Dublin, Ireland

Gilles Rode   Espace et Action, INSERM Unité 534, Bron, France

Yves Rossetti   Espace et Action, INSERM Unité 534, Bron, France

Gordon Shulman   Department of Psychology, Washington University School of Medicine, St Louis MO, USA

Peter Thier   Department of Cognitive Neurology, University of Tübingen, Tübingen, Germany

Alexander Tikhonov   Department of Cognitive Neurology, University of Tübingen, Tübingen, Germany

Edward Valenstein   Department of Neurology, University of Florida College of Medicine, Gainesville FL, USA

Giuseppe Vallar   Department of Psychology, University of Milano-Bicocca, Milan, Italy

Claire Wardak   Institut de Sciences Cognitives, CNRS, Bron, France

Robert Watson   Department of Neurology, University of Florida College of Medicine, Gainesville FL, USA

Section 1 Historical introduction

1.1 Spatial neglect

Kenneth M. Heilman, Robert T. Watson, and Edward Valenstein

Neglect is the failure to report, respond, or orient to novel or meaningful stimuli presented to the side opposite a brain lesion, when this failure cannot be attributed to either elemental sensory or motor defects (Heilman 1979). Many subtypes or forms of neglect have been described. These are usually distinguished by their presumed underlying mechanism or the distribution of the aberrant behavior. The presumed mechanism may involve deficits in attention, action–intention, or representation. The distribution may be spatial or personal. Spatial neglect may occur in three reference frames: body centered (egocentric), environmentally centered, and object centered (allocentric). Spatial neglect may occur in all three axes of space (horizontal, vertical, radial). These forms of neglect (i.e. attentional, intentional, representational, personal, spatial) are not mutually exclusive and a patient may have one or more forms of neglect. Patients may exhibit different behavioral manifestations of neglect at different times, and some never demonstrate certain manifestations.

This chapter will be limited to a discussion of the history and mechanisms underlying spatial neglect. Because of space limitations, we shall not discuss testing for spatial neglect, ipsilateral spatial neglect, right-left asymmetries of neglect, recovery, rehabilitation and treatment of spatial neglect. Those who would like to read on these topics should consult other chapters in this book and Heilman *et al.* (2003). There are other manifestations of the neglect syndrome that we will not fully discuss here. These include: sensory and motor extinction, personal neglect or asomatognosia, allesthesia, allokinesia, anosognosia, anosodiaphoria and limb akinesia or motor neglect.

Description and history

When patients with spatial neglect are asked to perform a variety of tasks in space, they neglect the hemispace contralateral to their lesion. For example, when asked to draw a picture of a flower, they may fail to draw the petals on the contralesional half of the flower, and they may place the flower on the ipsilesional side of the page. When asked to bisect a line, they commonly make their mark toward the ipsilesional side of the line. When asked to cancel or cross out stimuli distributed across a page they may fail to cross out lines on the side of the page that is opposite their hemispheric injury. These patients appear to be neglecting a portion of contralateral space. Neglect may also occur in internal space. Denny-Brown and Banker (1954) described a patient who could not describe from memory the details of the side of a room opposite her cerebral lesion. Bisiach and Luzzatti (1978) also described patients with neglect who were unable to recall left-sided details of a famous square in Milan. Whereas neglect is most severe for contralesional space, many patients with unilateral cerebral lesions will also demonstrate a milder neglect for stimuli in ipsilesional space (Albert 1973; Heilman and Valenstein 1979; Weintraub and Mesulam 1987). There are even reports of neglect that is more severe in ipsilateral than contralateral space (Kwon and Heilman 1991; Kim *et al.* 1999). In addition to horizontal neglect, neglect of lower vertical space, upper vertical space, and radial space have been reported (Rapcsak *et al.* 1988; Shelton *et al.* 1990). Mark and Heilman (1998) demonstrated that many patients with spatial neglect have a combination of horizontal, vertical, and radial neglect. Halligan and Marshall (1991*a*) reported a patient who had horizontal neglect when the stimuli were near the body, but did not have neglect when the stimuli were placed far from the body. In contrast, Vuilleumier *et al.* (1998) reported a patient with a right temporal hematoma who had neglect in far space but no neglect in near space. Neglect may be viewer centered (egocentric), object centered (allocentric), or environmentally centered. Viewer-centered neglect may be defined in relation to the position of the trunk, the head, or the eyes.

Spatial neglect has been called by a variety of names, including visual–spatial agnosia, unilateral spatial agnosia (Duke-Elder 1949), unilateral visual inattention (Allen 1948), amorphosynthesis (Denny-Brown and Banker 1954), hemi-inattention (Weinstein and Friedland 1977), unilateral neglect (Hecean and Albert 1978), and hemispatial neglect (Heilman 1979). In this chapter we have elected to call this disorder spatial neglect because it is not an agnosia and because this term does not imply a specific mechanism. In addition, as we shall discuss, neglect is not always unilateral or limited to hemispace.

Several authors (Battersby *et al.* 1956; Gainotti *et al.* 1972) have attributed the original description of neglect to Holmes (1918), but Holmes actually reported six patients with disturbed visual orientation from bilateral lesions. Both Holmes (1918) and Poppelreuter (1917) often discussed disorders of attention, but these discussions primarily addressed the extinction phenomena. According to Halligan and Marshall (1993) the first description of this disorder may have been by Hughlings Jackson who in 1876 observed a patient with a right posterior temporal lesion who, when having his visual acuity tested with a Snellen visual acuity chart, '. . . began to read at the lower right corner and read backwards'. The patient also occasionally failed to read letters on the left side of words. In 1883 Anton reported four patients with right hemisphere lesions who neglected activities and objects in the left half of space. The first person to use the term neglect (*Vernachlässigung*) was probably Pineas (1931) who described a woman who was unaware of extrapersonal space after a right hemisphere lesion. Brain (1941) also described three patients who had visual disorientation limited to homonymous half-fields not caused by defects in visual acuity. There were two aspects of this visual disorientation: patients were impaired in localizing targets in contralateral space, but they were also 'agnosic' for the left side of space and acted as if that side of space was not present. Paterson and Zangwill (1944), McFie *et al.* (1950), and Denny-Brown and Banker (1954) demonstrated that patients with unilateral inattention (spatial neglect) not only had visual disorientation limited to a half-field but also omitted material on one side of drawings and failed to eat from one side of their plate.

Mechanisms underlying contralateral spatial neglect

Sensory deficits

Battersby *et al.* (1956) thought that neglect in humans resulted from decreased sensory input superimposed on a background of decreased mental function. Sprague *et al.* (1961) concluded that neglect was caused by loss of patterned sensory input to the forebrain, particularly to the neocortex. Eidelberg and Schwartz (1971) similarly proposed that neglect was a passive phenomenon due to quantitatively asymmetrical sensory input to the two hemispheres.

Although hemianopia may enhance the symptoms of spatial neglect, hemianopia by itself cannot entirely account for this deficit, because some patients with hemispatial neglect do not have hemianopia (McFie *et al.* 1950) and some patients with hemianopia do not demonstrate hemispatial neglect. Further evidence against the visual sensory postulate is that patients with visual spatial neglect may also have spatial neglect in other modalities such as auditory and tactile (Làdavas and Pavani 1998). In addition, whereas most sensory systems project primarily to the contralateral hemisphere the distribution of neglect is spatial and as mentioned above, neglect can be object (allocentric), environmentally, or viewer centered (egocentric).

Hemispatial deficits

Another argument against the sensory hypothesis is that spatial neglect is predominantly viewer centered (Heilman and Valenstein 1979) and is thus independent of the afferent pathways used to gain information about the environment. For example, the left side of objects may be neglected in either visual field, and tactile exploration or action in the left half of space may be impaired regardless of the hand used. The interruption of a sensory pathway or its cerebral terminus (deafferentation) could not account for this behavior. This observation also suggests that each hemisphere is organized not only to receive information from the contralateral visual field and arm but also to mediate awareness or action in the opposite hemispace (Heilman 1979; Bowers and Heilman 1980).

Hemispace is a complex construct which can be defined according to several frames of reference including eye position, head position, or trunk position. With the eyes and head facing directly ahead, the hemispaces defined by these three reference systems are congruent. In other situations, however, they may become incongruent. If the eyes are directed to the far right, for example, the left visual field falls in large part in the right hemispace, as defined by the head and body midline. Similarly, if the head and eyes are turned far to the right, left head and eye hemispace can both be in right body hemispace. There is evidence to suggest that both head and body hemispace are of importance in determining the symptoms of hemispatial neglect (Heilman and Valenstein 1979; Bowers and Heilman 1980).

Studies of normal people support the hypothesis that each hemisphere is organized to interact with stimuli in contralateral hemispace. If normal subjects fix their gaze at a midline object, keep their right arm in right hemispace and their left arm in left hemispace, and receive stimuli delivered to their right visual half-field, they will respond more rapidly with their right hand than with their left hand. Similarly, if stimuli are delivered to their left visual half-field, they will respond more rapidly with their left hand than with their right hand (Anzola *et al.* 1977). These results can be explained by an anatomical pathway transmission model: the reaction time is longer when the hand opposite the stimulated field responds because in this situation information must be transmitted between hemispheres, and this transmission takes more time than when information can remain intrahemsipheric. However, if the subject's hands are crossed so that the left hand is in right hemispace and the right hand is in left hemispace, the faster choice reaction times are made by the hand positioned in the same side of space as the stimulus (Anzola *et al.* 1977), even though in this situation the information must cross the corpus callosum. Clearly, a pathway transmission model cannot explain these crossed-arm results. Cognitive theorists have attributed this crossed-hand stimulus–response compatibility effect to a 'natural' tendency to respond to a lateralized stimulus with the hand that is in a corresponding spatial position (Craft and Simon 1970). Alternatively, each hemisphere may be important for preparing actions (intending) in the contralateral hemispatial field independent of which hand is used to respond (Heilman 1979; Heilman and Valenstein 1979). According to this hemispatial hypothesis, when each hand works in its own hemispace, the same hemisphere mediates both the sensorimotor system and the intentional system; however, when a hand works in the opposite hemispace, different hemispheres mediate the sensorimotor and intentional systems.

If the cerebral hemispheres are organized hemispatially, a similar compatibility may exist between the visual half-field in which a stimulus is presented and the side of hemispace in which the visual half-field is aligned. Our group (Bowers *et al.* 1981) has found a hemispace-visual half-field compatibility suggesting that each hemisphere may not only be important for intending (preparing action) in the contralateral hemispatial field, independent of hand, but may also be important for attending or perceiving stimuli in contralateral hemispace independent of the visual field to which these stimuli are presented.

According to this attentional-intentional spatial hypothesis, when each hand works in its own spatial field, the same hemisphere mediates both the sensorimotor systems and the attentional-intentional systems. When a hand operates in the opposite spatial field, however, the hemisphere contralateral to that hand controls the sensorimotor apparatus, whereas the hemisphere ipsilateral to the hand mediates spatial attention and intention. Under these conditions, the sensorimotor and attentional-intentional system must communicate through the corpus callosum. When patients with callosal disconnection bisect lines in opposite hemispace, each hand errs by gravitating toward its 'own' (compatible) hemispace (Heilman *et al.* 1984; Goldenberg 1986). These behavioral studies in humans, as well as microelectrode studies in alert monkeys (Lynch 1980), support the hypothesis that the brain is hemispatially organized. Each hemisphere mediates attention and intention in contralateral viewer-centered hemispace independent of the sensory hemifield or the extremity used.

To determine if patients with neglect have a body-centered hemispatial deficit, we required patients with left-sided neglect to identify a letter at either the right or left end of a line before bisecting the line. The task was given with the lines placed in either right, center, or left hemispace. Even when subjects were required to look to the left before bisecting a line, ensuring that they saw the entire line, performance was significantly better when the line was placed in the right hemispace than when it was in the left hemispace (Heilman and Valenstein 1979) These observations indicate that patients with spatial neglect have a hemispatial defect rather than a hemifield or hemanopic defect.

Several neuropsychological mechanisms have been hypothesized to account for this hemispatial deficit, including deficits in attention, intention, and representation. These will be discussed in the following sections.

Attentional hypothesis

It has often been said that everyone knows what attention is, but no one can fully define it. Perhaps this is because attention is a mental process rather than a thing. Brains have a limited capacity to process stimuli. Under many circumstances, the brain receives more afferent stimuli than it can possibly process. In addition to external stimuli, humans can activate internal representations. The processing of these internal representations may further tax a limited capacity system and reduce a person's ability to process afferent stimuli. Since organisms, including humans, have a limited processing capacity, they need a means to triage incoming information. Attention is the mental process that permits humans to triage afferent input.

Normally triage depends on the potential importance of the incoming information to the organism. Significance is determined by two major factors: goals or sets, and biological drives or needs. Stimuli that are important for a person's goals, sets, needs, or drives will be triaged at a higher level than irrelevant stimuli.

In order to triage stimuli, organisms must direct their attention to significant stimuli and away from irrelevant stimuli. There are at least two means to direct attention: by sensory modality, and by spatial location. One sensory modality may be attended over others. For example, visual information can be attended rather than information carried by touch or audition. Spatial location can be used to direct attention either between sensory modalities or within a sensory modality.

Some of the first references in the neglect syndrome literature referred to defects of attention. Poppelreuter (1917) introduced the word inattention. Brain (1941) and Critchley (1966) were also strong proponents of this view. However, Bender and Furlow (1944, 1945) challenged the attentional theory; they felt that inattention could not be important in the pathophysiology of the syndrome because neglect could not be overcome by having the patient 'concentrate' on the neglected side. After Bender and Furlow's papers there was little interest in the attentional hypothesis of neglect until about three decades ago when Kinsbourne (1970), Heilman and Valenstein (1972) and Watson *et al.* (1973, 1974) again postulated an attention-arousal hypothesis to account for neglect. These authors argued that the sensory and perceptual hypotheses could not explain all cases of neglect, since lesions outside the traditional sensory pathways often produced neglect. Evoked potential studies in animals with unilateral neglect have demonstrated a change in late waves (that are known to be influenced by changes in attention and stimulus significance) but not in the early (sensory) waves (Watson *et al.* 1977). Furthermore, neglect is often multimodal and therefore cannot be explained by a defect in any one sensory modality.

At least five attentional hypotheses have been proposed to explain spatial neglect:

(1) spatial unawareness or inattention;
(2) ipsilesional spatial attentional bias;
(3) extinction of simultaneous stimuli;
(4) inability to disengage from stimuli in ipsilesional space;
(5) reduced vigilance or premature habituation.

These five hypotheses are not necessarily mutually exclusive.

Spatial unawareness

The spatial unawareness or inattention hypothesis states that patients with, for example, left hemispatial neglect fail to act in left hemispace because they are unaware of stimuli in left hemispace. Alternatively, with less severe inattention they may be aware of stimuli in contralesional space but, because they are inattentive, stimuli in left hemispace may appear to have a reduced magnitude. In the cancellation task, for example, patients with neglect fail to cancel targets in left hemispace because they are unaware of them. In the line bisection task they are unaware of a portion of the left side of the line and only bisect the portion of line of which they are aware. Alternatively, because they are inattentive to the contralesional side of the line, this segment appears to be smaller than it actually is and they bisect the line to the right of center to create two segments that appear equal. There are several observations supporting this unawareness–inattention hypothesis. The severity of left-sided neglect may be decreased by instructions to attend to a contralesional stimulus, and increased by instructions to attend to an ipsilesional stimulus (Riddoch and Humphreys 1983). These instructions may modify attention in a 'top-down' manner. The severity of neglect may also be modified by novelty. Novelty may influence attention in a 'bottom-up' manner. Butter *et al.* (1990) showed that novel stimuli presented on the contralesional side reduced the severity of spatial neglect. Cues may also be intrinsic to the stimulus. Kartsounis and Warrington (1989) have shown that neglect is less severe when drawing meaningful pictures than when drawing meaningless pictures.

Ipsilesional spatial attentional bias

When patients with spatial neglect explore an array they often start their exploration on the ipsilesional side. For example, on the cancellation task, patients with left-sided neglect often begin to search for targets on the right side of the page (normal people who read European languages usually begin on the left). Làdavas *et al.* (1990) demonstrated that patients with right parietal lesions have shorter reaction times to right-sided stimuli than to left-sided stimuli, providing evidence of an attentional bias. Kinsbourne (1970) posited that each hemisphere attends to the opposite space. In order for people to shift their attention, the hemisphere that is engaged in an attentive process must inhibit the opposite hemisphere's attentional systems. Thus, when one hemisphere is injured, the other becomes hyperactive, and attention is biased contralaterally (to ipsilesional hemispace) and one is unaware of stimuli in contralesional hemispace. Heilman and Watson (1977) agree with Kinsbourne's notion that there is an ipsilesional bias, but they believe that the bias is not induced by absolute hyperactivity. If, normally, each hemisphere orients attention in a contralateral direction and one hemisphere (e.g. the right) is hypoactive, there will also be an ipsilesional (e.g. right) attentional bias. A seesaw or teeter-totter may tilt one way because one child is either too heavy (hyperactive hypothesis of Kinsbourne (1970)) or the other child is too light (hypoactive hypothesis of Heilman and Watson (1977)).

Support for the hypoactive (versus Kinsbourne's hyperactive) hemisphere hypothesis comes from both behavioral and physiological studies. Làdavas *et al.* (1990) found that attentional shifts between vertically aligned stimuli were slower when stimuli were in left (contralesional) hemispace than when they were in right (ipsilesional) hemispace. This slowing cannot be explained by the hyperactive hemisphere hypothesis, which predicts only slowing in the horizontal axis (i.e. left directional shifts of attention should be slower than right shifts). Physiological studies using EEG (Heilman 1979) and positron emission tomography (PET) (Fiorelli *et al.* 1991) have shown that patients with neglect have reduced activation of both hemispheres, with the injured hemisphere being less activated than the uninjured one.

Capacity-obscuration hypotheses

Hemispheric damage may not only induce an ipsilateral bias, but may also reduce attentional capacity. Many patients with spatial neglect also demonstrate a phenomenon called sensory extinction. These patients are able to correctly detect unilateral stimuli both contralateral and ipsilateral to their lesion, but when presented with bilateral simultaneous stimuli they often fail to report contralesional stimuli. This phenomenon was first noted by Loeb (1885) and Oppenheim (1885) in the tactile modality, and by Anton (1899) and Poppelreuter (1917) in the visual modality. It may also be seen in the auditory modality (Bender 1952; Heilman *et al.* 1970). A patient may have extinction in several modalities (multimodal extinction) or in one modality. Although extinction is most severe when the stimulus presented to the side contralateral to the lesion is paired with a stimulus on the other side, extinction may also occur when both stimuli are on the same side, even when they are both ipsilateral to the lesion (Rapcsak *et al.* 1987). Extinction (unawareness of contralesional stimuli in the presence of simultaneous ipsilesional stimuli) and spatial neglect are dissociable; thus it is doubtful that all forms of spatial neglect can be caused by extinction. However, an extinction-like phenomenon, which we shall term obscuration, may account for some of the signs of spatial neglect. Unlike extinction, where there is unawareness of the contralesional stimulus, with obscuration there is a reduction in the perception of stimulus magnitude. Recently, Riestra and coworkers (2001) gave patients an alternative form of the Landmark test (Harvey *et al.* 1995) where a small gap divides a line into two unequal segments. The subject is requested to report which side has either the longer or the shorter segment. Subjects with left spatial neglect underestimated the contralesional (left) segment. In a second test, the same line segments were given sequentially instead of simultaneously. Now the subjects performed just like normal controls, suggesting that in these subjects competition for limited attentional resources induced the systematic bias observed in the Landmark test. The mechanisms by which competition for limited resources reduces the perception of magnitude is unknown. Several hypotheses have been proposed, including suppression mediated by transcallosal inhibition (Nathan 1946; Reider 1946) or asymmetric inhibition of thalamic relay nuclei by the nucleus reticularis (Heilman *et al.* 1993). (A more detailed discussion of the mechanisms of extinction is given by Heilman *et al.* (2003).)

Ipsilesional attentional disengagement disorder

Posner *et al.* (1984) proposed a three-stage model of attention. When people are called upon to shift their attention, they must first disengage attention from the stimulus to which they are currently attending, move attention to the new stimulus, and then engage that stimulus. Posner hypothesis of spatial neglect is similar to that of Kinsbourne, but is couched in different terms. Posner posited that patients neglect contralesional space because they cannot disengage from ipsilesional space. Posner *et al.* (1984) studied patients with parietal lesions by providing visual cues signaling which side of extrapersonal space the imperative (reaction time) stimulus would appear. The cues could be either valid, indicating the side on which the stimulus would actually appear, or invalid, when the imperative stimulus appears on the side opposite that indicated by the cue. In normal subjects valid cues reduce reaction times and invalid cues increase reaction times. Posner and coworkers found that, in patients with parietal lobe lesions, invalid cues indicating that the reaction time stimulus is to appear ipsilesionally resulted in abnormal prolongation of reaction times to contralesional stimuli. These results suggest that one of the functions of the parietal lobe is to disengage attention and patients may have spatial neglect because they cannot disengage from right-sided (ipsilesional) stimuli.

Mark *et al.* (1988) tested Posner's disengagement hypothesis and Kinsbourne's bias hypothesis of spatial neglect by comparing the performance of patients on a traditional cancellation task, where the subject marks each detected target with a pen (but does not remove it), with an experimental cancellation test where the subject erases the detected targets. If a target is erased, the subject should have no difficulty in disengaging from the target. In addition, erasing targets should also systematically reduce an attentional bias. Mark and coworkers observed that on the standard cancellation task, subjects with neglect would first start cancelling targets on the side of the sheet that is ipsilateral to their lesion (right side). Although they could disengage from specific targets, they often returned to these targets and cancelled them again. When erasing targets, patients' performance improved (they erased more targets); however, they continued to neglect some targets on the left. These observations suggest a bias rather than a problem with stimulus accounts for abnormal performance. The bias hypothesis accounts for the distribution of neglect but does not explain why subjects still failed to cancel left-sided targets in the erase paradigm. One could argue that bias is in part a 'top-down' process and, while right-sided stimuli are more likely to 'draw' attention than left-sided stimuli, even in the absence of right-sided stimuli the subject with left neglect continues to have a right-sided attentional bias and is unable to move attention fully leftward.

Defective vigilance or enhanced habituation

Chatterjee *et al.* (1992) requested that a patient with left-sided neglect on standard cancellation tasks alternately cancel targets on the right and left side of an array. Using this procedure, the patient was able to overcome her right-sided bias, but she did not cancel more targets. Instead, she now neglected targets in the center of the array. This result suggests that, in addition to an ipsilateral spatial attentional bias manifested on the traditional cancellation task, she may have become inattentive to stimuli because she had a rapid loss of vigilance or rapid habituation. A person's vigilance is a function of the brain's arousal, and patients with neglect have reduced arousal (Heilman *et al.* 1978; Heilman 1979; Storrie-Baker 1997). Patients with neglect most often have parietal lesions (Heilman *et al.* 1983*a*; Vallar and Perani 1986), and Mennemeier *et al.* (1994) demonstrated that parietal lesions are also associated with inappropriately rapid habituation.

Anatomical and physiological basis of attentional deficits

Unilateral neglect in humans and monkeys can be induced by lesions in many different brain regions. These include neocortical areas such as the temporoparietal–occipital junction and the dorsolateral frontal lobe (Critchley 1966; Heilman *et al.* 1970, 1983*a*; Heilman and Valenstein 1972; Vallar and Perani 1986), limbic areas such as the cingulate gyrus (Heilman and Valenstein 1972; Watson *et al.* 1973; Leibovitch *et al.* 1998), and subcortical areas such as the thalamus (Watson and Heilman 1979; Watson *et al.* 1981; Karussis *et al.* 2000), the basal ganglia (Sakashita 1991; Vallar and Perani 1986; Damasio *et al.* 1980), and the mesencephalic reticular formation (Watson *et al.* 1974). We have proposed that inattention is induced by dysfunction in a corticolimbic–reticular formation network (Heilman and Valenstein 1972; Watson *et al.* 1973, 1981; Heilman 1979). Mesulam (1981) has made a similar proposal. We shall briefly review the evidence for this attentional model.

Arousal

To process information, the cortex has to be in a physiological state of readiness, called arousal. The mesencephalic–diencephalic reticular system mediates arousal. Stimulation of the mesencephalic reticular formation is associated with behavioral arousal and also with desynchronization of the EEG, a physiological measure of arousal (Moruzzi and Magoun 1949). In humans, the performance of attention-demanding tasks increases the activation of the mesencephalic reticular formation and the thalamic intralaminar nuclei as determined by positron emission tomography (Kinomura *et al.* 1996). Unilateral stimulation of the reticular activating system induces greater EEG desynchronization in the ipsilateral than in the contralateral hemisphere (Moruzzi and Magoun 1949). Whereas bilateral lesions of the mesencephalic reticular formation result in coma (in monkeys and cats), discrete unilateral lesions result in profound sensory neglect (Reeves and Hagaman 1971; Watson *et al.* 1974).

Influence of the mesencephalic reticular formation on the cortex

Many neurons that ascend from the mesencephalic reticular activating system and its environs are monoaminergic. The area of the mesencephalon stimulated by Moruzzi and Magoun (1949) contains ascending catecholamine systems, including the noradrenergic system which projects diffusely from the locus ceruleus to the cortex. Although this norepinephrine (noradrenaline) system would appear to be ideal for mediating cortical arousal (Jouvet 1977), destruction of most of the locus ceruleus neither has a profound effect on behavioral arousal nor changes EEG patterns (Jones *et al.* 1977).

Although unilateral injury to the dopaminergic system may induce neglect because dopamine is critical for mediating intention (see the following section on intention), dopamine does not appear to be important in arousal because blockade of dopamine synthesis or of dopamine receptors does not appear to affect EEG desynchronization (Feeney and Wier 1979).

Acetylcholine appears to have a more promising role in the mediation of arousal. Shute and Lewis (1967) described an ascending cholinergic reticular formation. Stimulation of the mesencephalic reticular activating system not only induces the arousal response but also increases the rate of acetylcholine release from the neocortex (Kanai and Szerb 1965). Acetylcholine makes some neurons more responsive to sensory input (McCormick and Williamson 1989). Cholinergic agonists induce neocortical desynchronization, while antagonists abolish desynchronization (Bradley 1968). It is believed that cholinergic projections from the nucleus basalis are responsible for increasing neuronal responsivity (Sato *et al.* 1987). The nucleus basalis receives a projection from the peripeduncular area of the mesencephalon, which in turn receives a projection from the cuneiform area of the mesencephalon (Arnault and Roger 1987). Thus, mesencephalic stimulation may influence cortical cholinergic activity via the nucleus basalis. Unilateral interruption of the basal forebrain's cholinergic projections to the neocortex may induce inattention to contralateral stimuli (Bushnell *et al.* 1998).

The mesencephalic reticular activating system may also influence the cortex by diffuse polysynaptic projections (Scheibel and Scheibel 1967). Steriade and Glenn (1982) found that the centralis lateralis and paracentralis thalamic nuclei project to widespread cortical regions.

Cortical influence on the reticular system

Sensory information that reaches the cortex is relayed through specific thalamic nuclei. The nucleus reticularis thalami, a thin reticular nucleus enveloping the thalamus, projects to the thalamic relay nuclei and appears to inhibit thalamic relay to the cortex (Scheibel and Scheibel 1966). The mesencephalic reticular activating system also projects to the nucleus reticularis. Rapid mesencephalic reticular activating system stimulation or behavioral arousal inhibits the nucleus reticularis and is thereby associated with enhanced thalamic transmission to the cerebral cortex (Singer 1977). Hence, unilateral lesions of the mesencephalic reticular formation may induce neglect not only because the cortex is unprepared for processing sensory stimuli in the absence of arousal mediated by the mesencephalic reticular formation, but also because the thalamic sensory relay nuclei are being inhibited by the nucleus reticularis.

Lesions of thalamic relay nuclei or of the primary sensory cortex induce a sensory defect rather than neglect. Primary cortical sensory areas project to the unimodal association cortex which synthesizes modality-specific information and store modality specific representations. Thus, lesions of the unimodal association cortex may induce perceptual deficits in a single modality (e.g., apperceptive agnosia). Modality-specific association areas may also detect stimulus novelty (modelling) (Sokolov 1963). When a stimulus is neither novel nor significant, corticofugal projections to the nucleus reticularis may allow habituation to occur by selectively inhibiting thalamic relay. When a stimulus is novel or significant, corticofugal projections might inhibit the nucleus reticularis and thereby allow the thalamus to relay additional sensory input. This capacity for selective control of sensory input is supported by a study revealing that stimulation of specific areas within the nucleus reticularis related to specific thalamic nuclei (e.g. nucleus reticularis lateral geniculate, nucleus reticularis medial geniculate, or nucleus reticularis ventrobasal complex) results in abolition of corresponding (visual, auditory, or tactile) cortical evoked responses (Yingling and Skinner 1977). Physiological imaging studies reveal that selectively attending to tactile stimuli may activate the primary (somesthetic) cortex (Meyer *et al.* 1991). This activation may be mediated by corticofugal projections that inhibit the inhibition that the nucleus reticularis exerts on thalamic relay nuclei such as the ventral posterior lateral.

There are many different association areas in the visual system, but in general areas located in ventral occipital–temporal regions are important in processing the visual properties of objects (the 'what' system), whereas visual association areas in dorsal (superior) occipital-parietal regions are important in processing the spatial position of stimuli (the 'where' system) (Haxby *et al.* 1991). Patients with ventral ('what' system) lesions may be impaired in recognizing objects (visual object agnosia) and faces (prosopagnosia). In contrast, patients with dorsal ('where' system) lesions may have problems locating objects in space (e.g. optic ataxia). Unimodal association areas converge upon polymodal association areas. In the monkey, these are the prefrontal cortex (periarcuate, prearcuate, and orbitofrontal) and both banks of the superior temporal sulcus (Pandya and Kuypers, 1969). Unimodal association areas may also project directly to the caudal inferior parietal lobule or, alternatively, may reach the inferior parietal lobule after a synapse in polymodal convergence areas (e.g. prefrontal cortex and both banks of the superior temporal sulcus) (Mesulam *et al.* 1977). Polymodal convergence areas may subserve cross-modal associations and polymodal sensory synthesis. Polymodal sensory synthesis may also be important in 'modelling' (detecting stimulus novelty) and detecting significance. In contrast with the unimodal association cortex that projects to specific parts of the nucleus reticularis and thereby gates sensory input in one modality, these multimodal convergence areas may have a more general inhibitory action on the nucleus reticularis and provide further arousal after cortical analysis. These convergence areas may also project directly to the mesencephalic reticular formation, which may induce a general state of arousal because of diffuse multisynaptic connections to the cortex, or increase thalamic transmission via connections with the nucleus reticularis, as discussed above, or both. Evidence that polymodal areas of cortex modulate arousal comes from neurophysiological studies showing that stimulation of select cortical sites induces a generalized arousal response. These sites in monkeys include the frontal prearcuate region and both banks of the superior temporal sulcus, i.e. the precursor of the human's inferior parietal lobe (Segundo *et al.* 1955). When similar sites are ablated, there is EEG evidence of ipsilateral hypoarousal (Watson *et al.* 1977a).

Determining stimulus significance

Although determination of stimulus novelty may be mediated by the sensory association cortex, stimulus significance is determined in part by the needs by the organism (motivational state). Limbic system input into brain regions important for determining stimulus significance might provide information about biological needs. Since the frontal lobes play a critical role in goal-mediated behavior and in developing sets, the frontal lobes might provide input about needs related to goals that are neither directly stimulus dependent nor motivated by an immediate biological need.

Polymodal (e.g. superior temporal sulcus) and supramodal (inferior parietal lobule) areas have prominent limbic and frontal connections. Polymodal cortices project to the cingulate gyrus (a portion of the limbic system), and the cingulate gyrus projects to the inferior parietal lobule. The prefrontal cortex, superior temporal sulcus, and inferior parietal lobule have strong reciprocal connections. The posterior cingulate cortex (Brodmann's area 23) has more extensive connections with polymodal association areas (prefrontal cortex and superior temporal sulcus) and the inferior parietal lobule than does the anterior cingulate cortex (Brodmann's area 24) (Vogt *et al.* 1979; Baleydier and Maugierre 1980). These connections provide an anatomical substrate by which motivational states (e.g. biological needs, sets, and long-term goals) may influence stimulus processing.

In concert with the anatomical hypothesis discussed above, investigators have defined the properties of neurons in the parietal lobe of the monkeys (Mountcastle *et al.* 1975, 1981; Goldberg and Robinson 1977; Robinson *et al.* 1978; Lynch 1980; Motter and Mountcastle 1981; Bushnell *et al.* 1981). Unlike single cells in the primary sensory cortex, the activity of many parietal neurons correlates best with stimuli or responses of importance to the animal, while similar stimuli or responses that are unimportant are associated with either no change or a lesser change in neuronal activity (Colby and Goldberg 1999).

Investigations identified parietal neurons that responded to visual stimuli of biological signi-ficance, aversive as well as rewarding, suggesting activity that might mediate selective attention (Goldberg and Robinson 1977; Robinson *et al.* 1978). Some neurons were active with fixation of non-moving stimuli, some only when the animal was tracking a moving stimulus, and some responded only when stimuli were moving in a specific direction. Most had receptive fields in the contralateral visual field (i.e. they responded only to stimuli in a portion of the contralateral visual field), but other neurons had large receptive fields, sometimes spanning both visual fields (Mountcastle *et al.* 1981).

More recent neurophysiological research has revealed a striking specialization of parietal sub-regions related to spatial organization (Colby and Goldberg 1999). Neurons in inferior parietal lobule will respond equally to a stimulus if the response is an eye movement toward the stimulus or a bar press without visual fixation (Colby *et al.* 1996). Because many of the neurons in these regions respond differentially to objects that are of significance to the organism, lesions in these areas can reduce awareness of objects in far or near space, suggesting an anatomical and physio-logical basis for the spatial direction of attention. Therefore damage to these areas may result in various distributions of hemispatial neglect. This may be relevant to the production of spatially restricted forms of the neglect syndrome in humans, for example the reports of horizontal neglect in near but not far space (Halligan and Marshall 1991) and of neglect for far but not near space (Vuilleumier *et al.* 1998).

Habituation

Evidence that polymodal parietal cortex may be important in enhancing thalamic transmission, by inhibiting the inhibitory thalamic reticular nucleus, comes from the observation that patients with Balint's syndrome from biparietal lesions note that visual stimuli, unless moving, disappear after a few seconds. Mennemeier *et al.* (1994) suggested and provided support for the hypothesis that visual stimuli disappear because the parietal lobes can no longer inhibit this inhibitory nucleus and visual gating occurs. These authors also suggested that, whereas the parietal lobes inhibit the inhibitory thalamic reticular nucleus and thereby enhance stimulus transmission, the frontal lobes excite the inhibitory nucleus reticularis, diminish transmission, and promote habituation. To test this hypothesis they studied visual habituation using the Troxlar paradigm. In this paradigm the subject looks at a central fixation point and notes when a dot on the right or left of this fixation point fades from vision. Mennemeier and coworkers found that there was enhanced habituation (rapid fading) contralateral to parietal lesions and delayed habituation contralateral to frontal lesions.

Summary of attentional model

The mesencephalic–diencephalic reticular system mediates arousal, and unilateral attentional neglect follows unilateral mesencephalic reticular activating system lesions because the mesen-cephalic reticular formation does not prepare the cortex for sensory processing and/or because it no longer inhibits the ipsilateral nucleus reticularis, which then inhibits thalamic transmission of sensory input to the cortex. Corticothalamic collaterals from parietal association cortex to the nucleus reticularis may serve attentional orienting, and collaterals from the frontal cortex to the nucleus reticularis may serve habituation. Unilateral lesions of multimodal sensory convergence areas that project to the mesencephalic reticular activating system and nucleus reticularis, such as the inferior parietal lobe, induce contralateral inattention because the subject cannot be aroused by or process contralateral stimuli. To attend selectively to a biologically significant stimulus one must recognize the stimulus and know its spatial location. The sensory association systems that mediate 'what' and 'where' sensory analysis converge in the inferior parietal cortex. Biological significance is determined by immediate needs or drives mediated by portions of the limbic system such as the cingulate gyrus, or by long-term goals and sets mediated by dorsolateral frontal lobes. The inferior parietal lobe, cingulate gyrus and dorsolateral frontal lobe are all highly intercon-nected, and, with the reticular (arousal) systems, form an attentional network. A lesion affecting any one of these modules or the connections between them (Burcham *et al.* 1997) can result in unilateral neglect.

Motor intentional hypothesis

In monkeys, lesions of both the temporal–parietal cortex (Heilman *et al.* 1970) and the dorsolateral frontal lobes (Welch and Stuteville 1958) produce neglect. Because monkeys with frontal lesions were not weak but did not respond to contralesional stimuli, Welch and Stuteville assumed that they had sensory neglect. However, Watson *et al.* (1978*b*) posited that the failure to interact with a stimulus, even in the absence of weakness, could be caused by a failure to respond—an action-intentional disorder. To test this hypothesis they wanted to dissociate afferent from efferent processes and thus trained the monkeys to respond to a stimulus on one side with a movement of the contralateral limb (crossed-response task). After a dorsolateral frontal lesion, the animals correctly responded to a stimulus on the contralesional side with an ipsilesional response; however, when stimulated ipsilesionally the animals failed to make a contralesional response.

The action–intention hypothesis of spatial neglect states that while patients may be aware of stimuli in contralateral hemispace, they fail to act on these stimuli. Just as there are several forms of attentional deficits that have been proposed to explain spatial neglect, there are also several forms of intentional deficits that parallel their attentional counterparts. These include the following:

(1) a failure to act in contralesional space (hemispatial akinesia);
(2) an ipsilesional spatial intentional bias (directional hypokinesia);
(3) an inability to disengage from stimuli in ipsilesional space (motor perseveration);
(4) reduced ability to sustain an action in or toward contralesional hemispace (directional impersistence).

Like their attentional counterparts, these four hypotheses are not necessarily exclusive of each other or of the attentional hypotheses discussed above.

Hemispatial akinesia

De Renzi *et al.* (1970) asked blindfolded patients with spatial neglect to manually search a maze for a target. The subjects failed to explore the left side of the maze. When using the tactile modality to explore, one can only attend to stimuli in a new spatial position after one has moved. Therefore, the failure to explore the left (contralesional) side of the maze cannot be attributed to an attentional deficit and may provide evidence for a hemispatial action-intentional deficit. However, De Renzi and coworkers thought that this abnormal behavior was induced by a representational deficit. Unfortunately, their study could not discriminate between these alternative mechanisms.

Heilman and Valenstein (1979) asked patients to read a letter on the left side of a line prior to bisecting the line. This strategy ensures that the subjects were aware of the entire line. Despite using this strategy, patients did better when the line was in right (ipsilesional) rather than left (contralesional) hemispace, suggesting a reduced ability to act in contralesional hemispace. Although patients were able to see the leftward limits of the line when attempting to bisect lines in right space, the attentional bias may be less than when attempting to bisect them in left space, and in this study Heilman and Valenstein did not dissociate intentional from attentional deficits.

To investigate whether defective hemispatial attention or intention was primarily responsible for the abnormal performance of patients with spatial neglect, Coslett *et al.* (1990) asked patients to bisect lines that they only saw displayed on a TV monitor connected to a video camera focused on the patient's hand and the line. Using this technique, motor action (intention) and sensory feedback (attention) could be dissociated such that the action could take place in left hemispace but the feedback could take place in right hemispace, or vice versa. Independent of the position of the line, two of the four subjects improved when the monitor was moved from left (contralesional) to right (ipsilesional) hemispace, suggesting that their primary disturbance was spatial inattention. The two other subjects were not improved by moving the monitor into right hemispace but were primarily affected by the hemispace in which the action took place, performing better when the line was in right (ipsilesional) rather than in left (contralesional) hemispace, suggesting that they had primarily a motor-intentional deficit. The two patients who had primarily intentional neglect had frontal lesions and those with attentional neglect had parietal lesions. Tegner and Levander (1991) used a 90° mirror to dissociate intentional (premotor) from attentional spatial neglect and replicated the study by Coslett *et al.* (1990).

Directional hypokinesia and intentional (motor) bias

Acutely following a stroke, patients with neglect have what has been termed a gaze palsy. For example, after a right hemisphere stroke their eyes are often deviated to the right. Although this is called a gaze palsy, many of these patients move their eyes fully to the left to verbal command. Thus, this eye deviation is not a palsy or paresis but rather a directional gaze bias. This gaze bias may be related to either contralesional inattention or a directional (ipsilesional) motor bias. If the patients close their eyes so that there is no afferent input and then open them, the gaze bias is present immediately, suggesting that what is termed a gaze palsy is really a directional motor intentional bias—a form of directional hypokinesia.

To investigate whether patients with neglect have a similar directional motor bias with their arms, Heilman *et al.* (1983*a*) tested subjects with left-sided spatial neglect and normal controls by asking them to close their eyes, point their right index finger to their sternum, and then point to an imaginary spot in space in the midsagittal plane (perpendicular to the middle of their chest). The patients with neglect pointed to the right of midline, whereas the controls pointed slightly to its left. Because this task did not require visual or somesthetic input from left hemispace, the defective performance could not be attributed to hemispatial inattention or an attentional bias, but again suggested a motor intentional bias. Heilman *et al.* (1985) also tested the ability of patients with left-sided hemispatial neglect to move a lever toward or away from the side of their lesion. Patients with neglect had a directional motor bias and needed more time to initiate movements toward the neglected left hemispace than toward the right (ipsilesional) hemispace. These asymmetries were not found in brain-lesioned controls without neglect. This directional hypokinesia may be related to a motor-intentional bias or to an inability for the motor-intentional system to disengage from the right.

The work of Bisiach *et al.* (1990) also supports the idea that spatial neglect can be associated with a motor-intentional bias. They used a loop of string stretched around two pulleys. The string was positioned horizontally, with one pulley on the left and the other on the right. An arrow was attached to the top segment of string. Subjects with neglect and control subjects were asked to place the arrow midway between the two pulleys. In the congruent condition, the subject held the arrow on the upper string to move it. In the incongruent condition, the subject displaced the lower string laterally, which moved the arrow in the opposite direction. If neglect was caused by a directional hypokinesia, the error in the congruent and incongruent conditions should be in opposite directions. Six of thirteen subjects showed a significant reduction of neglect in the incongruent condition, suggesting that they had a significant motor-intentional bias. These patients had predominantly frontal lesions.

Na *et al.* (1998b) attempted to dissociate attentional and intentional aspects of neglect by having subjects view their performance of a line bisection task on a video monitor. Subjects could not view the workspace directly. The task was displayed on the monitor either normally or right–left reversed. If neglect were primarily attentional, the subjects' performance would be influenced by the monitor display of the task and one would expect that when the monitor image was right–left reversed, subjects would reverse the direction of line bisection error. In contrast, the performance of patients with intentional spatial neglect should be influenced primarily by the motor aspects of the task, and they should continue to bisect lines toward the right in the image-reversed condition, even though on the monitor this is displayed as a leftward bisection. This technique allows investigation of the relative contribution of attentional and intentional biases in the same subject. For example, if a patient reverses his or her deviation in the reversed-display condition, but the deviation is less than it was in the normal display condition, this suggests an attentional bias, with some lesser contribution of a rightward intentional bias. Using this apparatus Na *et al.* (1998b) found that most patients with spatial neglect had both intentional and attentional biases, but in patients with frontal lesions the intentional bias dominated whereas the attentional bias was dominant in patients with temporal-parietal lesions. The finding of mixed attentional and intentional bias is consistent with the idea that the networks subserving attention and intention influence one another. Anatomically, the parietal and frontal lobes are involved in both networks. Support of this postulate also comes from Mattingley *et al.* (1998), who demonstrated that the parietal lobe serves a sensorimotor interface.

Ipsilesional intentional disengagement disorder

Unfortunately, this hypothesis of hemispatial neglect has not been fully evaluated. In addition, the distinction between this hypothetical mechanism and the ipsilesional motor (intentional) bias discussed above is not entirely clear. For example, directional hypokinesia, in which subjects take longer to initiate a response to contralesional than ipsilesional stimuli, may be related to either an ipsilateral motor bias or an inability to disengage from ipsilateral stimuli. A stronger argument for the failure to disengage intentionally from ipsilesional space is the observation that when performing the cancellation task about 40 per cent of subjects repeatedly cancel the same target (Na *et al.* 1999).

Directional impersistence

Motor impersistence is the inability to sustain an act. It is the intentional equivalent of defective vigilance. It can be demonstrated in a variety of body parts, including the limbs, eyes, eyelids, jaw, and tongue. Like akinesia, it may also be directional (Kertesz *et al.* 1985) or hemispatial (Roeltgen *et al.* 1989).

One possible explanation of abnormal performance on the cancellation test is that patients fail to persist in searching for left-sided targets. To test this hypothesis Womack and Heilman (in preparation) tested a patient with left-sided neglect on a cancellation in two conditions. The control condition was the routine cancellation test. The experimental condition was designed to overcome impersistence. After the subject cancelled a target the stimulus sheet was covered to give the subject a chance to 'rest and recover' and was then uncovered again so that the patient could cancel the next target. The patient's performance in the second condition was much better than in the first. This improvement could not be explained by hemispatial or directional unawareness or hypokinesia, an attentional or intentional bias, a disengagement deficit, or a representational memory deficit. These results appear to support the directional impersistence hypothesis; however, it is possible that the rest period may also have delayed habituation.

Anatomical and physiological mechanisms

The region of the arcuate gyrus (periarcuate region) in monkeys contains the frontal eye field. Stimulation of the frontal eye field elicits contralateral eye movement, head rotation, and pupillary dilation resembling attentive orienting (Wagman and Mehler 1972). The connections of the periarcuate region are important in understanding its possible role in motor activation or intention. The periarcuate region has reciprocal connections with the auditory, visual, and somesthetic association cortex (Chavis and Pandya 1976). Evoked potential studies have confirmed this as an area of sensory convergence (Bignall and Imbert 1969). The periarcuate region is also reciprocally connected with the cortex on the banks of the superior temporal sulcus, another site of multimodal sensory convergence, and with the cortex on the banks of the intraparietal sulcus, an area of somatosensory and visual convergence. There are also connections with the prearcuate cortex. The periarcuate cortex has reciprocal connections with subcortical areas: the paralamellar portion of dorsomedial nucleus and the adjacent centromedian–parafascicularis complex (Kievet and Kuypers 1977; Akert and Von Monakow 1980). Just as the periarcuate region is transitional in architecture between agranular motor cortex and granular prefrontal cortex, the paralamellar–centromedian–parafascicularis complex is situated between the medial thalamus, which projects to the granular cortex, and the lateral thalamus, which projects to the agranular cortex. Projections to the mesencephalic reticular formation (Kuypers and Lawrence 1967), as well as nonreciprocal projections to the caudate, also exist. Lastly, the periarcuate region also receives input from the limbic system, mainly from the anterior cingulate gyrus (Baleydier and Mauguiere 1980).

The neocortical sensory association and sensory convergence area connections provide the frontal lobes with information about external stimuli that may call the individual to action. Limbic connections (from the anterior cingulate gyrus) may provide the frontal lobe with motivational information. Connections with the mesencephalic reticular formation may be important in arousal.

Because the dorsolateral frontal lobe has sensory association cortex, limbic, and reticular formation connections, it would appear to be an ideal candidate for mediating a response to a stimulus to which the subject is attending. While this area may not be critical for mediating how to respond (e.g. providing instruction for the spatial trajectory and temporal patterns), it may control when one responds. There is evidence from physiological studies to support this hypothesis. Recordings from single cells in the posterior frontal arcuate gyrus reveal responses similar to those of the superior colliculus, a structure also important in oculomotor control (Goldberg and Bushnell 1981). These visually responsive neurons show enhanced activity time-locked to the onset of stimulus and preceding eye movement. This differs from inferior parietal lobule neurons which respond to visual input independent of behavior; an inferior parietal lobule neuron whose activity enhances in a task that requires a saccade also enhances with tasks that do not require a saccade. Therefore the inferior parietal lobule neurons seem to be responsible for selective spatial attention, which is independent of behavior, and any neuron that is enhanced to one type of behavior will also be enhanced to others (Bushnell *et al.* 1981). However, the frontal eye-field neurons are linked to behavior, but only to movements that have motivational significance. Responses to other stimulus modalities (e.g. audition) may be controlled by an adjacent group of neurons in the arcuate gyrus (Whittington and Hepp-Reymond 1977).

The dorsolateral frontal lobe has extensive connections with the centromedian–parafascicularis, one of the 'nonspecific' intralaminar thalamic nuclei. Nonsensory or motor-intentional neglect has also been reported in monkeys after centromedian–parafascicularis lesions (Watson *et al.* 1978) and in a patient with an intralaminar lesion (Bogousslavsky *et al.* 1986). An akinetic state (akinetic mutism) is seen with bilateral centromedian–parafascicularis lesions in humans (Mills and Swanson 1978). We have postulated a possible role for the centromedian–parafascicularis in behavior (Watson *et al.* 1981). This role is based on behavioral, anatomical, and physiological evidence that the centromedian–parafascicularis and the periarcuate cortex are involved in mediating responses to meaningful stimuli.

Neuropharmacology of intentional disorders

Much evidence suggests that dopaminergic neurons mediate aspects of intention. Intentional deficits are prominent in patients with Parkinson's disease, which is characterized pathologically by degeneration of ascending dopaminergic neurons. In animals, unilateral lesions in these pathways (Marshall *et al.* 1971) and unilateral destruction of the dopaminergic system by a toxin (Schneider *et al.* 1992), cause unilateral neglect. In contrast, stimulation of dopamine pathways reinforces ongoing behavior (Olds and Milner 1954; Corbett and Wise 1980).

Three related dopaminergic pathways have been defined. The nigrostriatal pathway originates in the pars compacta of the substantia nigra (SN), and projects to the neostriatum (caudate and putamen). The mesolimbic pathway originates principally in the ventral tegmental area of the midbrain (area A10), just medial to the substantia nigra, and terminates in the limbic areas of the basal forebrain (nucleus accumbens septi and olfactory tubercle). The mesocortical pathway originates principally in dopaminergic neurons located more laterally in the midbrain (areas A8 and A9) and projects to the frontal and cingulate cortex (Ungerstedt 1971*a*; Lindvall *et al.* 1974; Williams and Goldman-Rakic 1998).

Ascending dopaminergic fibers course through the lateral hypothalamus in the median forebrain bundle. Bilateral lesions in the lateral hypothalamus of rats induce an akinetic state (Teitelbaum and Epstein 1962). Unilateral lesions of the lateral hypothalamus cause unilateral neglect. These rats transiently circle toward the side of their lesion; after they recover to the point where spontaneous activity appears symmetrical, they still tend to turn toward their lesioned side when stimulated (e.g. by pinching their tails) and they fail to respond to sensory stimuli delivered to the contralateral side (Marshall *et al.* 1971). There is considerable evidence that lateral hypothalamus lesions cause neglect by damaging dopaminergic fibers passing through the hypothalamus. Neglect occurs with 6-hydroxydopamine (6-OHDA) lesions of the lateral hypothalamus that damage dopaminergic fibers relatively selectively (Marshall *et al.* 1974), but not with kainic acid lesions that damage cell bodies but not fibers of passage (Grossman *et al.* 1978). Unilateral damage to the same dopaminergic fibers closer to their site of origin in the midbrain also causes unilateral neglect (Ljungberg and Ungerstedt 1976; Marshall 1979). Conversely, unilateral stimulation in the area of ascending dopaminergic fibers (Arbuthnott and Ungerstedt 1975) or of the striatum (Pycock 1980) causes animals to turn away from the side of stimulation, as if they are orienting to the opposite side.

Lesions of the ascending dopaminergic pathways affect the areas of termination of these pathways in at least two ways. First, degeneration of dopamine-containing axons depletes these areas of dopamine. Marshall (1979) has shown that the neglect induced in rats by ventral tegmental 6-OHDA lesions is proportional to the depletion of dopamine in the neostriatum and, to a lesser extent, in the olfactory tubercle and nucleus accumbens. Second, the target areas attempt to compensate for the depletion of dopaminergic afferents by increasing their responsiveness to dopamine. This is mediated, at least in part, by an increase in the number of dopaminergic receptors (Heikkila *et al.* 1981), which correlates with behavioral recovery from neglect (Neve *et al.* 1982).

Changes in dopaminergic innervation and in dopaminergic receptor sensitivity and number can explain many effects of pharmacological manipulation in animals with unilateral lesions of the ascending dopaminergic pathways. Such lesions result in degeneration of dopaminergic axon terminals on the side of the lesion. Therefore, drugs such as L-dopa or amphetamines which increase the release of dopamine from normal dopaminergic terminals will cause more dopamine to be released on the unlesioned side than on the lesioned side, resulting in orientation or turning toward the lesioned side (Ungerstedt 1971*b*, 1974). Several days after the lesion, when dopaminergic receptor concentration on the side of the lesion begins to increase, drugs that directly stimulate dopaminergic receptors, such as apomorphine, cause the animal to turn away from the side of the lesion (Ungerstedt 1971*b*, 1974). Although rats have been used in most studies, lesions that probably involve the ascending dopaminergic systems have also induced unilateral neglect in cats (Hagamen *et al.* 1977) and monkeys (Deuel 1980; Apicella *et al.* 1991).

The evidence summarized above indicates the importance of dopaminergic pathways in mediating intention. Although the neglect induced by lateral hypothalamus or ventral tegmental area lesions has been called 'sensory' neglect or inattention, rats trained to respond to unilateral stimulation by turning to the side opposite the side of stimulation respond well to stimulation of their 'neglected' side (the side opposite the lesion) but fail to turn when stimulated on their 'normal' side (Hoyman *et al.* 1979). This paradigm is similar to that used by Watson *et al.* (1978), and demonstrates that lesions in ascending dopaminergic pathways cause a defect of intention.

The striatum, which receives dopaminergic innervation from the substantia nigra, projects to globus pallidus, which in turn has output to three major regions (Fonnum and Walaas 1979; Grofova 1979). It projects to the subthalamic nucleus, which projects back to the internal segment of the globus pallidus. It projects to the thalamus, as part of the striato-pallidal-thalamo-cortical-striatal loop described above. It also projects to the intralaminar nuclei of the thalamus (Mehler 1966). In addition, the striatum also projects back to the to the substantia nigra, in part providing feedback to dopaminergic neurons, but also connecting the striatum with the targets of substantia nigra projections—the intralaminar nuclei of the thalamus, the superior colliculus, and portions of the reticular formation (Anderson and Yoshida 1977; Herkenham 1979; Dalsass and Krauthamer 1981). The intralaminar thalamus, the superior colliculus, and the mesencephalic reticular formation are all areas which have been implicated in the mediation of attention and in which lesions can induce unilateral neglect. It appears likely that striatal input into these areas, regulated in part by activity in the ascending dopaminergic pathways, provides information about the intentional state of the organism.

The frontal neocortex and cingulate cortex receive dopaminergic input from the ventral tegmental area of the midbrain and adjacent areas (Brown *et al.* 1979; Williams and Goldman-Rakic 1998), and the entire neocortex projects strongly to the striatum. This corticostriatal projection is largely glutaminergic (Divac *et al.* 1977). Stimulation in the motor or visual areas of the cat's cortex causes a release of dopamine in the striatum (Nieoullon *et al.* 1978). However, 6-OHDA lesions of the mesial prefrontal cortex in rats resulted in an increase of both striatal dopamine content and striatal dopaminergic receptor concentration after 30 days (Pycock *et al.* 1980). Rats with unilateral frontal cortical ablations may turn toward the side of their lesion, and amphetamines initially increase this turning (Avemo *et al.* 1973). After a week, amphetamines induce contralateral turning, while apomorphine causes turning toward the side of the lesion (i.e. the opposite of the pharmacological effects seen after unilateral lesions of the ascending dopaminergic pathways). Rats subjected to a previous unilateral 6-OHDA lesion of the ascending dopaminergic pathways and then a unilateral frontal lesion initially reverse their direction of spontaneous turning, but do not change their turning response to amphetamine or apomorphine (Crossman *et al.* 1977). Monkeys that have recovered from neglect induced by unilateral frontal arcuate lesions do not show asymmetrical behavior when given L-dopa, amphetamine, haloperidol, scopolamine, physostigmine, or bromocriptine, but do show dramatic turning toward the side of their lesion when given apomorphine (Valenstein *et al.* 1980). This turning is blocked by prior administration of haloperidol. Following unilateral frontal lesions, rats demonstrated contralateral neglect which was reversed by the dopamine agonist apomorphine (Corwin *et al.* 1986). This apomorphine-induced reduction of neglect was blocked by the prior administration of the dopamine blocker spiropiridol. Rats who had neglect induced by ablation of the frontal cortex recover; however, a selective D1 blocker administered to these animals can again induce neglect (Vargo *et al.* 1989). Humans with neglect have also been treated with dopamine agonists. Electrophysiological studies of striatal neurons reveal short latency responses to stimuli that are novel or signal reward (meaningful) (Schultz 1998; Redgrave *et al.* 1999). These neurons also fire in relation to the preparation, initiation, or execution of movements that are related to significant stimuli (Schultz *et al.* 2000). These studies provide evidence that the activity of the dopaminergic system is related to the regulation of actions that are triggered by significant stimuli.

Fleet *et al.* (1987) treated two neglect patients with bromocriptine, a dopamine agonist. Both showed dramatic improvements. Subsequently, other investigators have also shown that dopamine agonist therapy may be helpful in the treatment of neglect (Geminiani *et al.* 1998; Hurford *et al.* 1998). In addition, Geminiani *et al.* found that dopaminergic agonist treatment helped both the sensory-attentional and motor-intentional forms of spatial neglect. However, Barrett *et al.* (1999) and Grujic *et al.* (1998) found that, in some patients, dopamine agonist therapy increased rather than decreased the severity of neglect. Barrett *et al.* suggested that the paradoxical effect seen in their patient, who had striatal injury, may be related to involvement of the basal ganglia. In patients with striatal injury, dopamine agonists may be unable to activate the striatum on the injured side but instead activate the striatum on the uninjured side, thereby increasing the ipsilesional orientation bias.

Representational and memory hypotheses

Anterograde deficits

After a hemispheric injury patients with spatial neglect may have trouble recalling perceived stimuli presented in contralesional hemispace—an anterograde memory deficit. They may also be impaired at recalling contralesional stimuli that were learned before the stroke—a retrograde deficit. The anterograde memory deficit has been reported in several modalities. For example, we randomly presented consonants through earphones to patients on either the neglected or non-neglected side and asked subjects with spatial neglect to report the stimulus either immediately or after a distraction-filled interval. We found that distraction induced more of a memory deficit for stimuli presented to the contralesional ear than those presented to the ipsilesional ear (Heilman *et al.* 1974). In the visual modality Samuels *et al.* (1971) tested patients with right parietal lesions and found a similar phenomenon, but unfortunately they did not evaluate their subjects for neglect.

In theory, a memory deficit that results in a subject not fully recalling the presence or magnitude of a stimulus could induce neglect in tasks such as picture-copying, cancelling stimuli distributed on a page, or bisecting lines. To test this hypothesis, Reistra *et al.* (2001) presented pre-bisected lines to patients with spatial neglect and asked them which segment was shorter. Unlike the original Landmark test (Harvey *et al.* 1995) where a vertical mark divides the line into two segments, in this test a gap divided the line into two segments. When the two segments were presented sequentially not only did the subjects perform better than when they were presented simultaneously, but also their performance was no different from that of control subjects, suggesting that in these subjects, with this testing paradigm, a contralesional anterograde memory defect could not account for their spatial neglect.

Retrograde deficits

Denny-Brown and Banker (1954) reported a patient who could not describe from memory the details of the side of a room that was opposite to her cerebral lesion. Bisiach and Luzzatti (1978) asked two patients with neglect to recall details of a square in Milan from one perspective. These patients were unable to recall left-sided details. They then asked them to recall details of the same famous square from the opposite perspective (the other side of the square) and the patients had trouble recalling details that were on the left from this perspective (but were on the right from the first perspective). Denny-Brown and Banker's observations as well as Bisiach and Luzzati's descriptions suggest that patients can have a deficit in body-centered hemispatial memory or imagery. Bisiach attributed this deficit to destruction of the representation of left space stored in the right hemisphere. More recently Bisiach and coworkers have modified this hemispatial representational hypothesis and now suggest that with spatial neglect the representation of space is distorted ('anisometry') (see Chapter 4.1). Destruction or distortion of a representation may account not only for a deficit in imagery and memory but also for spatial neglect. The construct of attention derives from the knowledge that the human brain has a limited capacity to process information simultaneously. Therefore the organism must select what stimuli to process. Except for stimuli that will be attended regardless of significance, such as unexpected moving objects, loud sounds, or bright lights, attention is directed in a 'top-down' fashion. Therefore knowledge or representations must direct the selection process. There are at least two representations that are needed to perform a spatial task: a representation of the target independent of its position in space, and a representation of the environment. Because patients with left-sided spatial neglect are able to detect target stimuli on the right side in a cancellation task, their failure to detect stimuli on the left cannot be attributed to a loss of the representation of the target. If the knowledge of left space is stored in the right hemisphere and these representations are destroyed, attention may not be fully directed to left space because the person has no knowledge of this space. In a similar fashion, mental representations may also direct action. The number of independent actions one can perform simultaneously is also limited. Therefore, just as one selects stimuli to process, one must also select actions to perform. There are at least two pieces of knowledge that guide action—how to move, and where to act. Since patients with spatial neglect know how to act in ipsilesional space, their failure to act in contralesional space cannot be attributed to a loss of the 'how' representation, but if knowledge of contralesional space is lost, one may fail to act in or toward that portion of space. Thus, both intentional and attentional defects may be induced by a representational defect.

The loss of a representation (knowledge) of one-half of space should be manifested by all the signs we discussed: an attentional deficit, an intentional deficit, a memory deficit, and an imagery deficit. Unless a patient has all these deficits, hemispatial neglect cannot be attributed to a loss of the spatial representation. In the clinic we see patients who have primarily a motor-intentional disorder as well as others who have primarily a sensory-attentional disorder. Not all patients with neglect have imagery defects and some patients with imagery defects do not have hemispatial neglect (Guariglia *et al.* 1993). Therefore, a representational deficit cannot account for all types of spatial neglect. A representational defect also cannot account for the attentional and intentional biases we have discussed. However, there are patients who are severely inattentive to contralesional stimuli, fail to explore contralesional space, and have a profound contralesional spatial memory defect. Although these patients may have defects in multiple systems, their representation for contralesional space may be destroyed so that they no longer know of its existence.

Possible mechanisms for spatial memory deficits

William James (1890) noted that 'an object once attended will remain in the memory whilst one inattentively allowed to pass will leave no trace behind.' The relationship of attention-arousal to learning has received considerable interest (Eysenck 1976). For example, direct relationships have been found between phasic skin conductance response amplitude during learning and accuracy of immediate and delayed recall (Stelmack *et al.* 1983). As discussed above, spatial neglect may be associated with an attention-arousal deficit. Stimuli presented in the hemispace contralateral to a hemispheric lesion may receive less attention and be associated with less arousal than stimuli presented in ipsilateral hemispace. Because these stimuli are poorly attended and do not induce arousal, they may be poorly encoded and thereby induce a hemispatial anterograde memory deficit.

Based on their demonstration that patients with spatial neglect have a hemispatial retrograde amnesia, Bisiach *et al.* (1979) posited that the mental representation of the environment is structured topographically and is mapped across the brain such that the mental picture of the environment (e.g. the square in Milan) can be split between the two hemispheres (like the projection of a real scene) so that the left side of the square is mapped on the right side of the brain and the right side of the square on the left side of the brain. Thus, with right-hemisphere damage there is a representational disorder for the left half of this image. There are at least two other reasons why one side of a mental image could not be envisioned: the representation may have been intact but could not be activated so that an image was not formed; the full image was formed, but one portion of this image was not attended and thus not fully inspected. If, as suggested by Bisiach, the representation is destroyed, attentional manipulation should not affect retrieval, but if patients with neglect have either a activational or attentional deficit, attentional manipulation may affect retrieval. Meador *et al.* (1987) replicated Bisiach and Luzzatti's observations and also provided evidence that behavioral manipulations could affect performance. It has been shown that when normal subjects are asked to recall objects in space, they move their eyes to the position that the object occupied (Kahneman 1973). Although it is unclear why normal subjects move their eyes during this type of recall task, having patients move their eyes toward neglected hemispace may aid recall because the eye movement induces hemispheric activation, or helps direct attention, or both. Meador *et al.* (1987) asked a patient with left hemispatial neglect and defective left hemispatial recall to move his eyes to either right or left hemispace during recall. The patient's recall of left-sided detail was better when he was looking toward the left than toward the right. Further support of the attentional-activation hypothesis of representational neglect comes from the work of Guariglia *et al.* (1998) who demonstrated that somatosensory stimulation on the left side improves left-sided imagery disorders. Although these findings provide evidence that hemispatial retrograde amnesia may be induced by an exploratory-attentional deficit or an activation deficit, they do not differentiate between these possibilities. They also do not exclude the possibility that in other cases the representation may have been destroyed.

Exploratory hypothesis

Chedru *et al.* (1973) recorded eye movements of patients with left-sided spatial neglect and demonstrated a failure to explore the left side of space. This failure to explore could not be accounted for by paralysis, since these patients could voluntarily look leftward. Karnath *et al.* (1998) measured both head and eye movements and again demonstrated a rightward exploratory bias. If patients fail to explore the left side of a line, they may never learn the full extent of the line, bisecting only the portion they have explored. Similarly, if they do not fully explore the left side of a sheet, they may fail to cancel targets on the part of the sheet that they have failed to explore. However, deficits of exploration may be attributed to the attentional, intentional, or representational defects previously discussed.

Conclusions

Spatial neglect is a common and severely disabling neurobehavioral disorder induced by a variety of pathological processes. Studies have shown that patients with neglect are less likely to live independently than even patients with severe aphasia and a right hemiparesis. An understanding of the pathophysiology of neglect has allowed investigators to begin to develop some rational treatments for this disorder. When we started this research, more than three decades ago, no more than five papers were published in a year. Now, hundreds of important and exciting papers are published annually. Hopefully, this research will continue to improve our understanding and treatment of this behavioral disorder. Perhaps of equal or greater importance, the study of neglect has enabled investigators to understand the brain mechanisms underlying mental functions such as attention and intention. These functions are critical in all stages of life and are affected by many diseases and disorders, both developmental and acquired.

References

Akert, K. and von Monakow, K. H. (1980). Relationship of precentral, premotor, and prefrontal cortex to the mediodorsal and intralaminar nuclei of the monkey thalamus. *Acta Neurobiologica Experimentalis*, **40**, 7–25.

Albert, M. D. (1973). A simple test of visual neglect. *Neurology*, **23,** 658–64.

Allen, I. M. (1948) Unilateral visual inattention. *New Zealand Medical Journal*, **47**, 605–17.

Anderson, M. and Yoshida, M. (1977). Electrophysiological evidence for branching nigral projections to the thalamus and superior colliculus. *Brain Research*, **137**, 361–4.

Anton, G. (1899). Uber die Selbstwahrnehmung der Herderkrankungen des Gehirns durch den Kranken der Rindenblindheit und Rindentaubheit. *Archiv für Psychiatrie*, **32**, 86–127.

Anzola, G. P., Bertoloni, A., Buchtel, H. A., and Rizzolatti, G. (1977). Spatial compatibility and anatomical factors in simple and choice reaction time. *Neuropsychologia*, **15**, 295–302.

Apicella, P., Legallet, E., Nieoullon, A., and Trouche, E. (1991). Neglect of contralateral visual stimuli in monkeys with unilateral dopamine depletion. *Behavioural Brain Research*, **46**, 187–95.

Arbuthnott, G. W. and Ungerstedt, U. (1975). Turning behavior induced by electrical stimulation of the nigro-striatal system of the rat. *Experimental Neurology*, **27**, 162–72.

Arnault, P. and Roger, M. (1987). The connections of the peripeduncular area studied by retrograde and anterograde transport in the rat. *Journal of Comparative Neurology*, **258**, 463–78.

Avemo, A., Antelman, S., and Ungerstedt, U. (1973). Rotational behavior after unilateral frontal cortex lesions in the rat. *Acta Physiologica Scandinavica Supplementum*, **396**, 77.

Baleydier, C. and Mauguiere, F. (1980). The duality of the cingulate gyrus in monkey— neuroanatomical study and functional hypothesis. *Brain*, **103**, 525–54.

Barrett, A. M., Crucian, G. P., Schwartz, R. L., and Heilman, K. M. (1999). Adverse effect of dopamine agonist therapy in a patient with motor-intentional neglect. *Archives of Physical Medicine and Rehabilitation*, **80**, 600–3.

Battersby, W. S., Bender, M. B., and Pollack, M. (1956). Unilateral spatial agnosia (inattention) in patients with cerebral lesions. *Brain*, **79**, 68–93.

Bender, M. B. (1952). *Disorders of perception*. C. C. Thomas, Springfield, IL.

Bender, M. B., and Furlow, C. T. (1944). Phenomenon of visual extinction and binocular rivalry mechanism. *Transactions of the American Neurological Association*, **70**, 87–93.

Bender, M. B. and Furlow, C. T. (1945). Phenomenon of visual extinction and homonymous fields and psychological principals involved. *Archives of Neurology and Psychiatry*, **53**, 29–33.

Bignall, K. E. and Imbert, M. (1969). Polysensory and cortico-cortical projections to frontal lobe of squirrel and rhesus monkey. *Electroencephalography and Clinical Neurophysiology*, **26**, 206–15.

Bisiach, E. and Luzzatti, C. (1978). Unilateral neglect of representational space. *Cortex*, **14**, 29–133.

Bisiach, E., Luzzatti, C., and Perani, D. (1979). Unilateral neglect, representational schema and consciousness. *Brain*, **102**, 609–18.

Bisiach, E., Geminiani, G., Berti, A., and Rusconi, M. L. (1990). Perceptual and premotor factors of unilateral neglect. *Neurology*, **40**, 1278–81.

Bogousslavsky, J., Miklossy, J., Deruaz, J. P., Regli, F., and Assai, G. (1986). Unilateral left para-median infarction of thalamus and midbrain: a clinico-pathological study. *Journal of Neurology, Neurosurgery and Psychiatry*, **49**, 686–94.

Bowers, D. and Heilman, K. M. (1980). Effects of hemispace on tactile line bisection task. *Neuropsychologia*, **18**, 491–8.

Bowers, D., Heilman, K. M., and Van Den Abell, T. (1981). Hemispace–visual half field compatibility. *Neuropsychologia*, **19**, 757–65.

Bradley, P. B. (1968). The effect of atropine and related drugs on the EEG and behavior. *Progress in Brain Research*, **28**, 3–13.

Brain, W. R. (1941). Visual disorientation with special reference to lesions of the right cerebral hemisphere. *Brain* **64**: 224–72.

Brown, R. M., Crane, A. M., and Goldman, P. S. (1979). Regional distribution of monamines in the cerebral cortex and subcortical structures of the rhesus monkey: concentrations and *in vivo* synthesis rates. *Brain Research*, **168**, 133–50.

Burcham, K. J., Corwin, J. V., Stoll, M. L., and Reep, R. L. (1997). Disconnection of medial agranular and posterior parietal cortex produces multimodal neglect in rats. *Behavioural Brain Research*, **86**, 41–47.

Bushnell, M. C., Goldberg, M. E., and Robinson, D. L. (1981). Behavioral enhancement of visual responses in monkey cerebral cortex. I: Modulation of posterior parietal cortex related to selected visual attention. *Journal of Neurophysiology*, **46**, 755–772.

Bushnell, P. J., Chiba, A. A., and Oshiro, W. M. (1998). Effects of unilateral removal of basal forebrain cholinergic neurons on cued target detection in rats. *Behavioural Brain Research*, **90**, 57–71.

Butter, C. M., Kirsch, N. L., and Reeves, G. (1990). The effect of lateralized dynamic stimuli on unilateral spatial neglect following right hemisphere lesions. *Restorative Neurology and Neuroscience*, **2**, 39–46.

Chatterjee, A., Mennemeier, M., and Heilman, K. M. (1992). Search patterns and neglect: a case study. *Neuropsychologia*, **30**, 657–72.

Chavis, D. A. and Pandya, D. N. (1976). Further observations on corticofrontal connections in the rhesus monkey. *Brain Research*, **117**, 369–86.

Chedru, F., Leblanc, M., and Lhermitte, F. (1973). Visual searching in normal and braindamaged subjects. *Cortex* **9**: 94–111.

Colby, C. L. and Goldberg, M. E. (1999). Space and attention in parietal cortex. *Annual Review of Neuroscience*, **22**, 319–49.

Colby, C. L., Duhamel, J.-R., and Goldberg, M. E. (1996). Visual, presaccadic and cognitive activation of single neurons in monkey lateral intraparietal area. *Journal of Neurophysiology*, **76**, 2841–52.

Corbett, D. and Wise, R. A. (1980). Intracranial self-stimulation in relation to the ascending dopaminergic systems of the midbrain: moveable electrode mapping study. *Brain Research*, **185**, 1–15.

Corwin, J. V., Kanter, S., Watson, R. T., Heilman, K. M., Valenstein, E., and Hashimoto, A. (1986). Apomorphine has a therapeutic effect on neglect produced by unilateral dorsomedial prefrontal cortex lesions in rats. *Experimental Neurology*, **36**, 683–98.

Coslett, H. B., Bowers, D., Fitzpatrick, E., Haws, B., and Heilman, K. M. (1990). Directional hypokinesia and hemispatial inattention in neglect. *Brain*, **113**, 475–86.

Craft, J. and Simon, J. (1970). Processing symbolic information from a visual display: interference from an irrelevant directional clue. *Journal of Experimental Psychology*, **83**, 415–20.

Critchley, M. (1966). *The Parietal Lobes*. New York: Hafner.

Crossman, A. R., Sambrook, M. A., Horwitz, M., and Ritter, W. (1977). The neurological basis of motor asymmetry following unilateral 6-hydroxydopamine lesions in the rat: the effect of motor decortication. *Journal of Neurological Science*, **34**, 407–14.

Dalsass, M. and Krauthamer, G. M. (1981). Behavioral alterations and loss of caudate modulation in the CM–PF complex of the cat after electrolytic lesions of the substantia nigra. *Brain Research*, **208**, 67–79.

Damasio, A. R., Damasio, H., Chui, and H. C. (1980). Neglect following damage to frontal lobe or basal ganglia. *Neuropsychologia*, **18**, 123–32.

Denny-Brown, D. and Banker, B. Q. (1954). Amophosynthesis from left parietal lesions. *Archives of Neurology and Psychiatry*, **71**, 302–13.

De Renzi, E., Faglioni, P., and Scott, G. (1970). Hemispheric contribution to the exploration of space through the visual and tactile modality. *Cortex*, **1**, 410–33.

Deuel, R. K. (1980). Sensorimotor dysfunction after unilateral hypothalamic lesions in rhesus monkeys. *Neurology*, **30**, 358.

Divac, I., Fonnum, F., and Storm-Mathison, J. (1977). High affinity uptake of glutamate in terminals of corticostriatal axons. *Nature*, **266**, 377–8.

Duke-Elder, W. S. (1949). *Textbook of opthalmology*. Vol. 4, *The neurology of vision: motor and optical anomalies*. C. V. Mosby, London.

Eidelberg, E. and Schwartz, A. J. (1971). Experimental analysis of the extinction phenomenon in monkeys. *Brain*, **94**, 91–108.

Eysenck, M. W. (1976). Arousal, learning and memory. *Psychological Bulletin*, **83**, 389–404.

Feeney, D. M. and Wier, C. S. (1979). Sensory neglect after lesions of the substantia nigra and lateral hypothalamus: differential severity and recovery of function. *Brain Research*, **178**, 329–46.

Fiorelli, M., Blin, J., Bakchine, S., LaPlane, D., and Baron, J. C. (1991). PET studies of cortical diaschisis in patients with motor hemi-neglect. *Journal of Neurological Science*, **104**, 135–42.

Fleet, W. S., Valenstein, E., Watson, R. T., and Heilman, K. M. (1987). Dopamine agonist therapy for neglect in humans. *Neurology*, **37**, 1765–71.

Fonnum, F. and Walaas, I. (1979). Localization of neurotransmitter candidates in neostriatum. In *The neostriatum* (ed. I. Divac and R. G. E. Oberg), pp. 53–69. Pergamon Press, Oxford.

Geminiani, G., Bottini, G., and Sterzi, R. (1998). Dopaminergic stimulation in unilateral neglect. *Journal of Neurology, Neurosurgery and Psychiatry*, **65**, 344–7.

Gainotti, G., Messerli, P., and Tissot, R. (1972). Qualitative analysis of unilateral and spatial neglect in relation to laterality of cerebral lesions. *Journal of Neurology, Neurosurgery and Psychiatry*, **35**, 545–50.

Goldberg, M. E. and Bushnell, M. C. (1981). Behavioral enhancement of visual responses in monkey cerebral cortex. II: Modulation in frontal eye fields specifically related saccades. *Journal of Neurophysiology*, **46**, 773–87.

Goldberg, M. E., and Robinson, D. C. (1977). Visual responses of neurons in monkey inferior parietal lobule: the physiological substrate of attention and neglect. *Neurology*, **27**, 350.

Goldenberg, G. (1986). Neglect in a patient with partial callosal disconnection. *Neuropsychologia*, **24**, 397–403.

Grofova, I. (1979). Extrinsic connections of neostriatum. In *The neostriatum* (ed. I. Divac and R. G. E. Oberg ed.), pp. 37–51. Pergamon Press, Oxford.

Grossman, S. P., Dacey, D., Halaris, A. E., Collier, T., and Routtenberg, A. (1978). Aphagia and adipsia after preferential destruction of nerve cell bodies in the hypothalamus. *Science*, **202**, 537–9.

Grujic, Z., Mapstone, M., Gitelman, D. R., *et al.* (1998). Dopamine agonists reorient visual exploration away from the neglected hemispace. *Neurology*, **51**, 1395–8.

Guariglia, C., Padovani, A., Pantano, P., and Pizzamiglio, L. (1993). Unilateral neglect restricted to visual imagery. *Nature*, **364**, 237.

Guariglia, C., Lippolis, G., and Pizzamiglio, L. (1998). Somatosensory stimulation improves imagery disorders in neglect. *Cortex*, **34**, 233–41.

Hagamen, T. C., Greeley, H. P., Hagamen, W. D., and Reeves, A. G. (1977). Behavioral asymmetries following olfactory tubercle lesions in cats. *Brain Behavior and Evolution*, **14**, 241–50.

Halligan, P. W. and Marshall, J. C. (1991). Left neglect for near but not far space in man. *Nature*, **350**, 498–500.

Halligan, P. W. and Marshall, J. C. (1993). The history and clinical presentation of neglect. In *Unilateral neglect: clinical and experimental studies* (ed. I. H. Robertson and J. C. Marshall). Lawrence Erlbaum, Hillsdale, NJ, pp. 3–25.

Harvey, M., Milner, A. D., and Roberts, R. C. (1995). An investigation of hemispatial neglect using the Landmark Task. *Brain and Cognition*, **27**, 59–78.

Haxby, J. V., Grady, C. L., Horwitz, B., *et al.* (1991). Dissociation of object and spatial visual processing pathways in human extrastriate cortex. *Proceedings of the National Academy of Sciences of the United States of America*, **88**, 1621–5.

Hecean, H. and Albert, M. L. (1978). *Human neuropsychology*. Wiley, New York.

Heikkila, R. E., Shapiro, B. S., and Duvoisin, R. C. (1981). The relationship between loss of dopamine nerve terminals: striatal [3H]spiroperidol binding and rotational behavior in unilaterally 6-hydroxdopamine-lesioned rats. *Brain Research*, **211**, 285–307.

Heilman, K. M. (1979). Neglect and related disorders. In *Clinical neuropsychology* (ed. K. M. Heilman and E. Valenstein), pp. 268–307. Oxford University Press, New York.

Heilman, K. M. and Valenstein, E. (1972). Frontal lobe neglect in man. *Neurology*, **22**, 660–4.

Heilman, K. M. and Valenstein, E. (1979). Mechanisms underlying hemispatial neglect. *Annals of Neurology*, **5**, 166–70.

Heilman, K. M. and Watson, R. T. (1977). The neglect syndrome—a unilateral defect of the orienting response. In *Lateralization in the nervous system* (ed. S. Hardned, R. W. Doty, L. Goldstein, J. Jaynes, and G. K. Thamer). Academic Press, New York, pp. 285–302.

Heilman, K. M., Pandya, D. N., and Geschwind, N. (1970). Trimodal inattention following parietal lobe ablations. *Transactions of the American Neurological Association*, **95**, 259–61.

Heilman, K. M., Watson, R. T., and Schulman, H. (1974). A unilateral memory deficit. *Journal of Neurology, Neurosurgery and Psychiatry*, **37**, 790–3.

Heilman, K. M., Schwartz, H. F., Watson, R. T. (1978) Hypoarousal in patients with the neglect syndrome and emotional indifference. *Neurology*, **28**, 229–32.

Heilman, K. M., Bowers, D., and Watson, R. T. (1983*a*). Performance on hemispatial pointing task by patients with neglect syndrome. *Neurology*, **33**, 661–4.

Heilman, K. M., Valenstein, E., and Watson, R. T. (1983*b*). Localization of neglect. In *Localization in neurology* (ed. A. Kertesz), pp. 471–92. Academic Press, New York.

Heilman, K. M., Bowers, D., and Watson, R. T. (1984). Pseudoneglect in patients with partial callosal disconnection. *Brain*, **107**, 519–32.

Heilman, K. M., Bowers, D., Coslett, H. B., Whelan, H., and Watson, R. T. (1985). Directional hypokinesia: prolonged reaction times for leftward movements in patients with right hemisphere lesions and neglect. *Neurology*, **35**, 855–60.

Heilman, K. M., Watson, R. T., and Valenstein, E. (1993). Neglect and related disorders. In *Clinical neuropsychology* (3rd edn) (ed. K. M. Heilman and E. Valenstein), pp. 279–336. Oxford University Press, New York.

Heilman, K. M., Watson, R. T., and Valenstein E. (2003). Neglect and related disorders. In *Clinical neuropsychology* (4th edn) (ed. K. M. Heilman and E. Valenstein). Oxford University Press, New York.

Herkenham, M. (1979). The afferent and efferent connections of the ventromedial thalamic nucleus in the rat. *Journal of Comparative Neurology*, **183**, 487–518.

Holmes, G. (1918). Disturbances of vision from cerebrel lesions. *British Journal of Ophthalmology*, **2**, 253–384.

Hoyman, L., Weese, G. D., and Frommer, G. P. (1979). Tactile discrimination performance deficits following neglect-producing unilateral lateral hypothalamic lesions in the rat. *Physiology and Behavior*, **22**, 139–47.

Hurford, P., Stringer, A. Y., and Jann, B. (1998). Neuropharmacologic treatment of hemineglect. *Archives of Physical Medicine and Rehabilitation*, **79**, 346–9.

James, W. (1890). *The principles of psychology*, Vol. 2. Holt, New York.

Jones, B. E., Harper, S. T., and Halaris, A. E. (1977). Effects of locus coeruleus lesions upon cerebral monoamine content, sleep-wakefullness and the response to amphetamines in the cat. *Brain Research*, **124**, 473–96.

Jouvet, M. (1977). Neuropharmacology of the sleep waking cycle. In *Handbook of psychopharmacology* (ed. L. L. Iverson, S. D. Iverson, and S. H. Snyder). pp. 233–293. Plenum Press, New York.

Kahneman, D. (1973). *Eye movement attention and effort*. Prentice-Hall, Englewood Cliffs, NJ.

Kanai, T. and Szerb, J. C. (1965). Mesencephalic reticular activating system and cortical acetylcholine output. *Nature*, **205**, 80–2.

Karnath, H-O., Niemeier, M., and Dichgans, J. (1998). Space exploration in neglect. *Brain*, **121**, 2357–67.

Kartsounis, L. D. and Warrington, E. K. (1989). Unilateral visual neglect overcome by ones implicit in stimulus arrays. *Journal of Neurology, Neurosurgery and Psychiatry*, **52**, 1253–9.

Karussis, D., Leker, R. R., and Abramsky, O. (2000). Cognitive dysfunction following thalamic stroke: a study of 16 cases and review of the literature. *Journal of Neurological Science*, **172**, 25–9.

Kertesz, A., Nicholson, I., Cancelliere, A., Kassa, K., and Black, S. E. (1985). Motor impersistence: a right-hemisphere syndrome. *Neurology*, **35**, 662–6.

Kievet, J., and Kuypers, H. G. J. M. (1977). Organization of the thalamo-cortical connections to the frontal lobe in the rhesus monkey. *Experimental Brain Research*, **29**: 299–322.

Kim, M., Na, D. L., Kim, G. M., Adair, J. C., Lee, K. H., and Heilman K. M. (1999). Ipsilesional neglect: behavioural and anatomical features. *Journal of Neurology, Neurosurgery and Psychiatry*, **67**, 35–8.

Kinomura, S., Larsson, J., Gulyas, B., and Roland, P. E. (1996). Activation by attention of the human reticular formation and thalamic intralaminar nuclei. *Science*, **271**, 512–15.

Kinsbourne, M. (1970). A model for the mechanism of unilateral neglect of space. *Transactions of the American Neurological Association*, **95**, 143.

Kuypers, H. G. J. M. and Lawrence, D. G. (1967). Cortical projections to the red nucleus and the brain stem in the rhesus monkey. *Brain Research*, **4**, 151–88.

Kwon, S. E. and Heilman, K. M. (1991). Ipsilateral neglect in patient following a unilateral frontal lesion. *Neurology*, **41**, 2001–4.

Làdavas, E. and Pavani, F.(1998). Neuropsychological evidence of the functional integration of visual, auditory and proprioceptive spatial maps. *Neuroreport*, **9**, 1195–2000.

Làdavas, E., Petronio, A., and Umiltà, C. (1990). The deployment of visual attention in the intact field of hemineglect patients. *Cortex*, **26**, 307–12.

Leibovitch, F. S., Black, S. E., Caldwell, C. B., Ebert, P. L., Ehrlich, L. E., and Szalai, J. P. (1998). Brain–behavior correlations in hemispatial neglect using CT and SPECT: the Sunnybrook Stroke Study. *Neurology*, **50**, 901–8.

Lindvall, O., Bjorklund, A., Morre, R. Y., and Stenevi, U. (1974). Mesencephalic dopamine-neurons projecting to the neocortex. *Brain Research*, **81**, 325–31.

Ljungberg, T. and Ungerstedt, U. (1976). Sensory inattention produced by 6-hydroxydopamine-induced degeneration of ascending dopamine neurons in the brain. *Experimental Neurology*, **53**, 585–600.

Loeb, J. (1885). Die elementaren Storunger eirfacher functionennach oberflachlicher umschriebener Verletzung des Grosshirns. *Pflugers Archiv für die gesamte Physiologie des Menschen und der Tiere*, **37**, 51–6.

Lynch, J. C. (1980). The functional organization of posterior parietal association cortex. *Behavioral and Brain Sciences*, **3**, 485–534.

McCormick, D. A. and Williamson, A. (1989). Convergence and divergence of neurotransmitter action in human cerebral cortex. *Proceedings of the National Academy of Sciences of the United States of America*, **86**, 8098–102.

McFie, J., Piercy, M. F., and Zangwell, O. L. (1950). Visual spatial agnosia associated with lesions of the right hemisphere. *Brain*, **73**, 167–90.

Mark, V. W. and Heilman, K. M. (1998). Diagonal spatial neglect. *Journal of Neurology, Neurosurgery and Psychiatry*, **65**, 348–52.

Mark, V. W., Kooistra, C. A., and Heilman, K. M. (1988). Hemispatial neglect affected by nonneglected stimuli. *Neurology*, **38**, 1207–11.

Marshall, J. F. (1979). Somatosensory inattention after dopamine-depleting intracerebral 6-OHDA injections: spontaneous recovery and pharmacological control. *Brain Research*, **177**, 311–24.

Marshall, J. F., Turner, B. H., and Teitelbaum, P. (1971). Sensory neglect produced by lateral hypothalamic damage. *Science*, **174**, 523–5.

Marshall, J. F., Richardson, J. S., and Teitelbaum, P. (1974). Nigrostriatal bundle damage and the lateral hypothalamic damage. *Journal of Comparative and Physiological Psychology*, **87**, 808–30.

Mattingley, J. B., Husain, M., Rorden, C., Kennard, C., and Driver, J. (1998). Motor role of human inferior parietal lobe revealed in unilateral neglect patients. *Nature*, **392**, 179–82.

Meador, K., Hammond, E. J., Loring, D. W., Allen, M., Bowers, D., and Heilman, K. M. (1987). Cognitive evoked potentials and disorders of recent memory. *Neurology*, **37**, 526–9.

Mehler, W. R. (1966). Further notes of the center median nucleus of Luys. In *The thalamus* (ed. D. P. Purpura and M. D. Yahr), pp. 109–22. Columbia University Press, New York.

Mennemeier, M. S., Chatterjee, A., Watson, R. T., Wertman, E., Carter, L. P., and Heilman, K. M. (1994). Contributions of the parietal frontal lobes to sustained attention and habituation. *Neuropsychologia*, **32**, 703–16.

Mesulam, M. M. (1981). A cortical network for directed attention and unilateral neglect. *Annals of Neurology*, **10**, 309–25.

Mesulam, M., Van Hesen, G. W., Pandya, D. N., and Geschwind, N. (1977). Limbic and sensory connections of the inferior parietal lobule (area PG) in the rhesus monkey: a study with a new method for horseradish peroxsidase histochemistry. *Brain Research*, **136**, 393–414.

Meyer, E., Ferguson, S. S. G., Zarorre, R. J., *et al.* (1991). Attention modulates somatosensory cerebral blood flow response to vibrotactile stimulation as measured by positron emission tomography. *Annals of Neurology*, **29**, 440–3.

Mills, R. P. and Swanson, P. D. (1978). Vertical oculomotor apraxia and memory loss. *Annals of Neurology*, **4**, 149–53.

Moruzzi, G. and Magoun, H. W. (1949). Brainstem reticular formation and activation of the EEG. *Electroencephalography and Clinical Neurophysiology*, **1**, 455–73.

Motter, B. C. and Mountcastle, V. B. (1981). The functional properties of the light sensitive neurons of the posterior parietal cortex studied in waking monkeys: foveal sparing and opponent vector organization. *Journal of Neuroscience*, **1**, 3–26.

Mountcastle, V. B., Lynch, J. C., Georgopoulos, A., Sakata, H., and Acuna, C. (1975). Posterior parietal association cortex of the monkey: command function from operations within extrapersonal space. *Journal of Neurophysiology*, **38**, 871–908.

Mountcastle, V. B., Anderson, R. A., and Motter, B. C. (1981). The influence of attentive fixation upon the excitability of the light sensitive neurons of the posterior parietal cortex. *Journal of Neuroscience*, **1**, 1218–45.

Na, D. L., Adair, J. C., Kim, G. M., Seo, D. W., Hong, S. B., and Heilman, K. M. (1998*a*). Ipsilateral neglect during intracarotid amobarbital test. *Neurology*, **51**, 276–9.

Na, D. L., Adair, J. C., Williamson, D. J., Schwartz, R. L., Haws, B., and Heilman, K. M. (1998*b*). Dissociation of sensory-attentional from motor-intentional neglect. *Journal of Neurology, Neurosurgery and Psychiatry*, **64**, 331–8.

Na, D. L., Adair, J. C., Kang, Y., Chung, C. S., Lee, K. H., and Heilman, K. M. (1999). Motor perseverative behavior on a line cancellation task. *Neurology*, **52**, 1569–76.

Nathan, P. W. (1946). On simultaneous bilateral stimulation of the body in a lesion of the parietal lobe. *Brain*, **69**, 325–34.

Neve, K. A., Kozlowski, M. R., and Marshall, J. F. (1982). Plasticity of neostriatal dopamine receptors after nigrostriatal injury: relationship to recovery of sensorimotor functions and behavioral supersensitivity. *Brain Research*, **244**, 33–44.

Nieoullon, A., Cheramy, A., and Glowinski, J. (1978). Release of dopamine evoked by electrical stimulation of the motor and visual areas of the cerebral cortex in both caudate nuclei and in the substantia nigra in the cat. *Brain Research*, **15**, 69–83.

Olds, J. and Milner, P. (1954). Positive reinforcement produced by electrical stimulation of septal area and other regions of the rat brain. *Journal of Comparative and Physiological Psychology*, 47: 419–427.

Oppenheim, H. (1885). Ueber eine durch eine klinisch bisher nicht verwertete Untersuchungs-methode ermittelte Form der Sensibitats-storung bei einseitigen Erkrankunger des Grosshirns. *Zentralblatt für Neurologie*, **4**, 529–33. (Cited by Benton, A. L. (1956). Jacques Loeb and the method of double stimulation. *Journal of the History of Medical and Allied Science*, **11**, 47–53.)

Pandya, D. M., and Kuypers, H. G. J. M. (1969). Cortico-cortical connections in the rhesus monkey. *Brain Research*, **13**, 13–36.

Paterson, A. and Zangwill, O. L. (1944). Disorders of visual space perception associated with lesions of the right cerebral hemisphere. *Brain*, **67**, 331–58.

Pineas, H. (1931). Ein Fall von räumlicher Orientierungsstörung mit Dyschirie. *Zeitschrift für die Gesamte Neurologie und Psychiatrie*, **133**, 180–95.

Poppelreuter, W. L. (1917). *Die psychischen Schadigungen durch Kopfschuss Krieg im 1914–1916: die Storungen der niederen und hoheren Leistkungen durch Verletzungen des Oksipitalhirns*, Vol. 1. Leopold Voss, Leipzig. (Cited by Critchley, M. (1949). *Brain*, **72**, 540.)

Posner, M. I., Walker, J., Friedrich, F. J., and Rafal, R. D. (1984). Effects of parietal lobe injury on covert orienting of visual attention. *Journal of Neuroscience*, **4**, 163–87.

Pycock, C. J. (1980). Turning behavior in animals. *Neuroscience*, **5**, 461–514.

Rapcsak, S. Z., Watson, R. T., and Heilman, K. M. (1987). Hemispace–visual field interactions in visual extinction. *Journal of Neurology, Neurosurgery and Psychiatry*, **50**, 1117–24.

Rapcsak, S. Z., Cimino, C. R., and Heilman, K. M. (1988). Altitudinal neglect. *Neurology*, **38**, 277–81.

Redgrave, P., Prescott, T. J., and Gurney, K. (1999). Is the short-latency dopamine response too short to signal reward error? *Trends in Neuroscience*, **22**, 146–51.

Reeves, A. G. and Hagamen, W. D. (1971). Behavioral and EEG asymmetry following unilateral lesions of the forebrain and midbrain of cats. *Electroencephalography and Clinical Neurophysiology*, **39**, 83–6.

Reider, N. (1946). Phenomena of sensory suppression. *Archives of Neurology and Psychiatry*, **55**, 583–90.

Riddoch, M. J., and Humphreys, G. (1983). The effect of cueing on unilateral neglect. *Neuropsychologia*, **21**, 589–99.

Riestra, A. R., Crucian G. P., Burks, D. W., Womack K. B., and Heilman, K. M. (2001). Extinction, working memory, and line bisection in spatial neglect. *Neurology*. **57**: 147–9.

Robinson, D. L., Goldberg, M. E., and Stanton, G. B. (1978). Parietal association cortex in the primate sensory mechanisms and behavioral modulations. *Journal of Neurophysiology*, **41**, 910–32.

Roeltgen, M. G., Roeltgen, D. P., and Heilman, K. M. (1989). Unilateral motor impersistence and hemispatial neglect from a striatal lesion. *Neuropsychiatry, Neuropsychology, and Behavioral Neurology*, **2**, 125–35.

Sakashita, Y. (1991). Visual attentional disturbance with unilateral lesions in the basal ganglia and deep white matter. *Annals of Neurology*, **30**, 673–7.

Samuels, I., Butters, N., and Goodglass, H. (1971). Visual memory defects following cortical limbic lesions: effect of field of presentation. *Physiology and Behavior*, **6**, 447–52.

Sato, H., Hata, Y., Hagihara, K., and Tsumoto, T. (1987). Effects of cholinergic depletion on neuron activities in the cat visual cortex. *Journal of Neurophysiology*, **58**, 781–94.

Scheibel, M. E. and Scheibel, A. B. (1966). The organization of the nucleus reticularis thalami: a Golgi study. *Brain Research*, **1**, 43–62.

Scheibel, M. E. and Scheibel, A. B. (1967). Structural organization of nonspecific thalamic nuclei and their projection toward cortex. *Brain*, **6**, 60–94.

Schneider, J. S., McLaughlin, W. W., and Roeltgen, D. P. (1992). Motor and nonmotor behavioral deficits in monkeys made hemiparkinsonian by intracarotid MPTP infusion. *Neurology*, **42**, 1565–72.

Schultz, W. (1998). Predictive reward signal of dopamine neurons. *Journal of Neurophysiology*, **80**, 1–27.

Schultz, W., Tremblay, L., and Hollerman, J. R. (2000). Reward processing in primate orbitofrontal cortex and basal ganglia. *Cerebral Cortex*, **10**, 272–84.

Segundo, J. P., Naguet, R., and Buser, P. (1955). Effects of cortical stimulation on electrocortical activity in monkeys. *Neurophysiology*, **1B**, 236–45. .

Shelton, P. A., Bowers, D., and Heilman, K. M. (1990). Peripersonal and vertical neglect. *Brain*, **113**, 191–205.

Shute, C. C. D., and Lewis, P. R. (1967). The ascending cholinergic reticular system, neocortical olfactory and subcortical projections. *Brain*, **90**, 497–520.

Singer, W. (1977). Control of thalamic transmission by corticofugal and ascending reticular pathways in the visual system. *Physiological Reviews*, **57**, 386–420.

Sokolov, Y. N. (1963). *Perception and the conditioned reflex*. Pergamon Press, Oxford.

Sprague, J. M., Chambers, W. W., and Stellar, E. (1961). Attentive, affective and adaptive behavior in the cat. *Science*, **133**, 165–73.

Stelmack, R. M., Plouffe, L. M., and Winogron, H. W. (1983). Recognition memory and the orienting response: an analysis of the encoding of pictures and words. *Biological Psychology*, **16**, 49–63.

Steriade, M. and Glenn, L. (1982). Neocortical and caudate projections of intralaminar thalamic neurons and their synaptic excitation from the midbrain reticular core. *Journal of Neurophysiology*, **48**, 352–70.

Storrie-Baker, H. J., Segalowitz, S. J., Black, S. E., McLean, J. A., and Sullivan, N. (1997). Improvement of hemispatial neglect with cold-water calorics: an electrophysiological test of the arousal hypothesis of neglect. *Journal of the International Neuropsychological Society*, **3**, 394–402.

Tegner, R. and Levander, M. (1991). Through a looking glass: a new technique to demonstrate direction hypokinesia in unilateral neglect. *Brain*, **114**, 1943–51.

Teitelbaum, P. and Epstein, A. N. (1962). The lateral hypothalamic syndrome: recovery of feeding and drinking after lateral hypothalamic lesions. *Psychological Review*, **69**, 74–90.

Ungerstedt, U. (1971*a*). Striatal dopamine release after amphetamine or nerve degeneration revealed by rotational behavior. *Acta Physiologica Scandinavica, Supplementum*, **82**, 49–68.

Ungerstedt, U. (1971*b*). Post-synaptic supersensitivity of 6-hydroxydopamine induced degeneration of the nigro-striatal dopamine system in the rat brain. *Acta Physiologica Scandinavica, Supplementum*, **82**, 69–93.

Ungerstedt, U. (1974). Brain dopamine neurons and behavior. In *Neurosciences*, Vol. 3 (ed. F. O. Schmidt and F. G. Woren), pp. 695–703. MIT Press, Cambridge, MA.

Valenstein, E., van den Abell, T., Tankle, R., and Heilman, K. M. (1980). Apomorphine-induced turning after recovery from neglect induced by cortical lesions. *Neurology*, **30**, 358.

Vallar, G. and Perani, D. (1986). The anatomy of unilateral neglect after right-hemisphere stroke lesions: a clinical/CT-scan correlation study in man. *Neuropsychologia*, **24**, 609–22.

Vargo, J. M., Richard-Smith, M., and Corwin, J. V. (1989). Spiroperidol reinstates asymmetries in neglect in rats recovered from left or right dorsomedial prefrontal cortex lesions. *Behavioral Neuroscience*, **103**, 1017–27.

Vogt, B. A., Rosene, D. L., and Pandya, D. N. (1979). Thalamic and cortical afferents differentiate anterior from posterior cingulate cortex in the monkey. *Science*, **204**, 205–7.

Vuilleumier, P., Valenza, N., Mayer, E., Reverdin, A., and Landis, T. (1998). Near and far visual space in unilateral neglect. *Annals of Neurology*, **43**, 406–10.

Wagman, I. H., and Mehler, W. R. (1972). Physiology and anatomy of the cortico-oculomotor mechanism. *Progress in Brain Research*, **37**, 619–35.

Watson, R. T. and Heilman, K. M. (1979). Thalamic neglect. *Neurology*, **29**, 690–4.

Watson, R. T., Heilman, K. M., Cauthen, J. C., and King, F. A. (1973). Neglect after cingulectomy. *Neurology*, **23**, 1003–7.

Watson, R. T., Heilman, K. M., Miller, B. D., and King, F. A. (1974). Neglect after mesencephalic reticular formation lesions. *Neurology*, **24**, 294–8.

Watson, R. T., Andriola, M., and Heilman, K. M. (1977*a*). The EEG in neglect. *Journal of Neurological Science*, **34**, 343–8.

Watson, R. T., Miller, B. D., and Heilman, K. M. (1977*b*). Evoked potential in neglect. *Archives of Neurology*, **34**, 224–7.

Watson, R. T., Miller, B. D., and Heilman, K. M. (1978). Nonsensory neglect. *Annals of Neurology*, **3**, 505–8.

Watson, R. T., Valenstein, E., and Heilman, K. M. (1981). Thalamic neglect: the possible role of the medial thalamus and nucleus reticularis thalami in behavior. *Archives of Neurology*, **38**, 501–7.

Weinstein, E. and Friedland, R. (1977). *Hemi-inattention and hemispheric specialization*. Raven Press, New York.

Weintraub, S. and Mesulam, M. M. (1987). Right cerebral dominance in spatial attention: further evidence based on ipsilateral neglect. *Archives of Neurology*, **44**, 621–5.

Welch, K. and Stuteville, P. (1958). Experimental production of neglect in monkeys. *Brain*, **81**, 341–7.

Whittington, D. A. and Hepp-Reymond, M. C. (1977). Eye and head movements to auditory targets. *Neuroscience Abstracts*, **3**, 158.

Williams, S. M. and Goldman-Rakic, P. S. (1998). Widespread origin of the primate mesofrontal dopamine system. *Cerebral Cortex*, **8**, 321–45.

Yingling, C. D. and Skinner, J. E. (1977). Gating of thalamic input to cerebral cortex by nucleus reticularis thalami. In *Progress in clinical neurophysiology*, Vol. 1 (ed. J. E. Desmedt), pp. 70–96. Karger, New York.

Section 2 Neural bases of neglect

2.1 Functional anatomy of attention and neglect: from neurons to networks

Marsel Mesulam

Orienting toward new and interesting events, searching for targets embedded among distractors and the mental scanning of internally represented scenes are among the manifestations of spatial attention. The neurological syndrome of hemispatial neglect reflects a major disruption in this area of functioning. Traditional textbooks refer to hemispatial neglect as a 'parietal syndrome'. However, clinical reports show that nearly identical clinical deficits can arise not only after parietal lobe damage but also after lesions in the frontal lobes, cingulate gyrus, striatum and thalamus. This chapter aims to show that these areas comprise a large-scale network subserving spatial attention (Fig. 1), that hemispatial neglect is a syndrome of the network as a whole, and that the complexity of this network is commensurate with the clinical heterogeneity of the neglect syndrome.

Left versus right

Clinical evidence based on thousands of patients shows that contralesional neglect is more frequent, severe, and lasting after right-hemisphere lesions than after equivalent lesions in the left hemisphere. In keeping with these clinical reports, unilateral intracarotid amytal injections lead to contrainjectional visual neglect and tactile extinction only after the inactivation of the right hemisphere (Meador *et al.* 1988; Spiers *et al.* 1990). A simple model based on a right-hemisphere specialization for spatial attention can account for this asymmetry (Fig. 2).

According to this model, the left hemisphere directs attention predominantly to the contralateral right side of space, whereas the right hemisphere directs attention to both sides of space. Therefore unilateral left-hemisphere lesions are not expected to cause much neglect for the right since the ipsiversive attentional functions of the right hemisphere are likely to take over. However, right-hemisphere lesions are expected to trigger severe left neglect since the left hemisphere has no substantial ipsiversive attentional functions. Experiments based on evoked potentials, transcranial magnetic stimulation, and functional imaging have supported this model (Desmedt 1977; Heilman and Van Den Abell 1979; Corbetta *et al.* 1993; Oyachi and Ohtsuka 1995; Gitelman *et al.* 1996). This model also predicts that lesions of the corpus callosum should not cause spatial neglect, that unilateral right hemisphere lesions should also cause some ipsilesional neglect, and that naturalistic settings where attention is symmetrically distributed to both sides of space should cause a greater engagement of the right hemisphere. All these expectations have been confirmed (Gazzaniga 1987; Weintraub and Mesulam 1987; Gitelman *et al.* 1999; Kim *et al.* 1999).

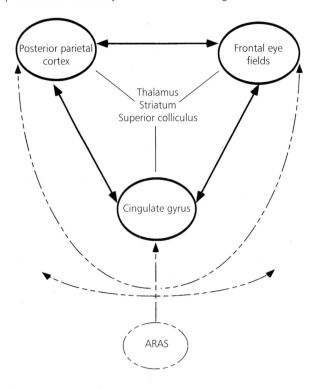

Figure 1 The attentional network: ARAS, ascending reticular activating system.

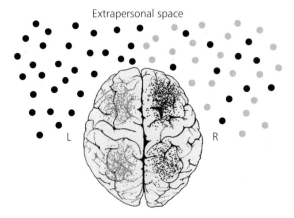

Figure 2 Model of right-hemisphere dominance for spatial attention.

Even in individuals with right-hemisphere dominance for language, neglect usually arises only after right-hemisphere inactivation, suggesting that the right-hemisphere specialization for directed attention may be more tightly conserved than the left-hemisphere specialization for language (Spiers *et al.* 1990). Rarely, right-sided neglect may occur after a unilateral left-hemisphere lesion in a right-handed patient. However, the most striking instances of right hemineglect have been described in patients with bilateral injury to the brain (Weintraub *et al.* 1996).

Posterior parietal cortex

Small lesions confined to parietal cortex rarely cause conspicuous neglect. Persistent and severe neglect in the context of parietal lobe damage almost always indicates a large lesion with considerable subcortical extension. Neglect-causing parietal lesions have been reported in many different parts of posterior parietal cortex. The single most common lesion site in these patients tends to be located in the inferior parietal lobule (Vallar 2001).

Functional imaging studies in neurologically intact subjects show that tasks of covert visuospatial attention (Corbetta *et al.* 1993; Nobre *et al.* 1997), tactile exploration (Gitelman *et al.* 1996), oculomotor search (Gitelman *et al.*, 2002), and auditory localization (Zatorre *et al.* 1999) elicit cortical activation in the superior and inferior parietal lobules, the banks of the intraparietal sulcus and, less frequently, medial parietal cortex in the precuneus. The one component of the posterior parietal cortex that is most consistently activated by all these tasks lies within the banks of the intraparietal sulcus and in its immediate vicinity. This region may constitute an all-purpose parietal core of the attentional network. Adjacent parts of posterior parietal cortex may make more specialized contributions to spatial attention. For example, functional imaging experiments suggest that the superior parietal lobule may mediate the shifting of the attentional focus (especially to moving targets), whereas the inferior parietal lobule may be involved in focalizing and fixating attention (Vandenberghe *et al.* 2001). A separate temporoparietal junctional area may mediate the detection of targets in unattended locations (Corbetta *et al.* 2000).

In the monkey, damage to the inferior parietal lobule causes contralesional extinction and reaching deficits, whereas damage that involves the banks of the immediately adjacent superior temporal sulcus causes neglect of contralesional stimuli (Lynch and McLaren 1989; Watson *et al.* 1994). Ingenious experiments, based on the recording of individual neurons in awake and behaving macaque monkeys, show that posterior parietal areas collectively display two properties of critical importance for shifting attention from one extrapersonal target to the other.

1. They form a representation of the external space based on motivational salience rather than on shape, color, or object identity.
2. They enable the mapping of 'kinetic plans' for exploring, grasping, and foveating salient events. Many of these neurons display both sensory and motor contingencies, explaining why so many manifestations of unilateral neglect resulting from parietal lesions reflect a breakdown of sensory–motor integration rather than an isolated disruption of perception or movement.

Area LIP, located in the lateral bank of the intraparietal sulcus, is known as the 'posterior eye field' because of its critical role in coordinating eye movements. It is closely interconnected with the frontal eye fields (FEF) and the superior colliculus, triggers saccadic eye movements in response to microstimulation, and gives directionally tuned responses prior to saccadic eye movements directed to visual targets or their remembered sites (Andersen 1995). In the monkey, Brodmann area (BA) 7a of posterior parietal cortex, located on the surface of the inferior parietal lobule, is monosynaptically interconnected with LIP. In comparison with LIP, the neurons in BA 7a have fewer connections with FEF, give fewer presaccadic responses, and do not trigger saccadic eye movements upon stimulation (Snyder *et al.* 1998*b*). Even in the absence of any head and eye movements, the response of these neurons to the onset of a light spot was much more vigorous when reward was made contingent on the detection of subsequent dimming (Bushnell *et al.* 1981). Therefore these neurons may play a major role in encoding a map of salience which can be used by LIP to generate plans for action.

Neurons in 7a and LIP participate not only in tasks that require an actual or intended overt movement of the attentional focus but also in tasks based on covert shifts of attention where there are no head or eye movements. Many of these neurons respond to cues which predict the location of a subsequent target. The subsequent appearance of a target excites area 7a neurons only if it is at a location different from that of the cue (Robinson *et al.* 1995; Steinmetz 1998). The lack of response to targets located at the same site as the cue indicates that these neurons are more closely involved in shifting the attentional focus than in registering the presence or location of a significant event.

Groups of neurons in areas LIP and 7a can encode spatial position in a head-centered frame of reference by combining retinotopic information with information about eye position (Andersen *et al.* 1985). Some of these neurons can also use proprioceptive information related to head position to create a body-centered representation and vestibular information to create a world-centered representation (Andersen 1995). There are even some neurons which encode events in world-centered coordinates based on environmental landmarks (Andersen *et al.* 1997). These experiments show that posterior parietal neurons can map salient events in multiple frames of reference. Damage to these neurons may account for the multi-coordinate manifestations of neglect.

Neurons medial and posterior to LIP, in a region known as the parietal reach region, fire during visually guided arm movements and may play a role in manual grasping and tactile exploration in a manner that is analogous to the role of LIP in visual search and gaze (Snyder *et al.* 1998*a*). Damage to an analogous region of the human brain may be responsible for the hypokinesia, intentional neglect, and tactile exploration deficits in patients with neglect. These observations suggest that the brain does not have a unitary 'spatial map'. Instead, posterior parietal cortex contains multiple mappings of behaviorally salient events in terms of the strategies that would be needed to make them targets of foveation, grasping or covert attentional shifts. If there is a sensory 'representation' in parietal cortex, it appears to be encoded in terms of strategies aimed at shifting the focus of attention to a behaviorally relevant target.

The temporo-occipito-parietal area

Extrapersonal events and the observer can move with respect to each other. Therefore the neural mechanisms that direct attention to external targets must be sensitive to motion. In the macaque, motion-sensitive neurons are located in the banks of the superior temporal sulcus, in areas known as MT (V5), MST, and FST. In the cat, the reversible inactivation of an area equivalent to MT (V5) causes severe contralesional visual neglect (Payne *et al.* 1996). Tasks of covert attentional shifts (especially when based on endogenous cognitive cues) have led to activations at the confluence of the temporal, parietal, and occipital lobes, within the most posterior aspects of the middle temporal gyrus (Gitelman *et al.* 1999; Kim *et al.* 1999). This activation falls within a region designated MT+ which probably includes the human homologs of MT (V5), MST and FST (DeYoe *et al.* 1996). In one patient, damage confined to this region led to left-sided target cancellation deficits even 4 years after the cerebrovascular accident (Hasselbach and Butter 1997). Our experience indicates that this area is more active during covert shifts of attention, when there is an inferred movement of the attentional focus across the extrapersonal space, than during overt search behaviors, when the eyes and the attentional focus move together (Gitelman *et al.* 1999; Gitelman *et al.*, 2002).

The frontal eye fields

Numerous clinical reports have shown that lesions confined to the right frontal lobe can cause contralesional neglect. The critical frontal area responsible for the neglect syndrome has been difficult to identify. Some authors have implicated the region of the FEF, and others the inferior frontal gyrus (Mesulam 1981; Daffner *et al.* 1990; Husain and Kennard 1996).

Functional imaging experiments based on tasks of spatial attention have reported activation in the region of the FEF, usually extending into adjacent premotor and prefrontal cortex (Corbetta *et al.* 1993; Nobre *et al.* 1997; Gitelman *et al.* 1999; Kim *et al.* 1999; Gitelman *et al.*, 2002). This activation occurs even during covert shifts of attention when real-time monitoring has confirmed the absence of eye movements and when potentially confounding factors, such as working memory, intense foveal fixation, inhibition of eye movements, and the conditional (go–no-go) aspects of the task have been controlled (Gitelman *et al.* 1999, 2000).

The activation of the FEF region has also been noted in nonvisual tasks of spatial attention based on auditory localization and manual search (Gitelman *et al.* 1996; Zatorre *et al.* 1999). Therefore the FEF participation in spatial attention is not contingent on the presence of visual processing or motor output. The FEF areas involved in spatial attention overlap with the areas that mediate saccadic eye movements (Corbetta *et al.* 1998; Nobre *et al.* 2000). However, this overlap is partial. In fact, the FEF displays a functional mosaic wherein nonattentional saccadic eye movements are represented most laterally, ocular search most medially, and covert attentional shifts in between the two (Gitelman *et al.*, 2002).

As opposed to the FEF of the monkey which is located in the posterior part of BA 8, the human FEF is located in BA 6 at the junction of the precentral and superior frontal sulci (Barbas and Mesulam 1981; Darby *et al.* 1996; Paus 1996). In the macaque monkey, lesions in the area of the FEF have been known to result in marked contralateral neglect (Watson *et al.* 1978). The FEF of the monkey is interconnected with posterior parietal cortex, peristriate and inferotemporal cortex, the cingulate gyrus, other premotor and prefrontal areas, the dorsomedial and medial pulvinar nuclei of the thalamus, and the superior colliculus (Barbas and Mesulam 1981). These projections provide direct access to pathways that control the head, eye, and limb movements necessary for visual scanning and other search behaviors. Up to 51 per cent of all extra-frontal neurons projecting into the caudal portion of the FEF are located in unimodal visual association areas in the peristriate and inferotemporal regions (Barbas and Mesulam 1981). Parts of the frontal eye fields also receive auditory input, and this connection may mediate orientation to auditory stimuli (Barbas and Mesulam 1981).

The FEF and the superior colliculus contain units that could be considered command neurons for eye movements, and combined lesions in both of these areas yield a severe depression of contralaterally directed saccades (Schiller *et al.* 1979). In the monkey, FEF neurons give a burst of activity just before a saccade to a behaviorally relevant target or to its remembered site. Thus, as in the case of LIP, with which it is tightly interconnected, the FEF can play a crucial role in foveating and visually exploring behaviorally relevant visual targets.

Premotor neurons located just posterior to the FEF may also participate in spatial attention. Ventrally situated premotor areas can encode the egocentric location of objects, even after the light is turned off, in a way that may underlie the ability to reach toward or avoid objects in the dark (Graziano *et al.* 1997). Dorsally situated premotor neurons respond to cues that reorient the attentional focus and the direction of limb movements (Kermadi and Boussaoud 1995). The numerous premotor areas posterior to FEF may mediate attention-related reaching and grasping behaviors directed to objects in near space, whereas the FEF may be more closely involved in mediating orienting and exploratory behaviors directed to visual and auditory events in far space.

The FEF projection to the superior colliculus arises predominantly from saccade-related neurons, none of which have purely visual activity, whereas the LIP projection to the superior colliculus comes predominantly from neurons with visual activity, none of which have exclusively saccade-related activity (Paré and Wurtz 1997). Therefore it appears that the FEF signal conveys a more advanced sensory-to-motor transformation and may exert a greater top-down influence upon the collicular encoding of eye movements (Segraves and Goldberg 1987; Paré and Wurtz 1997). Neurons with exclusively sensory responses to stimuli are more common in LIP, whereas neurons that display exclusively presaccadic discharges are more common in the FEF. Although this information appears to imply that LIP is more 'sensory' and FEF is more 'motor,' both areas support sensory–motor integration which explains why frontal as well as parietal lesions can lead to neglect syndromes with sensory as well as motor manifestations.

The cingulate gyrus

Patients who develop neglect on the basis of lesions confined to the cingulate gyrus are rare (Heilman *et al.* 1983). However, functional imaging studies in neurologically normal subjects engaged in tasks of covert shifts of attention, overt oculomotor exploration, and manual search have consistently shown cingulate activation (Nobre *et al.* 1997; Gitelman *et al.* 1999; Kim *et al.* 1999). Imaging experiments suggest that the cingulate component of the attentional network may have two functionally segregated sectors, an anterior one in BA 24/32 and a posterior one in BA 23/29/30. The posterior sector appears to mediate the redirection of anticipatory attention toward extrapersonal sites where behaviorally significant events are expected to occur (Small *et al.* 2001). The anterior cingulate focus does not display such a relationship and is likely to mediate other aspects of attentional deployment, such as performance monitoring, response selection, or target detection (Mesulam *et al.* 2001).

In monkeys, unilateral lesions of the cingulum bundle and adjacent cingulate cortex result in contralateral somatosensory extinction (Watson *et al.* 1973). Monosynaptic connections link the cingulate gyrus to the FEF, BA 7a, and perhaps also the superior colliculus (Mesulam *et al.* 1977; Barbas and Mesulam 1981; Künzle 1995). Neurons in the dorsal part of the anterior cingulate fire in response to behaviorally relevant cues and during the planning and execution of reaching movements (Olson *et al.* 1993). Neurons of the posterior cingulate gyrus fire tonically during steady gaze at a rate determined by the direction of the preceding eye movement and the current angle of the eye in the orbit (Olson *et al.* 1993). These neurons seem to be monitoring (or resetting) rather than controlling directional shifts of visual attention.

Subcortical structures

Unilateral neglect in the human has been reported after lesions of the thalamus (Watson and Heilman 1979; Cambier *et al.* 1980; Schott *et al.* 1981; Rafal and Posner 1987). In some patients the medial dorsal and medial pulvinar nuclei were at the focus of the neglect-causing thalamic lesion. Such lesions can induce distal hypometabolism (diaschisis) in the cortical components of the attentional network (Fiorelli *et al.* 1991). Functional imaging during tasks of attentional shifts has shown activations in the ventral lateral nucleus and at the junction of the medial pulvinar and mediodorsal nuclei of the thalamus (Gitelman *et al.* 1999).

In the monkey, the receptive fields of neurons in the medial pulvinar nucleus are quite large. These neurons are sensitive to changes in behavioral relevance and may help to encode visual salience by increasing the signal-to-noise ratio (Petersen *et al.* 1985; Robinson 1993). Functional imaging suggests that the pulvinar nucleus may serve a similar purpose in the human brain (LaBerge and Buchsbaum 1990; Morris *et al.* 1997). The medial pulvinar is the major thalamic nucleus for BA 7a, whereas the mediodorsal nucleus provides the major thalamic input to the FEF. However, both thalamic nuclei project to FEF, BA 7a, and the cingulate gyrus (Mesulam *et al.* 1977; Barbas and Mesulam 1981).

Unilateral striatal damage has also been associated with contralateral neglect (Luria *et al.* 1966; Damasio *et al.* 1980; Healton *et al.* 1982). Functional imaging has shown caudate and putaminal activation during overt and covert shifts of spatial attention (Gitelman *et al.* 1999;

Gitelman *et al.*, 2002). Unilateral Parkinson's disease, especially on the right, leads to manifestations of contralesional neglect (Ebersbach *et al.* 1996). Striatal dysfunction induced by interrupting the dopaminergic nigrostriatal pathway yields contralateral neglect in monkeys (Miyashita *et al.* 1995). Some neurons in the caudate and putamen of the macaque monkey are preferentially activated by cues which direct spatial attention, whereas others participate in the spatial organization of oculomotor and limb movements (Kermadi and Joseph 1995; Miyashita *et al.* 1995).

The intermediate layers of the superior colliculus play a critical role in initiating eye movements, foveating visual targets, and releasing ocular fixation when a new target must be foveated (Dorris *et al.* 1997). The superior colliculus receives input directly from the retina, primary visual cortex, LIP, and the FEF, and perhaps also from the cingulate gyrus (Künzle 1995). Its intermediate (oculomotor) layers receive partially overlapping input from the FEF and LIP (Selemon and Goldman-Rakic 1988). Lesions of the superior colliculus can lead to contralesional neglect in the cat (Sprague and Meikle 1965). Functional imaging in humans shows significantly greater superior colliculus activation during oculomotor search behaviors than during saccadic eye movements that have a low attentional load (Gitelman *et al.*, 2002).

Several functional imaging studies had detected cerebellar activation even in tasks of covert attentional shifts, suggesting that the cerebellum may play an important role in spatial attention. However, an experiment which employed stringent controls for movements involved in the task failed to show cerebellar activation associated with covert shifts of attention (Gitelman *et al.* 1999). This is consistent with studies which show that cerebellar lesions do not cause deficits in covert shifts of attention (Yamaguchi *et al.* 1998). However, the cerebellum could conceivably play a more important role in tasks that involve active search (Gitelman *et al.*, 2002).

Components of the ascending reticular activating system, such as the intralaminar thalamic nuclei, the brainstem raphe nuclei, the nucleus locus ceruleus, the ventral tegmental area–substantia nigra, and the nucleus basalis project to each cortical component of the attentional network. Unilateral lesions in the intralaminar nuclei, the ventral tegmental tract, and even in the mesencephalic reticular formation trigger contralateral neglect in the rat, cat, and monkey (see Mesulam (1999) for a review).

Dissociations and subtypes: is there parietal versus frontal neglect?

The symptoms and signs of neglect are so numerous that no individual patient is likely to manifest them all. Dissociations among the behavioral components are the rule rather than the exception. Despite the overwhelming evidence which now links both posterior parietal cortex and the FEF to sensory–motor integration, traditional neurology still tends to associate the parietal lobe with 'sensory' function and the frontal lobe with 'motor' function. Therefore a relatively attractive hypothesis has revolved around the possibility that 'parietal neglect' might be predominantly perceptual whereas 'frontal neglect' might be predominantly motor. Several studies have shown that 'perceptual' tasks, such as extinction and line bisection, are more likely to be associated with parietal lesions whereas 'motor' tasks, such as target cancellation, are more likely to be associated with frontal lesions (see Mesulam (1999) for a review). However, other studies have not been able to confirm such functional segregations within the attentional network (Mattingley *et al.* 1998).

The frontal and parietal components of the attentional network subserve a level of sensory–motor integration where the boundaries between action and perception become blurred. At a behavioral level, sensory representations are necessary for guiding exploration, and exploration is necessary for updating representations (Droogleever-Fortuyn 1979; Mesulam 1981). At a physiological level, parietal and FEF neurons have motor as well as sensory fields.

Thus both parietal and frontal lesions would be expected to yield neglect syndromes with sensory–representational as well as motor–exploratory components. Furthermore, the strong inter-connectivity between the frontal and parietal components of the attentional network raises the possibility that damage to one may induce distal dysfunction in the other through the process of diaschisis. This would further reduce the possibility of seeing anatomically segregated subtypes of neglect even though the primary lesion sites themselves may display functional specializations. Therefore a narrow sensory versus motor dichotomy in relationship to parietal versus frontal lesions is unlikely and has not been supported by either animal or human studies on neglect.

A neural network for the distribution of spatial attention

The internal organization of the network shown in Fig. 1 was explored in the macaque brain by injecting two different retrogradely transported fluorescent tracers, one in the FEF and the other in the region of the intraparietal sulcus and BA 7a (Morecraft *et al.* 1993). The results showed that these two epicenters of the attentional network were interconnected not only with each other and the cingulate gyrus, but also with an identical set of 12 additional areas in the premotor, lateral prefrontal, orbitofrontal, lateral and inferior temporal, parahippocampal, and insular cortex. All these areas appear to participate in the coordination of spatial attention. However, the FEF, posterior parietal cortex, and cingulate gyrus play a more critical role than the others since they are the only sites where damage consistently leads to contralesional neglect. The fact that the FEF and posterior parietal cortex are interconnected with an identical set of cortical areas suggests that the attentional network can support parallel distributed processing. Through this computational architecture, the attentional network can execute a very rapid survey of a vast informational landscape related to motivational salience, spatial representations, and motor strategies (Mesulam 1999). Attention can thus be shifted adaptively from one site to another according to behavioral relevance.

Assigning an identifiable 'task' to each component of this network raises the specter of anthro-pomorphism but serves a heuristic purpose. Thus the posterior parietal component (centered around the intraparietal sulcus but including parts of the inferior and superior parietal lobules and perhaps the MT+ region in parieto-occipito-temporal cortex) may provide a mental representa-tion of salient events in multiple coordinates. The dual role of the parietal component might be to create a dynamic representation of salience and to compute provisional strategies (or plans) for shifting attention from one salient target to the other. Posterior parietal cortex would seem to play its key role in spatial attention as a critical gateway for linking distributed channels of spatially relevant information with each other and with channels of motor output related to orient-ing, reaching, grasping, and searching behaviors. When the parietal component of the attentional network is destroyed, the individual input and output channels may remain quite intact but they cannot be integrated into a coherent template for sustaining flexible shifts of spatial attention.

The frontal component of the attentional network (centered around the FEF but including adjacent premotor and perhaps prefrontal cortices) might play its critical role in the attentional network by converting plans and intentions into specific motor sequences that shift the focus of attention. There is no single set of spatial codes upon which all kinetic strategies for exploration, foveation, and grasping converge. Instead, there are multiple circuits, each specialized for specific input–output relationships related to looking, grasping, searching, etc. The parietal and frontal components provide gateways for accessing and coordinating these circuits. They also constitute 'bottlenecks' where lesions have the most severe impact on the integrity of directed attention. It might be said that the posterior parietal cortex sculpts a salience- and trajectory-based template of the extrapersonal space, whereas the FEF selects and sequences the individual acts needed to navigate and explore the resultant landscape. The role of the cingulate component is the least well understood. As a limbic component of the attentional network, the cingulate gyrus may play a critical role in identifying the motivational relevance of extrapersonal events, sustaining the level of effort during the execution of attentional tasks and modulating the spatial distribution of anticipatory biases.

Conclusions

The evidence reviewed above has led to the hypothesis that spatial attention is organized at the level of a distributed large-scale network revolving around three cortical components, each of which supports a slightly different neural representation of the extrapersonal space. Each of these components serves a dual purpose: it provides a local network for regional neural computations and also a nodal point for the linkage of distributed information. The cortical components of the network shown in Fig. 1 are interconnected with each other and with key subcortical areas in the striatum, thalamus, superior colliculus, and reticular activating system. Any task of spatial attention, regardless of input or output modality, activates many, if not all, of these components (Fig. 3). Therefore spatial attention is less likely to represent the sequentially additive product of perception, motivation, and search than the emergent (i.e. relational) quality of the network as a whole.

The components of the attentional network can collectively specify whether and how an event in extrapersonal space will attract covert attentional shifts, orientation, foveation, manual grasp, and overt search behaviors. This network is likely to control the top-down (executive) modulation of more downstream sensory and motor areas where the work of spatial attention becomes initiated. Damage to any network component or to its interconnections can potentially elicit neglect behaviors. Lesions within the network are likely to cause multimodal neglect, whereas lesions that disconnect it from specific sensory or motor areas could yield modality-specific neglect syndromes. The complexity of the network shown in Fig. 1 and the variability of lesion sites are likely to account for the clinical heterogeneity of hemispatial neglect.

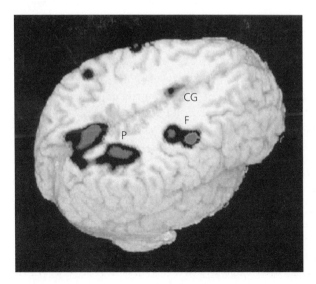

Figure 3 Functional imaging of covert shifts of spatial attention in one subject with functional magnetic resonance imaging. All three cortical components of the attentional network are activated. Furthermore, there is more activation in the right hemisphere even though the subject is symmetrically shifting attention to the left and the right. CG, cingulate; F, frontal; P, parietal. (Courtesy of Darren Gitelman M.D.)

Acknowledgements

This work was supported in part by NS 30863 from the National Institute of Neurological Diseases and Stroke.

References

Andersen, R. A. (1995). Encoding of intention and spatial location in the posterior parietal cortex. *Cerebral Cortex*, **5**, 457–69.

Andersen, R. A., Essick, G. K., and Siegel, R. M. (1985). Encoding of spatial location by posterior parietal neurons. *Science*, **230**, 456–8.

Andersen, R. A., Snyder, L. H., Bradley, D. C., and Xing, J. (1997). Multimodal representation of space in the posterior parietal cortex and its use in planning movements. *Annual Reviews of Neuroscience*, **20**, 303–30.

Barbas, H. and Mesulam M. M. (1981). Organization of afferent input to subdivisions of area 8 in the rhesus monkey. *Journal of Comparative Neurology*, **200**, 407–31.

Bushnell, M. C., Goldberg, M. E., and Robinson, D. L. (1981). Behavioral enhancement of visual responses in monkey cerebral cortex. 1: Modulation in posterior parietal cortex related to selective visual attention. *Journal of Neurophysiology*, **46**, 755–71.

Cambier, J., Elghozi, D., and Strube, E. (1980). Lésion du thalamus droit avec syndrome de l'hémisphère mineur. Discussion du concept de négligence thalamique. *Revue Neurologique*, **136**, 105–16.

Corbetta, M., Akbudak, E., Conturo, T. E., *et al.* (1998). A common network of functional areas for attention and eye movements. *Neuron*, **21**, 761–73.

Corbetta, M., Kincade, J. M., Ollinger, J. M., McAvoy, M. P., and Shulman, G. L. (2000). Voluntary orienting is dissociated from target detection in human posterior parietal cortex. *Nature Neuroscience*, **3**, 292–7.

Corbetta, M., Miezin, F. M., Shulman, G. L., and Petersen, S. E. (1993). A PET study of visuospatial attention. *Journal of Neuroscience*, **13**, 1202–26.

Daffner, K. R., Ahern, G. L., Weintraub, S., and Mesulam, M. M. (1990). Dissociated neglect behavior following sequential strokes in the right hemisphere. *Annals of Neurology*, **28**, 97–101.

Damasio, A. R., Damasio, H., and Chui, H. C. (1980). Neglect following damage to frontal lobe or basal ganglia. *Neuropsychologia*, **18**, 123–32.

Darby, D. G., Nobre, A. C., Thangaraj, V., Edelman, R. R., Mesulam, M.-M., and Warach S. (1996). Cortical activation in the human brain during lateral saccades using EPISTAR functional magnetic resonance imaging. *NeuroImage*, **3**, 53–62.

Desmedt, J. E. (1977). Active touch exploration of extrapersonal space elicits specific electrogenesis in the right cerebral hemisphere of intact right handed man. *Proceedings of the National Academy of Sciences of the United States of America*, **74**, 4037–40.

DeYoe, E., Carman, G. J., Bandettini, P., *et al.* (1996). Mapping striate and extrastriate visual areas in human cerebral cortex. *Proceedings of the National Academy of Sciences of the United States of America*, **93**, 2382–6.

Dorris, M. C., Paré, M., and Munoz, D. P. (1997). Neuronal activity in monkey superior colliculus related to the initiation of saccadic eye movements. *Journal of Neuroscience*, **17**, 8566–79.

Droogleever-Fortuyn, J. (1979). On the neurology of perception. *Clinical Neurology and Neurosurgery*, **81**, 97–107.

Ebersbach, G., Trottenberg, T., Hattig, H., Schelosky, L., Schrag, A., and Poewe, W. (1996). Directional bias of initial visual exploration: a symptom of neglect in Parkinson's disease. *Brain*, **119**, 79–87.

Fiorelli, M., Blin, J., Bakchine, S., Laplane, D., and Baron, J. C. (1991). PET studies of cortical diaschisis in patients with motor hemi-neglect. *Journal of Neurological Science*, **104**, 135–142.

Gazzaniga, M. S. (1987). Perceptual and attentional processes following callosal section in humans. *Neuropsychologia*, **25**, 119–33.

Gitelman, D. R., Alpert, N. M., Kosslyn, S. M., *et al.* (1996). Functional imaging of human right hemispheric activation for exploratory movements. *Annals of Neurology*, **39**, 174–9.

Gitelman, D. R., Nobre, A. C., Parrish, T. B., *et al.* (1999). A large-scale distributed network for spatial attention: further anatomical delineation based on stringent behavioural and cognitive controls. *Brain*, **122**, 1093–1106.

Gitelman, D. R., Parrish, T. B., LaBar, K. S., and Mesulam, M.-M. (2000). Real-time monitoring of eye movements using infrared video-oculography during functional magnetic resonance imaging of the frontal eye fields. *NeuroImage*, **11**: 58–65.

Gitelman, D. R., Parrish, T. B., Friston, K. J., and Mesulam, M.-M. (2002). Functional anatomy of visual search, regional segregations within the frontal eye fields and effective connectivity of the superior colliculus. *NeuroImage*, **15**: 970–82.

Graziano, M. S. A., Hu, X. T., and Gross, C. G. (1977). Coding the locations of objects in the dark. *Science*, **277**, 239–41.

Hasselbach, M. and Butter, C. M. (1997). Ipsilesional displacement of egocentric midline in neglect patients with, but not in those without, extensive right parietal damage. In *Parietal lobe contributions to orientation in 3D space* (ed. P. Thier and H.-O. Karnath), pp. 579–95. Springer-Verlag, Heidelberg.

Healton, E. B., Navarro, C., Bressman, S., and Brust, J. (1982). Subcortical neglect. *Neurology*, **32**, 776–8.

Heilman, K. M. and Van Den Abell, T. (1979). Right hemispheric dominance for mediating cerebral activation. *Neuropsychologia*, **17**, 315–21.

Heilman, K. M., Watson, R. T., Valenstein, E., and Damasio, A. R. (1983). Localization of lesions in neglect. In *Localization in neuropsychology* (ed. A. Kertesz), pp. 455–70. Academic Press, New York.

Husain, M. and Kennard, C. (1996). Visual neglect associated with frontal lobe infarction. *Journal of Neurology*, **243**, 652–7.

Kermadi, I. and Boussaoud, D. (1995). Role of the primate striatum in attention and sensorimotor processes: comparison with premotor cortex. *NeuroReport*, **6**, 1177–81.

Kermadi, I. and Joseph, J. P. (1995). Activity in the caudate nucleus of monkey during spatial sequencing. *Journal of Neurophysiology*, **74**, 911–33.

Kim, Y.-H., Gitelman, D. R., Nobre, A. C., Parrish, T. B., LaBar, K. S., and Mesulam, M.-M. (1999). The large scale neural network for spatial attention displays multi-functional overlap but differential asymmetry. *NeuroImage*, **9**, 269–77.

Künzle, H. (1995). Regional and laminar distribution of cortical neurons projecting to either superior or inferior colliculus in the hedgehog tenrec. *Cerebral Cortex*, **5**, 338–52.

LaBerge, D. and Buchsbaum, M. S. (1990). Positron emission tomographic measurements of pulvinar activity during an attention task. *Journal of Neuroscience*, **10**, 613–19.

Luria, A. R., Karpov, B. A., and Yarbuss, A. L. (1966). Disturbances of active visual perception with lesions of the frontal lobes. *Cortex*, **2**, 202–12.

Lynch, J. C. and McLaren, J. W. (1989). Deficits of visual attention and saccadic eye movements after lesions of parietooccipital cortex in monkeys. *Journal of Neurophysiology*, **61**, 74–90.

Mattingley, J. B., Husain, M., Rorden, C., Kennard, C., and Driver, J. (1998). Motor role of human inferior parietal lobe revealed in unilateral neglect patients. *Nature*, **392**, 179–82.

Meador, K. J., Loring, D. W., Lee, G. P., *et al.* (1988). Right cerebral specialization for tactile attention as evidenced by intracarotid sodium amytal. *Neurology*, **38**, 1763–6.

Mesulam, M.-M. (1981). A cortical network for directed attention and unilateral neglect. *Annals of Neurology*, **10**, 309–25.

Mesulam, M.-M. (1999). Spatial attention and neglect, parietal, frontal, and cingulate contributions to the mental representation and attentional targeting of salient extrapersonal events. *Philosophical Transactions of the Royal Society of London, Series B*, **354**, 1325–46.

Mesulam, M.-M., Van Hoesen, G. W., Pandya, D. N., and Geschwind, N. (1977). Limbic and sensory connections of the inferior parietal lobule (area PG) in the rhesus monkey, a study with a new method for horseradish peroxidase histochemistry. *Brain Research*, **136**, 393–414.

Mesulam, M.-M., Nobre, A. C., Kim, Y.-H., Parrish, T. B., and Gitelman, D. R. (2001). Heterogeneity of cingulate contributions to spatial attention. *NeuroImage*, **13**: 1065–72.

Miyashita, N., Hikosaka, O., and Kato, M. (1995). Visual hemineglect induced by unilateral striatal dopamine deficiency in monkeys. *NeuroReport*, **6**, 1257–60.

Morecraft, R. J., Geula, C., and Mesulam, M.-M. (1993). Architecture of connectivity within a cingulo-fronto-parietal neurocognitive network for directed attention. *Archives of Neurology*, **50**, 279–84.

Morris, J. S., Friston, K. J., and Dolan, R. J. (1997). Neural responses to salient visual stimuli. *Proceedings of the Royal Society of London, Section B*, **264**, 769–775.

Nobre, A. C., Sebestyen, G. N., Gitelman, D. R., Mesulam, M.-M., Frackowiak, R. S. J., and Frith, C. D. (1997). Functional localization of the system for visuospatial attention using positron emission tomography. *Brain*, **120**, 515–33.

Nobre, A. C., Gitelman, D. R., Dias, E. C., and Mesulam, M.-M. (2000). Covert visual spatial orienting and saccades, overlapping neural systems. *NeuroImage*, **11**, 210–16.

Olson, C. R., Musil, S. Y., and Goldberg, M. E. (1993). Posterior cingulate cortex and visuospatial cognition, properties of single neurons in the behaving monkey. In *Neurobiology of cingulate cortex and limbic thalamus: a comprehensive handbook* (ed. B. A. Vogt and M. Gabriel), pp. 366–80. Birkhäuser, Boston, MA.

Oyachi, H. and Ohtsuka, K. (1995). Transcranial magnetic stimulation of the posterior parietal cortex degrades accuracy of memory-guided saccades in humans. *Investigative Ophthalmology and Visual Science*, **36**, 1441–9.

Paré, M. and Wurtz, R. H. (1997). Monkey posterior parietal cortex neurons antidromically activated from superior colliculus. *Journal of Neurophysiology*, **78**, 3493–7.

Paus, T. (1996). Location and function of the human frontal eye-field: a selective review. *Neuropsychologia*, **34**, 475–83.

Payne, B. R., Lomber, S. G., Geeraerts, S., van der Gucht, E., and Vandenbussche, E. (1996). Reversible visual hemineglect. *Proceedings of the National Academy of Sciences of the United States of America*, **93**, 290–4.

Petersen, S. E., Robinson, D. L., and Keys, W. (1985). Pulvinar nuclei of the behaving rhesus monkey: visual responses and their modulation. *Journal of Neurophysiology*, **54**, 867–86.

Rafal, R. D. and Posner M. I. (1987). Deficits in human visual spatial attention following thalamic lesions. *Proceedings of the National Academy of Sciences of the United States of America*, **84**, 7349–53.

Robinson, D. L. (1993). Functional contributions of the primate pulvinar. *Progress in Brain Research*, **95**, 371–80.

Robinson, D. L., Bowman, E. M., and Kertzman, C. (1995). Covert orienting of attention in macaques. II: Contribution of parietal cortex. *Journal of Neurophysiology*, **74**, 698–712.

Schiller, P. H., True, S. D., and Conway, J. L. (1979). Effects of frontal eye field and superior colliculus ablations on eye movements. *Science*, **206**, 590–2.

Schott, B., Laurent, B., Mauguiere, F., and Chazot, G. (1981). Négligence motrice par hematome thalamique droit. *Revue Neurologique*, **137**, 447–55.

Segraves, M. A. and Goldberg, M. E. (1987). Functional properties of corticotectal neurons in the monkey's frontal eye field. *Journal of Neurophysiology*, **58**, 1387–1419.

Selemon, L. D. and Goldman-Rakic, P. D. (1988). Common cortical and subcortical targets of the dorsolateral prefrontal and posterior parietal cortices in the rhesus monkey, evidence for a distributed neural network subserving spatially guided behavior. *Neuroscience*, **8**, 4049–68.

Small, D. M., Gitelman, D. R., Gregory, M. D., Nobre, A. C., Parrish, T., and Mesulam, M.-M. (2001). The posterior cingulate gyrus and anticipatory shifts of spatial attention. *NeuroImage*, **13**, S360.

Snyder, L. H., Batista, A. P., and Andersen, R. A. (1998*a*). Change in motor plan, without a change in the spatial locus of attention, modulates activity in posterior parietal cortex. *Journal of Neurophysiology*, **79**, 2814–19.

Snyder, L. H., Grieve, K. L., Brotchie, P., and Andersen, R. A. (1998*b*) Separate body- and world-referenced representations of visual space in parietal cortex. *Nature*, **394**, 887–91.

Spiers, P. A., Schomer, D. L., Blume, H. W., *et al.* (1990). Visual neglect during intracarotid amobarbital testing. *Neurology*, **40**, 1600–6.

Sprague, J. M. and Meikle, T. H., Jr (1965). The role of the superior colliculus in visually guided behavior. *Experimental Neurology*, **11**, 115–46.

Steinmetz, M. A. (1998). Contributions of posterior parietal cortex to cognitive functions in primates. *Psychobiology*, **26**, 109–18.

Vallar, G. (2001). Extrapersonal visual unilateral spatial neglect and its neuroanatomy. *NeuroImage*, **14**, S52–8.

Vandenberghe, R., Gitelman, D. R., Parrish, T., and Mesulam, M.-M. (2001). Functional specialisation in parietal cortex. *NeuroImage*, **13**: 368.

Watson, R. T. and Heilman, K. M. (1979). Thalamic neglect. *Neurology*, **29**, 690–4.

Watson, R. T., Heilman, K. M., Cauthen, J. C., and King, F. A. (1973). Neglect after cingulectomy. *Neurology*, **23**, 1003–7.

Watson, R. T., Miller, B. D., and Heilman, K. M. (1978). Nonsensory neglect. *Annals of Neurology*, **3**, 505–8.

Watson, R. T., Valenstein, E., Day, A., and Heilman, K. M. (1994). Posterior neocortical systems subserving awareness and neglect. *Archives of Neurology*, **51**, 1014–21.

Weintraub, S. and Mesulam, M.-M. (1987). Right cerebral dominance in spatial attention. Further evidence based on ipsilateral neglect. *Archives of Neurology*, **44**, 621–5.

Weintraub, S., Daffner, K. R., Ahern, G., Price, B. H., and Mesulam, M.-M. (1996). Right sided hemispatial neglect and bilateral cerebral lesions. *Journal of Neurology, Neurosurgery and Psychiatry*, **60**, 342–4.

Yamaguchi, S., Tsuchiya, H., and Kobayashi, S. (1998). Visuospatial attention shift and motor responses in cerebellar disorders. *Journal of Cognitive Neuroscience*, **10**, 95–107.

Zatorre, R. J., Mondor, T. A., and Evans, A. C. (1999). Auditory attention to space and frequency activates similar cerebral systems. *NeuroImage*, **10**, 544–54.

2.2 Neglect in monkeys: effect of permanent and reversible lesions

Claire Wardak, Etienne Olivier, and Jean-René Duhamel

Behavioral changes referred to as 'unilateral neglect' and sharing some similarities with deficits observed in humans after right parietal lobe damage were described in nonhuman primates more than a century ago (Bianchi 1895). Early studies combined the surgical ablation of the cortex in the frontal lobe (Welch and Stuteville 1958) with simple observational methods that revealed distinctive changes in behavior in the few hours or days following the lesion, for example deviation of the eyes and head toward the side of the lesion, disregard for contralesional visual stimuli in the absence of definite hemianopia, and unwillingness to use the arm opposite to the lesion in the absence of hemiparesis. A similar approach was also used in more theoretically motivated investigations which focused on the characteristics of tactile extinction (Schwartz and Eidelberg 1968) or on the distinction between sensory and motor aspects of neglect (Valenstein et al. 1982).

However, despite obvious analogies between human and monkey neglect, there is still considerable debate as to whether there exists a genuine monkey analog of human neglect, and whether similar lesions produce comparable functional impairments in both species. Indeed, parallels drawn between the monkey and human forms of neglect somehow fell short of expectations because the deficits in monkeys were initially observed after frontal rather than parietal lobe lesions. In addition, neglect reported in monkeys was comparatively mild and short-lived (Kennard and Ectors 1938; Welch and Stutteville 1958). Although neglect in humans has been shown to occur after frontal lobe damage (Heilman et al. 1971) and although later studies have also reported neglect in monkeys after parietal lobe lesions (Deuel and Regan 1985), differences between human and monkey neglect is an unsettled issue. As for its seemingly more benign and transient expressions in monkeys, different explanations have been put forward including the specialization of human right hemisphere for visuospatial functions, which could hamper the degree of cortical plasticity, and the size of lesions which in humans often match large cerebral vascular territories and frequently produce extensive damage not only to the cortex but also to the underlying white matter. This is probably a more significant factor than might be assumed on first analysis. Clinicians who have the opportunity to observe patients with small parietal lesions in the acute stage of their injury typically report neglect symptoms which vanish within a few days, much like in monkeys following lesions restricted to the cortical grey matter. In contrast, most of the patients that are included in neuropsychological investigations of neglect are recruited, for obvious medical and practical reasons, several weeks or months, sometimes years, following the injury. Therefore the persistence of significant and stable manifestations of neglect after a prolonged recovery period could be related to the extent of white matter damage. This hypothesis is further supported by the work of Gaffan and Hornak (1997), who were able to produce lasting neglect in monkeys with minimal damage to cortex by using strategically placed lesions in the white matter.

In conclusion, if the primary purpose of conducting lesion experiments in monkeys is to mimic the features of human neglect by targeting brain regions homologous to those which are damaged in neglect patients, restricted cortical ablations or reversible inactivation may not represent an ideal approach because lesion size and underlying mechanisms are unlikely to be identical. However, if one wishes to address the question of how a given brain area contributes to the cognitive operations thought to be altered in neglect, animal experiments constitute a highly useful tool. Moreover, with reversible inactivation techniques, it is now possible to mimic an acute lesion state and to study its effects on behavioral tasks before any major cerebral reorganization begins to take place. In a rapidly evolving field, with growing evidence supporting similar modular principles of functional cortical organization in both humans and monkeys, fine-grained lesion experiments are likely to provide valuable insight into the functional homologies, as well as possible divergence, between the two species regarding the brain structures responsible for space representation, attention, and multisensory integration.

In this chapter we shall review results from permanent and reversible lesion experiments in monkeys and discuss these in the light of current knowledge of the anatomical and functional organization of the parietal and frontal cortices. We first briefly establish the current anatomical and functional background with respect to which monkey lesion experiments have to be interpreted.

The functional organization of monkey parietal and frontal cortex

The parietal lobe of the macaque monkey contains a number of functional subdivisions which have been defined on the basis of multiple criteria including cytoarchitectonic features, connectivity patterns, and neuronal responses characteristics. The brain map shown in Fig. 1(a) clearly suggests that the parietal lobe cannot be reduced to a single function. This is also true of the frontal cortex, which contains several premotor areas in its caudal portion and higher-order areas more rostrally. Parietal and frontal areas are interconnected in a systematic manner and establish connections with several subcortical structures involved in arousal, motivation, memory, sensory processing, and motor control. In-depth review of the anatomy and physiology of the frontal and parietal cortices can be found elsewhere (Rizzolatti et al. 1998; Colby and Golberg 1999), and we shall only briefly describe the cortical areas which have been implicated in spatial attention and orientation behaviors, and which have been targeted by lesion experiments. Figure 1(b) has been compiled from published lesion experiments and illustrates the variety of lesion sites associated with neglect. Each outline corresponds to a single lesion experiment. As can be seen from the areas of maximum overlap (the darker shades of gray), the most frequently targeted locations are the periarcuate region in the frontal lobe and the inferior parietal lobule, which is bounded by the intraparietal and the superior temporal sulci. A frontal lesion spanning the two banks of the arcuate sulcus and part of the convexity cortex would typically compromise both a major eye movement region, the frontal eye field (FEF) and portions of several premotor areas. In the parietal lobe, the extent of cortex which is typically ablated encompasses about half a dozen different functional areas. Single-cell recording experiments have highlighted the high degree of functional specialization within each of these areas.

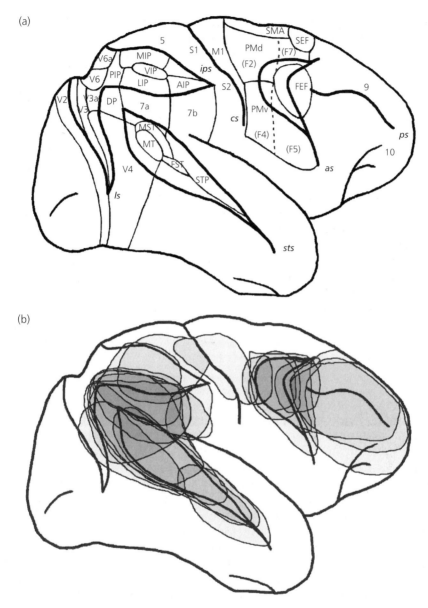

Figure 1 Representation of a macaque cerebral hemisphere with the arcuate, intraparietal, superior temporal, and lunate sulci (thick lines) opened up. (a) Boundaries of major functional subdivisions within the frontal and the parietal lobe: *ps*, principal sulcus; *as*, arcuate sulcus; *cs*, central sulcus; *ips*, intraparietal sulcus; *sts*, superior temporal sulcus; *ls*, lunate sulcus. (b) Outlines of the variety of ablations performed in the experiments cited in the text; gray shading indicates the degree of overlap, across these studies, between the lesion sites within the parietal or the frontal lobes that are associated with neglect (redrawn from 17 studies).

Parietal cortex

The superior parietal lobule is principally involved in somatosensory processing and motor aspects of arm and hand movements (area 5), but also participates in visuomotor processes (area MIP (Colby and Duhamel 1991); area V6A (Galletti *et al.* 1996, 1999)). Area 7b (or PF) in the anterior portion of the inferior parietal lobule is also strongly related to somatosensory processing, although subpopulations of neurons respond to both visual and somatic stimuli (Hyvärinen 1981; Graziano and Gross 1995). The posterior region of the inferior parietal lobule contains a number of functionally distinct areas which are part of the dorsal visual processing stream. Early studies reported mainly on the properties of cells located in the exposed surface of the posterior parietal lobe (area 7a or PG), and a wide range of response types were described: visual activity in relation to static or moving stimuli, activity related to attention, fixation, and saccadic and smooth pursuit eye movements (for a review of the early work see Hyvärinen (1981)). Several other areas are hidden within the depth of the superior temporal and intraparietal sulci. Located laterally to area 7a in the posterior portion of the superior temporal sulcus, areas MT and MST are crucial cortical relays for the processing of visual motion. Both areas have been studied extensively in relation to object- and ego-motion perception, smooth pursuit eye movements, and attention to moving stimuli (Tanaka *et al.* 1986; Komatsu and Wurtz 1988; Treue and Maunsell 1996; Duffy 1998). Area FST is defined anatomically, but its functional specificity is unknown. More anteriorly, the superior temporal polysensory area (STP) contains neurons responding to stimuli in one or several sensory modalities: visual, tactile, and auditory (Bruce *et al.* 1981; Hikosaka *et al.* 1988). Neurons in this area can also respond to complex stimuli such as particular body parts or 'biological' motion (Perett *et al.* 1982). In the intraparietal sulcus, the lateral intraparietal area (LIP) is involved in visual attention and saccadic eye movement planning (Barash *et al.* 1991*a,b*; Colby *et al.* 1996). Response modulations that are contingent upon task-related behavioral requirements, in the absence of changes in the physical characteristics of sensory stimuli, are often used as neural markers for covert processing related to attention and intention. LIP neurons, for example, show enhanced responses when visual stimuli appearing in their receptive field are targets of eye movements, but also during sustained attention to peripheral stimuli in the absence of eye movements (Colby *et al.* 1996). Similar attentional effects have previously been described in area 7a (Robinson *et al.* 1978). Both areas have also been shown to carry signals related to attention reorienting (Robinson *et al.* 1995; Steinmetz and Constantinidis 1995). The ventral intraparietal area (VIP) is located in the fundus of the intraparietal sulcus and is characterized by a different set of response characteristics. VIP neurons respond to visual, tactile, vestibular, and auditory information (Colby *et al.* 1993; Bremmer *et al.* 1997; Duhamel *et al.* 1998; Schlack *et al.* 2000), and show strong sensitivity to objects in near peripersonal space. The anterior intraparietal area (AIP) and the medial intraparietal area (MIP) are involved in visuomotor transformations for hand-grasping and arm-reaching movements respectively (Sakata *et al.* 1995; Johnson *et al.* 1996).

Frontal cortex

The premotor cortex contains several subfields associated with eye, mouth, hand, and limb movements. Results from single-cell recording investigations in monkeys suggest that these areas are important for higher-order aspects of movement selection, preparation, and initiation. Furthermore, several studies have shown a contribution of the premotor cortex to attentional processing of sensory stimuli and to spatial integration of multisensory information. Visual and saccade-related activities are found in the FEF (Goldberg and Bruce 1985), the supplementary eye field (SEF) (Schall 1991), and the principal sulcus (Boch and Goldberg 1989; Funahashi *et al.* 1991). In the FEF, subsets of neurons respond to visual stimuli with very short latency and could participate in the attentional selection of targets for a saccadic eye movements (Goldberg and Bushnell 1981). Genuine responsiveness to visual stimuli independent of, or in the absence of, overt motor responses have also been found in areas not directly involved in oculomotor functions. In the ventral premotor cortex in particular, cells responding during the execution of a specific movement also discharge in response to the mere presentation of the object which will be the target of the motor response, or to a visual stimulus in the vicinity of the relevant body segment (Fogassi *et al.* 1996; Graziano *et al.* 1997). The dorsal premotor cortex (F2) also exhibits the capacity of responding to object presentation (Fogassi *et al.* 1999). Sensory responses are not limited to the visual modality, and single neurons can integrate visual, tactile, and even auditory information in a spatially congruent and complementary manner (Graziano and Gandhi 2000), suggesting that the premotor cortex plays a significant role in the selection of targets for specific behavioral goals.

Both the parietal and frontal cortices have subcortical projections to oculomotor centers, in particular the superior colliculus which is a subcortical structure important for multisensory integration (Wallace *et al.* 1996) and saccadic eye movements (Sparks 1986). Enhancement of visual activity in the superior colliculus was originally described as contingent upon the execution of ocular saccades (Goldberg and Wurtz 1972), but other studies have also observed response modulation during attentional tasks that did not require overt eye movements (Robinson and Kertzman 1995; Gattass and Desimone 1996). It is clear that the neuronal mechanisms for attention and orienting are distributed across this wide cortical and subcortical network, which may explain to some extent the transient nature of the deficits which occur following focal damage to the parietal or the frontal lobe. Yet it is also reasonable to assume that each area within this network has evolved in order to fulfil a specific function. Hypotheses regarding the distinctive functional characteristics of most of the parietal and frontal areas considered here remain tentative.

Ablation studies

Lesions in a number of brain structures can produce neglect in monkeys. The operational definition of neglect in monkeys mainly involves behavioral manifestations of reduced spatial exploration and inattention. Lesion studies have variously reported tendencies to search for food more on the ipsilesional than the contralesional side of space, to orient the eye, head, body ipsilesionally, to orient one of two bilateral visual or tactile stimuli to the ipsilesional, to ignore single contralesional visual or tactile stimuli, and to orient away from contralesional auditory stimuli. The lesion sites responsible for these deficits can be frontal (Welch and Stuteville 1958; Valenstein *et al.* 1987) or parietal (Heilman *et al.* 1971; Faugier-Grimaud *et al.* 1978, 1985; Deuel and Regan 1985; Lynch and McLaren 1989). These deficits, although similar to those observed in humans, tend to be rather short-lived, with full recovery reportedly occurring between 2 days and 2 weeks, and rarely more than a few months. A number of studies have made direct comparisons of the effects of frontal and parietal lesions using the same set of behavioral measures (Schwartz and Eidelberg 1968; Rizzolatti *et al.* 1985; Gaffan and Hornak 1997). In general, very similar deficits are reported after parietal or frontal lesions, with a tendency for more severe and longer-lasting deficits to occur following frontal lobe lesions, although Deuel and Farrar (1993) reported that contralesional tactile neglect and ipsilesional limb preference was more pronounced following a parietal lesion than after a frontal lesion. Comparisons of frontal and parietal lesions must be interpreted with caution, however, because the location and size of the lesions within each region vary considerably across studies and because the effects could depend to a large extent on the particular functional subregions included in the lesions, as illustrated in the previous section.

As in humans, unilateral neglect can occur as a result of subcortical lesions. Tactile extinction as well as lateralized orienting deficits toward stimuli in other sensory modalities have been reported following midbrain lesions (Eidelberg and Schwartz 1971; Watson *et al.* 1974). Unilateral lesions of the superior colliculus have clearly been shown to produce unilateral impairments in ocular or manual responses to visual stimuli (Schiller *et al.* 1980; Albano *et al.* 1982; Robinson and Kertzman 1995). Some of the behavioral deficits resulting from cortical lesions may in fact result from decreased activity in subcortical structures. Reduced oxygen metabolism (revealed by the 2-DG autoradiographic technique) is observed after parietal or frontal lesions in several subcortical structures, including the thalamus, basal ganglia, and superior colliculus, and in monkeys a return to normal metabolic levels follows recovery from neglect (Deuel 1987). Functional 'deafferent-ation' of the cortex can also produce neglect. In a provocative study, Gaffan and Hornak (1997) proposed an account of visual neglect which requires neither cortical nor subcortical damage. The combination of a post-chiasmatic unilateral section of the optic tract with a complete section of the forebrain commissures was found to produce more severe contralesional impairments in a visual search task than did individual or combined parietal and frontal lesions, or optic tract section alone. Thus the authors suggest that a cerebral hemisphere which is completely deprived of visual information, by cutting both intra- and inter-hemispheric routes, cannot generate and update con-tralateral space 'representation' and is thus unable to guide visual exploration. There are currently no reports of hemianopic split-brain human patients which corroborate this hypothesis; however, it suggests that the contribution of hemianopia and white matter involvement, which can be quite extensive following naturally occurring vascular lesion, should be evaluated carefully in relation to the severity and persistence of neglect symptoms in human patients. Interestingly, in Gaffan and Hornak's study, a lesion limited to the posterior part of the corpus callosum in association with a unilateral parietal leucotomy, thereby isolating the parietal lobe while preserving its cortical gray matter, was sufficient to produce deficits nearly as severe as the optic tract plus forebrain commissure section.

The evidence of neglect and the causative brain damage presented above suffer from a number of interpretation problems. Firstly, as already mentioned, the lesions are typically quite large and the rather broad spectrum of impairments reported in several studies could be due to simultaneous damage in multiple functional subsystems. Secondly, many of the tasks used do not allow us to characterize unambiguously the underlying functional impairment. For instance, care must be taken in using the presence of contralesional tactile or visual extinction to double stimuli, despite intact detection of single stimuli, as evidence of an attentional deficit since it has been argued that a mild sensory impairment can also produce a similar pattern (De Renzi et al. 1984). Another important issue, pointed out by Milner (1987), is that a failure to orient does not necessarily imply a failure to attend. The behavioral changes offered as signs of neglect often involve responding to a lateralized sensory event with an oriented motor act. Different experimental tools could be used to distinguish between attentional and intentional deficits. One approach is to measure reaction time with a simple non-lateralized button-press response. Another is to dissociate the side of sensory stimulation from that of the responding limb. This is the method adopted by Valenstein et al. (1982, 1987) whose seminal work demonstrated that monkeys trained to open a door with one hand in response to a stimulus applied to the opposite leg show a deficit which is related to the side of the response and not to the side of the stimulus, and this occurs after both parietal cortex and frontal cortex lesions. These results suggest that unilateral akinesia, an impairment in initiating movements of the contralesional limb and/or in the contralesional direction, is a prominent feature of neglect in monkeys.

Another general difficulty with interspecies comparisons is that it remains unclear which criteria need to be adopted in comparing human and monkey neglects. As more fine-grained behavioral dissociations are uncovered in humans, it may be necessary to adopt similarly sophisticated tasks in monkey. Quite often, experimenters will report having observed 'neglect' in experimental animals only when the equivalent of obvious bedside symptoms are readily observable. As is the case with humans, however, such tests have a low sensitivity, with the exception of large lesions or in the acute stage, and subtle signs of unilateral impairment can easily be overlooked. For example, in the study by Valenstein et al. (1987), the effects of frontal arcuate lesions were compared with those of a 'control' lesion located in the anterior superior temporal region. Simple observation revealed that, following a frontal lesion, monkeys 'ignored visual, auditory and somatosensory stimuli delivered to the neglected side', spontaneously preferred using the ipsilesional limb to reach for food, and displayed abnormal response times in a manual door-opening task. Monkeys who underwent a temporal lesion showed no clinical signs of neglect and were said to appear entirely normal. Histological reports of the temporal lobe lesion indicate that the ablated cortex included almost in its entirety the upper bank and the fundus of the anterior half of the superior temporal sulcus, corresponding to the superior temporal polysensory area (STP), a region connected with both the posterior parietal cortex and the FEF. Interestingly, although few lesion studies have been published on STP, there are at least two reports of impaired deficits in saccadic reaction time and smooth pursuit eye movements (Luh *et al.* 1986; Scalaidhe *et al.* 1995). Thus, although area STP may be less critical than the frontal cortex in limb movement initiation and general orienting, it could play a non-negligible role in visual attention and visuomotor functions. Within the frontal lobe, selective functional impairments have also been described as a function of lesion site. Neglect can be observed for stimuli within near peripersonal space but not for more distant stimuli following lesions in the postarcuate premotor cortex, while the reverse pattern occurs after lesions involving the FEF in the anterior bank of the arcuate sulcus (Rizzolatti *et al.* 1983). Such a distinction between orienting to near and far has also been shown to be relevant in human neglect (Berti and Frassinetti 2000).

Inactivation studies

Reversible inactivation offers the possibility of analyzing lesion effects on spatial attention and orienting in discrete brain areas that have been characterized electrophysiologically beforehand. Using muscimol, a $GABA_A$ agonist, Li *et al.* (1999) tested the effects of area LIP inactivation on visually- and memory-guided saccadic tasks. Saccade latency was slightly increased for contralesional targets in both tasks and saccade accuracy was impaired for memory-guided saccades. We also studied the effect of LIP inactivation on a variety of saccade tasks in order to test the hypothesis of a specific contribution of this area to attentional target selection (Wardak *et al.* 2001). In contrast with the study by Li *et al.*, we found no change in latency or accuracy on saccades to single targets. However, during saccades to intermixed double and single flashed stimuli, extinction and neglect were both present: on bilateral trials, the monkeys made saccades almost exclusively to the ipsilesional stimulus; on unilateral trials, they failed to initiate a saccade to about 40 per cent of the contralesional stimuli. Impairments were also observed in visual search. In this task, a target was presented along with three, seven, or fifteen radially arranged distractors in two conditions (pop-out and conjunction search) and monkeys were rewarded for foveating the target. In conjunction search only, finding contralesional targets required more time and more saccades than ipsilesional targets, and the ocular scanning strategy was ipsilesionally biased. In fact, in one animal this resulted in better search performance under inactivation for targets located in the ipsilesional side than for the same targets under normal conditions. Control injections were also made in the adjacent VIP and had no effect on any tasks. The presence of a significant attentional deficit in target selection, independent of saccade initiation or execution, strongly suggests that area LIP is one of the critical parietal sites for visuospatial attention, in agreement with single-cell recording data indicating that LIP neurons encode the saliency of visual stimuli (Gottlieb *et al.* 1998). To our knowledge, no other inactivation studies so far have addressed the issue of spatial attention in the parietal cortex. Inactivation of AIP in the anterior portion of the intraparietal sulcus has been investigated in relation to manual grasping, and produces selective deficits in hand shaping (Gallese *et al.* 1994).

Similar inactivation experiments in the FEF produce more clear-cut saccadic eye movement deficits. Sommer and Tehovnik (1997) investigated the effects of muscimol and lidocaine injections in three oculomotor tasks (delay task, step task, and fixation task) and found increased latency and poorer accuracy of contraversive saccades as well as difficulties in fixating a contralesional target. Dias and Segraves (1999) also reported deficits in saccades and fixation following muscimol injections in the FEF. Using a cooling method, Keating and Gooley (1988) found saccade latency and accuracy deficits, the severity and topography of which depended on the degree of cooling. Neglect for visual targets in the contralesional hemifield was also reported, although the authors do not explain how they assessed for this.

Inactivation experiments have also been conducted in other parts of the frontal cortex. Sommer and Tehovnik (1999) injected lidocaine in the dorsomedial cortex, presumably inactivating the SEF and part of the supplementary motor area (SMA). Oculomotor deficits were present, but were milder than those produced by FEF inactivation and affected the execution of saccade sequences rather than isolated eye movements. Posterior to the arcuate sulcus, the ventral premotor cortex (PMv) has been implicated in visuomotor transformations for hand movements. Schieber (2000) showed that PMv inactivation with muscimol biases motoric choice ipsilaterally when two objects are presented simultaneously on the left and right side (e.g. motor extinction), but he did not observe impairments in the execution of reaching and grasping movements. In contrast, Fogassi *et al.* (2001) observed deficits in hand shaping, very similar to those observed by Gallese *et al.* (1994) after AIP inactivations, as well as peripersonal neglect in the contralesional hemispace around the mouth, the arm, and the body.

All the above inactivation experiments studied the detection of objects in space in the context of motor tasks which also involve an oriented motor component, and therefore did not address specifically the question of spatial allocation of attention independent of response orientation. A few studies have investigated this issue using variants of the cued reaction time task introduced by Posner *et al.* (1984), in which a subject must respond, generally by pressing or releasing a bar, to the appearance of a peripheral stimulus which has been preceded by a cue presented on the same or the opposite side. Davidson and Marrocco (2000) recorded from single cells, in a region which encompassed areas 7a and LIP, to characterize attention-related neuronal activity during this cued reaction time task. They then injected scopolamine in order to block cholinergic transmission in the same portion of the parietal lobe. Compared with control conditions, monkeys showed a general increase in reaction time which was more pronounced for contralesional targets, and a reduced validity effect, defined as the difference in reaction time for validly and invalidly cued targets. Details of the interaction between side of the cue and side of the target are not reported, but the authors interpreted the effects as a deficit in covert orienting. Somewhat similar results have been reported after muscimol inactivation of the pulvinar, a large thalamic nucleus with strong connections to the parietal lobe. Petersen *et al.* (1987) observed that reaction times were impaired for invalidly cued contralateral targets but facilitated for invalidly cued ipsilesional targets, and suggested that the pulvinar participates in attention shifting. Inactivation of the superficial layers of the superior colliculus produces a global contralesional increase in reaction times but does not interfere with cue validity effects (Robinson and Kertzman 1995). Thus inactivating the parietal cortex, the pulvinar, or the superior colliculus can modify the processing of contralateral visual input, in agreement with a distributed neural circuit for the control of visual attention.

Conclusions

Cortical ablation studies in monkeys have shown that neglect can occur following lesions of either the periarcuate frontal and the inferior parietal regions. Such neglect recovers rapidly, which limits the usefulness of this approach for exploring the many different aspects of neglect and spatial attention revealed by neuropsychological investigations in humans. The rapid recovery of neglect could reflect a true difference in the cerebral organization of attention and space representation mechanisms between humans and monkeys, but it could also be related to secondary factors such as lesion size and extent of white matter damage. Reversible inactivation experiments offer an alternative approach to the study of neglect. These experiments have demonstrated that the inactivation of distinct parietal and frontal subregions can produce selective deficits in visual attention and in target and movement selection, largely confirming the functional role originally postulated for these areas on the basis of single-cell recording studies. However, much remains to be done in order to understand, on this scale of analysis, a number of important aspects of neglect which have been highlighted in studies of human patients, such as the preservation of pre-attentive processing, the relation between perceptual awareness and neglect, perceptual distortions of space, cross-modal links in spatial attention, and reference frames of neglect.

References

Albano, J. E., Mishkin, M., Westbrook, L. E., and Wurtz, R. H. (1982). Visuomotor deficits following ablation of monkey superior colliculus. *Journal of Neurophysiology*, **48**, 338–51.

Barash, S., Bracewell, R. M., Fogassi, L., Gnadt, J. W., and Andersen, R. A. (1991*a*). Saccade-related activity in the lateral intraparietal area. I: Temporal properties: comparison with area 7a. *Journal of Neurophysiology*, **66**, 1095–1108.

Barash, S., Bracewell, R. M., Fogassi, L., Gnadt, J. W., and Andersen, R. A. (1991*b*). Saccade-related activity in the lateral intraparietal area. II: Spatial properties. *Journal of Neurophysiology*, **66**, 1109–24.

Berti, A. and Frassinetti, F. (2000). When far becomes near: remapping of space by tool use. *Journal of Cognitive Neurosciences*, **12**, 415–20.

Bianchi, L. (1895). The functions of the frontal lobes. *Brain*, **18**, 497–522.

Boch, R. A. and Goldberg, M. E. (1989). Participation of prefrontal neurons in the preparation of visually guided eye movements in the rhesus monkey. *Journal of Neurophysiology*, **61**, 1064–84.

Bremmer, F., Duhamel, J.-R., Ben Hamed, S., and Graf, W. (1997). The representation of movement in near extrapersonal space in the macaque ventral intraparietal area (VIP). In *Parietal lobe contributions to orientation in 3D space* (ed. P. Thier and H.-O. Karnath), pp. 619–30. Springer-Verlag, Heidelberg.

Bruce, C., Desimone, R., and Gross, C. G. (1981). Visual properties of neurons in a polysensory area in superior temporal sulcus of the macaque. *Journal of Neurophysiology*, **46**, 369–84.

Colby, C. L. and Duhamel, J.-R. (1991). Heterogeneity of extrastriate visual areas and multiple parietal areas in the macaque monkey. *Neuropsychologia*, **29**, 517–37.

Colby, C. L., Duhamel, J.-R., and Goldberg, M. E. (1993). Ventral intraparietal area of the macaque: anatomic location and visual response properties. *Journal of Neurophysiology*, **69**, 902–14.

Colby, C. L., Duhamel, J.-R., and Goldberg, M. E. (1996). Visual, presaccadic and cognitive activation of single neurons in monkey lateral intraparietal area. *Journal of Neurophysiology*, **76**, 2841–2.

Colby, C. L. and Goldberg, M. E. (1999). Space and attention in parietal cortex. *Annual Review of Neuroscience*, **22**, 319–49.

Davidson, M. C. and Marrocco, R. T. (2000). Local infusion of scopolamine into intraparietal cortex slows covert orienting in rhesus monkeys. *Journal of Neurophysiology*, **83**, 1536–49.

De Renzi, E., Gentilini, M., and Pattacini, F. (1984). Auditory extinction following hemisphere damage. *Neuropsychologia*, **22**, 733–744.

Deuel, R. K. (1987). Neural dysfunction during hemineglect after cortical damage in two monkey models. In *Neurophysiological and neuropsychological aspects of spatial neglect* (ed. M. Jeannerod), pp. 315–34. Elsevier, Amsterdam.

Deuel, R. K. and Farrar, C. A. (1993). Stimulus cancellation by macaques with unilateral frontal or parietal lesions. *Neuropsychologia*, **31**, 29–38.

Deuel, R. K. and Regan, D. J. (1985). Parietal hemineglect and motor deficit in the monkey. *Neuropsychologia*, **23**, 305–14.

Duhamel, J.-R., Colby, C. L., and Goldberg, M. E. (1998). Ventral intraparietal of the macaque: congruent visual and somatic response properties. *Journal of Neurophysiology*, **79**, 126–36.

Dias, E. C. and Segraves, M. A. (1999). Muscimol-induced inactivation of monkey frontal eye field: effects on visually and memory-guided saccades. *Journal of Neurphysiology*, **81**, 2191–214.

Duffy, C. J. (1998). MST neurons respond to optic flow and translational movement. *Journal of Neurophysiology*, **80**, 1816–27.

Eidelberg, E. and Schwartz, A. S. (1971). Experimental analysis of the extinction phenomenon in monkeys. *Brain*, **94**, 91–108.

Faugier-Grimaud, S., Frenois, C., and Stein, D. G. (1978). Effects of posterior parietal lesions on visually guided behavior in monkeys. *Neuropsychologia*, **16**, 151–68.

Faugier-Grimaud, S., Frenois, C., and Peronnet, F. (1985). Effects of posterior parietal lesions on visually guided movements in monkeys. *Experimental Brain Research*, **59**, 125–38.

Fogassi, L., Gallese, V., Buccino, G., Craighero, L., Fadiga, L., and Rizzolatti, G. (2001). Cortical mechanism for the visual guidance of hand grasping movements in the monkey. A reversible inactivation study. *Brain*, **124**, 571–86.

Fogassi, L., Gallese, V., Fadiga, L., Luppino, G., Matelli, M., and Rizzolatti, G. (1996). Coding of peripersonal space in inferior premotar cortex (area F4). *Journal of Neurophysiology*, **76**, 141–57.

Fogassi, L., Raos, V., Franchi, G., Gallese, V., Luppino, G., and Matelli, M. (1999). Visual responses in the dorsal premotor area F2 of the macaque monkey. *Experimental Brain Research*, **128**, 194–9.

Funahashi, S., Bruce, C. J., and Goldman-Rakic, P. S. (1991). Neuronal activity related to saccadic eye movements in the monkey's dorsolateral prefrontal cortex. *Journal of Neurophysiology*, **65**, 1464-83.

Gaffan, D. and Hornak, J. (1997). Visual neglect in the monkey: representation and disconnection. *Brain*, **120**, 1647–57.

Gallese, V., Murata, A., Kaseda, M., Niki, N., and Sakata, H. (1994). Deficit in hand preshaping after muscimol injection in monkey parietal cortex. *NeuroReport*, **5**, 1525–9.

Galletti, C., Fattori, P., Battaglini, P. P., Shipp, S., and Zeki, S. (1996). Functional demarcation of a border between areas V6 and V6A in the superior parietal gyrus of the macaque monkey. *European Journal of Neurosciences*, **8**, 30–52.

Galletti, C., Fattori, P., Kutz, D. F., and Gamberini, M. (1999). Brain location and visual topography of cortical area V6A in the macaque monkey. *European Journal of Neurosciences*, **11**, 575–82.

Gattass, R. and Desimone, R. (1996). Responses of cells in the superior colliculus during performance of a spatial attention task in the macaque. *Revista Brasileira de Biologia*, **56**, 257–79.

Goldberg, M. E. and Bruce, C. J. (1985). Cerebral cortical activity associated with the orientation of visual attention in the rhesus monkey. *Vision Research*, **25**, 471–81.

Goldberg, M. E. and Bushnell, C. J. (1981). Behavioral enhancement of visual responses in monkey cerebral cortex. II: Modulation in frontal eye fields specifically related to saccades. *Journal of Neurophysiology*, **46**, 773–87.

Goldberg, M. E. and Wurtz, R. H. (1972). Activity of superior colliculus in behaving monkey. II: Effect of attention on neuronal responses. *Journal of Neurophysiology*, **35**, 560–74.

Gottlieb, J. P., Kusunoki, M., and Goldberg, M. E. (1998). The representation of visual salience in monkey parietal cortex. *Nature*, **391**, 481–4.

Graziano, M. S. and Gandhi, S. (2000). Location of the polysensory zone in the precentral gyrus of anesthetized monkeys. *Experimental Brain Research*, **135**, 259–66.

Graziano, M. S. A. and Gross C. G. (1995). The representation of extrapersonal space: a possible role for bimodal, visual–tactile neurons. In *The cognitive neurosciences* (ed. M. S. Gazzaniga), pp. 1021–34. MIT Press, Cambridge, MA.

Graziano, M. S. A., Xin Tian Hu, and Gross, C. G. (1997). Visuospatial properties of ventral premotor cortex. *Journal of Neurophysiology*, **77**, 2268–92.

Heilman, K. M., Pandya, D. N., Karol, E. A., and Geschwind, N. (1971). Auditory inattention. *Archives of Neurology*, **24**, 323–5.

Hikosaka, K., Iwai, E., Saito, H.-A., and Tanaka, K. (1988). Polysensory properties of neurons in the anterior bank of the caudal superior temporal sulcus of the macaque monkey. *Journal of Neurophysiology*, **60**, 1615–37.

Hyvärinen, J. (1981). Regional distribution of functions in parietal association area 7 of the monkey. *Brain Research*, **206**, 287–303.

Johnson, P. B., Ferraina, S., Bianchi, L., and Caminiti, R. (1996). Cortical networks for visual reaching: physiological and anatomical organization of frontal and parietal lobe arm regions. *Cerebral Cortex*, **6**, 102–19.

Keating, E. G. and Gooley, S. G. (1988). Saccadic disorders caused by cooling the superior colliculus or the frontal eye field, or from combined lesions of both structures. *Brain Research*, **438**, 247–55.

Kennard, M. A. and Ectors, L. (1938). Forced circling in monkeys following lesions of the frontal lobes. *Journal of Neurophysiology*, **1**, 45–54.

Komatsu, H. and Wurtz, R. H. (1988). Relation of cortical areas MT and MST to pursuit eye movements. I: Localization and visual properties of neurons. *Journal of Neurophysiology*, **60**, 580–603.

Li, C.-S. R., Mazzoni, P., and Anderson, R. A. (1999). Effect of reversible inactivation of macaque lateral intraparietal area on visual and memory saccades. *Journal of Neurophysiology*, **81**, 1827–38.

Luh, K. E., Butter, C. M., and Buchtel, H. A. (1986). Impairments in orienting to visual stimuli in monkeys following unilateral lesions of the superior sulcal polysensory cortex. *Neuropsychologia*, **24**, 461–70.

Lynch, J. C. and McLaren, J. W. (1989). Deficit of visual attention and saccadic eye movements after lesions of parietooccipital cortex in monkey. *Journal of Neurophysiology*, **61**, 74–90.

Milner, A. D. (1987). Animal models for the syndrome of spatial neglect. In *Neurophysiological and neuropsychological aspects of spatial neglect* (ed. M. Jeannerod), pp. 259–88. Elsevier, Amsterdam.

Perett, D. I., Rolls, E. T., and Caan, W. (1982). Visual responses to faces in the monkey temporal cortex. *Experimental Brain Research*, **47**, 329–42.

Petersen, S. E., Robinson, D. L., and Morris, J. D. (1987). Contributions of the pulvinar to visual spatial attention. *Neuropsychologia*, **25**, 97–105.

Posner, M. I., Walker, J. A., Friedrich, F. J., and Rafal, R. D. (1984). Effects of parietal lobe injury on covert orienting of visual attention. *Journal of Neuroscience*, **4**, 1863–74.

Rizzolatti, G., Luppino, G., and Matelli, M. (1998). The organization of the cortical motor system: new concepts. *Electroencephalography and Clinical Neurophysiology*, **106**, 283–96.

Rizzolatti, G., Matelli, M., and Pavesi, G. (1983). Deficits in attention and movement following the removal of postarcuate (area 6) and prearcuate (area 8) cortex in macaque monkeys. *Brain* **106**, 655–73.

Rizzolatti, G., Gentilucci, M., and Matelli, M. (1985). Selective spatial attention: one center, one circuit, or many circuits? In *Attention and Performance XI* (ed. M. I. Posner and O. S. M. Marin), pp. 251–65. Lawrence Erlbaum, London.

Robinson, D. L., Goldberg, M. E., and Stanton, G. B. (1978). Parietal association cortex in the primate: sensory mechanisms and behavioral modulations. *Journal of Neurophysiology*, **41**, 910–32.

Robinson, D. L., Bowman, E. M., and Kertzman, C. (1995). Covert orienting of attention in macaques. II: Contributions of parietal cortex. *Journal of Neurophysiology*, **74**, 698–712.

Robinson, D. L. and Kertzman, C. (1995). Covert orienting of attention in macaques III: Contributions of the superior colliculus. *Journal of Neurophysiology*, **74**, 713–21.

Sakata, H., Taira, M., Murata, A., and Mine, S. (1995). Neural mechanisms of visual guidance of hand action in the parietal cortx of monkey. *Cerebral Cortex*, **5**, 429–38.

Scalaidhe, S. P., Albright, T. D., Rodman, R. H., and Gross, C. G. (1995). Effects of superior temporal polysensory area lesions on eye movements in the macaque monkey. *Journal of Neurophysiology*, **73**, 1–19.

Schall, J. D. (1991). Neuronal activity related to visually guided saccades in the frontal eye fields of rhesus monkeys: comparison with supplementary eye fields. *Journal of Neurophysiology*, **66**, 559–79.

Schieber, M. H. (2000). Inactivation of the ventral premotor cortex biases the laterality of motoric choices. *Experimental Brain Research*, **130**, 497–507.

Schiller, P. H., True, S. D., and Conway, J. L. (1980). Deficits in eye movements following frontal eye-field and superior colliculus ablations. *Journal of Neurophysiology*, **44**, 1175–89.

Schlack, A., Sterbing, S., Hartung, K., Hoffmann, K.-P., and Bremmer, F. (2000). Auditory responsiveness in the macaque ventral intraparietal area (VIP). *Society of Neuroscience Abstracts*, **26**, 1064.

Schwartz, A. S. and Eidelberg, E. (1968). 'Extinction' to bilateral simultaneous stimulation in the monkey. *Neurology*, **18**, 61–8.

Sommer, M. A. and Tehovnik, E. J. (1997). Reversible inactivation of macaque frontal eye field. *Experimental Brain Research*, **116**, 229–49.

Sommer, M. A. and Tehovnik, E. J. (1999). Reversible inactivation of macaque dorsomedial frontal cortex: effects on saccades and fixations. *Experimental Brain Research*, **124**, 429–46.

Sparks, D. L. (1986). Translation of sensory signals into commands for control of saccadic eye movements: role of primate superior colliculus. *Physiological Review*, **66**, 118–71.

Steinmetz, M. A. and Constantinidis, C. (1995). Neurophysiological evidence for a role of posterior parietal cortex in redirecting visual attention. *Cerebral Cortex*, **5**, 448–56.

Tanaka, K., Hikosaka, K., Saito, H., Yukie, M., Fukada, Y., and Iwai, E. (1986). Analysis of local and wide-field movements in the superior temporal visual areas of the macaque monkey. *Journal of Neuroscience*, **6**, 134–44.

Treue, S. and Maunsell, J. H. (1996). Attentional modulation of visual motion processing in cortical areas MT and MST. *Nature*, **382**, 539–41.

Valenstein, E., Heilman, K. M., Watson, R. T., and Van Den Abell, T. (1982). Nonsensory neglect from parietotemporal lesions in monkeys. *Neurology*, **32**, 1198–1201.

Valenstein, E., Watson, R. T., Van den Abell, T., Carter, R., and Heilman, K. M. (1987). Response time in monkeys with unilateral neglect. *Archives of Neurology*, **44**, 517–20.

Wallace, M. T., Wilkinson, L. K., and Stein, B. E. (1996). Representation and integration of multiple sensory inputs in primate superior colliculus. *Journal of Neurophysiology*, **76**, 1246–66.

Wardak, C., Olivier, E., and Duhamel, J.-R. (2001). Saccadic target selection but no initiation or execution impairments following reversible inactivation of monkey lateral intraparietal cortex. *Society for Neuroscience Abstracts*, **27**, 348–348.5.

Watson, R. T., Heilman, K. M., Miller, B. D., and King, F. A. (1974). Neglect after mesencephalic reticular formation lesions. *Neurology*, **24**, 294–8.

Welch, K. and Stuteville, P. (1958). Experimental production of unilateral neglect in monkeys. *Brain*, **81**, 341–7.

2.3 Posterior parietal networks encoding visual space

Claudio Galletti and Patrizia Fattori

Clinical data on patients with cortical lesions suggest that the posterior parietal cortex (PPC) is involved in the representation of visual space (Bisiach and Luzzatti 1978; De Renzi 1982; Newcombe and Ratcliff 1989; Bisiach and Vallar 2000; Vallar 2001). After a stroke that involves the PPC, patients often find that their conception of space completely alters. The contralateral half of their visual space shrinks or sometimes completely disappears, the ipsilateral half may dilate, and the apparent positions of objects in the field of view may become jumbled up, even if each object can still be correctly recognized. Such patients are very inaccurate when attempting to reach out for things. They also tend to bump into objects when walking around in a room, even though they have correctly recognized them before starting to move.

On the whole, these impairments seem to be the result of two main deficits, one involving the cognitive reconstruction of the visual space (e.g. spatial neglect (Bisiach and Luzzatti 1978; Vallar and Perani 1986)) and the other the use of visuospatial information by the effectors in visually guided actions (optic ataxia (Perenin and Vighetto 1988; Nichelli 1999)). The neurophysiological counterpart of these clinical data is represented by the functional properties of PPC neurons, particularly of those involved in the encoding process of visual space. The aim of this chapter is to analyse and review the cellular mechanisms that are probably involved in the encoding process of visual space in physiological conditions.

Frames of reference of visual information

There are several lines of evidence indicating that the brain uses nonretinotopic representations of visual space. When the eyes move, for instance, the perceived visual world remains stable despite the movements of retinal images. Also, one can reach accurately to the location of visual targets independently of the location of the target image on the retinas (i.e. independent of eye, head, or body position). It seems likely that visuospatial information is provided to the brain in different frames of reference according to the different specific demands. Thus, for the cognitive reconstruction of visual space, the frame of reference should be centered on the objects present in the visual field (allocentric coordinates), while for the visual guiding of body actions it should be centered on the effector to be moved (body, arm, head, etc.) (egocentric coordinates). None of these frames of reference needs to be centered on the retina.

A typical visual neuron, exclusively sensitive to visual stimulation, is not able to encode visual space in a nonretinotopic frame of reference. The visual neuron collects visual information through

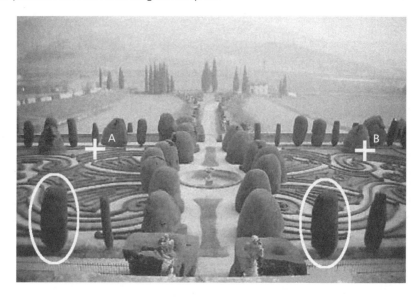

Figure 1 Retinotopic organization of visual RFs. The crosses marked A and B indicate two possible fixation points of a subject looking at the scene. The ovals indicate the two locations in the field of view of the RF of an hypothetical visual cell while the subject looks at A and B.

its receptive field (RF). The RF is like a window which is open in a particular part of the visual field according to its retinotopic location. When a subject is looking at a scene containing many different objects, and is gazing at one of these objects (e.g. A in Fig. 1), a given cell collects visual information from a given part of the visual field (oval in Fig. 1). As long as the eyes are still, the retinal locus of the object falling on the RF (a tree in the example in Fig. 1) corresponds to the spatial location of the object. However, when the subject changes the direction of gaze, the RF moves with the eyes, reaching another part of the visual field (e.g. B in Fig. 1). After gaze displacement, the cell informs us about what is happening in a new part of the visual field, and its activity is dependent on the kind of object falling on its RF. If the object is the same, as in the case shown in Fig. 1 (a tree), the cell continues to discharge at about the same frequency, no matter where the tree is located in the visual scene. In other words, as in everyday life the eye movements continually shift the location at which an image of an object strikes the retina, and a visual cell continually informs us about *which* object falls into its RF but does not inform us about *where* the object really is in space.

Gaze-dependent visual cells

To localize objects in space, the brain needs to combine information about the retinal position of the object image with information about the direction of gaze. Referring again to the example shown in Fig. 1, if the hypothetical cell shown there responded to the same object (the tree) with different discharge frequencies according to the direction of gaze (situations A and B respectively), we could infer that this cell is able to encode the spatial location of the object instead of simply recognizing the object itself.

Many cortical and subcortical structures of the brain contain neurons whose activity is influenced by the position of the eyes in the orbits, but only some of them contain visual neurons whose response to visual stimulation is modulated by the direction of gaze. Schlag and coworkers first reported a gaze modulation on visual responses in the intralaminar nuclei of the thalamus and superior colliculus of the cat (Peck *et al.* 1980; Schlag *et al.* 1980). Mountcastle and Andersen were the first to demonstrate that the visual RF of PPC neurons remained in retinotopic coordinates while the animal changed its direction of gaze, and the magnitude of cell response to the visual stimulation of the same retinotopic position was modulated by the gaze direction (Mountcastle 1981; Andersen and Mountcastle 1983). Since then, gaze-dependent visual neurons have been found in many structures of the brain, even outside the PPC, as summarized in Fig. 2.

According to the classic schema proposed by Ungerleider and Mishkin (1982), visual information leaves the visual cortex of the occipital pole by two main routes—a ventral route passing through the temporal lobe, involved in visual recognition of objects, and a dorsal route reaching the cortex of the parietal lobe, involved in visuospatial processing. It was originally proposed that the dorsal stream included only the inferior parietal lobule but, as Fig. 2 shows, we now know that the cortex hidden in the intraparietal sulcus and the cortex of the caudal part of the superior

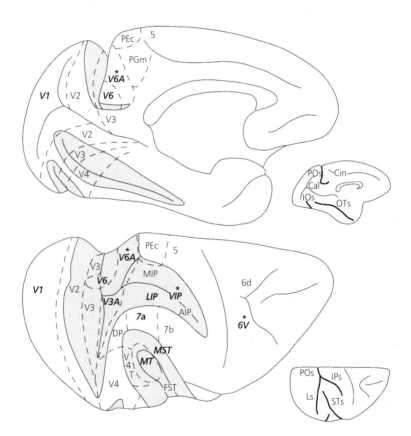

Figure 2 Cortical areas containing gaze-dependent visual cells or real-position cells. Medial (top) and dorsal (bottom) views of the left hemisphere of a macaque brain. The parieto-occipital (POs), inferior occipital (IOs), occipitotemporal (OTs), lunate (Ls), intraparietal (IPs), and superior temporal (STs) sulci, indicated by bold lines on the brain silhouettes on the right, are shown open (gray regions) to reveal the cortical areas hidden inside the sulci. Bold characters are used to indicate areas containing gaze-dependent visual cells (Andersen and Mountcastle 1983; Galletti and Battaglini 1989; Andersen *et al.* 1990; Boussaoud *et al.* 1993; Galletti *et al.* 1995; Bremmer *et al.* 1997, 1999; Trotter and Celebrini 1999); the asterisks indicate the cortical areas containing real-position cells (Fogassi *et al.* 1992, 1996; Galletti *et al.* 1993; Duhamel *et al.* 1997; Graziano and Gross 1998). Cin, cingulate sulcus; Cal, calcarine fissure.

parietal lobule are also involved in visuospatial processing. These regions of the brain include a large number of distinct cortical areas, and it is noteworthy that cells putatively able to encode the visual space (gaze-dependent visual cells) have been found in almost all the areas of the dorsal visual stream, from the primary visual cortex to the premotor cortex.

As discussed above, gaze-dependent visual cells are not able to inform us continually about what happens in the same spatial location of the visual field, regardless of eye movements. On the contrary, each cell of this type continually informs us about different spatial locations according to the direction of gaze. It has been suggested that information about single spatial locations could be extracted from the activity of the entire population of gaze-dependent visual cells of a given area in a distributed encoding system (Andersen *et al.* 1985; Galletti and Battaglini 1989). Unfortunately, this system creates some problems in the interpretation of cellular activity. For instance, as the RFs of PPC gaze-dependent visual cells are large and nonuniform in their visual responsiveness (Andersen and Mountcastle 1983), a change in their activity could be due to either a change in the direction of gaze, with the visual stimulus that remains within the same part of the large RF, or a displacement of the visual stimulus within the RF while the animal maintains fixation. This is not the case for the gaze-dependent visual cells of the prestriate area V3A, as their RFs are small (a few degrees) and have a uniform profile of excitability (Galletti and Battaglini 1989). When one of these cells discharges, it means that the visual stimulus is in a well-defined spatial location. However, as V3A cells are very sensitive to the orientation of the stimulus, a change in activity of these cells could be the result of a change in stimulus orientation rather than a change in the spatial location of the stimulus. In other words, gaze-dependent visual cells are not able to encode the visual space univocally, not even those with small and uniform RFs.

Real-position cells

Cells explicitly encoding the visual space do exist, but they seem to be present in only a few regions of the brain. Early studies, carried out in monkey area 6 (Gentilucci *et al.* 1983) and in the thalamic intralaminar nuclei and the PPC of the cat (Schlag *et al.* 1980; Pigarev and Rodionova 1988), showed that visual stimulations delivered in the same spatial location evoked similar neuronal responses regardless of gaze direction. Subsequent studies have demonstrated that the visual RFs of some cells in a restricted number of cortical areas (see asterisks in Fig. 2) were organized in craniotopic instead of retinotopic coordinates. The RFs of these cells do not move with the eyes, remaining anchored to the same spatial location regardless of the direction of gaze. Cells of this type (sometimes called 'real-position' cells) have been described in areas V6A (Galletti *et al.* 1993) and VIP (Duhamel *et al.* 1997) of the monkey PPC, and in area F4 (Fogassi *et al.* 1992, 1996; Graziano and Gross 1998) of the monkey premotor cortex. In the primary visual cortex of the monkey, Motter and Poggio (1990) described a phenomenon similar to the real-position behavior. They found that, during fixation, the RF of V1 cells did not follow the micromovements of the eyes, remaining perfectly still in the same spatial location regardless of eye movements.

Figure 3 shows the behavior of a real-position cell recorded in area V6A. The cell had a visual RF just below the fovea. The visual stimulation of the RF evoked a good response from the cell when the animal looked toward the bottom right part of its field of view (Fig. 3(a)). The stimulation of the same retinotopic position was not effective when the animal looked toward other spatial locations (Fig. 3(a)), but if the stimulus was on the bottom right part of its field of view, the cell was always strongly activated, no matter where it was looking (Fig. 3(b)). In other words, the RF of this cell did not move with the eyes and the cell encoded a specific part of the field of view regardless of eye movements.

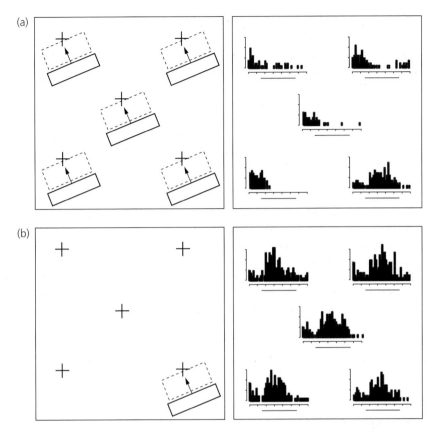

Figure 3 Neural responses of a 'real-position' cell to the visual stimulation of (a) the same retinotopic location or (b) the same spatial location, while the animal looked at five different screen positions. Each large square represents the 80° × 80° screen in front of the animal. The experimental paradigm is shown on the left, fixation-point locations on the screen are indicated by crosses; visual stimuli (full-line rectangles) were moved across the RF (broken-line rectangles) at a speed of 18°/s. The neural responses to visual stimulation are shown on the right; peristimulus time histograms of impulse sequences are reported at fixation point locations (the bold lines under the neural responses indicate the stimulation time; scales are 4 spikes per vertical division, and 300 ms per horizontal division).

Neurons of this type encode the visual space directly. Each real-position cell encodes a different spatial location according to the spatial coordinates of its visually responsive region. In contrast with gaze-dependent visual cells, the activity of real-position cells does not create any ambiguity of interpretation. If one of these cells discharges, it means that the object activating the cell is in a particular region of the visual space (that encoded by that particular cell).

The output of real-position cells could be used to direct movements toward visual targets, or to direct selective attention to relevant points in space for acquisition of stimuli in the immediate environment, either by gaze or manual reaching (Galletti et al. 1993, 1999). In this regard, it is worth noting that when one reaches toward a target that suddenly appears in the peripheral visual field, not only does the arm extend toward the object, but the eyes, head, and body also move in such a way that the image of the object falls on the fovea. The saccadic eye movement directed at the target is typically completed while the hand is still moving (Biguer et al. 1982). This means that during the execution of reaching movement, the target of movement changes its retinal location from the periphery to the fovea; nevertheless, the arm movement goes straight toward the target, as if the motor center controlling the movement 'knew' in advance the final position to be reached out in spatial coordinates. It has been suggested that area V6A could play an important role in all these visuomotor transformations (Galletti *et al.* 1999).

New concepts on visual RF organization

It is hard to believe that the RF of a visual cell does not move with the eyes, because the RF represents a part of the retina and so it *must* move with the eyes; however, in real-position cells, it does not move. To obtain this result, the part of the retina sensitive to the visual stimulation must continually change according to the direction of gaze, thus maintaining constant that part of the visual field explored by the RF. In other words, we have to admit that the real-position cells have an RF potentially as large as the whole visual field, with only part of the potential RF active at any given time, according to gaze direction, in order that visual information is always received from the same location in visual space.

It is worth noting that the 'remapping' of visual space described in area LIP of the monkey PPC (Duhamel *et al.* 1992) is a somewhat similar phenomenon. The RFs of visual cells in area LIP are retinotopically organized, but in some cases they shift to a different part of the visual field during fixation, just before a saccadic eye movement, and then return to the previous retinotopic location after the saccade. In other words, these visual cells have potentially large RFs including at least the two retinotopic positions occupied before and after the saccade. The potential RF of these cells probably also includes further different retinotopic positions around the original one, to account for different RF shifts according to saccade direction. The different parts of the potential RF of these cells become alternatively sensitive to the visual stimulation according to the direction of gaze and/or the impending saccade. Also in this case, as for real-position cells, the RF is not anchored to a fixed part of the retina. Rather, the region of retina that becomes active at a particular time is dictated by the oculomotor activity.

Data on bimodal neurons activated by visual and somatosensory stimulations support the view that the visual RF should no longer be seen as an expression of a fixed part of the retina. This type of neuron is sensitive to the visual stimulation of restricted regions of space around specific parts of the body. In the putamen and the premotor cortex, it has been demonstrated that the visual RF of bimodal neurons moves when the specific part of the body moves, remaining in register with it (Graziano and Gross 1993; Graziano *et al.* 1994, 1997). To obtain this result, the active region of the retina (the RF) cannot be fixed. It must be dictated by the somatosensory/skeletomotor activity, similarly to the active region of the retina of real-position cells, which is time by time dictated by the oculomotor activity. For some bimodal neurons, it has been demonstrated that the visual RF moves with the arm while the eyes are still and, conversely, does not move with the eyes when the upper limbs are still (Graziano *et al.* 1994, Graziano and Gross 1998). This means that in these neurons the active region of retina is time by time dictated by either oculomotor or skeletomotor activities. Such behavior has clear functional implications for the possible role that this type of cell can play in the visual guidance of actions.

From gaze-sensitive to real-position behavior

To change the retinotopic coordinates of visual RFs according to oculomotor or skeletomotor activities, the visual cells must receive signals relative to these motor activities as well as visual information from the retina. In agreement with this view, the oculomotor activity is largely represented in those PPC areas that include real-position cells and in area LIP (Andersen *et al.* 1990; Galletti *et al.* 1991, 1995; Bremmer *et al.* 1999), and the skeletomotor activity is largely represented in the ventral premotor cortex (Gentilucci *et al.* 1988; Graziano *et al.* 1994). It is also well known that in these cortical regions the sensori-motor interactions actually occur on single cells. In this respect, the gaze-dependent visual cells are typical examples of this interaction. What is still unknown is how the motor activities could dictate to the visual cells which part of the retina has to be activated.

Recently, a model has been proposed which suggests that strongly modulated gaze-dependent visual cells could automatically dictate to the real-position cells the retinal regions to be activated at a particular time, according to the direction of gaze (Galletti *et al.* 1995). A strongly modulated gaze-dependent visual cell is a cell whose RF is visually responsive only when the animal looks toward restricted regions of the visual field. When the animal looks elsewhere, the visual responsiveness of the RF suddenly decreases, and the RF itself is no longer responsive. These strongly modulated gaze-dependent visual cells resemble real-position cells in that they are activated only when the visual stimulation is delivered on a specific part of the visual field. However, unlike real-position cells, this specific part of the visual field is not always effective, regardless of gaze direction. Rather, its activation strictly depends on the direction of gaze.

The real-position behavior could be the result of the work of many strongly modulated gaze-dependent visual cells, as illustrated schematically in Fig. 4. Let us assume that we have five visual cells whose RFs are in different retinal locations (say, on the fovea and in the upper, lower, ipsilateral, and contralateral hemifields). Suppose also that the visual responsiveness of each cell is strongly modulated by gaze, in a different way for different cells, so that all of them are visually responsive *only* when the RF is in about the same spatial location in a head frame of reference (for instance, cell 1 when the animal looks down, cell 3 when it looks up, etc.). If this were the case, another cell receiving these five inputs would behave as a real-position cell, responding to visual stimulation delivered at the center of the screen regardless of eye position.

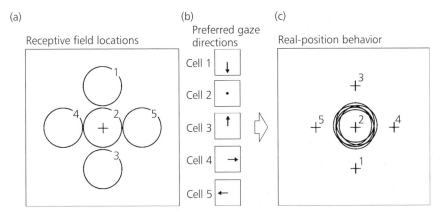

Figure 4 Schematic representation of the neural mechanism possibly involved in building up the real-position behavior. Squares and crosses as in Fig. 3. (a) Screen locations of the RFs of five hypothetical visual neurons (1–5) while the animal maintains fixation at the center of the screen. (b) Arrows indicate the preferred gaze directions of the five gaze-dependent visual cells shown in (a). The point at the center of the square for cell 2 indicates that the cell prefers the center of the screen, i.e. the RF is maximally responsive for the straight-ahead direction. (c) RF locations of the hypothetical neurons shown in (a) when the animal looks at the preferred screen positions for each cell (1–5). Note as in all cases, the RFs are in about the same spatial location, at the center of the screen.

Area V6A contains all the elements required to construct real-position cells according to the model described above, i.e. visual neurons with RFs in different retinal locations (Galletti *et al.* 1999) and strongly modulated gaze-dependent visual cells (Galletti *et al.* 1995). Moreover, area V6A also contains the real-position cells themselves (Galletti *et al.* 1993, 1996). The different cell categories are intermingled in restricted volumes of V6A cortex, as shown in Fig. 5. This cortical organization allows the interaction between cells of the network to occur through local circuits within V6A, conferring specific computational advantages to the nontopographic organization of this area (Galletti *et al.* 1999). According to this view, the apparent 'crude' retinotopic representation of V6A could actually be a 'refined' brain representation of visual space.

The cortical network we proposed for encoding spatial coordinates in V6A (Galletti *et al.* 1995) is closely related to the models proposed by other authors for PPC (Zipser and Andersen 1988; Pouget and Sejnowski 1997). All these models are based on the interaction between visual information and gaze direction. All of them predict the existence of output layer cells explicitly encoding the visual space but, as this type of cell was not found in the parietal area 7a, it was hypothesized that spatial coordinates in this area were only *implicitly* coded by the population of gaze-dependent visual cells. In contrast, parietal areas V6A and VIP do contain cells *explicitly* coding the visual space (Galletti *et al.* 1993, 1996; Duhamel *et al.* 1997) together with cells whose visual responsiveness is modulated by the direction of gaze (Galletti *et al.* 1995; Bremmer

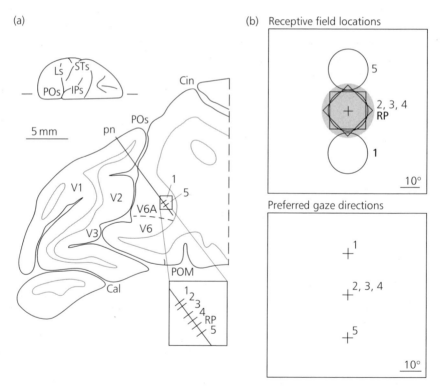

Figure 5 Functional properties of a cluster of V6A neurons containing a real-position cell. (a) Reconstruction of microelectrode penetration through area V6A. Numbers 1–5 along the electrode track indicate the locations of a cluster of neurons grouped around a real-position cell (RP). (b) RF locations and preferred gaze directions of the cluster of cells indicated in (a). The gray area is the screen location of the visually responsive region of the real-position cell. Other details are as in Fig. 4.

et al. 1999). Although, in principle, strongly modulated gaze-dependent cells are not critical for producing an explicit codification of the visual space (Pouget and Sejnowski 1997), it is known that V6A does contain many of these strongly modulated cells, sometimes with a clear Gaussian profile of excitation, together with neurons more linearly modulated by eye position (Galletti *et al.* 1995). We suggest that in V6A (and possibly in VIP) the gaze-dependent cells with a linear tuning profile of visual responsiveness represent the first elements where visual and oculomotor inputs interact; the gaze-dependent cells with a Gaussian profile could represent the second step in this functional chain, and the real-position cells the third step, as well as the output layer of the network.

Conclusions

Two mechanisms possibly encoding the visual space have been proposed in the PPC. One is distributed, retinotopically organized, and based on the activity of gaze-dependent visual cells, and the other is direct, nonretinotopically organized, and based on the activity of the so-called real-position cells.

We suggest that the interaction between visual and oculomotor signals, as they occur in gaze-dependent visual cells, represents the first step in the analysis of visual space occurring in almost all areas of the dorsal visual stream. The output of gaze-dependent visual cells could be further elaborated by other neurons (e.g. real-position cells) to compute the visuospatial transformations required to encode visual space explicitly. We cannot exclude the possibility that the output of gaze-dependent visual neurons is also used to compute more sophisticated visuospatial transformations, such as those required in the cognitional reconstruction of visual space.

So far, real-position cells have been found in the dorsal PPC (areas V6A and VIP) and in the ventral premotor cortex, i.e. in regions of the dorsal visual stream that are probably implicated in the visual guidance of actions. Area V6A is organized in cortical modules, well equipped for building up real-position cells from gaze-dependent visual cells. Each module could encode a different spatial location, and all of them together could represent a spatial map of the visual world in at least a head frame of reference.

Acknowledgements

This work was supported by Grants from Ministero dell'Università e della Ricerca Scientifica e Tecnologica, Italy.

References

Andersen, R. A. and Mountcastle, V. B. (1983). The influence of the angle of gaze upon the excitability of the light-sensitive neurons of the posterior parietal cortex. *Journal of Neuroscience*, **3**, 532–48.

Andersen, R. A., Essick, G. K., and Siegel, R. M. (1985). Encoding of spatial location by posterior parietal neurons. *Science*, **230**, 456–8.

Andersen, R. A., Bracewell, R. M., Barash, S., Gnadt, J. W., and Fogassi, L. (1990). Eye position effects on visual, memory, and saccade-related activity in areas LIP and 7a of macaque. *Journal of Neuroscience*, **10**, 1176–96.

Biguer, B., Jeannerod, M., and Prablanc, C. (1982). The coordination of the eye, head, and arm movements during reaching at a single visual target. *Experimental Brain Research*, **46**, 301–4.

Bisiach, E. and Luzzatti, C. (1978). Unilateral neglect of representational space. *Cortex*, **14**, 129–33.

Bisiach, E. and Vallar, G. (2000). Unilateral neglect in humans. In *Handbook of Neuropsychology* (2nd edn), Vol. 1 (ed. F. Boller, J. Grafman, and G. Rizzolatti), pp. 459–502. Elsevier, Amsterdam.

Boussaoud, D., Barth, T. M., and Wise, S. P. (1993). Effects of gaze on apparent visual responses of frontal cortex neurons. *Experimental Brain Research*, **93**, 423–34.

Bremmer, F., Ilg, U. J., Thiele, A., Distler, C., and Hoffmann, K. P. (1997). Eye position effects in monkey cortex. I. Visual and pursuit-related activity in extrastriate areas MT and MST. *Journal of Neurophysiology*, **77**, 944–61.

Bremmer, F., Graf, W., Ben Hamed, S., and Duhamel, J.-R. (1999). Eye position encoding in the macaque ventral intraparietal area (VIP). *Neuroreport*, **10**, 873–8.

De Renzi, E. (1982). *Disorders of space exploration and cognition*. Wiley, New York.

Duhamel, J.-R., Colby, C. L., and Goldberg, M. E. (1992). The updating of the representation of visual space in parietal cortex by intended eye movements. *Science*, **255**, 90–2.

Duhamel, J.-R., Bremmer, F., Ben Hamed, S., and Graf, W. (1997). Spatial invariance of visual receptive fields in parietal cortex neurons. *Nature*, **389**, 845–8.

Fogassi, L., Gallese, V., Di Pellegrino, G., *et al.* (1992). Space coding by premotor cortex. *Experimental Brain Research*, **89**, 686–90.

Fogassi, L., Gallese, V., Fadiga, L., Luppino, G., Matelli, M., and Rizzolatti, G. (1996). Coding of peripersonal space in inferior premotor cortex (area F4). *Journal of Neurophysiology*, **76**, 141–57.

Galletti, C. and Battaglini, P. P. (1989). Gaze-dependent visual neurons in area V3A of monkey prestriate cortex. *Journal of Neuroscience*, **9**, 1112–25.

Galletti, C., Battaglini, P. P., and Fattori, P. (1991). Functional properties of neurons in the anterior bank of the parieto-occipital sulcus of the macaque monkey. *European Journal of Neuroscience*, **3**, 452–61.

Galletti, C., Battaglini, P. P., and Fattori, P. (1993). Parietal neurons encoding spatial locations in craniotopic coordinates. *Experimental Brain Research*, **96**, 221–9.

Galletti, C., Battaglini, P. P., and Fattori, P. (1995). Eye position influence on the parieto-occipital area PO (V6) of the macaque monkey. *European Journal of Neuroscience*, **7**, 2486–501.

Galletti, C., Fattori, P., Battaglini, P. P., Shipp, S., and Zeki, S. (1996). Functional demarcation of a border between areas V6 and V6A in the superior parietal gyrus of the macaque monkey. *European Journal of Neuroscience*, **8**, 30–52.

Galletti, C., Fattori, P., Kutz, D. F., and Gamberini, M. (1999). Brain location and visual topography of cortical area V6A in the macaque monkey. *European Journal of Neuroscience*, **11**, 575–82.

Gentilucci, M., Scandolara, C., Pigarev, I., and Rizzolatti, G. (1983). Visual responses in the postarcuate cortex (area 6) of the monkey that are independent of eye position. *Experimental Brain Research*, **50**, 464–8.

Gentilucci, M., Fogassi, L., Luppino, G., Matelli, M., Camarda, R., and Rizzolatti, G. (1988). Functional organization of inferior area 6 in the macaque monkey. I. Somatotopy and the control of proximal movements. *Experimental Brain Research*, **71**, 475–90.

Graziano, M. S. and Gross, C. G. (1993). A bimodal map of space—somatosensory receptive fields in the macaque putamen with corresponding visual receptive fields. *Experimental Brain Research*, **97**, 96–109.

Graziano, M. S. and Gross, C. G. (1998). Visual responses with and without fixation, neurons in premotor cortex encode spatial locations independently of eye position. *Experimental Brain Research*, **118**, 373–80.

Graziano, M. S. A., Yap, G. S., and Gross, C. G. (1994). Coding of visual space by premotor neurons. *Science*, **266**, 1054–7.

Graziano, M.S,. Hu, X. T., and Gross, C. G. (1997). Visuospatial properties of ventral premotor cortex. *Journal of Neurophysiology*, **77**, 2268–92.

Motter, B. C. and Poggio, G. F. (1990). Dynamic stabilization of receptive fields of cortical neurons (VI) during fixation of gaze in the macaque. *Experimental Brain Research*, **83**, 37–43.

Mountcastle, V. B. (1981). Functional properties of the light-sensitive neurons of the posterior parietal cortex and their regulation by state controls: influence on excitability of interested fixation and the angle of gaze. In *Brain mechanisms of perceptual awareness and purposeful behavior* (ed. O. Pompeiano and C. A. Marsan), pp. 67–100. IBRO Series, Vol. 8. Raven Press, New York.

Newcombe, F. and Ratcliff, G. (1989). Disorders of visuospatial analysis. In *Handbook of neuropsychology*, Vol. 2 (ed. F. Boller and J. Grafman), pp. 333–56. Elsevier, Amsterdam.

Nichelli, P. (1999). Visuo-spatial and imagery disorders. In *Handbook of clinical and experimental neuropsychology* (ed. G. Denes and L. Pizzamiglio), pp. 453–77. Psychology Press, Hove.

Perenin, M. T. and Vighetto, A. (1988). Optic ataxia, a specific disruption in visuomotor mechanisms. I. Different aspects of the deficit in reaching for objects. *Brain*, **111**, 643–74.

Peck, C. K., Schlag-Rey, M., and Schlag, J. (1980). Visuo-oculomotor properties of cells in the superior colliculus of the alert cat. *Journal of Comparative Neurology*, **194**, 97–116.

Pigarev, I. N. and Rodionova, E. I. (1988). Neurons with visual receptive fields independent of the position of the eyes in cat parietal cortex. *Sensory Systems (Moscow)* **2**, 245–54.

Pouget, A. and Sejnowski, T. J. (1997). Spatial transformations in the parietal cortex using basis functions. *Journal of Cognitive Neuroscience*, **9**, 222–37.

Schlag, J., Schlag-Rey, M., Peck, C. K., and Joseph, J. P. (1980). Visual responses of thalamic neurons depending on the direction of gaze and the position of the target in space. *Experimental Brain Research*, **40**, 170–84.

Trotter, Y. and Celebrini, S. (1999). Gaze direction controls response gain in primary visual-cortex neurons. *Nature*, **398**, 239–42.

Ungerleider, L. G. and Mishkin, M. (1982). Two cortical visual systems. In *Analysis of visual behavior* (ed. D. J. Ingle, M. A. Goodale, and R. J. W. Mansfield), pp. 549–86. MIT Press, Cambridge, MA.

Vallar, G. (2001). Extrapersonal visual unilateral spatial neglect and its neuroanatomy. *NeuroImage*, **14**, S52–8.

Vallar, G. and Perani, D. (1986). The anatomy of unilateral neglect after right-hemisphere stroke lesions. A clinical/CT-scan correlation study in man. *Neuropsychologia*, **24**, 609–22.

Zipser, D. and Andersen, R. A. (1988). A back-propagation programmed network that simulates response properties of a subset of posterior parietal neurons. *Nature*, **331**, 679–84.

2.4 Cortical substrates of visuospatial awareness outside the classical dorsal stream of visual processing

Peter Thier, Thomas Haarmeier, Subhojit Chakraborty, Axel Lindner, and Alexander Tikhonov

A dominant theme guiding our thinking about the cortical processing of visual information in the primate cortex has been the concept of two distinct visual streams, one for object vision and the other one for spatial vision (Ungerleider and Mishkin 1982). This concept holds that starting from different compartments in area V1, the primary visual cortex, two largely separate visual pathways emerge. The first, subserving object vision, involves the more ventrally located areas of the occipital lobe and finally leads into the inferior temporal cortex. The second, for spatial vision, is based on the more dorsally located parts of the occipital lobe and feeds a number of areas in the parietal operculum or the intraparietal sulcus, which subserve as major substrates of visually guided behavior. While these two pathways adjoin each other in their more caudal parts, they diverge in their more rostral segments, embracing the cortex of the lateral sulcus and the neighboring superior temporal cortex, a region which is usually perceived as nonvisual and nonspatial cortex, contributing, among others, to the analysis of somatosensory and auditory stimuli. While there is no reason to dispute the major role that this part of cortex plays in the analysis of nonvisual and nonspatial material, a number of observations strongly suggest an additional role in spatial orientation. For example, a recent study illustrated that the superior temporal cortex is the neural substrate of spatial neglect in humans (Karnath *et al.* 2001). Spatial neglect is a lateralized disorder with a characteristic failure to react or respond to stimuli located on this side. The stimuli neglected may originate from different modalities. Thus it may not be surprising that the lateral sulcus and the neighboring superior temporal cortex play a profound role in space perception and spatial orientation. What is more surprising, however, is the fact that this contribution to spatial orientation seems to involve a significant contribution from vision, building on signals handed over from the classical dorsal stream of visual processing. Such a view was first suggested by Grüsser and coworkers (Grüsser *et al.* 1990*a*,*b*; Guldin and Grüsser 1998), who had been able to delineate a *vestibular* representation in a region in the posterior insula in the depths of the lateral sulcus. They termed this area the parieto-insular vestibular cortex (PIVC), congruent with the retroinsular area Ri-m as delineated by cytoarchitectonical criteria. While its name might suggest a monomodal representation of the sixth sense in the lateral sulcus, the detailed analysis of PIVC neurons carried out by Grüsser and coworkers had shown early on that it integrated vestibular and somatosensory as well as visual information in order to represent a subject's orientation with respect to an external frame of reference. The existence of a human equivalent of monkey area PIVC has, among others, been suggested by the demonstration of vestibular disturbances in a patient suffering from an acute lesion of her insular cortex (Brandt *et al.* 1994), as well as by PET scanning showing activation by caloric vestibular stimuli (Bottini *et al.* 1994, 2001). Tract tracing work carried out by Guldin (reviewed by Guldin and Grüsser (1998)) could demonstrate that the major source of afferents impinging on PIVC is the visual posterior sylvian area (VPS), located caudally of PIVC close to the posterior end of the lateral suclus, not too far away from the visual areas of the superior temporal sulcus (STS) (see Fig. 1(a) for orientation). Although vestibular signals seem to occur in VPS, the dominating modality is vision with the overwhelming majority of neurons being responsive to large field 'optokinetic' stimuli. Not unsurprisingly in view of its location in between PIVC and STS, the major input to VPS seems to originate from the medial superior temporal area (MST). Our own work suggests that VPS may be a major player in a network of visual areas, underlying visual space perception and our *subjective* sense of visuospatial stability. This conclusion is based on experiments, which we have carried out in order to find an answer to the question of how our brain is able to construct a stable representation of the visual world, despite the confounding effects that movement of the subject has on the visual stimuli impinging on our retinas.

Retinal image motion may result from motion of objects in the external world or, alternatively, from movement of our eyes relative to the external world. Of course, as long as we are moving around most of the time, both sources of image slip will be available, providing the formidable challenge to the visual system of distinguishing the component of retinal image motion resulting from motion in the external world from the one arising from ego motion. The reason is that only the former, and not the latter, should be perceived as visual motion. If this were not the case, our concept of a reassuringly stable world, through which we move and in which we act, would inevitably be lost. Smooth-pursuit eye movements may serve as a case in point. They allow us to stabilize the image of a selected object on or close to the fovea in order to make use of the advantages of foveal vision (Haarmeier and Thier 1999). The inevitable consequence is that the images of all other objects (the 'visual background') will, if stationary in the world, move at a speed corresponding to the speed of the pursuit eye movement carried out without, however, being perceived as moving.

Building on early suggestions by von Helmholtz (1910), the **inferential theory of motion perception** holds that our ability to distinguish between external stimuli and self-induced sensory stimuli is achieved by subtracting an internal reference signal, termed the *Willensanstrengung* (the effort of will) by von Helmholtz and the *Efferenzkopie* (the efference copy) by von Holst and Mittelstaedt (1950), from the sensory signal (Fig. 1(b)). Specifically, perceptual stability in the case of smooth-pursuit eye movements is accomplished by subtracting a copy of the eye movement motor command from the retinal motion signal (Wertheim 1994). If the two cancel each other, visual structures, which do not move, will be perceived as nonmoving even though their images move on the retina as a consequence of the eye movement. Our ability to compensate for the visual consequences of eye movements is a typical example of an invariance operation, releasing perception from the influence of confounding variables. Other examples of perceptual invariance, such as color constancy (i.e. our ability to perceive a constant object color despite changes in the wavelength composition of the light), have been shown to have a cerebrocortical basis. Therefore it was reasonable to consider the possibility that eye movement invariance might also have a cerebrocortical basis.

Our early work on the visual cortex of nonhuman primates (Erickson and Thier 1991; Ilg and Thier 1996) indicated that eye movement invariance must be an achievement of later stages of the visual hierarchy of cerebrocortical areas involved in the processing of visual motion (Fig. 1(b)). This was suggested by the fact that neurons in area 17, the primary visual cortex, and in the middle temporal area (MT), the prototypical motion processing area in the STS of the monkey

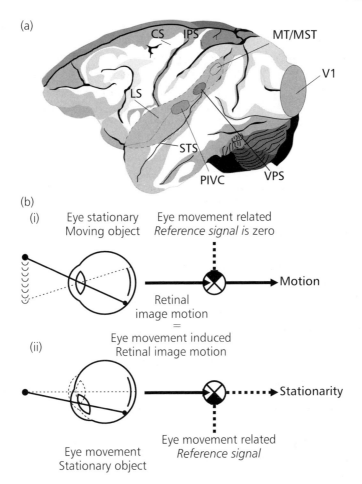

(a)

(b)

(i) Eye stationary   Eye movement related
Moving object   *Reference signal is zero*

Retinal
image motion
=
Eye movement induced
Retinal image motion

(ii)

Eye movement related
Reference signal

Eye movement
Stationary object

Figure 1 (a) Schematic view of the left hemisphere of the rhesus monkey with the sylvian (lateral) sulcus and parts of the superior temporal sulcus unfolded (gray, surrounded by dashed lines) to show the visual areas explored in the experiments of Erickson and Thier (1991), Ilg and Thier (1996), and Chakraborty and Thier (2000) as well as the parieto-insular vestibular cortex, a vestibular representation in the lateral sulcus discovered by Grüsser and coworkers (Guldin and Grüsser 1998). LS, lateral sulcus; CS, central sulcus; STS, superior temporal sulcus; IPS, intraparietal sulcus; PIVC, parieto-insular vestibular cortex. (b) Diagram of the inferential mechanism underlying vision during eye movements, capturing the essentials of the reafference principle (von Holst and Mittelstaedt 1950). (i) The eyes are stationary and the object moves in the external world, resulting in externally induced retinal image motion. In this situation the eye-movement-related reference signal is zero and the output of the element subtracting the reference signal from the retinal signal corresponds to the retinal image motion input. The interpretation of this result is object motion in the world. (ii) The eyes move while the object is stationary. In this case retinal image motion is exclusively due to the eye movement. Reafference in the terminology of von Holst and Mittelstaedt is cancelled by the nonzero reference signal. The interpretation of the zero output of the comparator is the stationarity of the object. (Part (a) adapted from Thier *et al.*, *NeuroImage*, **14**, S33–S39, (2001) by permission of Academic Press.)

brain, typically discharged invariably in response to smooth slow retinal image slip, irrespective of its source being object movement in the world or, alternatively, a smooth eye movement across a stationary object. On the other hand, a significant number of neurons in the posterior parietal area MST on the anterior bank of the STS seemed to differentiate between the two forms of retinal image stimulation, often responding selectively or at least much more strongly

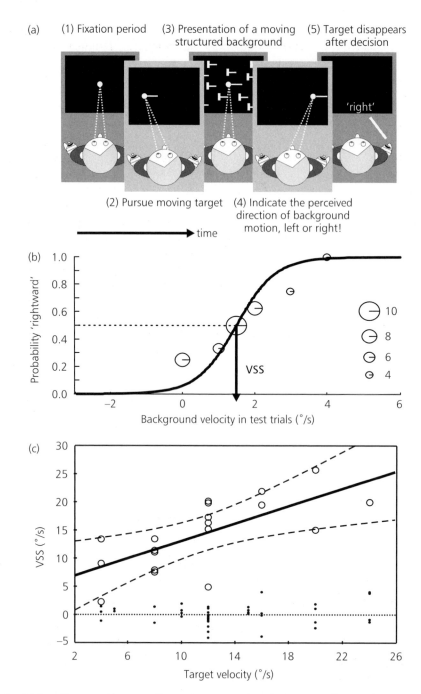

Figure 2 (a) Paradigm used to quantify motion perception during smooth-pursuit eye movements. The subject tracks a small dot which is initially stationary for a few hundred milliseconds, and then jumps to the left and from there moves to the right at a constant speed (of the order of 10°/s in most experiments). While the eyes are close to straight ahead, a large-field random-dot background, whose elements move coherently to the left or to the right, comes on for several hundred milliseconds. At the end of the pursuit trial, subjects have to indicate whether they perceived the background as moving to the left or to the right (two alternative forced choices). Eye movements are monitored with infrared optics in order to guarantee high-precision smooth-pursuit eye movement.

to externally induced image slip than to self-induced image slip. Very similar conclusions were suggested by a later study of visually evoked potentials in humans (Haarmeier and Thier 1998), whose presentation requires a preceding discussion of the psychophysical measurement of motion perception during eye movements and several key findings on human motion perception based on these techniques.

The basic task in all these later experiments was to carry out smooth-pursuit eye movements in one horizontal direction, usually to the right, across a large visual background (Fig. 2(a)). This background also moved along the horizontal, at a velocity which varied in magnitude and direction. At the end of each trial, subjects were required to indicate whether they had seen background movement to the right or to the left. Of course, this decision is easy if the background moves at high speed to the left or to the right. On the other hand, as shown in Fig. 2(b), if the speed is reduced, subjects' decisions become increasingly inconsistent as the velocity approaches the velocity of subjective stationarity (VSS). At the VSS, which is titrated by varying background velocity according to a staircase procedure, subjects guess, as indicated by 50 per cent left and 50 per cent right choices. They guess because the background has become *subjectively* stationary. Healthy subjects have a VSS which does not deviate much from physical stationarity (Fig. 2(c), dots). In other words, they perceive the background as being stationary when it is physically stationary despite the fact that the eye movement shifts the background image across the retina. According to the inferential theory of perception, at this VSS the reference signal encoding the eye movement is equal to the afferent signal, reflecting the velocity of the retinal image motion (Mack and Herman 1973; Wertheim 1994). Correspondingly, a VSS of zero reflects an ideal reference signal, with a magnitude which allows it to compensate fully for the effects of the eye movement.

Surprisingly, our psychophysical studies also showed that a very simple variation of the basic psychophysical paradigm allowed us to evoke predictable changes of the percept of eye-movement-induced visual motion (Haarmeier and Thier 1996, 1998; Haarmeier *et al.* 2001).

Figure 2 *Contd* (b) The percentage of 'rightward' decision of subjects is plotted as a function of the background velocity. Background stimuli moving at comparably high velocities (4°/s) to the right are always perceived as moving to the right. Physically stationary backgrounds (0°/s) were more often perceived as moving leftward than rightward. The turning point of the probit function fitted gives the velocity of subjective stationarity (VSS), i.e. the velocity leading to as many right as left decisions of the subject. The size of the different circles represents the number of presentations of a given background velocity. (c) Perception of smooth-pursuit induced visual motion in healthy controls (18 subjects, 50 individual measurements represented by dots, partially lying on top of each other) and patient RW (open circles). The plot shows the VSS as function of pursuit target velocity varied from 4 to 24°/s. In this and all other experiments discussed, pursuit target and background were presented on a 19-inch computer monitor at a viewing distance of 57 cm in a dark experimental room. The pursuit target was a red dot (diameter 10 min of arc) and the background subtended 27° × 27°of visual angle and consisted of 350 white dots (diameter 15 min of arc, local contrast 0.01). The background was presented for 300 ms at a time when the eyes were close to straight ahead. Target motion was always to the right. Positive values of VSS indicate background movement in the same direction as the eyes. The higher the VSS, the less the resulting retinal image slip velocity allowing the percept of stationarity and thus the less the ability to cope with self-induced visual motion. In the control subjects the VSS is always close to 0°/s. Hence perceived background motion is tightly related to visual motion in extrapersonal space, i.e. stationarity is preserved despite increasing retinal image shifts with growing target velocities. In RW, however, perceived motion reflects image movement on the retina. The linear regression (with 99 per cent confidence bands) suggests that RW is deprived of a sense of stationarity unless the background image is stabilized to some degree on the retina. Accordingly, he will experience an illusory background motion (*Filehne* illusion) of the order of the prevailing eye velocity. (Adapted from Haarmeier *et al.*, Nature, **389**, 489–52 (1997) by permission of Macmillan Magazines Ltd.)

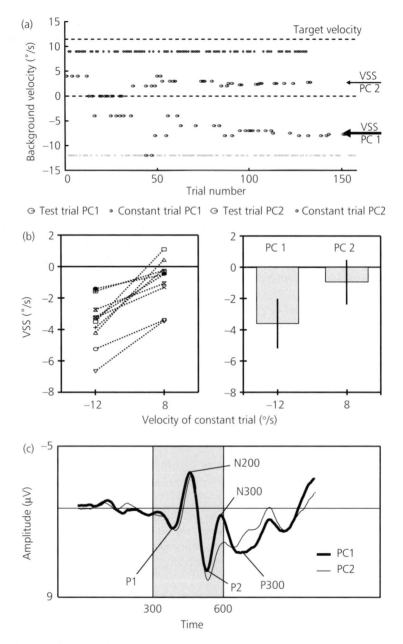

Figure 3 (a) Dependence of the VSS on the choice of the 'constant background' trial. Temporal sequences of background velocities are shown for a healthy subject, carrying out smooth-pursuit eye movements to the right at 12°/s. Each dot marks one trial as illustrated in Fig. 2(a). The temporal sequence of two experimental sessions is shown: PC1, full symbols characterizing the constant trial backgrounds and the test trial backgrounds; PC2, open symbols. In the first run, the 'constant trial' background moved at –12°/s (PC1); in the second run, it moved at 9°/s (PC2). (b) VSS as a function of the velocity of the 'constant trial' background for ten healthy subjects, represented by individual symbols (left panel) and their means/standard deviations (right panel). Negative velocities indicate the direction opposite to the eye movement. Smooth pursuit was to the right at 12°/s. The VSS depends on the choice of the 'constant trial' background. A velocity of –12°/s mimics a viewing condition in which the reference signal is too small, causing a compensatory increase of the reference signal and therefore a shift of the VSS towards stronger movement to the left

According to the inferential theory, an illusory movement of the physically stationary world in a direction opposite to the direction of smooth-pursuit eye movement would be perceived if the reference signal were too small. Conversely, false perception of movement of the world in the direction of the eye movement would result from a reference signal which was too large. If the inferential mechanism providing and using the reference signal were able to sense its insufficiencies, it would use such feedback information to increase the size of the reference signal gradually if it were too small and, conversely, to decrease it if it were inappropriately large. This is exactly what we found when we mimicked such imperfections by asking subjects to execute smooth pursuit across backgrounds moving at a high constant velocity ('constant background' trials). In these 'constant trials' there was a marked discrepancy between the velocity of executed eye movement and the expected size of the rotational retinal flow, resulting in the repeated perception of background motion, i.e. a deviation from the percept of a stable world. The VSS for rightward pursuit elicited by a target moving at 12°/s was determined for two conditions differing in the direction of background motion during constant trials relative to the eye movements chosen such as to simulate an inappropriately high and small reference signal, respectively. In the first condition (rf_too_large), background movement during constant trials was in the same direction as eye movements (8°/s), thereby substantially reducing the rotational retinal flow during pursuit. A reference signal that would encode the physical velocity of the eye movement (12°/s) would overcompensate the reduced retinal flow (12°/s − 8°/s = 4°/s), i.e. it would be inappropriately high. In the second condition, (rf_too_small), background movement during constant trials was opposite to the eye movements (12°/s) simulating, conversely, an underestimated reference signal.

The sequence of these constant background trials was occasionally interrupted by 'test' trials consisting of backgrounds whose velocity was determined by the staircase procedure needed to pinpoint the VSS. As suggested by the differential development of the staircase procedures shown in Fig. 3(a), representing an individual subject in the rf_too_large and rf_too_small conditions respectively, this manipulation indeed induces changes in motion perception consistent with an ecologically useful adaptation of the reference signal. This conclusion was first supported by a comparison of the VSSs for a group of 10 subjects tested in the rf_too_large and rf_too_small conditions and has since been replicated many times. In summary, these psychophysical experiments show that the perception of eye-movement-induced visual motion can be modified predictably by mimicking insufficiencies of the reference signal, prompting functionally useful changes of the reference signal. Control experiments exclude the possibility that the changes of motion perception are a simple consequence of motion adaptation (Haarmeier *et al.* 2001). In addition, the psychophysical responses of nonhuman primates are very similar to those of humans in experiments mimicking insufficiencies of the reference signal (Chakraborty 2001), suggesting that the visual system of nonhuman and human primates share a common inferential mechanism.

Our ability to associate qualitatively different percepts of motion with one and the same amount of eye-movement-induced retinal image slip is obviously an ideal tool to reveal those parts of cerebral cortex reflecting the subjective percept of self-induced visual motion rather than the

Figure 3 *Contd* (PC1, perceptual condition 1). Conversely, a velocity of +8°/s mimics a reference signal which is too large, inducing the opposite changes (PC2, perceptual condition 2). (c) Grand average VEPs for the O1 recording site based on five out of ten subjects who showed the strongest difference between the perceptual conditions PC1 (bold line) and PC2 (thin line). The responses are plotted for a 1000-ms period starting 300 ms before onset of the stationary background. The vertical gray column marks the period of background presentation. ((Part (a) reproduced from Thier *et al.*, *NeuroImage*, **14**, S33–S39 (2001) by permission of Academic Press. Parts (b) and (c) adapted from Haarmeier and Thier, *Journal of Cognitive Neuroscience*, **10**, 464–71 (1998) by permission of MIT Press.)

sensory signal conveyed by the retina. The first study based on this approach, alluded to earlier, was a study of visually evoked potentials (VEPs), picked up from the scalp with 12 surface electrodes (Haarmeier and Thier 1998). VEPs were produced by pursuit-induced slip of stationary backgrounds (share 25 per cent), presented randomly interleaved with the test backgrounds (share 25 per cent) needed to measure the VSS and a much larger number of constant backgrounds (share 50 per cent) required to modify the percept. The constant backgrounds came in two varieties in two subsequent blocks, giving rise to the different VSS values presented in Fig. 3(b). It is important to understand that the VEPs collected in these two subsequent blocks were based on stationary backgrounds only and that neither the constant nor the test trials contributed to the VEP. Since the eye movements did not differ between blocks, the size of self-induced retinal stimulation was the same. Figure 3(c) shows the grand average VEP waveforms for the O1 lead for a group of five out of ten subjects whose percept varied the most. The VEP responses are shown for a period of time centered on the presentation of the stationary background. The two curves superimposed are the averages for the two perceptually different conditions. The two waveforms are identical, independent of the percept of motion, for more than 200 ms. The first component which differed significantly between conditions was a negativity peaking at about 300 ms, denoted N300. Since its amplitude modulation correlated significantly with the perceptual differences between conditions, we take N300 as an electrophysiological correlate of the percept of visual motion. N300 was followed by P300, also differing between conditions but probably arising too late to be a direct reflection of the percept of motion. The fact that N300 followed an earlier N200, known to arise from the human MT/V5 complex (Bach and Ulrich 1994; Kubová et al. 1995) suggests that the generators of N300 are located upstream of MT/V5. We have recently obtained independent support for this notion from single-unit recording experiments in monkeys (Chakraborty and Thier 2000) and MEG recording experiments in humans, based on the same approach underlying the VEP experiments discussed earlier.

The work performed with awake behaving monkeys indicates that the neuronal substrates underlying our percept of motion seem to be concentrated in VPS, a region close to the caudal end of the lateral fissure (Fig. 1(b)) which is reciprocally interconnected with the parieto-insular-vestibular cortex (Guldin and Grüsser 1998; Grüsser et al. 1990a,b), both subserving as elements in a specialized cortical network underlying primates' subjective sense of spatial stability which supplements the visuomotor contributions of the posterior parietal components of the classical dorsal stream. In addition, our recent MEG recording experiments in humans suggest that medial parieto-occipital cortex, an area that has not yet been tested for percept-related activity in the monkey brain, may also contribute to our percept of visual motion during eye movements. Primary visual cortex and probably also the next early stages of the cortical processing of visual motion, up to and including area MT/V5, are ignorant of the percept of motion during eye movements. This is suggested by the lack of any significant percept-related influence on the early parts of the VEP response and the fact that, as discussed before, neurons in monkey area V1 usually do not distinguish between self-induced and externally induced retinal image slip, although it is very likely that the percepts affiliated with these two forms of retinal image slip will also differ in the monkey. We emphasize that this view is by no means invalidated by the observation of a few neurons in the early parts of the cortical visual system which may show subtle differences in their activity evoked by self-induced compared with externally induced visual motion (Galletti et al. 1984; Chakraborty and Thier 2000).

Further support for the notion of a representation of visual motion awareness in humans, excluding area 17, is provided by the case of patient RW (Haarmeier et al. 1997), who suffers from bilateral lesions involving large parts of dorsal extrastriate and posterior parietal cortex, while sparing area 17 (Fig. 4). RW has normal eye movements and normal vision if the eyes do not move. However, he is completely unable to compensate for the visual consequences of his

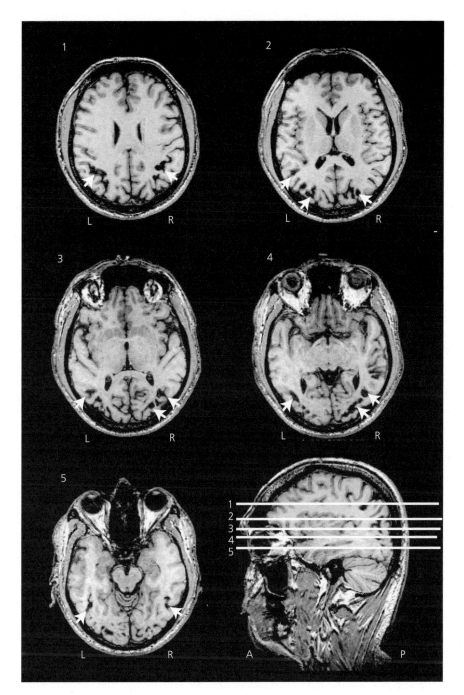

Figure 4 Magnetic resonance imaging of patient RW shows bilateral cyst-like widenings (arrows) of the sulci of the parietal and occipital lobes mainly affecting areas 18, 19, and possibly 37 on the lateral aspect of the hemispheres and areas 18 and 19 on the inferior aspect. In addition, cortex in and around the intraparietal suclus of the parietal lobes is involved. The lesions represent strictly cortical defects and local cortical atrophy with no signs of progression. Subcortical white matter and basal ganglia are intact. Although the lesional pattern does not allow a definitive pathogenetic assignment, post-hypoxic cortical laminar necrosis seems to be the most likely explanation. As a possible cause, RW had suffered from a severe pertussis infection in early childhood which had required artificial respiration. A, anterior; P, posterior; L, left; R, right. (Courtesy of the Department of Neuroradiology, University of Tübingen. Reprinted from Thier *et al.*, *NeuroImage*, **14**, S33–S39 (2001) by permission of Academic Press.)

smooth-pursuit eye movements. Instead of perceiving the image shifted across the retina by the eye movement as stationary, he perceives image movement. Lack of compensation for his smooth-pursuit eye movements is indicated by the fact that his velocity of subjective stationarity roughly equals his eye velocity (Fig. 2(c), open symbols). He perceives the world as stationary only if it is moved with the eyes, thereby stabilizing its image physically on the retina. Destabilizing the image of the world on the retina by moving the eyes jeopardizes his sense of visual stability and gives rise to complaints of severe dizziness. In accordance with this interpretation, dizziness immediately subsides if he closes his eyes or stops moving them.

In summary, our work clearly supports the notion that the perception of visual motion is based on an inferential mechanism involving a nonretinal reference signal capturing the visual consequences of the eye movement. Furthermore, it indicates that this inferential mechanism resides in rather 'late' parts of the cortical hierarchy of motion processing, sparing the early stages up to cortical area MT, and finally that disturbances of this mechanism may give rise to severe disturbances of vision and spatial orientation as exemplified by RW. In general, support for an inferential mechanism underlying motion perception residing in cortex strengthens the view that one important function of cerebral cortex is the extraction of invariances. The specific inferential mechanism we have discussed in this chapter applies to the problem of how to accomplish ego-motion-invariant motion perception. It is tempting to assume that functionally analogous mechanisms may pertain to other aspects of space perception and spatial awareness, for instance those confined to the position domain. That this may indeed be the case is suggested by the fact that lesions of cortex neighboring the immediate vicinity of the posterior lateral sulcus on the superior temporal gyrus seem to cause hemispatial neglect in humans and a syndrome reminiscent of hemispatial neglect in monkeys (Watson *et al.* 1994; Karnath *et al.* 2001).

References

Bach, M. and Ulrich, D. (1994). Motion adaptation governs the shape of motion-induced cortical potentials. *Vision Research*, **34**, 1541–7.

Bottini, G., Sterzi, R., Paulesu, E., *et al.* (1994). Identification of the central vestibular projections in man: a positron emission tomography activation study. *Experimental Brain Research*, **99**, 164–9.

Bottini, G., Karnath, H.-O., Vallar, G., *et al.* (2001). Cerebral representations for egocentric space: functional-anatomical evidence from caloric vestibular stimulation and neck vibration. *Brain*, **124**, 1182–96.

Brandt, T., Dieterich, M., and Danek, A. (1994). Vestibular cortex lesions affect the perception of verticality. *Annals of Neurology*, **35**, 403–12.

Chakraborty, S. (2001). Neuronal mechanisms underlying perceptual stability during smooth-pursuit eye movements. PhD Thesis, University of Tübingen.

Chakraborty, S. and Thier, P. (2000). A distributed neuronal substrate of perceptual stability during smooth-pursuit eye movements in the monkey. *Society of Neurscience Abstracts*, **26**, 674.

Erickson, R. G. and Thier, P. (1991). A neuronal correlate of spatial stability during periods of self-induced visual motion. *Experimental Brain Research*, **86**, 608–16.

Galletti, C., Squatrito, S., Battaglini, P. P., and Grazia-Maioli, M. (1984). 'Real-motion' cells in the primary visual cortex of macaque monkeys. *Brain Research*, **301**, 95–110.

Grüsser, O.-J., Pause, M., and Schreiter, U. (1990*a*). Localization and responses of neurons in the parieto-insular vestibular cortex of awake monkeys (*Macaca fascicularis*). *Journal of Physiology*, **430**, 537–57.

Grüsser, O.-J., Pause, M., and Schreiter, U. (1990*b*). Vestibular neurons in the parieto-insular cortex of monkeys (*Macaca fascicularis*): visual and neck receptor responses. *Journal of Physiology*, **430**, 559–83.

Guldin, W. O. and Grüsser, O.-J. (1998). Is there a vestibular cortex? *Trends in Neurosciences*, **21**, 254–9.

Haarmeier, T. and Thier, P. (1996). Modification of the *Filehne* illusion by conditioning visual stimuli. *Vision Research*, **36**, 741–50.

Haarmeier, T. and Thier, P. (1998). An electrophysiological correlate of visual motion awareness in man. *Journal of Cognitive Neuroscience*, **10**, 464–71.

Haarmeier, T. and Thier, P. (1999). Impaired analysis of moving objects due to deficient smooth pursuit eye movements. *Brain*, **122**, 1495–1505.

Haarmeier, T., Thier, P., Repnow, M., and Petersen, D. (1997). False perception of motion in a patient who cannot compensate for eye movements. *Nature*, **389**, 849–52.

Haarmeier, T., Bunjes, F., Lindner, A., Berret, E., and Thier, P. (2001). Optimzing visual motion perception during eye movements. *Neuron*, **32**, 527–35.

Ilg, U. and Thier, P. (1996). Inability of visual area V1 to discriminate between self-induced and externally-induced retinal image slip. *European Journal of Neuroscience*, **8**, 1156–66.

Karnath, H.-O., Ferber, S., and Himmelbach, M. (2001). Spatial awareness is a function of the temporal not the posterior parietal lobe. *Nature*, **411**, 950–3.

Kubová, Z., Kuba, M., Spekreijse, H. and Blakemore, C. (1995). Contrast dependence of motion-onset and pattern-reversal evoked potentials. *Vision Research*, **35**, 197–205.

Mack, A. and Herman, E. (1973). Position constancy during pursuit eye movements: an investigation of the *Filehne* illusion. *Quarterly Journal of Experimental Psychology*, **25**, 71–84.

Ungerleider, L. G. and Mishkin, M. (1982). Two cortical visual systems. In *Analysis of visual behavior* (ed. D. G. Ingle, M. A. Goodale, and R. J. Q. Mansfield), pp. 549–86. MIT Press, Cambridge, MA.

von Helmholtz, H. (1910). *Handbuch der physiologischen Optik*, Vol. 3. Leipzig, Voss.

von Holst, E. and Mittelstaedt, H. (1950). Das Reafferenzprinzip. *Naturwissenschaften*, **37**, 464–76.

Watson, R. T., Valenstein, E., Day, A., and Heilman, K. M. (1994). Posterior neocortical systems subserving swareness and neglect: neglect associated with superior temporal sulcus but not area 7 lesions. *Archives of Neurology*, **51**, 1014–21.

Wertheim, A. H. (1994). Motion perception during self-motion: the direct versus inferential controversy revisited. *Behavioural Brain Science*, **17**, 293–355.

Section 3 Frameworks of neglect

3.1 What is 'left' when all is said and done? Spatial coding and hemispatial neglect

Marlene Behrmann and Joy J. Geng

Moving one's eyes to view a fly sitting on one's forearm requires that one knows the spatial position of the fly. However, the process of spatial representation is fraught with problems. The tactile stimulation provided by the fly is initially registered in somatosensory cortex but the eye movement is executed to a position defined by the direction and distance from the current retinal position. Of course the sensory inputs, either visual or somatosensory, are subject to the inhomogeneities of their receptor surfaces with greater representation for the fovea in vision and for the fingers, lips, and tongue in touch, making correspondences between the modalities difficult. To complicate matters further, spatial location cannot be defined absolutely and therefore has to be described relatively, with respect to a reference frame with an origin and axes. How spatial position, defined in one modality and one set of coordinates, is represented and then translated to another set of coordinates has been the subject of numerous investigations, but still remains poorly understood.

One way of addressing these issues is to study the behavior of individuals who suffer from hemispatial neglect, a disorder in which the patients fail to orient towards or report information that appears on the contralateral side of space (McGlinchey-Berroth 1997; Driver and Mattingley 1998; Vallar 1998; Bisiach and Vallar 2000; Bartolomeo and Chokron 2001; Driver and Vuilleumier 2001). Neglect occurs most frequently following lesions to the inferior parietal lobule especially on the right (Bisiach and Vallar 1988; Stone *et al.* 1993; Vallar 1993, 1998; Milner 1997), and so we refer to neglect as 'left-sided' throughout this chapter. Patients with neglect may fail to notice objects on the left of a scene, may ignore words on the left of a page or food on the left of a plate, and typically omit to copy features on the left of a figure while preserving the corresponding features on the right. They may also show neglect of contralesional information in other sensory modalities, such as audition, somatosensation, and olfaction, and the deficit may even impair their ability to plan contralesional saccades or manual movements (Behrmann and Meegan 1998; Behrmann *et al.* 2001). Importantly, the failure to process contralateral information is not attributable to a primary sensory or motor problem. Rather, neglect is thought to occur because neurons in one hemisphere have predominant, although not exclusive, representation of the contralateral side; therefore, removing neurons impairs spatial representations for contralateral positions to a greater extent than those for ipsilateral positions (Pouget and Driver 2000; Rizzolatti *et al.* 2000; Cate and Behrmann 2002).

The specific question to be addressed is: When patients ignore information on the contralateral left, what is it left of? Furthermore, is the same form of spatial coding undertaken in different sensory modalities? By examining what coordinates are used to determine the midline such that information to the left of it is neglected, we may obtain an understanding of how spatial position is coded in parietal cortex and how cross-modal translation may occur. A number of potential reference frames can be used to define positions in space. These can be divided into two broad classes: objects and locations can be defined **egocentrically** (i.e. relative to the vantage point of the viewer) or **allocentrically** (i.e. from an extrinsic vantage point that is independent of the viewer's position). We start by reviewing the relevant neuropsychological findings that provide evidence for different reference frames, in both vision and other modalities, and then briefly review associated evidence from single-unit recording studies and functional imaging.

Neuropsychological evidence

Spatial reference frames

Egocentric reference frames

Many studies have examined spatial representations defined by an origin and axes aligned with the midline of (a) the eyes or vertical meridian of the visual field, (b) the head, (c) the trunk, and (d) the longitudinal axis of the limb that is involved in executing an action, such as the arm. To determine the role of different reference frames in coding spatial position, the experiments typically probe patients' ability to respond to a target that lies on the left or right of one midline which is rotated out of alignment from another. For example, to examine the individual contribution of a reference frame centered on the eyes, we recorded the latency and accuracy of saccades in neglect patients to targets presented individually at 5°, 10°, or 15° to the left or right of the midline of the eye or retinal axis (Behrmann *et al.* 2002*a,b*). In the baseline condition, the midline of the eyes was aligned with the midline of the head and trunk as well as the environment (i.e. subjects looked straight ahead) (Fig. 1(a)). In other conditions, the eyes were deviated to the right or left while the head, trunk and midline remained straight ahead (Figs 1(b) and 1(c)). In the baseline, the detection of the targets fell along a gradient with best performance on the right and poorest on the left (of all reference frames). When the midline of the eyes was rotated out of alignment with the other midlines, latency (and also accuracy to some extent) was affected by position defined relative to the eye: detection was good for targets to the right of the retinal axis and poor for targets to its left. Interestingly, there was further modulation of detection with the position of the eye in the orbit; when the eyes were deviated 15° to the right and the targets to the left of the fixation were sampled, neglect was significantly ameliorated compared with the same situation when the eyes were straight ahead. When the eyes were deviated to the left, there was no change in performance, probably because these targets (right of fixation) are already acquired well and there is no room for additional improvement. Support for retinocentric coding is also provided by many other studies (Kooistra and Heilman 1989; Nadeau and Heilman 1991; Duhamel *et al.* 1992; Vuilleumier *et al.* 1999) and consistent evidence for an influence of line-of-sight or orbital position has also been obtained in both humans (Bisiach *et al.* 1985) and animals (Andersen *et al.* 1985).

A spatial code defined with respect to the midline of the head is still somewhat controversial. Although Karnath *et al.* (1991) found no modulation of neglect with changes in head orientation in neglect patients, the combined influence of target defined retinally and modulated by orbital position reported above (Behrmann *et al.* 2002*b*) codes position with respect to the head, suggesting some contribution by the midline of the head. There is also support for a head-based reference frame in nonhuman primates (Brotchie *et al.* 1995). Evidence for coding with respect to the trunk midline is more robust. Karnath and colleagues, for example, have argued that the midline of the trunk (body-centered reference frame) plays a fundamental (perhaps exclusive) role, serving as the anchor or midline for dividing space into left and right (Karnath *et al.* 1991, 1993, 1996). In their study, there was significant amelioration of neglect when the patient's trunk was rotated

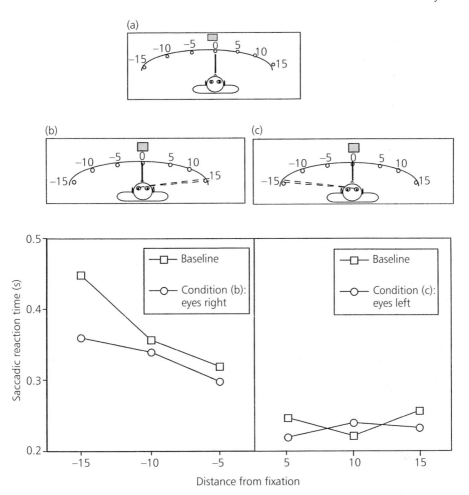

Figure 1 Schematic depiction of experiment on eye movements and reference frames. The subject is seated in an arc of LEDs with a speaker used to emit auditory signals to help elicit and maintain the subject's fixation. (a) Baseline condition with midline of eyes, head, and trunk aligned with the environmental midline. (b) Eyes right (ER) and (c) Eyes left (EL) with the midline of the eyes rotated 15° right or left but the midline of the head and trunk aligned with the environmental midline. The broken line indicates the position of the eyes and the solid line the position of the head and trunk. (Adapted from Behrmann et al. 2002b).

to the left compared with the baseline condition, although the neglect was not exacerbated by trunk rotations to the right, a result which they acknowledge is puzzling (see also Karnath (1997) for further discussion and consideration of vestibular and optokinetic variables, and Farnè et al. (1998) for a more general evaluation of these findings). Support for the role of the midline of the trunk is also obtained from studies by Chokron and Imbert (1993) and Beschin et al. (1997).

Rather less research has been done to evaluate the role of the position of the limb on neglect performance. In one tactile exploration study, Bisiach et al. (1985) manipulated the placement of the right limb such that the workspace of the limb either fell along the midline of the trunk or extended into the right side of space (as the board to be explored tactually was placed to the right). Performance did not differ in these conditions, suggesting that the limb coordinates are not crucial in affecting neglect (but for affirmative evidence in monkeys, see Graziano and Gross (1996)).

However, a recent study suggests that there may be some involvement of limb coordinates in neglect, although this may primarily involve the spatial position of the limbs in relation to each other. Aglioti *et al.* (1998) applied bilateral stimulation to the dorsum of the hands when the hands were placed either straight ahead (anatomical position) or one over the other. When the hands were crossed, the crossing could occur across the midline of the body or just in the right or in the left hemispace. Whereas extinction of the stimulus on the left-hand was prevalent in the anatomical position, in the crossed position there was both improved detection of the stimulus delivered to the left hand as well as poorer detection of the right-hand stimulus, and this was the case irrespective of whether the hands were positioned on the left, on the right, or across the midline of the trunk. These findings suggest that the spatial position of a tactile stimulus to one hand is coded with some sensitivity to the location of the other limb and is independent of the midsaggital plane of the trunk.

The studies reviewed thus far clearly point out the modulation of the severity of the neglect as a function of the midline of the trunk, the gaze angle or line-of-sight, and the position of the limb, and perhaps, albeit to a lesser extent, the midline of the head. Whether or not these various egocentric frames are truly separable from each other, and hence independent, or whether they are contingent on each other to varying degrees still remains to be determined.

Allocentric reference frames

Just as a number of different reference frames can be defined egocentrically and can influence performance differentially, so too can different allocentric reference frames. Most research has focussed on a reference frame defined with respect to the midline of a visual scene or environment, or on one defined with respect to the midline of individual objects or perceptual units in the scene.

The derivation of an environment-centered frame requires computations involving gravitational forces on the otolith organ of the vestibular system, visual input to define environmental landmarks with respect to gravity, and proprioceptive and tactile information to provide a sense of the body's posture in relation to gravity. Mennemeier *et al.* (1994) have argued that the environmental frame is perhaps the most important, and is even more salient than a viewer-based frame. Their conclusion is based on a line bisection study in which the environmental and body-centered frames were brought into opposition by rotating the subject's body in left, right, prone, and supine positions. The critical finding was that the patients' bisection errors were predicted better by the environmental than body-centered frames, leading the authors to conclude that environment coordinates dominate in coding spatial position.

In the last few years, considerable evidence has accumulated suggesting that spatial position may also be coded with respect to the midline of an individual object. The evidence comes from several studies showing that patients fail to report information appearing to the left of the object midline even when this information is located to the right of the midline of the viewer and/or the environment (Driver and Halligan 1991; Behrmann and Moscovitch 1994; Behrmann and Tipper 1994; Humphreys and Riddoch 1994*a*; Pavlovskaya *et al.* 1997; Young *et al.* 1990) (but see Farah *et al.* (1990) for contradictory evidence).

One of the earliest documented examples of object-based neglect is from patient NG, who had right-sided neglect and who failed to read the rightmost letters of a word. This was true when the word was presented vertically and in mirror-reversed format, and even when she was required to spell words backward (Caramazza and Hillis 1990*a,b*). Arguin and Bub (1993*a*) also showed that their patient's inability to report a target letter in a horizontal array of four elements depended on the object-relative position of the letter not the viewer-relative position. In a series of studies, Humphreys, Riddoch and their colleagues have also documented object-based neglect, showing that patients neglect letters positioned to the left of individual words

(Humphreys and Riddoch 1994*a,b*; Riddoch *et al.* 1995). Interestingly, these same patients show neglect for information on the right in multiple-stimulus displays simultaneous with the object-based effects, providing support for accounts that posit the involvement of multiple spatial frames and coding between as well as within objects (see Haywood and Coltheart (2000) and Subbiah and Caramazza (2000) for a discussion of neglect dyslexia and other object-based neglect findings).

Although all the studies cited above use letters or words as stimuli, object-based neglect has also been reported in studies that use other types of stimuli. For example, Young *et al.* (1990) reported that their patient performed poorly at identifying the left half of chimeric faces even when the faces were presented upside down and the relative left chimera occupied a position on the right side of space, again suggesting that the left of the object is disadvantaged even when it appears on the right of the viewer. The studies of Pavlovskaya *et al.* (1997) and Grabowecky *et al.* (1993) used geometric shapes and showed that information falling to the left of the center of mass of an object was less well detected than information appearing to the right. These data presuppose a computation of a center of mass that is specific to the object, the subsequent determination of the object midline, and the neglect of information to the left of this midline (Driver and Halligan 1991; Driver *et al.* 2002, 1994; Karnath and Niemeier 1992). The failure to orient towards and process the left half of the chimera is also evident in eye movements. Walker and Findlay (1996) reported that their patient RR restricted his fixations to the right side of an individual object. This object-based pattern could not be attributed to the failure to fixate the left of a display as RR could scan both the left and right of scenes and could also make left saccades when the left half of an object was presented in his left visual field (Walker and Findlay 1996; Walker and Findlay 1997).

The existence of an object-centered representation has not gone without challenge. Driver and colleagues (Driver 1999; Driver and Pouget 2000), for example, have suggested that there is no need to invoke a reference frame that is tied to an individual object. Rather, they have argued that the left and right of an object may be coded solely from one's initial egocentric (and viewpoint dependent) encounter with the object. The claim is that when an object is viewed, left and right are assigned in a purely egocentric manner in accordance with the strength of an underlying attentional gradient (Driver 1999) (for additional evidence of an attentional gradient, see Kinsbourne (1993)). A similar claim is made by Pouget and Sejnowski in their modelling work (Pouget and Sejnowski 1997*a,b*; Pouget *et al.* 1999); because the left of the object always appears at the poorer end of the gradient relative to the right of the object, in both absolute and relative egocentric space, the ipsilesional information will always dominate over the contralesional information, which will then be neglected.

This view suggests that object-centered coding is not necessary and that the same pattern of data may be obtained by simply assuming an egocentric gradient. Indeed, Mozer (2002) has conducted simulations of so-called object-centered neglect in the context of a computational model MORSEL, which assigns spatial position purely egocentrically (by virtue of a retinotopic attentional gradient) and does not have any object-centered representation. He shows that this implementation can account for a host of object-centered neglect effects (Driver and Halligan 1991; Arguin and Bub 1993*a*; Driver *et al.* 1994; Pavlovskaya *et al.* 1997). In all these cases, the left of the object always appears further left than the object right, both absolutely and relatively, and so is less activated.

An experimental paradigm in which the left of the object does not always appear further left than the right of the object can also reveal neglect (Behrmann and Tipper 1994, 1999; Tipper and Behrmann 1996). In one such paradigm (Fig. 2), a barbell appears on a screen with the left and right circles colored blue or red (the color remains constant for a single subject but is counterbalanced across subjects). In the first (static) condition, a position on the right or left is probed and this position is both right and left in both viewer and object coordinates and serves as

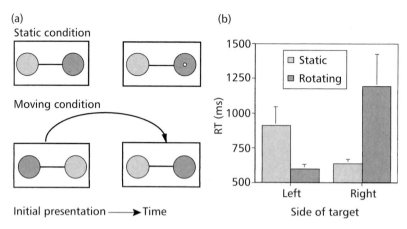

Figure 2 (a) Depiction of the static and rotating conditions in the barbell paradigm with identical final displays. One circle of the barbell was colored red and the other was colored blue. (b) Mean reaction time for four patients with neglect to detect the target on the left and right in the static and moving conditions. Note that, because a fifth subject made so many errors, his data are not included here in the RT analysis, but they reveal the same pattern with accuracy as the dependent measure. (Adapted from Behrmann and Tipper 1994.)

a baseline against which to compare performance in the second condition. In the critical rotating condition, the barbell is previewed and then undergoes a rotation of 180° so that the left, defined by the barbell, appears on the right of the viewer, and the right of the barbell appears on the left of the viewer. When a spatial position on the viewer-defined right or left is probed, both accuracy and speed of detection are influenced by whether this position occupies a right or left position, defined by the object. Thus, when the probe appears on the viewer's right but is on the left of the barbell (which rotated into that side), detection is poorer than when the position is both viewer- and object-right. Similarly, when the probe appears on the viewer's left, detection is better when the position occupies the right of the barbell (which rotated in) compared with when it is both viewer- and object-left.

In this experiment, because the left of the barbell does not fall further left than the right, a simple egocentric gradient cannot obviously account for the data. Instead, Mozer (2002) simulated the findings in the following way. When the barbell appears initially, the activation of the left and right is set by the strength of the egocentric gradient. As the barbell turns, because of the hysteresis of the system, the initial activation is pulled along with it and, through covert attention, is carried to the new location. Probing the new location then yields poor performance even when the probe appears on the right as the activation associated with that location has been carried there by the covert tracking of the moving barbell. According to Mozer, these simulations demonstrate that the results of the barbell studies do not necessarily implicate object-based representations (see Chapter 3.2 for further discussion of these issues and an approach to dealing with the egocentric versus object-centered issue).

An outstanding question is what mechanism would allow for the representation of the object and its parts under conditions of misorientation. When objects are translated in the picture plane, the left of the object always remains to the relative left of the right of the object, but this is not true when objects are rotated. Two potential processes have been suggested to deal with rotated objects. As described above, Mozer (2002) suggests that covert attentional tracking represents the left and right of a stimulus, initially defined egocentrically, as the objects rotate. The second suggested process is mental rotation; Buxbaum et al. (1996) have suggested that, in the case of misoriented stimuli, the stimulus is first normalized to its upright orientation through mental rotation and then the relative left is neglected. This implies that an egocentric gradient can still explain the empirical results; in the case of the barbell, the patients transform the rotated barbell to its canonical upright position and then neglect the left of the 'upright' barbell (i.e. now defined gravitationally or egocentrically). They base their claim on the fact that they only obtained object-centered results when they specifically instructed a neglect patient to perform the mental transformation on the barbell paradigm.

However, both proposed mechanisms appear to encounter problems. With regard to covert tracking explanations, it is now well established that patients with neglect have problems directing covert (and overt) attention contralesionally (Arguin and Bub 1993*b*; Posner *et al.* 1984). Functional imaging studies have also shown that the right parietal region plays a critical role in directing attention to the left (Corbetta *et al.* 1993; Nobre *et al.* 1997); after damage to this region, as in the case of neglect, attentional monitoring, either covert or overt, would be compromised. There is also the problem of how such a tracking system might operate when stimuli are static and do not need to be tracked, for example when a stimulus is displayed inverted as in the faces study by Young *et al.* (1990) or the words study by Caramazza and Hillis (1990*a*). In these cases, there is no opportunity for covert attention to carry the activation of the egocentric gradient along with it. It is precisely under such conditions that one might invoke a process of normalization via mental rotation.

However, the involvement of mental rotation to account for the results is itself problematic. Unlike Buxbaum *et al.* (1996), Behrmann and Tipper (1994, 1999) did not explicitly instruct the patients to perform mental rotation and yet they still obtained the critical pattern of results. Moreover, nothing in the demands of the task (simple light detection) would have prompted patients to engage in what is generally considered to be an effortful time-consuming process. Furthermore, it has been repeatedly demonstrated that the right parietal lobe plays a critical role in mental rotation (Alivasatos and Petrides 1997; Tagaris *et al.* 1997) and that, when it is damaged, mental rotation is significantly impaired (Farah and Hammond 1988). Because the neglect patients typically have extensive damage to parietal cortex, it is unlikely that they are capable of exploiting mental rotation processes. Therefore it is unlikely that object-centered effects emerge from covert attentional tracking or from normalizing via mental rotation; instead, an object-centered reference frame may exist, potentially in tandem with a reference frame that is defined by the viewer (Behrmann and Plaut 2002) (see also Chapter 3.2).

Support for a representation of spatial position, defined with respect to the midline of an individual object, has also been obtained from studies with animals. Olson and colleagues obtained recordings of single neurons in monkeys who were required to move their eyes to the left or right of objects (Olson and Gettner 1995; Olson *et al.* 1999; Olson 2001). Interestingly, the results showed that neurons in the supplementary eye field, a premotor area in frontal cortex, as well as in parietal cortex participate selectively when the monkey is planning to make an eye movement to the left of an object while other neurons are activated when the monkey plans an eye movement to the right of an object. This object-based directional selectivity occurs regardless of the direction of the eye movement required and the retinal position of the object, regardless of the exact visual features of the object, and regardless of whether the monkey was specifically following an object-centered instruction. These results point directly to a neural mechanism which might be responsible for locating positions in an object-based reference frame. Damage to neurons with object-left spatial selectivity would then give rise to the object-based neglect that is revealed by the patients (see Chapter 2.2 for a review of spatial representation studies in monkeys).

Cross-modal neglect

The question of which reference frames are compromised in hemispatial neglect has largely been investigated within single modalities, and in fact has been addressed almost exclusively in the visual modality. However, evidence for cross-modal representations has been documented in behavioral psychophysics as well as in monkey physiology. Driver and Spence (1998), for example, have shown in a number of studies that attending to a stimulus in one modality can attract attention to stimuli from other modalities in that location. Similarly, bimodal neurons sensitive to visual and somatosensory information have been found in association areas such as premotor and parietal cortex (Graziano *et al.* 1994; Colby and Goldberg 1999). Furthermore, these neurons have receptive fields tied to shared arm centered reference frames (Làdavas *et al.* 1998) (see also Chapter 3.4).

In an early study of cross-modal extinction, Mattingley *et al.* (1997*a,b*) found cross-modal extinction both when a contralesional tactile stimulus was coupled with an ipsilesional visual stimulus and in the reverse condition. In this study, the patient's hands were occluded from view, but the visual stimulus was presented near the hand, just above the occluder. Extinction was more severe in the cross-modal condition than in the unimodal visual condition, but less severe than in the unimodal tactile condition. This asymmetry suggests that there are overlapping as well as discrete areas of representation for different modalities within an interactive network.

A host of recent studies have elucidated the cross-modal effects well. For example, the extent of the extinction appears to depend on the exact location of the visual stimulus, with greater extinction when the visual stimulus is presented near the body (di Pellegrino *et al.* 1997; Làdavas *et al.* 2000; Maravita *et al.* 2000). The extinction is reduced when the visual stimulus appears near the contralesional hand. However, the mere presence of a visual stimulus in the vicinity of a passive hand, without vision of the hand, does not seem to be sufficient (Rorden *et al.* 1999; di Pellegrino and Frassinetti 2000; Làdavas *et al.* 2000), although proprioceptive information via movement of the arm does contribute significantly when vision is dissociated (Làdavas *et al.* 1997; Vaishnavi *et al.* 2001). These results reinforce the notion that cross-modal effects are produced by an interaction between converging visual and tactile stimuli and used to build multidimensional representations of a single action, object, or sensation.

One question that follows from these studies in extinction patients is why cross modal effects occur if the areas containing cross-modal neurons are damaged. Intriguing suggestions come from functional magnetic resonance imaging (fMRI) studies by Macaluso *et al.* (2000*a,b*; 2002). They presented flashing light-emitting diode (LED) stimuli near the left or right hand while maintaining central fixation. LED stimulation occurred either alone or with a tactile vibration delivered to the right hand. Although the lingual gyrus is generally considered to be a unimodal sensory area, the authors found stronger activation in the left lingual gyrus in response to right visual stimulation when simultaneous tactile stimulation occurred. Conversely, there was a nonsignificant reduction in right lingual gyrus when left LEDs were accompanied by right tactile stimulation. These findings suggest that feedback from multimodal association areas to primary sensory areas may act to support processing of a single spatial location when multiple modalities present converging information.

Therefore the studies with extinction patients can be thought of as reflecting a competitive interaction between both primary sensory and association areas representing disparate locations in space. Although only visuotactile studies have been discussed so far, other cross-modal effects have also been found (Làdavas and Pavani 1998; Bertelson *et al.* 2000). Information from multiple sensory sources that converge can increase the likelihood of attention being distributed to that location. Thus the competitive strength of a particular stimulus is increased when multiple sources of information support its presence. When the right parietal network is damaged, cross-modal sensory information on the ipsilesional side can cause extinction via the distributed network of activation in primary sensory and association areas. Similarly, cross-modal contralesional information can help support weak representations in another modality.

Functional imaging and spatial reference frames

Insight into the neural mechanisms involved in the computation of spatial reference frames has also been gained from recent studies using positron emission tomography and fMRI. The studies that have compared the neural bases of egocentric and allocentric reference frames most directly use the same visual stimuli but require different judgments in the two conditions (Fink *et al.* 2000*a*). For example, Galati *et al.* (2000) asked participants to determine whether a vertical bar, which intersected a horizontal line, was located to the left or right of their subjective midline (egocentric) or the midpoint of the horizontal line (object). As a nonspatial control, subjects were asked to determine whether the color of the vertical bar was lighter or darker than that of the horizontal bar. Their results showed that both spatial tasks activated a common network of frontoparietal areas, including the right posterior parietal and right frontal premotor cortex (Brodmann areas 7 and 6 respectively), but that the activation in the object judgment task was much less extensive (only 12 per cent of that in the egocentric condition).

Similar findings from other studies have found additional areas such as left inferior parietal, dorsolateral prefrontal cortex, cerebellar vermis, bilateral precuneus, and bilateral superior parietal cortex to be activated by both egocentric and allocentric tasks (Faillenot *et al.* 1997; Fink *et al.* 1997; Creem *et al.* 2001). Similar areas of activation have been found in PET studies comparing reaching or grasping with perceptual matching (Faillenot *et al.* 1997; Honda *et al.* 1998) and line bisection in near compared with far space (Weiss *et al.* 2000). These results suggest that this network is involved in action-oriented processing.

Areas of activation when object conditions are subtracted from egocentric conditions include right inferior temporal gyrus, bilateral cuneus, and extensive frontal areas, as well as those described above (Fink *et al.* 1997; Creem *et al.* 2001). Areas unique to object conditions include extrastriate, bilateral occipital, lingual gyrus, right hippocampal, inferior occipitotemporal, and inferior parietal cortex (Fink *et al.* 1997; Honda *et al.* 1998; Creem *et al.* 2001). Fink *et al.* (2000*b*) investigated object-based spatial representations further by contrasting one- and two-dimensional objects. Participants were asked to determine whether a line was correctly bisected (Landmark task) or if a dot was located in the center of a square (Squaremark task). The interesting finding was expressed in an interaction implicating the right intraparietal sulcus in the Landmark task and the lingual gyrus bilaterally in the Squaremark task. The authors suggest that both areas are preferentially activated in response to object-based spatial processing, but that more ventral stream areas are recruited when an object forms a better *gestalt*. Both egocentric and object-based tasks have resulted in greater right-hemisphere activation (Vallar *et al.* 1999; Fink *et al.* 2000*a*).

While a frontoparietal network appears to be involved in egocentric and object-based reference frames, it is still unclear what role the parietal lobe plays in creating a coherent perceptual representation of spatial information. Lumer and colleagues (Lumer *et al.* 1998; Lumer and Rees 1999) have proposed that perception is dependent on the covariation of activation between multiple areas. Using binocular rivalry to dissociate subjective perception and sensory input, Lumer and colleagues found that extrastriate (Brodmann area 18/19) activation reflected changes in subjective perception of rivalrous stimuli, whereas activation in striate cortex did not. Consistent with this, activation in fusiform and temporal gyri was correlated with extrastriate activation when face and motion stimuli were used. Additionally, bilateral superior and inferior parietal cortex, right superior frontal cortex, and middle and inferior frontal gyrus activation were correlated with extrastriate activation, but only inferior parietal and inferior frontal regions were significantly more correlated during rivalry than during stable viewing.

These data suggest that a network of areas, operating in synchrony, is responsible for the experience of perceiving one stimulus to the exclusion of others. In particular, the frontoparietal network (predominantly in the right hemisphere) may mediate switching between perceptual experiences (Rees 2001). Lumer and colleagues suggest that although switches in binocular rivalry are not spatial, they do involve the selection of a subset of available information over other subsets. It may be that frontoparietal areas are involved in both object-centered and egocentric spatial processing because this network is integral for the selection of spatial reference frames. This selection naturally interacts with the competitive strength of stimuli represented within each frame. The winner of the competition is then further processed by functionally specialized areas, which give rise to the emergent perception of a stimulus within a particular reference frame.

Further evidence supporting the notion of an integrative network including frontal and parietal areas being involved in selective perception comes from imaging and ERP data with extinction patients. The critical comparisons in these studies are (a) between bilateral stimulus trials in which the left stimulus is extinguished and those in which only one right visual field stimulus is present, and (b) between bilateral stimulus trials in which the left stimulus is extinguished and those in which both stimuli are detected. In the first case, perceptual report is the same but sensory information differs; in the second, sensory information is identical, but perceptual report differs. The interesting finding is that while some activation is preserved in the first comparison, a more extensive network of activation occurs when the left stimulus is reported (Marzi et al. 2000; Rees et al. 2000; Vuilleumier et al. 2001). For example, Vuilleumier et al. (2001) found preserved fMRI activation in right V1 and bilateral postero-inferior temporal areas when faces in the left-visual field (LVF) were extinguished, but right V1, bilateral cuneus and fusiform gyrus, and left superior parietal cortex activation when the LVF face was reported as seen. Similarly, in their event-related potential (ERP) data, extinguished faces elicited normal early N1 and face-specific N170 activity, but only seen faces elicited P1 and P190 activity (although P190 may have been associated with eye movements specific to that condition). Thus, less competitive stimuli may become extinguished when neural information representing that stimulus is not synchronized in multiple areas at once.

Imaging studies offer fertile ground for understanding how networks within the brain may inter-act to produce the experience of a coherent spatial visual world (Bottini et al. 2001). Understanding how different regions of human parietal cortex map onto better understood monkey models of parietal areas promises to bring greater understanding to the contribution of this area to visuomotor function and representations of objects in space (Culham and Kanwisher 2001).

Concluding comments

The focus of this chapter has been on brain–behavior correspondences in the domain of spatial representation. The data from neuropsychological studies, fMRI studies, and neurophysiological investigations with nonhuman primates have been presented. While there is general convergence and agreement between these studies, the questions posed at the outset are far from being answered. Although we know that multiple spatial reference frames are used for coding spatial position, we do not know how these are coordinated to subserve integrated behavior. And, although we know that there is some cross-modal coding which might facilitate translation among different sensory modalities, much work remains to be done to understand exactly how this is achieved. There are also many issues which have not been addressed here. This chapter has focused exclusively on reference frames coding left and right, but similar questions apply with regard to other spatial dimensions such as up–down (vertical) and near–far (radial). It is known, for example, that some patients show 'altitudinal neglect' in which they omit more information from the upper than the lower portion of the array (Shelton et al. 1990) or vice versa (Butter et al. 1989; Halligan and Marshall 1989; Nichelli et al. 1993; Mennemeier et al. 1994; Pitzalis et al. 1997). Performance may also differ along the radial dimension, with some patients showing personal neglect (Guariglia and Antonucci 1992; Beschin and Robertson 1997; Peru and Pinna 1997) and others showing neglect for peripersonal space (Halligan and Marshall 1991; Mennemeier *et al*. 1992) or extra-personal space (Bisiach *et al*. 1986; Cowey *et al*. 1994). What spatial reference frames are used for coding space in the altitudinal and radial direction remain to be determined. Finally, how these different representations mediate outputs and action requires further investigation and exploration.

Acknowledgements

This work was supported by grants from the National Institutes of Mental Health to MB (MH54246) and from the National Defense Science and Engineering Fellowship to JJG.

References

Aglioti, S., Smania, N., and Peru, A. (1998). Frames of reference for mapping tactile stimuli in brain-damaged patients. *Journal of Cognitive Neuroscience*, **11**, 67–79.

Alivasatos, B. and Petrides, M. (1997). Functional activation of the human brain during mental rotation. *Neuropsychologia*, **35**, 111–18.

Andersen, R. A., Essick, G. K., and Siegel, R. M. (1985). Encoding of spatial location by posterior parietal neurons. *Science*, **230**, 456–8.

Andersen, R. A., Snyder, L. H., Li, C.-S., and Stricanne, B. (1993). Coordinate transformations in the representation of spatial information. *Current Opinion in Neurobiology*, **3**, 171–6.

Arguin, M., and Bub, D. (1993*a*). Evidence for an independent stimulus centered spatial reference frame from a case of visual hemineglect. *Cortex*, **29**, 349–57.

Arguin, M., and Bub, D. N. (1993*b*). Modulation of the directional attention deficit in visual neglect by hemispatial factors. *Brain and Cognition*, **22**, 148–60.

Bartolomeo, P. and Chokron, S. (2001). Levels of impairment in unilateral neglect. In *Handbook of neuropsychology*, Vol. 4 (ed. F. Boller and J. Grafman), pp. 67–98. North-Holland, Amsterdam.

Behrmann, M. and Meegan, D. (1998). Goal-directed action in hemispatial neglect. *Consciousness and Cognition*, **7**, 381–409.

Behrmann, M. and Moscovitch, M. (1994). Object-centered neglect in patients with unilateral neglect: Effects of left–right coordinates of objects. *Journal of Cognitive Neuroscience*, **6**, 1–16.

Behrmann, M. and Plaut, D. C. (2001). The interaction of spatial reference frames and hierarchical object representations: evidence from figure copying in hemispatial neglect. *Cognitive, Affective and Behavioral Neuroscience*, **1**, 307–329.

Behrmann, M. and Tipper, S. P. (1994). Object-based attentional mechanisms: evidence from patients with unilateral neglect. In *Attention and performance. XV: Conscious and nonconscious information processing* (ed. C. Umilta and M. Moscovitch), pp. 351–75. MIT Press, Cambridge, MA.

Behrmann, M. and Tipper, S. P. (1999). Attention accesses multiple reference frames: evidence from neglect. *Journal of Experimental Psychology: Human Perception and Performance*, **25**, 83–101.

Behrmann, M., Ghiselli-Crippa, T., and Di Matteo, I. (2001). Impaired initiation but not execution of contralesional saccades in hemispatial neglect. *Behavioral Neurology*, **13**, 1–16.

Behrmann, M., Ghiselli-Crippa, T., Sweeney, J., Dimatteo, I., and Kass, R. (2002). Mechanisms underlying spatial representation revealed through studies of hemispatial neglect. *Journal of Cognitive Neuroscience*, **14**, 272–90.

Bertelson, P., Pavani, F., Làdavas, E., Vroomen, J., and de Gelder, B. (2000). Ventriloquism in patients with unilateral visual neglect. *Neuropsychologia*, **38**, 1634–42.

Beschin, N. and Robertson, I. H. (1997). Personal versus extrapersonal neglect: a group study of their dissociation using a clinically reliable test. *Cortex*, **33**, 379–84.

Beschin, N., Cubelli, R., Della Sala, S., and Spinazzola, L. (1997). Left of what? The role of egocentric coordinates in neglect. *Journal of Neurology, Neurosurgery and Psychiatry*, **63**, 483–9.

Bisiach, E. and Vallar, G. (1988). Hemineglect in humans. In *Handbook of neuropsychology*, Vol. 1 (ed. In F. Boller and J. Grafman), pp. 195–222. North-Holland, Amsterdam.

Bisiach, E. and Vallar, G. (2000). Unilateral neglect in humans. In *Handbook of neuropsychology* (2nd edn), pp. 459–502, Vol. 1 (ed. F. Boller and J. Grafman). North-Holland, Amsterdam.

Bisiach, E., Capitani, E., and Porta, E. (1985). Two basic properties of space representation in the brain. *Journal of Neurology, Neurosurgery and Psychiatry*, **48**, 141–4.

Bisiach, E., Perani, D., Vallar, G., and Berti, A. (1986). Unilateral neglect: personal and extra-personal. *Neuropsychologia*, **24**, 759–67.

Bottini, G., Karnath, H.-O., Vallar, G., *et al.* (2001). Cerebral representations for egocentric space. *Brain*, **124**, 1182–96.

Brotchie, P. R., Andersen, R. A., Snyder, L. H., and Goodman, S. J. (1995). Head position signals used by parietal neurons to encode locations of visual stimuli. *Nature*, **375**, 232–5.

Butter, C. M., Evans, J., Kirsch, N., and Kewman, D. (1989). Altitudinal neglect following traumatic brain injury: a case report. *Neuropsychologia*, **25**, 135–46.

Buxbaum, L. J., Coslett, H. B., Montgomery, M. W., and Farah, M. J. (1996). Mental rotation may underlie apparent object-based neglect. *Neuropsychologia*, **34**, 113–26.

Caramazza, A. and Hillis, A. E. (1990a). Spatial representation of words in the brain implied by studies of a unilateral neglect patient. *Nature*, **346**, 267–9.

Caramazza, A., & Hillis, A. E. (1990b). Levels of representation, co-ordinate frames and unilateral neglect. *Cognitive Neuropsychology*, **13**, 391–446.

Cate, A. and Behrmann, M. (2002). Hemispatial neglect: spatial and temporal influences. *Neuropsychologia*, in press.

Chokron, S. and Imbert, M. (1993). Egocentric reference and asymmetric perception of space. *Neuropsychologia*, **31**, 267–75.

Colby, C. L. and Goldberg, M. E. (1999). Space and attention in parietal cortex. *Annual Review of Neuroscience*, **22**, 319–49.

Corbetta, M., Miezin, F. M., Shulman, G. L., and Petersen, S. E. (1993). A PET study of visusospatial attention. *Journal of Neuroscience*, **13**, 1202–26.

Cowey, A., Small, M., and Ellis, S. (1994). Left visuo-spatial neglect can be worse in far than near space. *Neuropsychologia*, **32**, 1059–66.

Creem, S. H., Downs, T. H., Snyder, A. P., Downs, J. H., III, and Proffitt, D. R. (2001). Egocentric versus object-relative spatial judgment tasks elicit differences in brain activity. Presented at the Society for Cognitive Neuroscience, New York.

Culham, J. and Kanwisher, N. G. (2001). Neuroimaging of cognitive functions in human parietal cortex. *Current Opinion in Neurobiology*, **11**, 157–63.

di Pellegrino, G. and Frassinetti (2000). Direct evidence from parietal extinction of enhancement of visual attention near a visible hand. *Current Biology*, **10**, 1475–7.

di Pellegrino, G., Làdavas, E., and Farnè, A. (1997). Seeing where your hands are. *Nature*, **388**, 730.

Driver, J. (1999). Egocentric and object-based visual neglect. In *The hippocampal and parietal foundations of spatial behavior* (eds. N. Burgess, K. J. Jeffery, and J. O'Keefe), pp. 67–89. Oxford University Press, Oxford.

Driver, J. and Halligan, P. W. (1991). Can visual neglect operate in object-centered coordinates: An affirmative study. *Cognitive Neuropsychology*, **8**, 475–96.

Driver, J. and Mattingley, J. B. (1998). Parietal neglect and visual awarenes. *Nature Neuroscience*, **1**, 17–22.

Driver, J. and Pouget, A. (2000). Object-centered visual neglect, or relative egocentric neglect. *Journal of Cognitive Neuroscience*, **12**, 542–5.

Driver, J., and Spence, C. (1998). Crossmodal attention. *Current Opinions in Neurobiology*, **8**, 245–53.

Driver, J. and Vuilleumier, P. (2001). Perceptual awareness and its loss in unilateral extinction. *Cognition*, **79**, 39–88.

Driver, J., Baylis, G. C., and Rafal, R. D. (1992). Preserved figure-ground segregation and symmetry perception in visual neglect. *Nature*, **360**, 73–5.

Driver, J., Baylis, G. C., Goodrich, S., and Rafal, R. D. (1994). Axis-based neglect of visual shape. *Neuropsychologia*, **32**, 1353–65.

Duhamel, J. R., Goldberg, M. E., Fitzgibbons, E. J., Sirigu, A., and Grafman, J. (1992). Saccadic dysmetria in a patient with a right frontoparietal lesion: the importance of corollary discharge for accurate spatial behavior. *Brain*, **115**, 1387–1402.

Faillenot, I., Toni, I., Decety, J., Gregoire, M. C., and Jeannerod, M. (1997). Visual pathways for object-oriented action and object recognition: functional anatomy with PET. *Cerebral Cortex*, **7**, 77–85.

Farah, M. J. and Hammond, K. M. (1988). Mental rotation and orientation-invariant object recognition: dissociable processes. *Cognition*, **29**, 29–46.

Farah, M. J., Brunn, J. L., Wong, A. B., Wallace, M., and Carpenter, P. (1990). Frames of reference for the allocation of spatial attention: evidence from the neglect syndrome. *Neuropsychologia*, **28**, 335–47.

Farnè, A., Ponti, F., and Làdavas, E. (1998). In search of biased egocentric reference frames in neglect. *Neuropsychologia*, **36**, 611–23.

Fink, G. R., Dolan, R. J., Halligan, P. W., Marshall, J. C., and Frith, C. D. (1997). Space-based and object-based visual attention: shared and specific neural domains. *Brain*, **120**, 2013–28.

Fink, G. R., Marshall, J. C., Weiss, P. H., *et al.* (2000*a*). Line bisection judgments implicate right parietal cortex and cerebellum as assessed by fMRI. *Neurology*, **54**, 1324–31.

Fink, G. R. Marshall, J. C., Weiss, P. H., Shah, N. J., Toni, I., Halligan, P. W., and Zilles, K. (2000*b*). 'Where' depends on 'what': A differential functional anatomy for position discrimination in one- versus two-dimensions. *Neuropsychologia*, **38**, 1741–8.

Galati, G., Lobel, E., Vallar, G., Berthoz, A., Pizzamiglio, L., and Le Bihan, D. (2000). The neural basis of egocentric and allocetric coding of space in humans: a functional magnetic resonance study. *Experimental Brain Research*, **133**, 156–64.

Grabowecky, M., Robertson, L. C., and Treisman, A. (1993). Preattentive processes guide visual search: evidence from patients with unilateral visual neglect. *Journal of Cognitive Neuroscience*, **5**, 288–302.

Graziano, M. and Gross, C. G. (1996). Multiple pathways for processing visual space. In *Attention and Performance XVI* (eds. T. Inui and J. L. McClelland), pp. 181–207. Bradford Book, MIT Press, Cambridge, MA.

Graziano, M. S. A., Yap, G. S., and Gross, C. G. (1994). Coding of visual space by premotor neurons. *Science*, **266**, 1054–7.

Guariglia, C. and Antonucci, G. (1992). Personal and extrapersonal space: A case of neglect dissociation. *Neuropsychologia*, **30**, 1001–9.

Halligan, P. W. and Marshall, J. C. (1989). Is neglect (only) lateral? A quadrant analysis of line cancellation. *Journal of Clinical and Experimental Neuropsychology*, **11**, 793–8.

Halligan, P. W. and Marshall, J. C. (1991). Left neglect for near but not far space in man. *Nature*, **350**, 498–500.

Haywood, M., and Coltheart, M. (2000). Neglect dyslexia and the early stages of visual word recognition. *Neurocase*, **6**, 33–43.

Honda, M., Wise, S. P., Weeks, R. A., Deiber, M. P., and Hallett, M. (1998). Cortical areas with enhanced activation during object-centred spatial information processing: a PET study. *Brain*, **121**, 2145–58.

Humphreys, G. W. and Riddoch, M. J. (1994*a*). Attention to within-object and between-object spatial representations: Multiple sites for visual selection. *Cognitive Neuropsychology*, **11**, 207–41.

Humphreys, G. W. and Riddoch, M. J. (1994*b*). Separate coding of space within and between perceptual objects: Evidence from unilateral visual neglect. *Cognitive Neuropsychology*, in press.

Karnath, H.-O. (1997). Neural encoding of space in egocentric coordinates. In *Parietal lobe contributions to orientation in 3D space* (ed. P. Thier and H.-O. Karnath), pp. 497–520. Springer-Verlag, Berlin.

Karnath, H.-O. and Niemeier, M. (2002). Task-dependent differences in the exploratory behaviour of patients with spatial neglect. *Neuropsychologia*, **40**, 1577–85.

Karnath, H.-O., Schenkel, P., and Fisher, B. (1991). Trunk orientation as the determining factor of the contralateral deficit in the neglect syndrome and as the physical anchor of the internal representation of body orientation in space. *Brain*, **114**, 1997–2014.

Karnath, H.-O., Christ, K., and Hartje, W. (1993). Decrease of contralateral neglect by neck muscle vibration and spatial orientation of the trunk midline. *Brain*, **116**, 383–96.

Karnath, H.-O., Fetter, M., and Dichgans, J. (1996). Ocular exploration of space as a function of neck proprioceptive and vestibular input—observations in normal subjects and patients with spatial neglect after parietal lesions. *Experimental Brain Research*, **109**, 333–42.

Kinsbourne, M. (1993) Orientational bias model of unilateral neglect: Evidence from attentional gradients within hemispace. In *Unilateral neglect: Clinical and Experimental Studies* (eds. I. H. Robertson and J. C. Marshall). pp. 63–86. Lawrence Erlbaum, Hove, UK.

Kooistra, C. A. and Heilman, K. M. (1989). Hemispatial visual inattention masquerading as hemianopia. *Neurology*, **39**, 1125–27.

Làdavas, E. and Pavani, F. (1998). Neuropsychological evidence of the functional integration of visual, auditory, and proprioceptive spatial maps. *NeuroReport*, **9**, 1195–1200.

Làdavas, E., Berti, A., Ruozzi, E., and Barboni, F. (1997). Neglect as a deficit determined by an imbalance between multiple spatial representations. *Experimental Brain Research*, **116**, 493–500.

Làdavas, E., di Pellegrino, G., Farnè, A., and Zeloni, G. (1998). Neuropsychological evidence of an integrated visuotactile representation of peripersonal space in humans. *Journal of Cognitive Neuroscience*, **10**, 581–9.

Làdavas, E., Farne, A., Zeloni, G., and di Pellegrino, G. (2000). Seeing or not seeing where your hands are. *Experimental Brain Research*, **131**, 458–67.

Lumer, E. D., Friston, K. J., and Rees, G. (1998). Neural correlates of perceptual rivalry in the human brain. *Science*, **280**, 1930–34.

Lumer, E. D., and Rees, G. (1999). Covariation of activity in visual and prefrontal cortex associated with subjective visual perception. *Proceedings of the National Academy of Sciences*, **96**, 1669–73.

McGlinchey-Berroth, R. (1997). Visual information processing in hemispatial neglect. *Trends in Cognitive Sciences*, **1**, 91–7.

Macaluso, E., Frith, C., and Driver, J. (2000a). Selective spatial attention in vision and touch: unimodal and multimodal mechanisms revealed by PET. *Journal of Neurophysiology*, **83**, 3062–75.

Macaluso, E., Frith, C. D., and Driver, J. (2000b). Modulation of visual cortex by crossmodal spatial attention. *Science*, **289**, 1206–8.

Macaluso, E., Frith, C. D., and Driver, J. (2002). Supramodal effects of covert spatial orienting triggered by visual or tactile events. *Journal of Cognitive Neuroscience*, **14**, 389–401.

Maravita, A., Spence, C., Clarke, K., Husain, M., and Driver, J. (2000). Vision and touch through the looking glass in a case of crossmodal extinction. *NeuroReport*, **11**, 3521–6.

Marzi, M., Girelli, M., Mimussi, C., Smania, N., and Maravita, A. (2000). Electrophysiological correlates of conscious vision: evidence from unilateral extinction. *Journal of Cognitive Neuroscience*, **12**, 869–77.

Mattingley, J. B., David, G., and Driver, J. (1997a). Pre-attentive filling in of visual surfaces in parietal extinction. *Science*, **275**, 671–4.

Mattingley, J. B., Driver, J., Beschin, N., and Robertson, I. H. (1997b). Attentional competition between modalities: Extinction between touch and vision after right hemisphere damage. *Neuropsychologia*, **35**, 867–80.

Mennemeier, M., Wertman, E., and Heilman, K. M. (1992). Neglect of near peripersonal space. *Brain*, **115**, 37–50.

Mennemeier, M., Chaterjee, A., Watson, R. T., Wertman, E., Carter, L. P., and Heilman, K. M. (1994). Contributions of the parietal and frontal lobes to sustained attention and habituation. *Neuropsychologia*, **32**, 703–16.

Milner, A. D. (1997). Neglect, extinction, and the cortical streams of visual processing. In *Parietal lobe contributions to orientation in 3D space* (ed. P. Thier and H. O. Karnath), pp. 3–22. Springer-Verlag, Berlin.

Mozer, M. C. (2002). Frames of reference in unilateral neglect and spatial attention: A computational perspective. *Psychological Review*, **109**, 156–85.

Nadeau, S. E. and Heilman, K. M. (1991). Gaze dependent hemianopia without hemispatial neglect. *Neurology*, **41**, 1244–50.

Nichelli, P., Venneri, A., Pentore, R., and Cubelli, R. (1993). Horizontal and vertical neglect dyslexia. *Brain and Language*, **44**, 264–83.

Nobre, A. C., Sebestyen, G. N., Gittleman, D. R., Mesulam, M. M., Frackowiak, R. S. J., and Frith, C. D. (1997). Functional localization of the system for the visuospatial attention using positron emission tomography. *Brain*, **120**, 515–33.

Olson, C. (2001). Object-based vision and attention in primates. *Current Opinion in Neurobiology*, **11**, 171–9.

Olson, C. R. and Gettner, S. N. (1995). Object-centered directional selectivity in the macaque supplementary eye field. *Nature*, **269**, 985–8.

Olson, C. R., Gettner, S. N., and Tremblay, L. (1999). Representation of allocentric space in the monkey frontal lobe. In *Spatial functions of the hippocampal formation and parietal cortex* (ed. N. Burgess, K. Geffrey, and J. O'Keefe), pp. 359–80. Oxford University Press.

Pavlovskaya, M., Glass, I., Soroker, N., Blum, B., and Groswasser, Z. (1997). Coordinate frame for pattern recognition in unilateral spatial neglect. *Journal of Cognitive Neuroscience*, **9**, 824–34.

Peru, A. and Pinna, G. (1997). Right personal neglect following a left hemisphere stroke: A case report. *Cortex*, **33**, 585–90.

Pitzalis, S., Spinelli, D., and Zoccolotti, P. (1997). Vertical neglect: behavioral and electrophysiological data. *Cortex*, **33**, 679–88.

Posner, M. I. *et al*. (1984).

Pouget, A. and Driver, J. (2000). Relating unilateral neglect to the neural coding of space. *Current Opinion in Neurobiology*, **10**, 242–9.

Pouget, A. and Sejnowski, T. J. (1997*a*). Lesion in a basis function model of parietal cortex: comparison with hemineglect. In *Parietal lobe contributions to orientation in 3D space* (ed. P. Thier and H.-O. Karnath), pp. 521–38. Springer-Verlag, Berlin.

Pouget, A., and Sejnowski, T. J. (1997*b*). Spatial transformations in the parietal cortex using basis functions. *Journal of Cognitive Neuroscience*, **9**, 222–37.

Rees, G. and Lavie, N. (2001). What can functional imaging reveal about the role of attention in visual awareness? *Neuropsychologia*, **12**, 1343–53.

Rees, G., Wojciulik, E., Clarkje, K., Husain, M., Frith, C., and Driver, J. (2000). Unconscious activation of visual cortex in the damaged right hemisphere of a parietal patient wth extinction. *Brain*, **123**, 1624–33.

Riddoch, M. J., Humphreys, G. W., Luckhurst, L., Burroughs, E., and Bateman, A. (1995). 'Paradoxical neglect': spatial representations, hemisphere-specific activation and spatial cueing. *Cognitive Neuropsychology*, **12**, 569–604.

Rizzolatti, G., Berti, A., and Gallese, V. (2000). Spatial neglect: Neurophysiological bases, cortical circuits and theories. In *Handbook of neuropsychology* (ed. F. Boller and J. Grafman). North-Holland, Amsterdam, 503–530.

Rorden, C., Heutink, J., Greenfield, E., and Robertson, I. H. (1999). When a rubber hand 'feels' what the real hand cannot. *NeuroReport*, **10**, 135–8.

Shelton, P. A., Bowers, D., and Heilman, K. M. (1990). Peripersonal and vertical neglect. *Brain*, **113**, 191–205.

Stone, S. P., Halligan, P. W., and Greenwood, R. J. (1993). The incidence of neglect phenomena and related disorders in patients with an acute right or left hemisphere stroke. *Age and Ageing*, **22**, 46–52.

Subbiah, I. and Caramazza, A. (2000). Stimulus-centered neglect in reading and object recognition. *Neurocase*, **6**, 13–30.

Tagaris, G. A., Kim, S. G., Strupp, J. P., Andersen, P., Ugurbil, K., and Georgopolous, A. P. (1997). Mental rotation studied by functional magnetic resonance imaging at high field (4 Tesla): Performance and cortical activation. *Journal of Cognitive Neuroscience*, **9**, 419–32.

Tipper, S. P. and Behrmann, M. (1996). Object-centred not scene-based visual neglect. *Journal of Experimental Psychology: Human Perception and Performance*, **22**, 1261–78.

Vaishnavi, S., Calhoun, J., and Chatterjee, A. (2001). Binding personal and peripersonal space: Evidence from tactile extinction. *Journal of Cognitive Neuroscience*, **13**, 181–9.

Vallar, G. (1993). The anatomical basis of spatial hemineglect in humans. In *Unilateral neglect: clinical and experimental studies* (ed. I. Robertson and J. C. Marshall), pp. 27–59. Lawrence Erlbaum, Hove.

Vallar, G. (1998). Spatial hemineglect in humans. *Trends in Cognitive Sciences*, **2**, 87–96.

Vallar, G. (1999). Spatial frames of reference and somatosensory processing: A neuropsychological perspective. In *The Hippocampal and Parietal Foundations of Spatial Cognition* (eds. N. Burgess and K. J. Jeffery), Oxford University Press, New York.

Vuilleumier, P., Valenza, N., Mayer, E., Perrig, S., and Landis, T. (1999). To see better when looking more to the right: effects of gaze direction and frames of spatial coordinates in unilateral neglect. *Journal of the International Neuropsychological Society*, **5**, 75–82.

Vuilleumier, P., Sagiv, N., Hazeltine, E., *et al.* (2001). Neural fate of seen and unseen faces in visuospatial neglect: a combined event-related functional MRI and event-related study. *Proceedings of the National Academy of Sciences of the United States of America*, **98**, 3495–500.

Walker, R. and Findlay, J. M. (1996). Saccadic eye movement programming in unilateral neglect. *Neuropsychologia*, **34**, 493–508.

Walker, R. and Findlay, J. M. (1997). Eye movement control in spatial- and obect-based neglect. In *Parietal lobe contributions to orientation in 3D space* (ed. P. Thier and H. O. Karnath), pp. 201–18. Springer-Verlag, Berlin.

Weiss, P. H., Marshall, J. C., Wunderlich, G., *et al.* (2000). Neural consequences of acting in near versus far space: a physiological basis for clinical dissociations. *Brain*, **123**, 2531–41.

Young, A. W., De Haan, E. H., Newcombe, F., and Hay, D. C. (1990). Facial neglect. *Neuropsychologia*, **28**, 391–415.

3.2 The exploration of space and objects in neglect

Matthias Niemeier and Hans-Otto Karnath

To interact successfully with our environment we need information about the positions of the stimuli surrounding us. The positions of such stimuli may be coded in two ways—in coordinates relative to the observer, or in coordinates that use an external anchor independent of the observer's position. The first type of spatial coordinates is called **egocentric**. For example, retina-, head-, or trunk-centered reference frames serve as such egocentric systems. The other type of coordinates is termed **allocentric**. When allocentric coordinates center on a single object, they are termed **object-centered** coordinates.

Studies from different research areas have provided evidence that the brain uses both egocentric and object-centered coordinates to code spatial locations of stimuli. Neurophysiological studies recording from single units in monkeys have found cortical areas that provide the brain with information about stimulus locations in egocentric coordinates (Andersen *et al.* 1985; Duhamel *et al.* 1992; Galletti *et al.* 1993; Brotchie *et al.* 1995; Duhamel *et al.* 1997) as well as in object-centered coordinates (Olson and Gettner 1995, 1999). Studies of human visual attention also have reported evidence for information processing in both reference systems. Some of these studies have regarded attention as a process for selecting stimuli from particular patches of the visual field, like a spotlight or a zoom lens (Eriksen and Schultz 1979; Posner 1980; Broadbent 1982). In other words, these concepts have assumed that attention acts in an egocentric reference system. However, other studies have demonstrated that selection processes are influenced by the visual features of the presented display (Duncan 1984; Kramer and Jacobson 1991; Tipper *et al.* 1991; Egly *et al.* 1994; Scholl *et al.* 2001). This suggests that attention also has access to object-centered representations of stimuli.

Disturbed egocentric and object-centered mechanisms also seem to be involved in the neuropsychological syndrome of neglect. The characteristic failure of neglect patients to explore the side of space contralateral to the lesion has been described as occurring not only with respect to egocentric reference frames, i.e. relative to the position of the patient's body or parts thereof, but also relative to object-centered coordinates. For example, when Gainotti *et al.* (1972) asked neglect patients to copy an array of line-drawn objects, they found that some patients completely ignored the objects contralesional to their body but copied objects located on the ipsilesional side, whereas others copied objects on both sides of the body midline but neglected the contralesional side of each object. While the first deficit could be described best in terms of egocentric (here, trunk-centered) coordinates, the latter has been interpreted as evidence for 'object-centered neglect'.

Further examples of egocentric and object-centered neglect symptoms come from studies on reading (Kartsounis and Warrington 1989; Riddoch *et al.* 1990; Karnath and Huber 1992) and on patients' exploratory eye movements. Patients with neglect (predominantly after right brain lesions) were described as performing eye movements that were almost exclusively confined to the egocentric right side and led to neglect of left-sided information in complex visual scenes (Karnath 1994) or in the whole visual surroundings (Karnath *et al.* 1998). Different from such behavior, Walker and Findlay (1997) reported a patient who made left saccades to locate objects to the left of the display's midline, but restricted most of his fixations to the right side of individual objects. The authors concluded that this patient had a deficit in orienting his attention within an object-based frame of reference, while being less impaired at orienting between objects.

Several other experiments have aimed at investigating object-centered symptoms in neglect patients (see Chapter 3.1). To study these effects systematically, independent of egocentric aspects, a number of paradigms have been developed which can be largely divided into two groups. They either present stimuli at different rotation angles around an object-centered axis (Caramazza and Hillis 1990; Farah *et al.* 1990; Driver and Halligan 1991; Young *et al.* 1992; Behrmann and Moscovitch 1994; Behrmann and Tipper 1994, 1999; Driver *et al.* 1994; Buxbaum *et al.* 1996; Tipper and Behrmann 1996; Hillis and Rapp 1998) or use different kinds of visual segmentation or grouping effects (Farah *et al.* 1989; Driver *et al.* 1992; Young *et al.* 1992; Arguin and Bub 1993; Marshall and Halligan 1994; Pavlovskaya *et al.* 1997).

In a study employing segmentation, Farah *et al.* (1989) found that neglect patients were more likely to ignore the contralesional side of the same stimulus array when the stimuli were superimposed onto two vertical figures that divided the array into a left and a right half than when there were two horizontal figures underlying the array. This demonstrates that visual segmentation processes influence the disturbed neural mechanisms underlying neglect. As another strategy to segment the presented display into different parts, Driver *et al.* (1992) employed figure-ground perception. The neglect patient tested in this study was better able to memorize an identically shaped vertical line when it formed the right border of an object than when it was the left side of an object. Thus the neglect symptoms were found to vary as a function of object-centered coordinates.

The same conclusion can be drawn from studies presenting stimulus arrays that are rotated into different orientations. For example, Driver *et al.* (1994) tachistoscopically presented a figure consisting of a row of three equilateral triangles diagonally running down from the top right or the top left side of the display. The task was to detect a gap that always occurred at the same position in egocentric coordinates, namely in the upper edge of the central triangle. However, the gap's position in object-centered coordinates varied depending on whether the row of triangles was running down from the top right or the top left. This had a crucial influence on the performance of the neglect patients. When the gap appeared in the left half of the object, the patients ignored it more often than when it appeared on the object's right side.

Instead of employing static stimuli in different orientations, Behrmann and Tipper (Behrmann and Tipper 1994, 1999; Tipper and Behrmann 1996) used a barbell-shaped object that rotated on a screen (see Chapter 3.1). They interpreted their results as evidence for neglect arising in an object-centered reference frame. Moreover, they found that neglect patients exhibited object-centered and egocentric effects simultaneously when the rotating barbell was combined with two separate non-moving stimuli appearing on either side of the screen (Behrmann and Tipper 1999). From this latter result they concluded (a) that the visual array must have been represented in two independent reference systems, i.e. the barbell object in object-centered coordinates and the two non-moving boxes in egocentric coordinates, and (b) that both reference systems must have been disturbed in the neglect patients.

Object-centered effects explained in the framework of egocentric neglect

The studies cited above show that both segmentation and rotation of stimuli have an influence on neglect symptoms which can be described in object-centered coordinates. But does this prove that these effects indeed originate from a disturbed object-centered reference system? In fact, different authors have pointed out that object-centered neglect symptoms might be explained by a disturbed 'purely' egocentric reference frame.

For example, Pouget and Sejnowski (1997) showed in computer simulations that many 'object-centered' effects that occur independent of the horizontal egocentric location of the stimulus might readily be expected in the absence of any knowledge about object-centered coordinates. The authors implemented a basis function network of units with retinotopic receptive fields whose activity was modulated by the orientation of the eyes relative to the head. To simulate cortical damage, they assumed a gradient of neuronal loss that linearly increased from the ipsilesional to the contralesional side for the network's representation of retinotopic and of eye-in-head positions (Pouget and Sejnowski 1997). The result was a disturbed, namely gradient- or ramp-shaped, distribution of salience across the egocentric horizontal dimension. (Salience was defined as the neuronal activity elicited by a stimulus at a certain location which in turn corresponded to the probability of attentional orienting to that location.) Thus, locations on the ipsilesional side of egocentric space were more salient than those on the contralesional side. Accordingly, the absolute salience that the model assigned to a single object varied with the object's egocentric location. However, in relative terms, the object's ipsilesional side was always more salient than its contralesional side. Consequently, the model accounted not only for egocentric neglect but also for effects resembling object-centered neglect—even if there was no explicit implementation of object-centered coordinates in the model.

Similar findings of such 'relative egocentric neglect' have been reported by Mozer (1999) while studying a lesioned version of his connectionist model MORSEL. In this study, Mozer assumed a disrupted attentional mechanism gating activity between a topographically (e.g. retinotopically) ordered feature map and a recognition network so that the transmission probability of detected features decreased monotonically with more contralesional positions. In effect, this resulted in an egocentric (in this case retina-centered) bias or a ramp-shaped distribution of salience similar to the curve postulated by Pouget and Sejnowski (1997). Like the latter model, MORSEL exhibited 'object-relative' as well as 'viewer-relative' neglect symptoms without representing any object-centered coordinates. What is more, the model showed responses similar to those observed in neglect patients when performing the rotating barbell task (Behrmann and Tipper 1994; Tipper and Behrmann 1996). This suggests that Behrmann and Tipper's results might be attributed to attentional tracking mechanisms of particular visual features in combination with the splitting of attentional focus.

However, even if the models of Pouget and Sejnowski (1997) and of Mozer (1999) show that object-centered effects emerge simply from disturbed distributions of salience applied to a raw retinal image, they do so only under certain conditions. To obtain neglect for the contralesional side of an object presented at different locations, in both models it is necessary to present this object without any visual distractors. To account for neglect on the object-centered left side of rotated objects, Mozer's (1999) model relies on visual input smoothly shifting across the feature map (so that attentional tracking can occur). In contrast, it appears to be difficult to reconcile the model with object-centered neglect symptoms obtained from static objects that have been rotated previously (Caramazza and Hillis 1990; Driver *et al.* 1994; Behrmann and Moscovitch 1994; Buxbaum *et al.* 1996; Hillis and Rapp 1998). Nevertheless, it has been suggested that these results are still compatible with a deficit in an egocentric reference frame, given that the system represents preprocessed visual stimuli rather than the raw retinal image (Buxbaum *et al.* 1996; Driver 1999; Driver and Pouget 2000).

But how could such preprocessed stimuli be represented in an egocentric reference frame? One solution would be a reference system which always veridically represents all visible stimuli in egocentric coordinates but enhances the stimuli that are currently relevant and/or inhibits all irrelevant stimuli. Such a concept—termed the **enhancement model**—would apply the respective segment of the disturbed salience distribution to the corresponding part of the retinal image containing the relevant stimuli (Driver and Pouget 2000). The model can explain object-centered neglect symptoms as observed for objects presented at different locations with or without distractors (Driver *et al.* 1992; Young *et al.* 1992; Arguin and Bub 1993; Marshall and Halligan 1994; Pavlovskaya *et al.* 1997). However, it still cannot account for neglect centered on objects that are rotated around an object-based axis (Caramazza and Hillis 1990; Farah *et al.* 1990; Driver and Halligan 1991; Young *et al.* 1992; Driver *et al.* 1994; Behrmann and Moscovitch 1994; Behrmann and Tipper 1994, 1999; Buxbaum *et al.* 1996; Tipper and Behrmann 1996; Hillis and Rapp 1998).

To reconcile these observations with a concept of a disrupted egocentric reference frame, one has to assume other forms of preprocessing that normalize the visual input with respect to egocentric location, orientation, or size. We shall call this type of model the **normalization model**. For example, Pouget and Sejnowski have proposed that preprocessing of the image could involve 'a normalization of the image for rotation—a form of mental rotation' (Pouget and Sejnowski 1997, p. 534). The view that mental rotation can be involved in the process of how neglect patients represent objects has been corroborated by Buxbaum *et al.* (1996). These authors demonstrated in a neglect patient that object-centered neglect symptoms for rotated objects occurred only when the patient was explicitly instructed to mentally rotate the display into its canonical orientation but not when asked to ignore the object's orientation. This suggests that preprocessing has access to 'higher' cortical areas associated with semantic representations. In addition to rotations, the normalization model could include other forms of preprocessing regarding the position and the size of objects. Thus, an object located in the egocentric periphery could be shifted to a central position of the representation and zooming mechanisms could scale the object to a standard size. However, it should be noted that normalization is also employed for transformations into an object-centered reference frame. Thus, an egocentric reference frame using normalization processes could closely resemble an object-centered coordinate system.

Task- and stimulus-dependent effects in the exploratory behavior of patients with neglect

We agree with the above position in that object-centered neglect symptoms result from an *egocentric* bias that induces an unattended contralesional and an attended ipsilesional side. The failure of the patients to explore the *contralesional* left side of an object cannot be determined by a purely allocentric system. *Ipsilesional* and *contralesional* sides have to be defined in egocentric terms. Neglect of an object's contralateral side does not occur with respect to an intrinsic allocentrically defined 'left side' irrespective of the object's actual orientation with respect to the patient. The 'left side' of an object that is neglected is defined by the patient's egocentric left.

However, the principle idea of the enhancement and the normalization models, namely to explain object-centered neglect with a deficit in a purely egocentric reference frame, has some problems. To illustrate this, we shall review experimental data reported on the spatial distribution of neglect patients' spontaneous exploratory behavior and then contrast these results with the predictions of the enhancement and the normalization models.

Several studies have shown that the pattern of exploratory movements is quite variable in neglect patients depending on the spatial extension of the array that should be explored. A bell-shaped exploration pattern has been observed along the horizontal dimension of space when neglect patients search for a stimulus in the surrounding scenery, while a ramp-shaped left-to-right gradient is obvious when exploring small arrays or single objects. In accordance with the latter observation, Behrmann *et al.* (1997) examined the exploratory eye movements of neglect patients when performing a visual search task in a small 45°-wide array of stimuli. The patients made more fixations and spent more time searching segments of the array further on the right such that the frequency distribution of horizontal eye positions monotonically increased from the left to the right side (Fig. 1(a)). Since eye movements and attentional mechanisms are closely related (Kowler *et al.* 1995; Schneider and Deubel 1995; Kustov and Robinson 1996), the results are in accordance with the classical view that neglect is associated with an attentional gradient or a ramp-shaped salience curve that monotonically increases from the contralesional to the ipsilesional side of space (Kinsbourne 1970, 1977).

However, when searching in substantially larger areas than those studied by Behrmann *et al.* (1997), neglect patients show quite different distributions of exploration behavior. Two studies investigated the exploratory movements of patients with neglect in wide-field scenery. The first study investigated the head and eye-in-head movements of neglect patients (Karnath *et al.* 1998). A random configuration of letters was presented on the inner surface of a sphere that surrounded the subjects in a horizontal range of ±140°, left and right of the body midline, requiring free exploratory eye and head movements. The patients were requested to search for a single (non-existent) target letter. No limitations, other than the patients' own anatomical constrains of eye-in-head and head-on-trunk movements, should steer the patients' exploratory behavior. Like healthy subjects, the patients with neglect explored space with head, eye-in-head, and eye-in-space or 'gaze' movements that were symmetrically distributed in a bell-shape around preferred orientations in space. However, in contrast with controls, these centers of exploration were shifted toward the right (Fig. 1(b)). The average horizontal position of gaze and head movements lay to the right of the body's mid-sagittal plane (gaze, c.40°; head, c.26°). The average eye-in-head position was to the right of the head midline (c.13°). The preferred orientations were located far away from the anatomical limits of horizontal gaze, head, and eye-in-head movements.

A second study made comparable observations concerning the tactile exploration of space in patients with neglect (Karnath and Perenin 1998). Here, subjects were seated in complete darkness and were instructed to explore the surface of a large table in front of them, using their right index finger, in search of a (non-existent) tactile target. The successive positions of the finger on the table were recorded. The study found that the whole distribution of neglect patients' exploratory hand movements was shifted toward the right. The median activity lay 18 cm to the right of the body's mid-sagittal plane (Fig. 1(c)). As with exploratory head and eye-in-head movements, the frequency of tactile exploration decreased toward the periphery of peripersonal space on the right and the left side.

Taken together, these studies suggest that, depending on the size of the field that should be explored, the spatial distribution of neglect behavior can be either bell-shaped or ramp-shaped. However, neither the predictions of the enhancement model nor the predictions of the normalization model can account for these experimental data. The enhancement model assumes that the visual display is always veridically represented in the egocentric reference frame and that those stimuli which are of current interest are enhanced. Consequently, if parts of such a representation are disturbed, as is assumed in patients with neglect, one should expect the dysfunction always to affect stimuli in the same part of space, independent of the visual stimulus configuration or the current task. When exploring an object appearing somewhere on the left side, the patient's behavior should correspond to the respective part of the salience curve on the left and when an

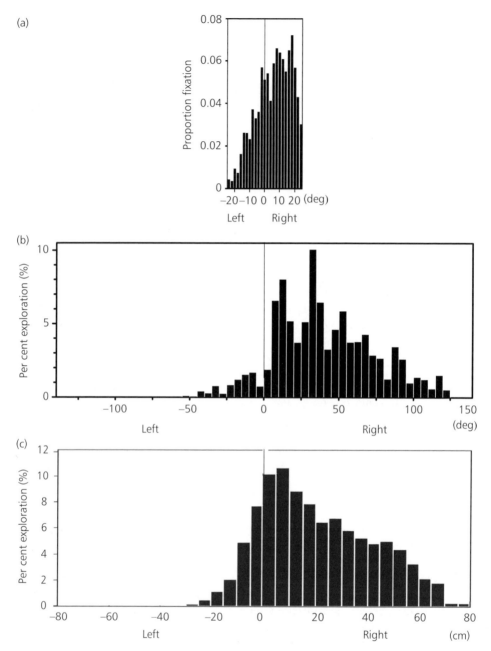

Figure 1 Spatial distribution of the exploratory behavior of patients with neglect while searching in areas of different horizontal extensions. (a) Percentage of visual search as a function of horizontal egocentric positions while counting target letters in a random array of letters located between −22.5° left and +22.5° right of the mid-sagittal plane. (b) Percentage of visual search as a function of horizontal egocentric coordinates during the exploration of a random letter array within a range of −140° left and +140° right of the mid-sagittal plane. (c) Percentage of tactile search as a function of horizontal (cartesian) coordinates. The neglect patients were blindfolded and asked to explore manually for a small target on a large table (160 cm × 80 cm). ((a) After Behrmann *et al.*, *Neuropsychologia*, **35**, 1445–58 (1997); (b) after Karnath *et al.*, *Brain*, **121**, 2357–67 (1998); (c) after Karnath and Perenin, *NeuroReport*, **9**, 2273–77 (1998).)

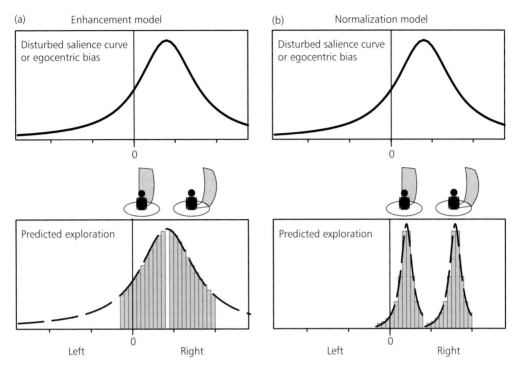

Figure 2   Predictions of the enhancement model and the normalization model for patients with neglect for a disturbed salience curve due to an affected representation of egocentric space (upper panels). (a) The 'enhancement model' assumes that the patient's behavior corresponds to the respective part of the salience curve. For a stimulus array located in the periphery of the contralesional side, it predicts a positive, increasing gradient of visual search (left-hand distribution in lower panel). However, for a stimulus array located in the periphery of the ipsilesional side, it predicts a negative *de*creasing gradient of visual search from the left to the right (right-hand distribution in lower panel). (b) The 'normalization model' assumes that every stimulus entering the reference frame is standardized. Thus, the same, total bell-shaped salience curve, is always applied to an object independent of its egocentric location (lower panel).

object appears on the right, the behavior should be associated with a segment of the salience curve on the right. Starting from a bell-shaped salience curve, for the full extent of the surroundings (Fig. 2(a), upper panel), the enhancement model predicts the following neglect behavior. For a stimulus array located in the periphery of the contralesional side, it predicts a positive increasing gradient of visual search (Fig. 2(a), left distribution in lower panel). However, for a stimulus array located in the periphery of the ipsilesional side, it predicts a negative *de*creasing gradient of visual search from the left to the right (Fig. 2(a), right distribution in lower panel). Although this prediction has never been tested directly, the consequences are bizarre. The model predicts that patients with neglect show a kind of 'negative neglect' for objects presented on the ipsilesional side with an attended left and an unattended right part.

In contrast, the normalization model assumes that every stimulus entering the reference frame is represented in a standardized way so that the reference frame always applies the same total salience curve to an object. Accordingly, one has to assume that the distribution of exploratory behavior of patients with neglect is proportionally similar, if not identical, when they explore objects of different types and of different spatial locations, orientations, and extensions (Fig. 2(b), lower panel). We expect the same salience curve regardless of whether the focus of attention concerns a very small object or a very large object, or concentrates on the whole surrounding scenery (e.g. when the subject searches for a particular object that he or she assumes to be located somewhere in the surroundings). Thus, in both cases, the distribution of salience should be *either* bell-shaped (as shown in Fig. 2(b) *or* ramp-shaped. However, the normalization model would not expect both curves.

A unifying concept to integrate object-centered and egocentric coordinates

Here, we suggest an alternative concept that avoids the above problems by combining the enhancement model with a normalization model. The model assumes a representation of visual input in two modes simultaneously:

(1)   in the veridical egocentric coordinates of the relevant stimulus;
(2)   in its normalized coordinates.

(Since the representation of a normalized stimulus is equivalent to an object-centered representation, in the following we shall term the normalized coordinates 'object-centered' coordinates.) We shall refer to this alternative concept as the **integrated space-object map** or **ISO-map**.

   To illustrate the basic idea behind this model, we shall only regard the horizontal dimension of the egocentric and the object-centered coordinates. Suppose that a person is sitting at a table and performing different tasks. When the task is 'to globally explore the table for all items on it' (Fig. 3, left panel), the table is the target of the subject's current action and thus the table is the 'object' actually represented in the ISO-map. Along the egocentric axis of the map, the table will be represented from −80° left of the subject's body midline to +80° on the right side. Along the

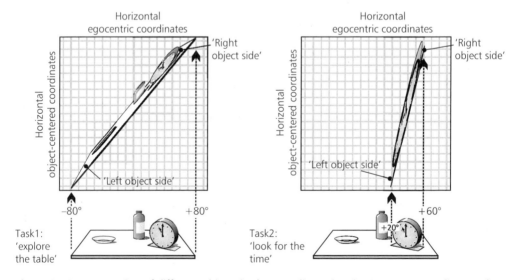

Figure 3   Representation of different objects in the two-dimensional ISO-map. Depending on the task assigned to the subject, the same physical stimuli are represented in the same egocentric but in different object-centered coordinates. Task 1 (left): when the task is, for example, to explore the whole table along the egocentric axis, the table is represented from −80° left of the subject's body midline to +80° on the right side; along the object-centered axis, the table is represented from the 'left object side' to the 'right object side'. Task 2 (right): when the clock is the target of current interest, it is represented between +20° and +60° in egocentric coordinates, and from its 'left side' to its 'right side' in object-centered coordinates.

object-centered axis, the table's left and right edges will be represented as the 'left object side' and the 'right object side' respectively.

Suppose further that, after exploring the whole table, the subject becomes interested in the clock standing on the right side. Accordingly, the clock is now the new target represented in the ISO-map (Fig. 3, right panel). In egocentric coordinates, the clock is coded between $+20°$ and $+60°$ on the right side. (Note that these egocentric coordinates are identical with those in the left panel of Fig. 3, since the clock did not move between tasks.) In contrast, along the object-centered axis, the clock's representation substantially changes. While in the first representation (Fig. 3, left panel), the clock was encoded as only part of the right side of the table in object-centered coordinates, it now spans the complete object-centered axis from the 'left object side' to the 'right object side' of the ISO-map (Fig. 3, right panel).

The ISO-map assigns salience values to each point of the represented object. We assume that in neglect this salience function is disturbed due to a cortical lesion affecting the neural substrate of the ISO-map. The distorted distribution of visual search is a consequence of this disturbance. As mentioned above, neglect patients show bell-shaped distributions of horizontal eye positions with the distribution peak shifted to the ipsilesional side when scanning large arrays (Figs 1(b) and 1(c)). In contrast, when exploring small arrays (Fig. 1(a)) or objects, these patients show ramp-shaped distributions increasing from the left to a maximum close to the right edge of the display. Given these two types of distributions, we assume that the disturbed salience function of the ISO-map is bell-shaped along its horizontal egocentric dimension (Fig. 4(a)) and ramp-shaped along its horizontal object-centered axis (Fig. 4(b)). The final three-dimensional (3D) salience function of the ISO-map is obtained by multiplying both dimensions and is illustrated in Fig. 4(c).

In the following, we use this final 3D salience function to examine the properties of the ISO-map model.[1] The salience curve that actually assigns to a target of action corresponds to a two-dimensional (2D) cross-section through the 3D salience function along the object's representation in the ISO-map. We determined different 2D cross-sections, i.e. the 2D salience curves assigned to different objects or search areas represented in the ISO-map of a neglect patient. In particular, we looked at the influence of size and position of the represented object in egocentric space. For large 'objects' represented in the map, the resulting salience curves are almost symmetrically bell-shaped with their maxima shifted ipsilesionally. This is illustrated in Fig. 5(a) for an object spanning a horizontal range from $-140°$ left to $+140°$ right of the body midline. For smaller objects (e.g. an object with a horizontal extension of $\pm20°$), the salience curve is found to be ramp-shaped (Fig. 5(a)). The salience curve assigned to an object with a horizontal extension of $\pm60°$ illustrates that there is a continuous transition from symmetrically bell-shaped to asymmetrically ramp-shaped curves (Fig. 5(a)).

---

[1] For simulating the disturbed 3D salience distribution in the ISO-map of a neglect patient, we combined a Gaussian of the egocentric (here, trunk-centered) position s_i multiplied by a linear ramp-shaped function of the object-centered location o_j (other asymmetric functions (e.g. exponentials and sigmoids) yielded similar model properties). The resulting function is as follows:

$$\text{salience}_{ij} = \beta \times o_j \times \frac{1}{\sqrt{2\pi \times \sigma^2}} \times \exp\left[-\frac{(s_i - \mu)^2}{2\sigma^2}\right]$$

To test the function we scaled the egocentric dimension from $-140°$ to $+140°$ left and right of the body. For the object-centered dimension a scale from zero to 100 per cent ('left object edge' versus 'right object edge') was taken. We examined the properties of the 3D function with a mean μ of $+35°$ and a standard deviation σ of $40°$ for the Gaussian. A slope of $\beta = 1$ was assumed for the linear component of the 3D function (actually, any value $\beta > 0$ could be assumed, since the model regards relative salience only). The resulting 3D curve is identical with the function given in Fig. 4(c).

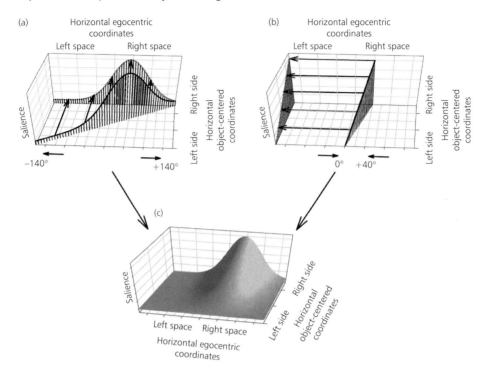

Figure 4 Extrapolation of the disturbed salience function in the ISO-map of a virtual neglect patient. The salience function is assumed to be (a) bell-shaped along its horizontal egocentric dimension, and (b) ramp-shaped along its horizontal object-centered axis. (c) The 3D salience function resulting from the multiplication of these two 2D curves.

Using the same disturbed 3D salience function we also determined the 2D salience curves of an object (width, 40°) at different egocentric locations up to +120° right of the body. We found an imbalance of salience always in favor of the right object half (Fig. 5(b)). Interestingly, however, with more ipsilesional object positions, the gradient became less steep and the width of the salience function expanded. In other words, the model predicts that the left–right asymmetry should improve (i.e. become less pronounced) with more ipsilesional positions of the objects. This latter finding is most interesting as it does not belong to the a priori properties of the ISO-map model.

A first study testing this prediction has recently been conducted (Niemeier and Karnath, in press). It investigated the visual exploratory behavior of neglect patients. On the basis of the ISO-map model, the authors constructed a saccade generation algorithm that directed the target location of each succeeding 'saccade', by a winner-take-all mechanism, to the most salient region of the represented object. Subsequently, the salience value of this fixated point was temporarily reduced, a mechanism known as 'inhibition of return' (Posner and Cohen 1984). Using this algorithm, exploratory eye movements were simulated under three conditions: scanning a large object almost surrounding the observer ('global' condition, object extending from −140° to +140°) and scanning a smaller object at two locations to the right of the mid-sagittal plane ('focus 1' condition, object extending from 0° to +40°; 'focus 2' condition, object extending from +40° to +80°). In a second step, the authors tested the predictions of the model examining the exploratory eye and head movements of four patients with neglect during these three visual search tasks. In fact, the neglect patients exhibited distributions of eye positions that closely matched those predicted by the ISO-map model. During the 'global' condition the distribution

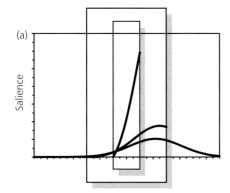

(a)

Salience

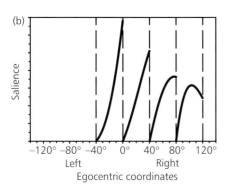

(b)

Salience

−120° −80° −40°　　0°　　40°　80°　 120°

Left　　　　　　　　　　 Right

Egocentric coordinates

Figure 5 Predicted normalized salience curves of different objects represented in the ISO-map as a function of egocentric (here, trunk-centered) coordinates. (a) The salience curves of objects of different horizontal width. For very large 'objects' represented in the ISO-map (here, the surrounding space within ±140° left and right of the body), the salience curve is bell-shaped. For smaller objects, e.g. between ±60° and ±20°, the salience curve is gradient-like. (b) The salience curve of an object (40° wide) presented at different locations in egocentric space. An imbalance of salience occurs in favor of the right half of the object regardless of its position. Nevertheless, with more ipsilesional positions, the width of the salience function expands.

of eye movements was bell-shaped with a peak shifted to the right side, whereas during the two 'focus' conditions the neglect patients exhibited ramp-shaped distributions of eye movements. Moreover, the patients' eye-movement data also confirmed the model's strongest prediction, i.e. that neglect symptoms ameliorate at more ipsilesional positions. The data thus complemented previous observations of reduced neglect symptoms for tasks performed on that side (Heilman and Valenstein 1979; Karnath *et al.* 1991; Schindler and Kerkhoff 1997).

As illustrated in the previous section, neither an enhancement model nor a normalization model can explain such results. Therefore it appears plausible that neglect is indeed associated with a disturbed representation that integrates egocentric and object-centered coordinates as suggested by the ISO-map model. Nevertheless, one may question whether it is inevitable to assume such a complex mechanism with a salience function combining two ipsilesional biases—a ramp-shaped object-centered bias and a bell-shaped egocentric bias. Maybe an ISO-map that is affected only along one of its dimensions could readily predict neglect behavior and could thus explain neglect in a simpler way?

In further simulations, we have looked at this possibility by studying the ISO-map for the case in which there is only one bias, along either its egocentric or its object-centered dimension, leaving the other dimension unaffected. It is not quite clear how the *unaffected* salience function might be shaped along its two horizontal dimensions. Here, we have chosen the simplest solution in that we assumed curves that are similar to the two affected curves but do not show a bias. For a curve along an 'intact' egocentric dimension we have assumed a broad bell-shaped curve with a maximum located in the straight-ahead direction, and for the 'intact' object-centered dimension we have chosen a uniform curve. Indeed, some experimental data on the exploratory behavior of healthy subjects corroborate these assumptions (Behrmann *et al.* 1997; Karnath and Perenin 1998; Karnath *et al.* 1998; Karnath and Niemeier 2002).

The version of the ISO-map with a disrupted egocentric dimension but a spared object-centered dimension is given in Fig. 6 (top panel). For this version of the ISO-map, we simulated the exploratory behavior of a neglect patient during the same three search tasks as used by Niemeier and Karnath (in press). For the 'global' search task, this ISO-map predicts a bell-shaped distribution of exploratory eye movements with a peak shifted to the right (Fig. 6, upper middle panel). The model also predicts left-sided neglect for the 'focus 1' task (object located between 0° and 40°) (Fig. 6, lower middle panel). For the 'focus 2' task (object located between 40° and 80°) (Fig. 6, bottom panel), this version of the ISO-map model predicts that neglect will 'switch' to the right

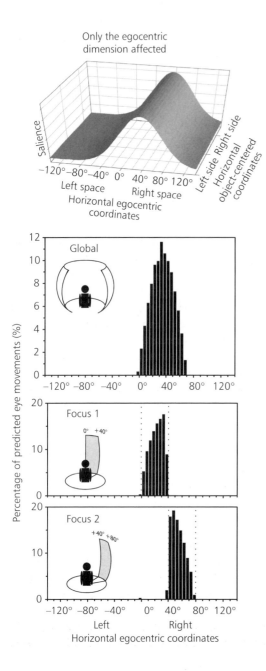

Figure 6 Predictions of the ISO-map model for a selectively affected egocentric dimension and a spared object-centered dimension. The top panel shows the 3D salience function. For the 'global' task (scanning a large object almost surrounding the observer), the model predicts a bell-shaped function that is shifted to the ipsilesional side. For the 'focus 1' task (scanning a smaller object located between 0° and 40° right of the mid-sagittal plane), left-sided neglect is predicted. However, for the 'focus 2' task (scanning a smaller object located between 40° and 80° right of the mid-sagittal plane), this version of the model predicts neglect for the object's right side.

side of the object, thus resembling what the 'enhancement model' would predict for such a task (Fig. 2(a)). However, experimental data are in conflict with this prediction. Neglect patients show an ipsilesional and not a contralesional bias even in this part of space.

We also examined a version of the ISO-map which had an affected object-centered dimension (ramp-shaped as before) but which now had an intact egocentric dimension. The salience function of this ISO-map is given in the upper panel of Fig. 7(a). Interestingly, for the two 'focus' conditions, this model predicts exploratory behavior similar to that generated by the simulation reported by Niemeier and Karnath (in press). Even for the 'global' condition, we find a bell-shaped distribution that is shifted to the right side (Fig. 7(a), upper middle panel). However, the width of this curve was almost as broad as that of the distribution predicted by an ISO-map that is intact both along its egocentric and its object-centered dimension (Fig. 7(b)). The latter result is at odds with previous findings showing marked differences in the width of the distributions of neglect patients compared with those of normal subjects (Karnath *et al.* 1998).

To conclude, for the configuration of the ISO-map that we propose in this chapter, it appears unlikely that only one of the two dimensions—the object-centered or the egocentric—is select-ively affected in neglect. Rather, our simulations suggest that both types of coordinates are simultaneously disturbed, suggesting that both coordinate systems might be closely connected in the brain.

How and where might the ISO-map be implemented in the brain?

The neurophysiological and the neurocomputational literature have demonstrated a significant interest in the question of how the brain represents spatial information in egocentric (in particular head- and trunk-centered) coordinates, basically suggesting three main approaches. Head-centered coordinates may be provided by gain fields of retinotopic neurons whose amplitude of activity varies with the orientation of the eyes relative to the head. Evidence for such a cortical network was first reported by Andersen *et al.* (1985) in the posterior parietal cortex. A recent study showed that these areas might also generate trunk-centered coordinates (Brotchie *et al.* 1995). Results from Duhamel *et al.* (1992) support another concept suggesting that the brain calculates head-centered coordinates with retinotopic maps that permanently update the visual field with each saccade. Related to this view, Henriques *et al.* (1998) proposed a 'conversion on command model'. According to this model, the brain normally represents the location of stimuli in retinotopic coordinates but transforms these coordinates into other egocentric coordinate systems when required for action. A third way to encode egocentric coordinates is to assume that neurons have head-centered receptive fields. In fact, recent data suggest the existence of such neurons in parietal areas (Galletti *et al.* 1993, Duhamel *et al.* 1997).

But what about object-centered coordinates? Olson and Gettner (1995, 1999) recorded from single cells in the supplementary eye fields of monkeys and observed neurons that were involved in saccades executed in specific directions. The activity of these neurons was differentially tuned depending on whether the monkey executed a saccade toward the left or the right end of a horizontal bar. This suggests that the supplementary eye field may code object-centered coordinates. As another possibility, information about object-centered coordinates could be provided by temporal areas. Chelazzi *et al.* (1993) showed that neurons in the inferior temporal cortex responded more strongly to a preferred stimulus when a subsequent saccade was executed toward this stimulus rather than to a distractor.

Finally, how might egocentric and object-centered coordinates be integrated as we suggest in our ISO-map model? Currently, only a few neurophysiological studies have dealt with this issue.

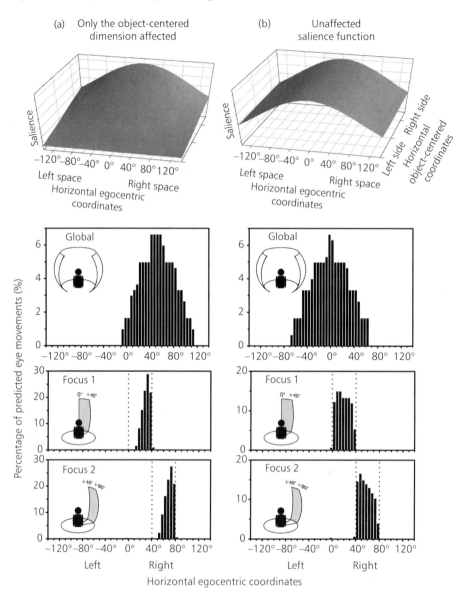

Figure 7 (a) Predictions of the ISO-map model for a selectively affected object-centered dimension and a spared egocentric dimension. The 3D salience function is shown in the top panel. This version of the model predicts a bell-shaped distribution that is shifted to the right side for the 'global' condition (scanning a large object almost surrounding the observer). Predominantly ramp-shaped distributions are predicted for the two 'focus' conditions (scanning a smaller object located either between 0° and 40° or between 40° and 80° right of the mid-sagittal plane). (b) Predictions of an intact ISO-map model in a virtual healthy subject.

Circumscribed lesions in monkey parietal cortex have been found to cause not only egocentric but also object-centered deficits (Olson and Gettner 1998). Also, single-unit recordings accounted for object-centered effects in the lateral intraparietal cortex, an area also involved in generating egocentric coordinates (Breznen *et al.* 1999; Sabes *et al.* 1999; Breznen and Andersen 2000).

These preliminary results corroborate the view that egocentric and object-centered coordinates might indeed be combined in one cortical area.

Karnath (2001) suggested that the superior temporal cortex might be a good candidate for one such area. The superior temporal cortex is located at the transition between the ventral and the dorsal streams of visual information processing (Ungerleider and Mishkin 1982; Ungerleider and Haxby 1994). Milner and Goodale (1995) asserted that the dorsal stream transforms the information about objects mainly into egocentric coordinates in order to control visually guided action. In contrast, the ventral stream embodies the enduring characteristics of objects in both egocentric and allocentric frameworks, promoting conscious awareness of the world.

The superior temporal cortex is known to receive polysensory inputs from both streams, thus representing a site for multimodal sensory convergence (Karnath 2001). Therefore lesions in this area are expected to cause behavioral disturbances involving the representation of object properties as well as their egocentric locations. In fact, both types of disturbance are observed in patients with neglect. Moreover, a recent study has revealed that it is the superior temporal cortex, and not the posterior parietal cortex or the junction area between the temporal, parietal, and occipital lobes (the so-called TPO junction), that is the cortical substrate of spatial neglect in humans (Karnath *et al.* 2001). Also in monkeys, comparable observations have been made in two studies investigating the behavioral consequences of superior temporal cortex lesions (Luh *et al.* 1986, Watson *et al.* 1994), but see Chapter 2.2.

This chapter has reviewed the evidence for disturbed egocentric and disturbed object-centered processes in neglect. Moreover, Karnath and Niemeier (2002) have shown that neglect patients can exhibit either object-centered or egocentric effects even within the same stimulus array, simply depending on the respective behavioral goal of the neglect patient. These results further favour the idea that object-centered as well as egocentric information is processed by the same or closely related brain structure(s). The ISO-map model suggests a way in which information from both coordinate systems might be integrated into one representation of the visual world.

However, for a more elaborate version of the ISO-map model, one has to take into account that this concept would comprise not just one horizontal object-centered and one horizontal egocentric axis, but would probably require six dimensions (i.e. two horizontal, two vertical, and two depth dimensions) to describe the 3D structure of an object in object-centered coordinates and its 3D relation with respect to the observer in egocentric coordinates. This could quickly lead to a combinatorial problem. To illustrate this, let us assume that the ISO-map is implemented by a neural network with one neuron corresponding to each combination of egocentric and object-centered positions. Even for a fairly coarse positional resolution with, say, 10 positions represented along each coordinate axis, this system would already require at least a million (10 to the power of six) neurons. A more economical implementation would be a network which nonlinearly combines egocentric and object-centered inputs, for example a network which multiplies egocentric by object-centered coordinates (which would actually provide exactly the same output properties as the solution above). For the same degree of positional resolution, such a model would only need 2000 neurons (i.e. $10 \times 10 \times 10$ neurons for both the egocentric and the object-centered coordinates).

Finally, this and the former solution represent only two extremes of a continuum of possible concepts. Any mixed model with neurons responding as predicted by the first or the second solution would be feasible. It remains an issue of future research to explore the neural representation of reference systems integrating both egocentric and object-centered spatial information. To conclude, the ISO-map model illustrates how egocentric and object-centered coordinates might be integrated in the brain to allow successful interaction with our environment.

Acknowledgements

This work was supported by grants from the Deutsche Forschungsgemeinschaft to H.-O. K. We are grateful to Simon Clavagnier, Denise Henriques, Eliana Klier, Julio Martinez-Trujillo, and Douglas Tweed for helpful discussions and comments on the manuscript.

References

Andersen, R. A., Essick, G. K., and Siegel, R. M. (1985). Encoding of spatial location by posterior parietal neurons. *Science*, **230**, 456–8.

Arguin, M. and Bub, D. N. (1993). Evidence for an independent stimulus-centered spatial reference frame from a case of visual hemineglect. *Cortex*, **29**, 349–57.

Behrmann, M. and Moscovitch, M. (1994). Object-centered neglect in patients with unilateral neglect: effects of left-right coordinates of objects. *Journal of Cognitive Neuroscience*, **6**, 151–5.

Behrmann, M. and Tipper, S. P. (1994). Object-based attentional mechanisms: evidence from patients with unilateral neglect. In *Attention and performance XV* (ed. C. Umiltà and M. Moscovitch), pp. 351–75. MIT Press, Cambridge, MA.

Behrmann, M. and Tipper, S. P. (1999). Attention accesses multiple reference frames: evidence from visual neglect. *Journal of Experimental Psychology: Human Perception and Performance*, **25**, 83–101.

Behrmann, M., Watt, S., and Barton, J. J. S. (1997). Impaired visual search in patients with unilateral neglect: an oculographic analysis. *Neuropsychologia*, **35**, 1445–58.

Breznen, B. and Andersen, R. A. (2000). Decoding of the population vector in LIP for object-centered saccades. *Society of Neuroscience Abstracts*, **26**, 668.

Breznen, B., Sabes, P. N., and Andersen, R. A. (1999). Parietal coding of object-based saccades: reference frames. *Society of Neuroscience Abstracts*, **25**, 1547.

Broadbent, D. E. (1982). Task combination and selective intake of information. *Acta Psychologica*, **50**, 253–90.

Brotchie, P. R., Andersen, R. A., Snyder, L. H., and Goodman, S. J. (1995). Head position signals used by parietal neurons to encode locations of visual stimuli. *Nature*, **375**, 232–5.

Buxbaum, L. J., Coslett, H. B., Montgomery, M. W., and Farah, M. J. (1996). Mental rotation may underlie apparent object-based neglect. *Neuropsychologia*, **34**, 113–26.

Caramazza, A. and Hillis, A. E. (1990). Spatial representation of words in the brain implied by studies of a unilateral neglect patient. *Nature*, **346**, 267–9.

Chelazzi, L., Miller, E. K., Duncan, J., and Desimone, R. (1993). A neural basis for visual search in inferior temporal cortex. *Nature*, **363**, 345–7.

Driver, J. (1999). Object-based and egocentric visual neglect. In *The hippocampal and parietal foundations of spatial cognition* (ed. N. Burgess, K. J. Jeffery and J. O'Keefe), pp. 67–89. Oxford University Press.

Driver, J. and Halligan, P. (1991). Can visual neglect operate in object-centered coordinates? An affirmative single case study. *Cognitive Neuropsychology*, **8**, 475–96.

Driver, J. and Pouget, A. (2000). Object-centered visual neglect, or relative egocentric neglect? *Journal of Cognitive Neuroscience*, **12**, 542–5.

Driver, J., Baylis, G. C., and Rafal, R. D. (1992). Preserved figure-ground segregation and symmetry perception in visual neglect. *Nature*, **360**, 73–5.

Driver, J., Baylis, G. C., Goodrich, S. J., and Rafal, R. D. (1994). Axis-based neglect of visual shapes. *Neuropsychologia*, **32**, 1353–65.

Duhamel, J. R., Colby, C. L., and Goldberg, M. E. (1992). The updating of the representation of visual space in parietal cortex by intended eye movements. *Science*, **255**, 90–2.

Duhamel, J. R., Bremmer, F., BenHamed, S., and Graf, W. (1997). Spatial invariance of visual receptive fields in parietal cortex neurons. *Nature*, **389**, 845–8.

Duncan, J. (1984). Selective attention and the organization of visual information. *Journal of Experimental Psychology: General*, **113**, 501–17.

Egly, R., Driver, J., and Rafal, R. D. (1994). Shifting visual attention between objects and locations: evidence from normal and parietal lesion subjects. *Journal of Experimental Psychology*, **123**, 161–77.

Eriksen, C. W. and Schultz, D. W. (1979). Information processing in visual search: a continuous flow conception and experimental results. *Perception and Psychophysics*, **25**, 249–63.

Farah, M. J., Brunn, J. L., Wallace, M. A., and Madigan, N. (1989). Structure of objects in central vision affects the distribution of visual attention in neglect. *Society of Neuroscience Abstracts*, **15**, 481.

Farah, M. J., Brunn, J. L., Wong, A. B., Wallace, M. A., and Carpenter, P. A. (1990). Frames of reference for allocating attention to space: evidence from the neglect syndrome. *Neuropsychologia*, **28**, 335–47.

Gainotti, G., Messerli, P., and Tissot, R. (1972). Quantitative analysis of unilateral spatial neglect in relation to lateralisation of cerebral lesions. *Journal of Neurology, Neurosurgery and Psychiatry*, **35**, 545–50.

Galletti, C., Battaglini, P. P. and Fattori, P. (1993). Parietal neurons encoding spatial locations in craniotopic coordinates. *Experimental Brain Research*, **96**, 221–9.

Heilman, K. M. and Valenstein, E. (1979). Mechanisms underlying hemispatial neglect. *Annals of Neurology*, **5**, 166–70.

Henriques, D. Y., Klier, E. M., Smith, M. A., Lowy, D., and Crawford, J. D. (1998). Gaze-centered remapping of remembered visual space in an open-loop pointing task. *Journal of Neuroscience*, **18**, 1583–94.

Hillis, A. E. and Rapp, B. (1998). Unilateral spatial neglect in dissociable frames of reference: a comment on Farah, Brunn, Wong, Wallace, and Carpenter (1990). *Neuropsychologia*, **36**, 1257–62.

Karnath, H.-O. (1994). Spatial limitation of eye movements during ocular exploration of simple line drawings in neglect syndrome. *Cortex*, **30**, 319–30.

Karnath, H.-O. (2001). New insights into the functions of the superior temporal cortex. *Nature Reviews Neuroscience*, **2**, 568–76.

Karnath, H.-O. and Huber, W. (1992). Abnormal eye movement behaviour during text reading in neglect syndrome: a case study. *Neuropsychologia*, **30**, 593–8.

Karnath, H.-O. and Niemeier, M. (2002). Task-dependent differences in the exploratory behaviour of patients with spatial neglect. *Neuropsychologia*, **40**, 1577–85.

Karnath, H.-O. and Perenin, M.-T. (1998). Tactile exploration of peripersonal space in patients with neglect. *NeuroReport*, **9**, 2273–77.

Karnath, H.-O., Schenkel, P., and Fischer, B. (1991). Trunk orientation as the determining factor of the 'contralateral' deficit in the neglect syndrome and as the physical anchor of the internal representation of body orientation in space. *Brain*, **114**, 1997–14.

Karnath, H.-O., Niemeier, M., and Dichgans, J. (1998). Space exploration in neglect. *Brain*, **121**, 2357–67.

Karnath, H.-O., Ferber, S., and Himmelbach, M. (2001). Spatial awareness is a function of the temporal not the posterior parietal lobe. *Nature*, **411**, 950–3.

Kartsounis, L. D. and Warrington, E. (1989). Unilateral visual neglect overcome by cues implicit in stimulus arrays. *Journal of Neurology, Neurosurgery and Psychiatry*, **52**, 1253–9.

Kinsbourne, M. (1970). A model for the mechanism of unilateral neglect of space. *Transactions of the American Neurological Association*, **95**, 143–6.

Kinsbourne, M. (1977). Hemi-neglect and hemisphere rivalry. *Advances in Neurology*, **18**, 41–9.

Kowler, E., Anderson, E., Dosher, B., and Blaser, E. (1995). The role of attention in the programming of saccades. *Vision Research*, **35**, 1897–1916.

Kramer, A. F. and Jacobson, A. (1991). Perceptual organization and focused attention: the role of objects and proximity in visual processing. *Perception and Psychophysics*, **50**, 267–84.

Kustov, A. A. and Robinson, D. L. (1996). Shared neural control of attentional shifts and eye movements. *Nature*, **384**, 74–7.

Luh, K. E., Butter, C. M., and Buchtel, H. A. (1986). Impairments in orienting to visual stimuli in monkeys following unilateral lesions of the superior sulcal polysensory cortex. *Neuropsychologia*, **24**, 461–70.

Marshall, J. C. and Halligan, P. W. (1994). The yin and the yang of visuo-spatial neglect: a case study. *Neuropsychologia*, **32**, 1037–57.

Milner, A. D. and Goodale, M. A. (1995). The visual brain in action. Oxford University Press, Oxford.

Mozer, M. C. (1999). Explaining object-based deficits in unilateral neglect without object-based frames of references. In *Progress in Brain Research*, **121**, 99–119.

Niemeier, M. and Karnath, H.-O. Simulating and testing visual exploration in spatial neglect based on a new model for cortical coordinate transformation. *Experimental Brain Research*, in press.

Olson, C. R. and Gettner, S. N. (1995). Object-centered direction selectivity in the macaque supplementary eye field. *Science*, **269**, 985–8.

Olson, C. R. and Gettner, S. N. (1998). Impairment of object-centered visison following lesions of macaque posterior parietal cortex. *Society of Neuroscience Abstracts*, **24**, 1140.

Olson, C. R. and Gettner, S. N. (1999). Macaque SEF neurons encode object-centered directions of eye movements regardless of the visual attributes of instructional cues. *Journal of Neurophysiology*, **81**, 2340–6.

Pavlovskaya, M., Glass, I., Soroker, N., Blum, B., and Groswasser, Z. (1997). Coordinate frame for pattern recognition in unilateral neglect. *Journal of Cognitive Neuroscience*, **9**, 824–34.

Posner, M. I. (1980). Orienting of attention. *Quarterly Journal of Experimental Psychology*, **32**, 3–25.

Posner, M. I. and Cohen, Y. (1984). Components of visual orienting. In *Attention and performance X* (ed. H. Bouma and D. Bouwhuis), pp. 531–56. Lawrence Erlbaum, Hove.

Pouget, A. and Sejnowski, T. J. (1997). Lesion in a basis function model of parietal cortex: comparison with hemineglect. In *Parietal lobe contributions to orientation in 3D space* (ed. P. Thier and H.-O. Karnath), pp. 521–38. Springer, Berlin.

Riddoch, J., Humphreys, G., Cleton, P., and Fery, P. (1990). Interaction of attentional and lexical processes in neglect dyslexia. *Cognitive Neuropsychology*, **7**, 479–517.

Sabes, P. N., Breznen, B., and Andersen, R. A. (1999). Parietal coding of object-based saccades: temporal aspects. *Society of Neuroscience Abstracts*, **25**, 1547.

Schindler, I. and Kerkhoff, G. (1997). Head and trunk orientation modulate visual neglect. *NeuroReport*, **8**, 2681–5.

Schneider, W. X. and Deubel, H. (1995). Visual attention and saccadic eye movements: evidence for obligatory and selective spatial coupling. In *Eye movement research* (ed. J. M. Findlay, R. Walker, and R. W. Kentridge), pp. 315–24. Elsevier, Amsterdam.

Scholl, B. J., Pylyshyn, Z. W., and Feldman, J. (2001). What is a visual object? Evidence from target merging in multiple object tracking. *Cognition*, **80**, 159–77.

Tipper, S. P. and Behrmann, M. (1996). Object-centered not scene-based visual neglect. *Journal of Experimental Psychology: Human Perception and Performance*, **22**, 1261–78.

Tipper, S. P., Driver, J., and Weaver, B. (1991). Short report: object-centered inhibition of return of visual attention. *Quarterly Journal of Experimental Psychology*, **43A**, 289–98.

Ungerleider, L. G. and Haxby, J. V. (1994). 'What' and 'where' in the human brain. *Current Opinion in Neurobiology*, **4**, 157–65.

Ungerleider, L.G. and Mishkin, M. (1982). Two cortical visual systems. In *Analysis of visual behavior* (ed. D. J. Ingle, M. A. Goodale, and R. J. W. Mansfield), pp. 549–86. MIT Press, Cambridge, MA.

Walker, R. and Findlay, J. M. (1997). Eye movement control in spatial and objec-based neglect. In *Parietal lobe contributions to orientation in 3D space* (ed. P. Thier and H.-O. Karnath), pp. 201–18. Springer, Berlin.

Watson, R.T., Valenstein, E., Day, A., and Heilman, K.M. (1994). Posterior neocortical systems subserving awareness and neglect. *Archives of Neurology*, **51**, 1014–21.

Young, A. W., Hellawell, D. J., and Welch, J. (1992). Neglect and visual recognition. *Brain*, **115**, 51–71.

3.3   Coding near and far space

Anna Berti and Giacomo Rizzolatti

In common language space is defined as 'the boundless, continuous expanse extending in all directions, within which all material things are contained' (*Webster's New World Dictionary of the American Language* 1974). This definition describes well the introspective idea that individuals have of space as something real, fixed, and unitary—a kind of 'container' in which objects are located.

Is this conventional view correct? Is there indeed a space center or a space circuit specifically devoted to space perception in the brain? There is now clear evidence that this is not the case. Historically, the work of Mountcastle *et al.* (1975) on posterior parietal cortex of the monkey was particularly influential in challenging the unitary view of space. These authors showed that in the monkey inferior parietal lobule there is a 'neural mechanism generating commands for selective attention to the immediate behavioral surround' for visual grasping of objects '. . . and for skilled co-ordinated actions of hand and eye' (Mountcastle 1976).

The notion of a space around individuals was expanded by Rizzolatti *et al.* (1981*a,b*, 1983). Based on their recording and lesion studies of the monkey premotor cortex, they proposed that the external space should be subdivided into two large sectors: **peripersonal** or **near space** and **far space**. Peripersonal space corresponds basically to the 'immediate peripersonal space'of Mountcastle (1976). It is space for arm and hand action. It extends around the body and is continuous with personal space. The neurons coding peripersonal space also code the body surface adjacent to it. (This notion of continuity between personal space and the space around the body was absent in Mountcastle's idea of an immediate behavioral surround.) Far space is the region in which oculomotor exploration occurs. It is also the space that can be reached by walking or running.

Other subdivisions of space have been proposed by Grusser (1983), Cutting and Vishton (1995), and Previc (1990, 1998) on various grounds. All these authors agree that the unitary idea of space is wrong and that the distinction between near space and far space is fundamental for understanding space perception and its deficits.

Space coding: anatomy and neurophysiological mechanisms

The classic view of how space is coded in the brain postulates the existence of a multipurpose space center located in the parietal lobe. Our object-directed actions are possible only when we have localized the spatial position of the objects that we want to act upon. It does not matter whether we intend to look at them, reach for them, or kick them.

The weakness of this position is immediately apparent when one examines the anatomical organization of the parietal lobe. If the parietal lobe were a multipurpose space center, its organization would be similar to that of a sorting station that receives convergent inputs from a series of areas and sends divergent outputs to a series of other areas. In fact, the parietal lobe comprises a large number of separate areas, whose connections with the occipital and frontal lobe and with subcortical centers are remarkably segregated (Godschalk *et al.* 1984; Petrides and Pandya 1984; Matelli *et al.* 1986; Cavada and Goldman-Rakic 1989; Andersen *et al.* 1990; 1997). This organizational pattern—a series of circuits working in parallel—is not compatible with any idea of a single multipurpose spatial map.

There is a functional segregation corresponding to the anatomical segregation of the parietal lobe. Evidence for this comes from a large number of neurophysiological studies, all showing that the various parietal areas have specific functional properties, with each area using sensory information for different motor purposes (Snyder *et al.* 1997; Rizzolatti *et al.* 1998; Colby and Goldberg 1999).

A good example of these different functional properties can be obtained by comparing the circuit formed by the lateral intraparietal area (LIP) and the frontal eye fields (FEFs), which is an oculomotor circuit, with that formed by the ventral intraparietal area (VIP) and the premotor area F4, which is a reaching circuit (Colby and Goldberg 1999; Rizzolatti *et al.* 2000).

Neurons in both these circuits respond to visual stimuli and discharge during movements. However, apart from these similarities, the neuronal properties of the two circuits are radically different. In the oculomotor circuit neurons respond to visual stimuli regardless of the distance of the stimulus from the individual being studied, their receptive fields are coded in retinal coordinates (i.e. the receptive field of each neuron has a specific position on the retina referred to the fovea), and the motor properties are exclusively related to eye movements (Andersen *et al.* 1997; Snyder *et al.* 1997; Colby and Godberg 1999). In contrast, in the somatomotor circuit most neurons are bimodal, responding to tactile and visual stimuli. They prefer three-dimensional visual objects with respect to simple light stimuli, they have receptive fields coded in body-part coordinates, and their motor activity is related to movement of body parts. Finally, and most importantly, in order to activate them, the visual stimuli should be presented within the animal's reach (i.e. in near or peripersonal space) (Gentilucci *et al.* 1983, 1988; Graziano and Gross 1995).

Particularly important is the different way in which the two circuits code space. In the oculomotor circuit, spatial information derives from neurons whose receptive fields are coded in retinal coordinates. The spatial position of an object is reconstructed by computing either the position of an object on the retina and the eye in the orbit (Zipser and Andersen 1988), or the impending saccade motor vectors (Bruce 1988; Goldberg and Bruce 1990). In contrast, in the reaching circuit space is coded in egocentric coordinates at a single neuron level. Receptive fields remain anchored to the body parts to which they are related, regardless of eye or body-part position (Gentilucci *et al.* 1983, 1988; Graziano and Gross 1995; Fogassi *et al.* 1996).

A further difference between these two systems is evident from lesion studies. Damage to LIP–FEF circuit produces, in addition to oculomotor deficits, preference for ipsilesional stimuli or even, in the case of large FEF lesions, unawareness for contralesional stimuli. In this last case, unawareness is particularly severe in far space. In contrast lesions of the VIP–F4 circuit result in inattention for stimuli presented contralateral to the brain damage, which is especially severe when stimuli are presented near the monkey's body and face.

It is important to stress that the severity of neglect in monkey experiments, especially recent ones, is rather modest (for a review see Chapter 2.2). This is probably because in modern studies, lesions are small, are limited to specific well-defined cortical areas, and leave the white matter beneath the ablated cortex intact. Thus the imbalance between opposite turning tendencies consequent to unilateral cortical damage (Kinsbourne 1993) and the hypoactivation of the hemisphere ipsilateral to the lesion that follows large cortical damage (Heilman *et al.* 1993) are minimal in monkey experimental neglect. Without these additional factors, the neglect symptomatology is much less severe and recovery is rapid and often almost complete.

A recent and very interesting development concerning space coding is the demonstration that near space is not static, but may expand in a dynamic way. Two sets of evidence point in this direction. One is related to the use of tools, and the other to the velocity of objects moving in the peripersonal space.

Iriki *et al.* (1996) recorded single neuron activity from the medial bank and the fundus of the intraparietal sulcus (IPS). They found that neurons in this region have passive properties similar to those of area F4, responding to tactile and visual stimuli presented in the peripersonal space. The tactile receptive fields are localized on the hand or on the arm and neck, and the visual receptive field occupies a rather large region around the tactile receptive field. When the arm moves, the visual receptive fields move with it. Iriki *et al.* (1996) trained monkeys to use a rake to retrieve food pellets and re-tested their neuron properties after they had learnt the task. The results showed that, after learning, the visual receptive field dramatically expanded and included the space around the tool as well as the space around the hand and arm. The expansion effect disappeared within few minutes of the monkey ceasing to use the tool. The authors proposed that, during raking, the monkey's body image expanded to incorporate the tool. As a consequence the peripersonal space also enlarged and included all the space within reach using the tool.

Further evidence that peripersonal space is not static has been provided by the experiments of Fogassi *et al.* (1996). They studied visual receptive fields located around the face in F4 neurons with stimuli moving towards the monkey at different speed. They found that, in most neurons, the outer border of the peripersonal visual receptive field expanded when the speed increased. This indicated that the peripersonal space in F4 is not a geometrical entity, where each position indicates a specific distance from the monkey, but a dynamic system that takes time into consideration. We shall discuss this important issue in the last section of this chapter.

Inference from monkey studies to human neglect

As shown in the previous section, monkey experiments indicate that space representation derives from the combined activity of several independent brain circuits. In view of the fundamental similarity between monkey and human brain organization, a logical inference is that the same should be true for humans. Do human studies support this view? If the hypothesis of multiple areas for space representation is correct, one would expect that a discrete lesion, impairing a specific human brain area, would affect the representation of specific space sectors.

Another question that monkey studies pose is whether peripersonal and far space are coded in humans by neuronal mechanisms similar to those found in the monkey. If this is the case one would expect that the same manipulations that affect space coding in monkeys would affect space coding of human patients when applied to them.

Evidence for separate mechanisms of near- and far-space representation

Until quite recently, it was tacitly assumed in neglect studies that neglect affects the entire con-tralesional space. The possibility that unawareness of stimuli could be limited either to the space surrounding the body or to the non-reachable space was not taken into account. Thus only near space was tested in clinical evaluation. Even now, neglect patients are usually examined with materials presented only in the space surrounding the body. However, following seminal studies in

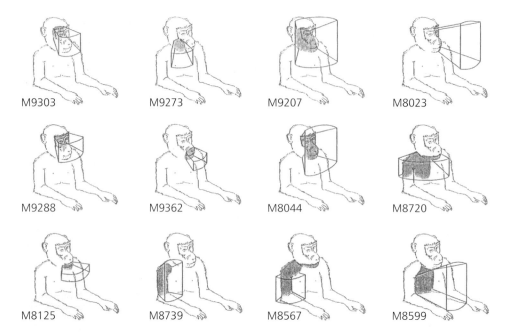

Figure 1 Coding of peripersonal space: examples of tactile and visual receptive fields of F4 bimodal neurons. The shaded areas show the tactile receptive fields, and the solids around different body parts indicate the visual receptive fields.

animals showing neglect limited to restricted space sectors (Rizzolatti *et al*. 1983), the possibility of a dissociation between near- and far-space neglect in humans has been considered.

Pizzamiglio *et al*. (1989) studied a group of patients with right brain damage using a modification of the Wundt–Jastrow illusion which had previously been proved to be sensitive to neglect (Massironi *et al*. 1988). In this illusion, two areas of the same extent and shape are arranged in such a way that normal subjects indicate one of the two areas as longer than the other. When orientation of the stimulus was subjectively perceived as directed to the left side, patients were not affected by the illusion and gave responses that were opposite to those given by normal subjects. Pizzamiglio and coworkers presented the stimulus both in near and far space and did not find a significant effect of distance on neglect patient's performance, i.e. they gave the same answers in both near- and far-space presentations. The authors commented that, although their conclusions were based on a negative finding, the strong association between neglect for near and far space suggested a unitary neural component for space representation.

The first evidence for a possible distinction between near- and far-space coding in man was found by Halligan and Marshall (1991). They described a patient, who, in addition to showing neglect in conventional tasks, demonstrated marked neglect when asked to bisect lines in near space using either an ordinary pen or a projection light pen. However, when the patient was asked to bisect lines presented in far space by means of a projection light pen, neglect was greatly reduced or even disappeared. These finding demonstrated, for the first time in humans, that space neglect can be restricted to a specific sector of the external world.

Cowey *et al*. (1994) described the opposite dissociation. They reported studies of five patients with right brain damage in whom neglect was more severe in far space than in near space. These dissociations were subsequently confirmed in other studies (Vuilleumier *et al*. 1998; Cowey *et al*. 1999; Frassinetti *et al*. 2001). The possibility of a double dissociation between far- and near-space neglect clearly demonstrates that in humans far and near space are separately coded by distinctive representations and that these representations can be selectively affected by a brain damage.

The studies in which dissociation between peripersonal and far space neglect was found used tasks, such as line bisection, which were not only perceptual, but also visuomotor. Because of the contrast with the earlier finding of Pizzamiglio *et al.* (1989), it was tentatively concluded that the motor component of the task was crucial for yielding asymmetry between far- and near-space neglect. However, a recent study by Pitzalis *et al.* (2001) has shown that this is not necessarily true. These authors also found a dissociation between near and far space in purely perceptual tasks. Therefore this finding supports the notion that, within a given space sector, the activity of the same brain circuit subserves both perceptual and visuomotor tasks.

Once it has been established that lesions can selectively affect near and far space, one may go deeper into the issue and consider whether peripersonal and far-space coding are sharply separated or whether they lie on a continuum. This issue was addressed by Cowey *et al.* (1999), using a line bisection test. Lines of different lengths were presented at six different distances from the body (25, 50, 100, 200, 300, and 400 cm) to patients affected by neglect. The authors assumed that the border between near- and far-space was located at 100 cm. The results showed that in five of the thirteen patients tested, there was an effect of line presentation distance, with neglect being more severe in far space than in near space. The performance impairment was achieved gradually, with no significant difference between individual steps. The only distance that significantly differed from all the others was that at 400 cm. The authors concluded that there was no evidence of a clear border between near and far space. An objection to this conclusion is that only one patient actually presented a smooth gradient going from near to far distances. All the others showed an abrupt change, although at different distances. Thus at present it is not possible to reach a definite conclusion on how near space switches to far space.

Anatomical and functional correlates of near- and far-space coding in humans

In principle, evidence on the anatomical correlates of peripersonal and far space in humans may be obtained from two sources—lesion studies and brain imaging experiments.

With regard to lesion studies, so far there has been no demonstration of an unequivocal association of specific brain regions with near- or far-space neglect. This lack of positive evidence is probably due to two main reasons: (a) no studies have been conducted with the specific aim of finding the anatomical basis of dissociation between far and near space in neglect; (b) the reported cases in which a clear-cut dissociation has been found are too few to allow significant neuroanatomical correlations.

An attempt to localize cortical areas active in tasks performed in near and far space in normal human volunteers was recently carried out by Weiss *et al.* (2000). Using positron emission tomography (PET), they instructed normal subjects to bisect lines or point to dots in near and far space. The results showed that actions performed in near and far space activated different brain areas. Near-space actions activated left dorsal occipital cortex, left intraparietal cortex, and left thalamus, whereas far-space actions activated the ventral occipital cortex bilaterally and the right medial temporal cortex. Although this result appears to suggest that near and far space are coded in different brain areas, it does not help much in defining areas in which lesions will produce near- or far-space neglect. Both of the patients so far described who presented neglect for near, but not far, space (Halligan and Marshall 1991; Berti and Frassinetti 2000) had damage to the right hemisphere and not to the left hemisphere, as predicted by the study of Weiss *et al.* (2000). However, as the authors themselves suggest, it is possible that the left-hemisphere activation they observed during near-space actions was due to the fact that more hand activity was required for the near-space task than the far-space task. Hence, as the tasks were performed using the right hand, the left hemisphere was activated.

Of greater relevance for the problem of the localization of the peripersonal space in humans is a recent functional MRI (fMRI) study in which the authors attempted to localize multimodal (tactile, auditory, and visual) cortical areas in humans (Bremmer *et al.* 2001). Tactile stimuli, moving visual stimuli located near the subject, and auditory stimuli producing the illusion of sound movement were presented. Several cortical areas related to different stimulus modalities were found to be activated by the stimuli. However, a multimodal convergence was found at only three sites: the depth of the IPS, the ventral premotor cortex, and the SII complex. Considering the type of stimuli used (which included tactile stimuli), the activated multimodal areas should include the areas coding peripersonal space. The data obtained fit this prediction. On the basis of their location (and properties) the area in the depth of IPS appears to be the homolog of area VIP in monkeys, while that located in the ventral premotor cortex should be the homolog of area F4. The final area that was activated in this study was SII complex. On the basis of the available evidence in monkeys, it is difficult to draw any firm conclusion on what role (if any) this multimodal area has in coding peripersonal space.

Further evidence that peripersonal space is subserved in humans by a system of bimodal neurons similar to that described in monkeys come from recent studies of patients with tactile extinction. Prompted by monkey data showing that F4 neurons respond to both tactile and visual stimuli delivered near the tactile receptive field, di Pellegrino *et al.* (1997) tested a patient who presented tactile extinction with both tactile and visual stimuli. The patient also showed cross-modal extinction, i.e. when a visual stimulus was presented near the ipsilesional right hand, a tactile stimulus delivered to the contralesional left hand was not perceived. The interesting finding was that when the visual stimulus was presented in exactly the same position but the patient's hand was placed behind his back, extinction was not observed. This showed that the visual stimulus had an effect on extinction only when it was presented in the space near the right hand (peripersonal space). This effect was also present when the arms were crossed, showing that the visual receptive field was anchored to the tactile receptive field of the hand. The existence of a visuotactile peripersonal space for faces has also been shown using a similar behavioral paradigm (Ladàvas *et al.* 1998).

Taken together, the neuropsychological and fMRI data reviewed above indicate the following:

- near and far space are differently coded in the human brain
- near space is coded in areas that appear to be the homologs of those coding peripersonal space in monkeys
- peripersonal space is implemented in a system of bimodal neurons which are responsible for the various effects of cross-modal extinction described above.

Modulation of near- and far-space representation by tool use

The modulation of peripersonal space by tool use described in monkeys has recently been demonstrated also in humans. Berti and Frassinetti (2000) asked a right-brain-damaged patient with neglect (patient PP) to bisect lines in near and far space. In near space, bisection was performed either by touching the midpoint of the line with the index finger of the right hand (reaching modality) or by indicating the midpoint of the line by means of a projection light-pen (pointing modality). In far space, the patient had to bisect the lines using either a 100-cm stick (reaching modality) or a projection light-pen (pointing modality). The dependent variable was the displacement error (in millimeters).

Patient PP had clear neglect in near space in many different tasks including line cancellation, reading, and line bisection. Line bisection in near space was affected when the patient had to perform the task by both reaching and pointing. When the lines were positioned in far space, neglect was much less severe or even absent when tested using the projection light-pen. However, when PP used the stick to bisect far lines, she showed a neglect in far space with a severity comparable to that in near space. Berti and Frassinetti (2000) explained this result by reference to the neurophysiological data reported by Iriki *et al.* (1996). As in monkeys, the use of a tool extended the body space, thus enlarging the peripersonal space to include all the space between the patient's body and the stimulus. In consequence, far space was remapped as near space but, because near-space representation was affected by neglect, neglect also became manifest during tool use in far space (see also Berti *et al.* (2001)).

The expansion of peripersonal space when tools are used was confirmed by Farnè and Làdavas (2000) and by Maravita *et al.* (2001) in studies of patients with cross-modal extinction, i.e. patients in whom a visual stimulus delivered close to the right hand extinguishes tactile stimulus delivered to the left hand. Cross-modal extinction was found to be reduced when the visual stimulus was placed distant from the hand, i.e. when the visual stimulus was no longer in near peripersonal space. However, when the patient held a stick in his or her hand, so that a right visual stimulus was now near the extremity of the stick, cross-modal extinction was again observed. Therefore it appears that, as in PP, holding the stick induced a remapping of space so that a far stimulus was treated as a peripersonal stimulus when presented near an extension of the patient's body. Maravita *et al.* (2001) also showed that the remapping effect was not present when the stick was lying near the patient's hand, but the patient was not touching it. This finding further indicates that the crucial factor for space remapping is that the tool becomes a prolongation of the subject's body.

Conclusions

The data reviewed above clearly show that there is no unitary representation of the space in the brain. Monkey studies and, more recently, human data indicate that different cortical areas code near and far space and that the neurophysiological mechanisms underlying space representation are different for the two space sectors.

While the dichotomy between near and far space is well proved, it is not immediately clear why evolution has kept the mechanisms of space representation separated, especially in view of the unity of the phenomenal experience of space perception. However, this becomes less mysterious if one admits that space representation is not a 'primary' brain function—space *per se* is not represented—rather, it derives from the activity of circuits whose primarily role is that of organizing actions with different effectors (e.g. an arm-reaching movement or a saccade) towards specific object location. All these circuits must compute space, but the computational constraints for programming actions with different effectors are different. Thus space is computed repetitively for different purposes. The joint activity of these sensory–motor circuits determines space awareness. Neurophysiological evidence proving this point was reviewed at the beginning of this chapter.

The link between space representation and motor system can be interpreted in two ways. The first view is that space is primarily 'sensorial' (e.g. visual) and the link with the motor system is secondary. According to this view the multiplicity of space representations would indicate only that the motor system requirements influence the space representation, but do not determine it. The opposite view is that space is primarily 'motor' (Rizzolatti *et al.* 1997). Space representation, during development, is constructed through action. Once the motor representation of space is consolidated, it is matched with sensory information that greatly enriches it and gives the introspective sensorial idea of perception of space that we all share.

The existence of a space around the body, anchored to the body parts and coded in the circuit that control body-part movements, appears to be a strong argument in favor of a motor origin of space. From the sensory perspective, there is no obvious reason why eyes with normal refraction and normal accommodation should select light stimuli coming exclusively from a space sector located around the body of the perceiver. Light stimuli that arrive from far locations should be equally effective. In contrast, the link between space around the body and body-part movements appears to be a logical arrangement if near-space representation derives from hand and head actions. Examination of the properties of neurons coding the peripersonal space in F4 gives further support to this view.

Let us examine their properties from the sensory and motor points of view. According to the first view the discharge of F4 neurons codes space 'visually'. This implies that, given a reference point, the neurons signal the location of objects using a cartesian or some other geometrical system. In contrast, according to the motor view, the discharge of F4 neurons does not code a specific spatial location, but codes 'potential motor actions' directed towards a particular spatial location. The term 'potential motor' refers to the fact that the activation of premotor neurons in F4 (and in other premotor areas as well) does not necessarily leads to an action. Rather, their activation *represents* an action that may or may not be executed (for a discussion of this concept see Rizzolatti *et al.* (1998)). According to the motor hypothesis, when a visual stimulus is presented in a given space location, it automatically evokes a potential motor action that maps the stimulus position in motor terms. The translation of potential motor actions into real actions 'validates' the neural representation and creates a space representation based on actions.

The tight temporal link between visual stimulus presentation and the onset of F4 neuron discharge, the response reliability, and the presence of what appear to be visual receptive fields can be considered as empirical evidence for the visual hypothesis. However, it should be noted that if, during development, a strict association is formed between motor actions and stimuli that elicit them, presentation of those stimuli may elicit the effects described above. Evidence in favor of a motor space has come from the study of properties of F4 neurons in response to moving stimuli. These data (Fogassi *et al.* 1996) show that the receptive field extension of F4 neurons increases in depth when the speed of an approaching stimulus increases. This finding cannot be accommodated by the visual hypothesis. Inherent in this last hypothesis is that each set of neurons, when activated, specifies object location in a rigorous geometrical way regardless of the temporal dimension of the stimulation. A locus 15 cm from the tactile receptive field should remain 15 cm from the tactile receptive field regardless of how the object reaches this position. In contrast, the motor space hypothesis predicts that the spatial map must have dynamic properties and therefore must vary according to the change in the object's spatial location with time. A stimulus that approaches an individual rapidly should elicit a faster response. Therefore space should be coded dynamically according to the motor requirements.

If one considers child development, there is little doubt that movements in space precede sensory information about space. Ecographic studies showed that even before birth babies have an extremely rich goal-directed motor activity. For example, hand movements reaching the face are already present at the eighth prenatal week. At 6 months, the fetus is able to bring its hand to the mouth and suck it. This indicates that a motor representation of directions in space is present well before birth (Butterworth and Harris 1994).

The sensory–motor condition of the infant at birth is extremely interesting. At birth, the child's movements become increasingly goal directed but obviously related to the space around the body. Very interestingly, the optical and motor situations are congruent. Because the crystalline lens is not fully functional, the focal distance is virtually fixed and the infant sees clearly only objects that are located about 20 cm from it. Far vision does not start to develop until the age of 3 months. The developmental advantage of the early visual condition is obvious. Because the depth of vision is limited to 20 cm, the infant can acquire a representation of peripersonal space (direction and depth) without needing to disentangle near from far stimuli. Therefore the infant can use its motor knowledge to construct the space associating the arm motor programs, developed before birth, first with the appearance of its hand in different spatial positions and then with objects present in the same positions. The observation of Piaget (1936) that at 3 months of age infants spend a large amount of time observing their hands is probably due to the necessity to calibrate peripersonal space according to an object of known dimension.

Not only the body-related peripersonal space, but also eye movements and especially eye convergence, develop during the first 3 months. Information on convergence, associated with that deriving from hand and head movements, gives infants richer information for constructing their peripersonal space. At 3 months, when peripersonal space is a coherent construct, maturation of the lens allows the infant to receive information from far space. Using peripersonal space representation as its initial spatial knowledge and correlating visual stimuli coming from far space with eye/head movements and later with body movements, the child starts to construct far space. However, no memory of this prolonged space construction remains, and to adults space appears as a 'boundless, continuous expanse extending in all directions'.

Acknowledgement

This work was supported by a MURST-PRIN grant to A.B. and G.R.

References

Andersen, R. A., Asanuma, C., Essick, G. K., and Siegel, R. M. (1990). Cortico-cortical connections of anatomically and physiologically defined subdivisions within the inferior parietal lobule. *Journal of Comparative Neurology*, **296**, 65–113.

Andersen, R. A., Snyder, L. H., Bradley, D. C., and Xing, J. (1997). Multimodal representation of space in the posterior parietal cortex and its use in planning movements. *Annual Review of Neuroscience*, **20**, 303–30.

Berti, A. and Frassinetti, F. (2000). When far becomes near: re-mapping of space by tool use. *Journal of Cognitive Neuroscience*, **12**, 415–20.

Berti, A., Smania, N., and Allport, A. (2001). Coding of far and near space in neglect patients. *NeuroImage*, **14**, S98–102.

Bremmer, F., Schlack, A., Shah, N. J., *et al.* (2001). Polymodal motion processing in posterior parietal and premotor cortex: a human fMRI study strongly implies equivalencies between humans and monkeys. *Neuron*, **29**, 287–296.

Bruce, C. J. (1988). Single neuron activity in the monkey's prefrontal cortex. In *Neurobiology of neocortex* (ed. P. Rakic and W. Singer), pp. 297–329. Wiley, Chichester.

Butterworth, G. and Harris, M. (1994). *Principles of developmental psychology*. Lawrence Erlbaum, Hove.

Cavada, C. and Goldman-Rakic, P. S. (1989). Posterior parietal cortex in rhesus monkey. I: Parcellation of areas based on distinctive limbic and sensory corticocortical connections. *Journal of Comparative Neurology*, **287**, 393–421.

Colby, C. L. and Goldberg, M. E. (1999). Space and attention in parietal cortex. *Annual Review of Neuroscience*, **22**, 319–349.

Cowey, A., Small, M., and Ellis, S. (1994). Left visuo-spatial neglect can be worse in far than in near space. *Neuropsychologia*, **32**, 1059–66.

Cowey, A., Small, M., and Ellis, S. (1999). No abrupt change in visual hemineglect from near to far space. *Neuropsychologia*, **37**, 1–6.

Cutting, J. E. and Vishton, P. M. (1995). Perceiving layout and knowing distances: The integration, relative potency, and contextual us of different information about depth. In *Handbook of perception and cognition*, Vol. 5 (ed. W. Epstein and S. Rogers), pp. 69–117. Academic Press, San Diego, CA.

di Pellegrino, G., Làdavas, E., and Farnè, A. (1997). Seeing where your hands are. *Nature*, **388**, 730.

Farnè, A. and Làdavas, E. (2000). E. Dynamic size-change of hand peripersonal space following tool use. *Neuroreport*, **11**, 1645–9.

Fogassi, L., Gallese, V., Fadiga, L., Luppino, G., Matelli, M., and Rizzolatti. (1996). Coding of peripersonal space in inferior premotor cortex (area F4). *Journal of Neurophysiology*, **76**, 141–57.

Frassinetti, F., Rossi, M., and Làdavas, E. (2001). Passive limb movements improve visual neglect. *Neuropsychologia*, **39**, 725–33.

Gentilucci, M., Scandolara, C., Pigarev, I. N., and Rizzolatti, G. (1983). Visual responses in the postarcuate cortex (area 6) of the monkey that are independent of eye position. *Experimental Brain Research*, **50**, 464–8.

Gentilucci, M., Fogassi, L., Luppino, G. Matelli, M., Camarda, R., and Rizzolatti, G. (1988). Functional organization of inferior area 6 in the macaque monkey. I. Somatotopy and the control of proximal movements. *Experimental Brain Research*, **71**, 475–90.

Godschalk, M., Lemon, R. N., Kuypers, H. G., and Ronday, H. K. (1984). Cortical afferents and efferents of monkey postarcuate area: an anatomical and electrophysiological study. *Experimental Brain Research*, **56**, 410–24.

Goldberg, M. E. and Bruce, C. J. (1990). Primate frontal eye fields. III: Maintenance of a spatially accurate saccade signal. *Journal of Neurophysiology*, **64**, 489–508.

Graziano, M. S. A. and Gross, C. G. (1995). The representation of extrapersonal space: possible role for bimodal, visual–tactile neurons. In *The cognitive neuroscience* (ed. M. Gazzaniga), pp. 1021–33. MIT Press, Cambridge, MA.

Grüsser, O. J. (1983). Multimodal structure of the extrapersonal space. In *Spatially oriented behavior* (ed. A. Hein and M. Jeannerod), pp. 327–52. Plenum Press, New York.

Halligan, P. and Marshall, J. M. (1991). Left neglect for near but not for far space in man. *Nature*, **350**, 498–500.

Heilman, K. M., Watson, R. T., Valenstein, E. (1993). Neglect and related disorders. In *Clinical neuropsychology* (3rd edn) (ed. K. M. Heilman and E. Valenstein), pp. 279–335. Oxford University Press.

Kinsbourne, M. (1993). Orientational bias model of unilateral neglect: evidence from attentional gradients within hemispace. In *Unilateral neglect: clinical and experimental studies* (ed. I. H. Robertson and J. C. Marshall), pp. 63–86. Lawrence Erlbaum, Hove.

Iriki, A., Tanaka, M., and Iwamura, Y. (1996). Coding of modified body schema during tool use by macaque post-central neurons. *Neuroreport*, **7**, 2325–30.

Làdavas, E., Zeloni, G., and Farnè, A. (1998). Visual peripersonal space centred on the face in humans. *Brain*, **121**, 2317–26.

Maravita, A., Husain, H., Clarke, K., and Driver, J. (2001). Reaching with a tool extends visual-tactile interactions into far space: evidence from cross-modal extinction. *Neuropsychologia*, **39**, 580–5.

Matelli, M., Camarda, R., Glickstein, M., and Rizzolatti, G. (1986). Afferent and efferent projections of the inferior area 6 in the macaque monkey. *Journal of Comparative Neurology*, **251**, 281–98.

Massironi, M., Antonucci, G., Pizzamiglio, L., Vitale, M. V., and Zoccolotti, P. (1988). The Wundt–Jastrow illusion in the study of spatial hemi-inattention. *Neuropsychologia*, **26**, 161–6.

Mountcastle, V. B. (1976). The word around us: neural command functions for selective attention. *Neurosciences Research Program Bulletin*, **14**, 1–47.

Mountcastle, V. B., Lynch, J. C., Georgopoulos, A., Sakata, H., and Acuna, C. (1975). Posterior parietal association cortex of the monkey: command functions for operations within extrapersonal space. *Journal of Neurophysiology*, **38**, 871–908.

Petrides, M. and Pandya, D. N. (1984). Projections to the frontal cortex from the posterior parietal region in the rheus monkey. *Journal of Comparative Neurology*, **228**, 105–116.

Piaget, J. (1936). *La naissance de l'intelligence chez l'enfant*. Delachauw et Niestlé, Neuchatel.

Pitzalis, S., Di Russo, F., Spinelli, D., and Zoccolotti, P. (2001). Influence of the radial and vertical dimension on lateral neglect. *Experimental Brain Research*, **136**, 281–94.

Pizzamiglio, L., Cappa, S., Vallar, G. *et al.* (1989). Visual neglect for far and near extra-personal space in humans. *Cortex*, **25**, 471–7.

Previc, F. H. (1990). Functional specialization in the lower and upper visual field in humans: Its ecological origin and neurophysiological implications. *Behavioral and Brain Sciences*, **13**, 559–66.

Previc, F. H. (1998). The neuropsychology of 3-D space. *Psychological Bulletin*, **124**, 123–64.

Rizzolatti, G., Scandolara, C., Matelli, M., and Gentilucci, M. (1981*a*). Afferent properties of peri-arcuate neurons in macaque monkeys. I: Somato-sensory responses. *Behavioral Brain Research*, **2**, 125–46.

Rizzolatti, G., Scandolara, C., Matelli, M., and Gentilucci, M. (1981*b*). Afferent properties of periarcuate neurons in macaque monkeys. II: Visual responses. *Behavioral Brain Research*, **2**, 147–63.

Rizzolatti, G., Matelli, M., and Pavesi, G. (1983). Deficits in attention and movement following he removal of postarcuate (area 6) cortex in macaque monkeys. *Brain*, **106**, 655–73.

Rizzolatti, G., Fadiga, L., Fogassi, L, and Gallese V. (1997). The space around us. *Science*, **277**, 190–1.

Rizzolatti, G., Luppino, G., and Matelli, M. (1998). The organization of the cortical motor system: new concepts. *Electroencephalography and Clinical Neurophysiology*, **106**, 283–96.

Rizzolatti, G., Berti, A., and Gallese, V. (2000). Spatial neglect: neurophysiological bases, cortical circuit and theories. In *Handbook of neuropsychology*, Vol. 1 (ed. F. Boller, J. Grafman, and G. Rizzolatti), pp. 503–37. Elsevier, Amsterdam.

Snyder, L. H., Batista, A. P., and Andersen, R. A. (1997). Coding of intention in the posterior parietal cortex. *Nature*, **386**, 122–3.

Vuilleumier, P., Valenza, N., Mayer, E., Reverdin, A., and Landis, T. (1998). Near and far visual space in unilateral neglect. *Annals of Neurology*, **43**, 406–10.

Weiss, P. H., Marshall, J. C., Wunderlich, G., *et al.* (2000). Neural consequences of acting in near versus far space: a physiological basis for clinical dissociations. *Brain*, **123**, 2531–41.

Zipser, D. and Andersen, R. A. (1988). A backpropagation programmed network that simulates response properties of a subset of posterior parietal neurons. *Nature*, **331**, 679–84.

3.4 Visual peripersonal space in humans

Elisabetta Làdavas

The processing of space is not unitary, but is divided among several brain areas, which code particular locations in space, and several coordinate systems. Contemporary neurophysiology has revealed brain areas that appear specialized for the coding of visual space surrounding the body (peripersonal space). This space is coded at the level of single neurons through the integration of sensory information from different modalities (for a review see Graziano and Gross (1998)). These neurons respond to both tactile and visual stimuli, provided that the visual stimulus is presented within the visual receptive field (RF) extending outward from the tactile RF of a given neuron (Rizzolatti *et al.* 1981; Duhamel *et al.* 1991; Graziano and Gross 1995; Iriki *et al.* 1996). Single-cell recording studies in monkeys have shown that this multimodal integration occurs in a number of cortical and subcortical structures. The premotor area PMv (approximately corresponding to area F4 (Rizzolatti *et al.* 1998)), the putamen, the post-central gyrus, and parietal areas 7b and VIP contain a relatively high number of bimodal neurons.

These bimodal cells have visual–tactile RFs predominantly distributed over the face, arm, hand, and upper part of the animal's body and they share some basic functional properties:

(1) visual and tactile RFs are in spatial register, i.e. visual RFs match the location of tactile RFs on the body surface;

(2) visual RFs have a limited extension in depth, being restricted to the space immediately surrounding the monkey's hand, face, or body;

(3) visual related activity shows a response gradient, i.e. the discharge decreases as the distance between visual stimulus and cutaneous RF increases;

(4) visual RFs operate in coordinate systems centered on body parts, i.e. they remain anchored to the tactile RFs of a given body part when this is moved, and their spatial location does not change when the eyes move.

Taken together, these properties indicate that ventral premotor cortex, parietal areas, and putamen form an interconnected system for integrated (visual–tactile) coding of peripersonal space centered on body parts (Colby *et al.* 1993; Fogassi *et al.* 1996a,b; Graziano *et al.* 1997; Duhamel *et al.* 1998).

One advantage of such body-part-centered coordinates is that sensory information about the location of the object can serve as a sensory input to the motor system concerned with movements toward objects in space. Therefore these neurons appear to form a sensory–motor interface, encoding the location of the target in the same spatial coordinate system that is used to control the arm or the head. Cells in the putamen, the VIP area, and the inferior area 6 (PMv) have motor functions as well as sensory functions. Indeed, the same neurons often have both sensory and motor activity and many of them respond only when the animal makes a voluntary movement (Rizzolatti *et al.* 1981; Alexander 1987; Fogassi *et al.* 1996*a*). The interesting point is that the neuron controlling body movements on the basis of cutaneous information can also control body movements on the basis of visual information. This could allow the neuron to localize the stimulus even when the skin is not stimulated and to produce an appropriate movement in response to it. Therefore these neurons can encode the distance and position from a body part to a nearby visual stimulus. Such information specifies the distance and direction the body part must move to reach or avoid the stimulus (Bruce 1990; Fogassi *et al.* 1996*b*). Thus, bimodal neurons with receptive fields located on the arm are useful for guiding the arm toward or away from nearby stimuli, and bimodal neurons with receptive fields located on the face are useful for guiding the head. This is a very important function because, even for a very 'simple' action such as avoiding a stimulus coming towards the face or the hand, reaching to grasp an object, or putting food into the mouth, it is necessary to know the position of the visual stimulus relative to the head, the hand, or both. Thus this information is most probably provided by the bimodal visuotactile neurons described in physiological studies.

Direct evidence for the notion that these areas encode the location of sensory stimuli and generate motor responses to such stimuli has been provided in a monkey study by Rizzolatti *et al.* (1983) in which lesions of PMv disrupted the animal's ability to avoid or to bite nearby visual stimuli. Surgical ablation of this area caused neglect only for the peripersonal space around the animals' mouth (peribuccal space), and abolished mouth grasping or licking responses to contralesional tactile and peripersonal visual stimuli.

Despite several single-cell studies, the representation of near space in humans has been little investigated. In this chapter we review evidence of the existence of a visual peripersonal space in humans that appears to be codified by an integrated visuotactile system. First, we review the evidence of the existence of the peripersonal space centered on the hand and on the face. Second, we describe the functional properties of this space, i.e. whether the spatial mapping between vision and touch which takes place in the peripersonal space is determined by a cross-modal interaction between vision and touch or whether it is also determined by the proprioceptive information related to the position of the body part. Finally, we address the dynamic aspect of the peripersonal space, i.e. whether this space is fixed or whether it can be expanded or reduced depending on the action performed in space.

Visual peripersonal space in humans

The existence of a peripersonal space in humans can be verified by studying patients with tactile extinction. Patients with unilateral brain lesion may fail to report a single stimulus presented on the contralesional side when a competing stimulus is presented simultaneously on the ipsilesional side, even though they can report either stimulus when it is presented alone. This phenomenon has been called 'extinction'.

Extinction has been attributed to unbalanced competition between simultaneous targets for access to a limited pool of attentional resources (Ward *et al.* 1994; Desimone and Duncan 1995). The unilateral damage of a brain area with a contralateral field representation determines a reduction of competitive weights assigned to stimuli in the affected field. As a consequence, stimuli presented in the contralesional space weakly activate that portion of space and therefore they are extinguished due to the competition with the stimuli presented in the intact ipsilesional space. It has been shown that extinction may occur within different sensory modalities (unimodal extinction): visual (Làdavas 1990; Ward *et al.* 1994; di Pellegrino and De Renzi 1995), auditory (De Renzi *et al.* 1984), and tactile (Bender 1952; Gainotti *et al.* 1989; Moscovitch and Behrmann 1994; Vallar *et al.* 1994). One interesting issue concerning extinction is whether the competition for selection operates across spatial representations based on different sensory modalities. More specifically, the question addressed is whether the antagonism between left and right space representations in one modality, which is the distinctive feature of extinction patients, can be modulated (i.e. reduced or exacerbated) by the activation of an intact spatial representation in a different modality. The prediction is that this phenomenon might occur only if the two different spatial representations interact with one another through mutual excitation or inhibition. When competition is biased in favor of the right tactile space representation, as the case of a patient with left tactile extinction, the activation of a right visual representation of space might produce a deficit even in the detection of a single left tactile stimulus (cross-modal visual–tactile extinction). This is because, owing to the activity of visuotactile bimodal neurons, a visual stimulus presented near the hand should be able to activate the somatosensory representation of that hand which will then compete with the somatosensory representation of the left hand. In contrast, a visual stimulus presented far from the hand, i.e. in the extrapersonal space, should not produce a cross-modal visual–tactile extinction because this sector of space is not coded by an integrated visuotactile system.

Visual peripersonal space centered on the hand

The existence of a visual peripersonal space has been shown by Làdavas *et al.* (1998*a*) in 10 right-brain-damaged (RBD) patients who suffered from reliable tactile extinction. In this experiment, a visual stimulus presented near the patient's ipsilesional hand (i.e. visual peripersonal space) inhibited the processing of a tactile stimulus delivered on the contralesional hand (cross-modal visuotactile extinction) to the same extent as did an ipsilesional tactile stimulation (unimodal tactile extinction). In striking contrast, less modulatory effects of vision on touch perception were observed when a visual stimulus was presented far from the space immediately around the patient's hand (i.e. extrapersonal space). Because extinction becomes manifest when there is a competition between two or more spatial representations, the simultaneous activation of somatosensory representation of the left hand by a tactile stimulus and of the right hand by a visual stimulus presented in the peripersonal space produces an extinction of those stimuli presented in the weaker representation, in this case that of the left hand. Instead, the same visual stimulus presented in the extrapersonal space induces an impressive reduction of cross-modal visual–tactile extinction. The weak modulatory effect of far visual stimuli on touch is consistent with single-neuron studies showing that visuotactile bimodal cells are less responsive when visual stimuli are administered far from the hand, i.e. in the extrapersonal space (Gentilucci *et al.* 1988; Graziano *et al.* 1994). In conclusion, the results of this study clearly showed the existence of a peripersonal space around the hand in humans. Moreover, the results of a single case study (di Pellegrino *et al.* 1997) seem to show that cross-modal visuotactile extinction is not modulated by the position of the hands in space. When a patient with tactile extinction was asked to cross the hands such that the left hand was in the right hemispace and the right hand in the left hemispace, a visual stimulus presented near the right hand (in the left space) extinguished tactile stimuli applied to the left hand (in right hemispace). This finding seems to suggest that, when the hand is moved, the peripersonal space remains anchored to the hand and therefore moves with it. Thus, it is possible to maintain that visual peripersonal space operates in coordinate systems centered on body parts.

Visual peripersonal space centered on the face

One interesting question is whether such peripersonal space also exists for other body parts. One body part which might be involved in the same mechanism is the face, and face-centered bimodal neurons have been identified in single-neuron studies. Again, as for the hand, visual stimuli delivered in the space near the ipsilesional side of the face in patients with tactile extinction extinguished tactile stimuli on the contralesional side (cross-modal visuotactile extinction) to the same extent as did an ipsilesional tactile stimulation (unimodal tactile extinction) (Làdavas et al. 1998b). However, when visual stimuli were delivered far from the face, visuotactile extinction effects were dramatically reduced. This is in accordance with single-neuron studies showing that visuotactile bimodal cells are less active when visual stimuli are administered far from the face, i.e. in the extrapersonal space (Gentilucci et al. 1988; Duhamel et al. 1991; Graziano and Gross 1994). Face-centered bimodal neurons have been shown to respond best to visual stimuli located in a spatial region 5 to 20 cm from the skin surface. These neurons can also be activated by visual stimuli located at greater distances but their response is substantially reduced (Duhamel et al. 1991, 1998; Graziano et al. 1994). Thus, bimodal neurons manifest varying responsiveness primarily as a function of the distance of the visual stimulus from the body surface, with their activation being higher at shorter distances. Therefore the strong cross-visuotactile extinction found when the visual stimulus is presented near the face and the mild cross-visuotactile extinction found when the visual stimulus is presented far from the face are fully compatible with the neurophysiological findings.

Thus, these studies suggest the existence of an integrated system controlling both visual and tactile inputs within peripersonal space around the face and the hand and show how this system is functionally separated from that controlling visual information in the extrapersonal space.

The relevance of the visual experience of the body part for the coding of peripersonal visual space

The relevance of sight of the hand for coding peripersonal space has been assessed by studies showing that only the visual experience of a body part produces cross-modal extinction or the feel–touch experience and the finding that peripersonal space can also be activated by sight of a rubber hand (see below). Moreover, it has recently been proved that sight of the hand, as well as being important for the feel–touch experience, enhances perception of visual stimuli presented in the peripersonal space (see below).

The visual experience of a body part produces cross-modal extinction and the feel–touch experience

Here evidence will be reported suggesting that the visual experience of the body can somehow 'boost' the signal strength to neuronal circuits associated with the feel–touch experience. The hands are continuously moved in space, and the brain has to compute their spatial position to update the visual mapping of the space surrounding the hand as posture changes. The position of the hand in space can be computed by the combined contribution of at least two pieces of sensory information, i.e. vision and proprioception (Rossetti et al. 1995). In the monkey, visual and proprioceptive cues about arm position converge on bimodal visual–tactile neurons, some of which also respond to peripersonal visual stimuli when the vision of the arm is presented to the monkey (Graziano et al. 1994). However, when information about arm position is provided by proprioception alone, the responsiveness of bimodal cells to peripersonal visual stimuli is substantially reduced (Graziano 1999) or even extinguished (MacKay and Crammond 1987), suggesting that visual information about a given body part might be more relevant than proprioceptive information.

In agreement with these neurophysiological data, a recent study conducted by Làdavas et al. (2000) on RBD patients with tactile extinction showed that proprioception alone is not sufficient to activate the representation of the hand-centered visual peripersonal space. In this study, visual stimuli were presented near to or far from the patient's ipsilesional hand while unseen tactile stimuli were concurrently delivered to the patient's contralesional hand. Sight of the ipsilesional hand could be either allowed or prevented. When sight of the hand was prevented, the amount of cross-modal extinction did not vary as a function of the distance of the visual stimulus from patients ipsilesional hand (i.e. near versus far). In other words, when hand position was specified only by means of proprioceptive cues, cross-modal extinction was not segregated in the peripersonal space. In contrast, when sight of the hand was allowed, tactile stimuli were more consistently extinguished by visual stimuli presented near the patient's ipsilesional hand than those presented far from it. These results demonstrate that the additional information provided by sight of the hand is necessary to find cross-modal effects segregated in the peripersonal space.

This finding is in accordance with that of Mattingley *et al.* (1997), who used a paradigm in many ways analogous to our own, and explains the lack of strong cross-modal links between vision and touch found by these authors. They studied the cross-modal interactions between vision and touch in three neurological patients suffering from both visual and tactile extinction, and found a mild cross-modal inhibitory effect when visual stimuli were presented either far from or near the ipsilesional hand, without any significant difference between the two conditions. However, in the study by Mattingley *et al.*, visual stimuli were always presented when the patient's view of the hand was obscured. Thus their results are consistent with our observation (Làdavas *et al.* 2000) that only a mild cross-modal inhibitory effect is obtained when patients cannot see their hands. In contrast, a strong cross-modal inhibitory effect is found only in the condition in which patients can see their hands being visually stimulated in the peripersonal space.

The notion that visual experience of a body part is linked with the feel–touch experience has also been confirmed in brain-damaged patients with dense hemisensory loss of the upper limb, without extinction or neglect (Halligan *et al.* 1996, 1997). These patients reported that they experienced a tactile sensation on the affected hand only if they were allowed to see the hand being touched by the experimenter. In one patient, an image on screen of the affected hand being touched produced reports of a tactile sensation, even if no real touch occurred (Halligan *et al.* 1997). A related phenomenon has been described in patients with phantom sensations. Visual, auditory, and olfactory phantom sensations have been reported after deafferentation of the corresponding sense organs, but the most obvious phantom phenomena are somesthetic in nature. Ramachandran and Rogers-Ramachandran (1996) have shown that the reflection of the normal arm in a vertical mirror generated a compelling visual perception of the missing arm in six arm amputees. This visual perception interacted with the somatic phantom sensation so effectively that patients reported vivid tactile sensations on the phantom when they viewed the experimenter touching the mirror image of their normal arm. This phenomenon can be explained by assuming that the virtual visual stimulus arising from the non-existing limb can activate the bimodal neurons that normally integrate tactile and visual inputs from that limb.

These findings suggest that visual information about hand position in space, as well as being necessary, can also be sufficient for mediating the integrated processing of visual–tactile input in the peripersonal space. This suggestion has been verified more directly in animal studies, as well as in patients with tactile extinction and in normal subjects by using the visual experience of a rubber hand.

The visual experience of a rubber hand produces cross-modal extinction and experience of feel touch

The responses of single neurons in area 5 while proprioceptive and visual information about arm position were independently manipulated have been assessed in animal studies (Graziano 1999).

In this investigation, the monkey's real arm was hidden from the view with a shield and a realistic fake arm was visible above the shield and placed either at the same location or at a different location from the monkey's own arm. It was found that many area 5 neurons were also modulated by the sight of the fake arm. To exclude an explanation of the findings in terms of changes in arousal or attentional cueing due to the sight of the fake arm, control experiments showed that neurons that responded to the sight of the arm were not affected by the sight of other visual objects (e.g. apple slices) placed at that location. Moreover, when the fake arm was placed backwards, such that the fingers were near the monkey's shoulder, area 5 neurons failed to respond to its position in space. Finally, when a left fake arm was attached to the right shoulder, visual modulation also vanished.

The hypothesis that the sight of a rubber hand might mediate the activation of corresponding visual peripersonal space representation has been recently verified also in humans (Farnè et al. 2000). To test this hypothesis, a group of RBD patients with tactile extinction were tested in two experimental settings using a cross-modal stimulation paradigm. In the first setting, visual stimuli were presented near or far from the patient's ipsilesional hand; in the second setting, visual stimuli were always presented far from the ipsilesional hand, which was placed behind the patient's back, but near a rubber hand that could be either visually aligned or misaligned with the patient's ipsilesional shoulder. In both situations, unseen tactile stimuli were delivered to the patient's contralesional hand. In patients with left tactile extinction, a visual stimulus presented near a right rubber hand which could be seen induced a strong cross-modal visual–tactile extinction, comparable to that obtained by presenting the same visual stimulus near the patient's right hand. Critically, this cross-modal effect was only found when the subject saw the rubber hand with a plausible posture relative to his or her own body (i.e. when it was aligned with the subject's right shoulder). In contrast, cross-modal extinction was strongly reduced when the rubber hand was arranged in an implausible posture (i.e. misaligned with respect to the subject's right shoulder). These results replicate the neurophysiological data and show that, owing to the dominance of vision over proprioception, the system coding peripersonal space can be deceived by the vision of a fake hand provided that its appearance looks plausible with respect to the subject's body.

In some circumstances, the visual bias of proprioception (Hay et al. 1965) can be strong enough to induce a healthy subject to perceive his or her hand in the position occupied by a rubber hand which can be seen (Botvinick and Cohen 1998, Pavani et al. 2000). Botvinick and Cohen (1998) demonstrated that after subjects looked at a rubber hand being stroked with a paintbrush, while receiving a synchronous stroke on their own hidden hand, they experienced the illusion that tactile sensations came from the seen rubber hand, which they felt as belonging to themselves. When required to indicate the felt position of their hidden hand they pointed towards the position of the rubber hand, showing that this illusion results from distorted proprioceptive information. Interestingly, Pavani et al. (2000) have shown that this illusory effect disappears when the subject sees the rubber hand in an implausible posture with respect to his or her own body, i.e. when it is not aligned with the shoulder.

All these studies show that, owing to this visual dominance over proprioception, a rubber hand appearing in a plausible posture relative to the subject's shoulder can deceive the integrated visual–tactile system in such a way that a visual stimulus, actually presented far from the subject's real hand, is processed as if it were in the peripersonal space. Although prima facie this deception could be considered rather surprising, it can be better understood as the result of a normal adaptive process. Since the visual response of monkeys' bimodal neurons do not change after repeated series of stimulation (Graziano et al. 1997), it has been suggested that their functional properties are hardwired, and the spatial correspondence between visual and tactile RFs can be calibrated through experience, perhaps within a critical period early in life (Salinas and Abbot 1995; Graziano et al. 1997). In the case of hand-centered bimodal neurons, the obvious crucial experience through which the spatial calibration is achieved consists in repeated exposure to visual stimuli approaching the hand, and vice versa. On almost all these occasions, both the visual stimulus and the hand are under visual control, and the felt position of the hand is congruent with its seen position. Thus, the deception operated by a rubber hand seems to reflect a sort of impenetrability of the integrated visual–tactile system to discrepant information provided by proprioception that, in Bayesian terms, will normally have little chance of being dissociated by vision.

The sight of the body part enhances perception of visual stimuli presented in the peripersonal space

One interesting question which needs to be addressed is whether the sight of the hand, as well as being important for the feel–touch experience, enhances perception of visual stimuli presented in the peripersonal space. Hari and Jousmaki (1996) were the first to report that motor reactions to visual stimuli were 20 to 40 ms faster when they fell on the reacting fingers than when they were a few centimeters away from them. Previous visual reaction time studies have missed this effect, evidently because the subjects in visual perception tasks typically react to stimuli presented on a screen and not on their bodies. This finding has recently been confirmed in a patient with left visual extinction (di Pellegrino and Frassinetti 2001). The patient's report of a contralesional visual target was considerably ameliorated when he placed his left hand adjacent to the spatial location of the left visual target. This effect was not a consequence of patient's hand acting as a spatial cue, because the presentation of a visual cue of the same size and shape as the hand at the hand's location did not reduce his level of extinction for the left visual stimulus. Importantly, the authors also noted that when patient's left hand was placed adjacent to the left visual stimulus but was hidden from his view, his visual extinction returned to previous levels. Therefore, it seems that the patient's visual extinction was only reduced when he could 'see' his hand in the left visual field.

So far we have stressed the relevance of the visual experience of the body part. However, there is one case in which cross-modal interactions between vision and touch in peripersonal space is modulated by a third modality (e.g. proprioception). As has been mentioned above, strong cross-modal effects between touch and vision in the peripersonal space have also been found centered on the face (Làdavas *et al.* 1998*b*), which is never under the subject's visual control. Thus, this seems to be a particular case in which the relevant information about the spatial location of the tactile receptive field may be mediated by proprioception. Because the face cannot be visually experienced by the subject, the characteristics of the bimodal cells responsible for coding visual peripersonal space centered on the face may be functionally different from those of bimodal neurons coding peripersonal space centered on the hand. Indeed, in the case of bimodal neurons with tactile receptive fields on the face, the best visual response is evoked by a stimulus approaching the body surface along a precise trajectory which would ideally bring the stimulus in contact with the tactile receptive field. Thus the main variable affecting neuron discharge in this case seems to be the direction of the approaching stimulus with respect to the tactile receptive field (Duhamel *et al.* 1998); in other words, these neurons are directionally selective. In contrast, in the case of bimodal neurons with tactile receptive fields on the hand, the best visual response is evoked by a stimulus approaching the seen hand. Thus, it seems that, as far as the role of proprioception is concerned, the characteristics of bimodal cells responsible for coding visual peripersonal space centered on the face may be functionally different from those of bimodal neurons coding peripersonal space centered on the hand.

Is peripersonal space fixed or dynamic?

An interesting question related to peripersonal space is whether the spatial extension of peri-hand space representation in humans is fixed or can be rapidly modified. The dynamic property of the visual peripersonal space has been investigated in a recent study by Farnè and Làdavas (2000). In this study, the authors tested the prediction that tool use could induce a transient elongation of hand-centered peripersonal space along the tool axis, i.e. the spatial extent of the representation of peri-hand visual space could be increased to incorporate the tool. To address this issue, the authors applied a cross-modal paradigm, well suited to revealing visual–tactile integration near the subject's hand, to a group of RBD patients with tactile extinction. Throughout the investigation, cross-modal visual–tactile extinction was assessed by presenting visual stimuli far from the patient's ipsilesional hand, corresponding to the distal edge of a rake held statically in the hand. The patient's performance was evaluated before tool use, immediately after using the tool for a period of 5 min, and after a rest period of a further 5 to 10 min. To exclude any possible confounding due to motor activity, cross-modal extinction was also assessed immediately after a 5-min period of pointing movements not involving the tool.

The authors found that cross-modal extinction was more severe after the patients used the rake to retrieve distant objects than when the rake was not used. Thus, they showed that visual peri-hand space has important dynamic properties; it can be expanded depending upon tool use. The evidence of an expansion of peri-hand space lasted for only few minutes after tool use. Cross-modal extinction was substantially reduced after a period of 5 to 10 min when the patient held the tool without being involved in any motor activity. After the rest period, the amount of cross-modal extinction was comparable to that obtained before tool use, suggesting that the spatial extension of the hand peripersonal space contracted towards the patient's hand. Finally, the study showed that the expansion of hand peripersonal space is strictly dependent upon the use of the tool, aimed at physically reaching distant objects, and does not merely result from directional motor activity. Cross-modal extinction, as assessed after patients performed pointing movements with their right hand towards distant objects, was entirely comparable to that obtained in the pre-tool-use condition. Therefore motor activity *per se* is not sufficient to expand peri-hand space. In contrast, the plasticity of peri-hand space seems to rely on the possibility of reaching objects located outside the hand reaching space. In conclusion, these results provide direct evidence that the representation of peri-hand space can be expanded along the tool axis to include its length and shows that re-mapping of far space as near space can be achieved through a re-sizing of the peri-hand area where visual–tactile integration occurs.

A similar re-coding of far visual stimuli as near ones has recently been observed in monkey single cells by using a long tool to connect the hand with a visual stimulus located in distant space (Iriki *et al.* 1996). Actually, the visual RFs of bimodal neurons studied by Iriki and colleagues were elongated after few minutes of tool use, and contracted towards the hand after a longer delay even if the monkey was still holding the rake. A phenomenon which can entirely be explained by the expansion of peri-hand space was recently reported by Berti and Frassinetti (2000) in a neglect patient affected by a selective deficit in the reaching space. Their result can be interpreted in terms of incorporation of a tool as a physical extension of the hand that it is due to an expansion of the visual–tactile integration area surrounding the hand (see Chapter 3.3).

A re-coding of far visual stimuli as near ones, leading to an increase in cross-modal tactile–visual interactions, has recently been observed in the behavior of neurological patients in a somewhat different context (Maravita *et al.* 2000). In a patient with tactile extinction, a visual event at the same far distance (in terms of the visual image) produced more cross-modal extinction when it was known to be the mirror reflection of an event near the true location of the patient's ipsilesional hand. A flash of light actually delivered close to the right hand, but appearing in far space because it was observed in a mirror, produced very similar effects to those produced by a light which was directly viewed near the hand in peripersonal space. In other words, this patient, when seeing his own hand in a mirror, activates a representation of the peripersonal space around that hand rather than the extrapersonal space suggested by the distant visual image in the mirror. Thus a mirror can be considered as a different kind of tool which allows objects located in far space to be treated as if they were close to the actual location of the patient's hand.

In summary, tools enable human beings, as well as other animals, to act on objects which cannot be reached directly with their hands. Acting on distant objects by means of a tool requires sensory information that is mainly provided by vision and touch. The expansion of the peri-hand area whereby vision and touch are integrated makes it possible to reach and manipulate far objects as if they were near the hand.

References

Alexander, G. E. (1987). Selective neuronal discharge in monkey putamen reflects intended direction of planned limb movements. *Experimental Brain Research*, **67**, 623–34.

Bender, M. B. (1952). *Disorders in perception*. C. C. Thomas, Springfield, IL.

Berti, A. and Frassinetti, F. (2000). When far becomes near, remapping of space by tool use. *Journal of Cognitive Neuroscience*, **3**, 415–20.

Botvinick, M. and Cohen, J. (1998). Rubber hands 'feel' touch that eyes see. *Nature*, **391**, 756.

Bruce, C. J. (1990). Integration of sensory and motor signals in primate frontal eye fields. In *From signal and sense: local and global order in perceptual maps* (ed. G. M. Edelman, W. E. Gall, and W. M. Cowan), pp. 261–314. Wiley–Liss, New York.

Colby, C. L., Duhamel, J. R., and Goldberg, M. E. (1993). Ventral intraparietal area of the macaque, anatomic location and visual properties. *Journal of Neurophysiology*, **69**, 902–14.

De Renzi, E., Gentilini, M., and Pattacini, F. (1984). Auditory extinction following hemisphere damage. *Neuropsychologia*, **22**, 1231–40.

Desimone, R. and Duncan, J. (1995). Neural mechanisms of selective visual attention. *Annual Review of NeuroscienceD*, **18**, 193–222.

di Pellegrino, G. and De Renzi, E. (1995). An experimental investigation on the nature of extinction. *Neuropsychologia*, **33**, 153–70.

di Pellegrino, G. and Frassinetti, F. (2001). Direct evidence from parietal extinction of enhancement of visual attention near a visible hand. *Current Biology*, **10**, 1475–7.

di Pellegrino, G., Làdavas, E., and Farnè, A (1997). Seeing where your hands are. *Nature*, **338**, 730.

Duhamel, J. R., Colby, C. L., and Goldberg, M. E. (1991). Congruent representation of visual and somatosensory space in single neurons of monkey ventral intra-parietal area (area VIP). In *Brain and space* (ed. J. Paillard), pp. 223–36. Oxford University Press, New York.

Duhamel, J. R., Colby, C. L., and Goldberg, M. E. (1998). Ventral intraparietal area of the macaque, congruent visual and somatic response properties. *Journal of Neurophysiology*, **79**, 126–36.

Farnè, A. and Làdavas, E. (2000). Dynamic size-change of hand peripersonal space following tool use. *NeuroReport*, **85**, 1645–9.

Farnè, A., Pavani, F., Meneghello, F., and Làdavas, E. (2000). Left tactile extinction following visual stimulation of a rubber hand. *Brain*, **123**, 2350–60.

Fogassi, L., Gallese, V., Fadiga, L., Luppino, G., Matelli, M., and Rizzolatti, G. (1996*a*). Coding of peripersonal space in inferior premotor cortex (area F4). *Journal of Neurophysiology*, **76**, 141–57.

Fogassi, L., Gallese, V., Fadiga, L., and Rizzolatti, G. (1996*b*). Space coding in inferior premotor cortex (area F4): facts and speculations. In *Neural bases of motor behaviour* (ed. F. Lacquaniti and P. Viviani), pp. 99–120. Kluwer, Dordrecht.

Gainotti, G., De Bonis, C., Daniele, A., and Caltagirone, C. (1989). Contralateral and ipsilateral tactile extinction in patients with right and left focal brain damage. *International Journal of Neuroscience*, **45**, 81–9.

Gentilucci, M., Scandolara, C., Pigarev, I. N., and Rizzolatti, G. (1983). Visual responses in the postarcuate cortex (area 6) of the monkey that are independent of eye position. *Experimental Brain Research*, **50**, 464–8.

Gentilucci, M., Fogassi, L., Luppino, G., Matelli, M., Camarda, R. M., and Rizzolatti, G. (1988). Functional organization of inferior area 6 in the macaque monkey. I: Somatotopy and the control of proximal movements. *Experimental Brain Research*, **71**, 475–90.

Graziano, M. S. (1999). Where is my arm? The relative role of vision and proprioception in the neuronal representation of limb position. *Proceedings of the National Academy of Sciences of the United States of America*, **96**, 10418–21.

Graziano, M. S. A. and Gross, C. G. (1994). Mapping space with neurons. *Current Directions in Psychological Science*, **3**, 164–7.

Graziano, M. S. A. and Gross, C. G. (1995). The representation of extrapersonal space, a possible role for bimodal, visuo-tactile neurons. In *The cognitive neurosciences* (ed. M. S. Gazzaniga), pp. 1021–34. MIT Press, Cambridge, MA.

Graziano, M. S. A. and Gross, C. G. (1998). Spatial maps for the control of movement. *Current Opinion in Neurobiology*, **8**, 195–201.

Graziano, M. S., Yap, G. S., and Gross, C. G. (1994). Coding visual space by premotor neurons. *Science*, **266**, 1054–7.

Graziano, M. S., Hu, X. T., and Gross, C. G. (1997). Visuospatial properties of ventral premotor cortex. *Journal of Neurophysiology*, **77**, 2268–92.

Halligan, P. W., Hunt, M., Marshall, J. C., and Wade, D. T. (1996). When seeing is feeling, acquired synaesthesia or phantom touch? *Neurocase*, **2**, 21–9.

Halligan, P. W., Marshall, J. C., Hunt, M., and Wade, D. T. (1997). Somatosensory assessment, can seeing produce feeling? *Journal of Neurology*, **244**, 199–203.

Hari, R. and Jousmaki, V. (1996). Preference of personal to extrapersonal space in a visuomotor task. *Journal of Cognitive Neuroscience*, **3**, 305–7.

Hay, J. C., Pick, H. L., and Ikeda, K. (1965). Visual capture produced by prism spectacles. *Psychonomic Science*, **2**, 215–16.

Iriki, A., Tanaka, M., and Iwamura, Y. (1996). Coding of modified body schema during tool use by macaque postcentral neurones. *NeuroReport*, **7**, 2325–30.

Làdavas, E. (1990). Selective spatial attention in patients with visual extinction. *Brain*, **113**, 1527–38.

Làdavas, E., di Pellegrino, G., Farnè, A., and Zeloni, G. (1998a). Neuropsychological evidence of an integrated visuotactile representation of peripersonal space in humans. *Journal of Cognitive Neuroscience*, **10**, 581–9.

Làdavas, E., Zeloni, G., and Farnè, A. (1998b). Visual peripersonal space centred on the face in humans. *Brain*, **121**, 2317–26.

Làdavas, E., Farnè, A., Zeloni, G., and di Pellegrino, G. (2000). Seeing or not seeing where your hands are. *Experimental Brain Research*, **131**, 458–67.

MacKay, W. A. and Crammond, D. J. (1987). Neuronal correlates in posterior parietal lobe of the expectation of events. *Behavioural Brain Research*, **24**, 167–79.

Maravita, A., Spence, C., Clarke, K., Husain, M., and Driver, J. (2000). Vision and touch through the looking glass in a case of crossmodal extinction. *NeuroReport*, **169**, 3521–6.

Mattingley, J. B., Driver, J., Beschin, N., and Robertson, I. H. (1997). Attentional competition between modalities, extinction between touch and vision after right hemisphere damage. *Neuropsychologia*, **35**, 867–80.

Moscovitch, M. and Behrman, M. (1994). Coding of spatial information in the somatosensory system, evidence from patients with neglect following parietal lobe damage. *Journal of Cognitive Neuroscience*, **6**, 151–5.

Pavani, F., Spence, C., and Driver, J. (2000). Visual capture of touch, out-of-the-body experiences with rubber gloves. *Psychological Science*, **11**, 353–9.

Ramachandran, V. S. and Rogers-Ramachandran, D. (1996). Synaesthesia in phantom limbs induced with mirrors. *Proceedings of the Royal Society of London*, **263**, 377–86.

Rizzolatti, G., Scandolara, C., Matelli, M., and Gentilucci, M. (1981). Afferent properties of periarcuate neurons in macaque monkeys. II: Visual responses. *Behavioral and Brain Science*, **2**, 147–63.

Rizzolatti, G., Matelli, M., and Pavesi, G. (1983). Deficits in attention and movement following the removal of postarcuate (area 6) cortex in macaque monkey. *Brain*, **106**, 655–73.

Rizzolatti, G. *et al.* (1998).

Rossetti, Y., Desmurget, M., and Prablanc, C. (1995). Vectorial coding of movement, vision, proprioception or both? *Journal of Neurophysiology*, **74**, 457–63.

Salinas, E. and Abbot, L. F. (1995). Transfer of coded information from sensory to motor networks. *Journal of Neuroscience*, **15**, 6461–74.

Smania, N. and Aglioti, S. (1995). Sensory and spatial components of somaesthesic deficits following right brain damage. *Neurology*, **45**, 1725–30.

Vallar, G., Rusconi, M. L., Bignamini, L., Geminiani, G., and Perani, D. (1994). Anatomical correlates of visual and tactile extinction in humans: a clinical CT scan study. *Journal of Neurology, Neurosurgery and Psychiatry*, **57**, 464–70.

Ward, R., Goodrich, S., and Driver, J. (1994). Grouping reduces visual extinction, neuropsychological evidence for weight linkage in visual selection. *Visual Cognition*, **1**, 101–29.

Section 4 Perceptual and motor factors

4.1   Space anisometry in unilateral neglect

Edoardo Bisiach, Marco Neppi-Mòdona, and Raffaella Ricci

In a recent series of experiments, neglect patients reproduced horizontal extents on either side of a perceived or remembered extent (the 'model'). We shall describe these experiments and comment on their results, except for those investigations in which the patients were only asked to generate contralesional extents. The results of the latter investigations have unquestionable points of interest, but their explanatory potential is less complete.

In what follows, the abbreviations LE and RE will designate respectively left (contralesional) and right (ipsilesional) extensions generated by experimental subjects as a percentage of the extent that they had to reproduce. The terms 'contralesional over-extension' and 'contralesional under-extension' will always tacitly imply the qualifier 'relative'. In fact, they will not refer to absolute lengths but to the ratio of contralesional to ipsilesional extension.

Initial studies

The results of the first experiment in the series (Bisiach *et al.* 1994) are summarized in Table 1. In repeated trials, two left-neglect patients (AF and AS), both with a contralesional visual field defect (VFD), were asked to bisect a horizontal line 150 mm long and then mark the endpoints of a virtual line of that length with reference to its midpoint, printed in the middle of a sheet of paper (see Bisiach *et al.* (1994) for details). AF was examined and re-examined during three sessions at intervals of several days. In the second task, both patients consistently showed contralesional over-extension (LE/RE > 1), although the difference between LE and RE was not significant in the second session with patient AF.

Table 1 LE and RE as percentages of the extent that subjects were asked to reproduce

	%LE	%RE	LE/RE
Patient AF			
Session 1	90.52	47.25	1.92*
Session 2	97.07	75.47	1.29
Session 3	142.44	48.37	2.94*
Patient AS	96.27	79.37	1.21*

Asterisks indicate significant differences between LE and RE.
Data from Bisiach *et al.* (1994).

The experiment was replicated (as a part of a larger investigation) on 10 patients with left neglect and 10 right-brain-damaged patients without neglect (Bisiach *et al.* 1996). The results are reported in Table 2. Group means showed contralesional over-extension in neglect patients and contralesional under-extension in patients without neglect. Significant contralesional over-extension was found in five patients with neglect and one patient without neglect. Significant contralesional under-extension was found in one patient with neglect and six patients without neglect.

The results of a further experiment (Chokron *et al.* 1997) deserve particular attention. In that experiment, two left-neglect patients with no VFD were required to construct the right half of a line from the given left half or vice versa. The half-lines presented were 25, 75, or 100 mm long. With both subjects, the authors found a significant under-construction of the right half of the line and a significant over-construction of the left half. This result was more evident with longer half-lines. The interesting feature of the experiment was that patients constructed the missing half of each line on a computer screen by key pressing. This did not involve lateral hand movements and therefore prevented any confounding effect of what Heilman *et al.* (1985) called 'unilateral directional hypokinesia'.

Nico *et al.* (1999) investigated the influence of body-centered coordinates on the reproduction of horizontal extents in 10 left-neglect patients, 10 right-brain-damaged patients without neglect, and 10 age-matched healthy controls (Table 3). Subjects had to mark the missing endpoint of 150-mm virtual lines of which the midpoint and the left or right endpoints were shown. The task

Table 2 LE and RE as percentages of the extent that subjects were asked to reproduce

	%LE	%RE	LE/RE
10N+	113.09	101.59	1.11
10N−	85.45	91.80	0.93

	Left bias	No bias	Right bias
N+	5	4	1
N−	1	3	6

N+, neglect present; N−, neglect absent.
Data from Bisiach *et al.* (1996).

Table 3 LE and RE as percentages of the extent that subjects were asked to reproduce

	%LE	%RE	LE/RE
10 C			
Left hemispace	96.40	98.63	0.98
Center	97.96	97.31	1.01
Right hemispace	100.07	94.92	1.05
10 N−			
Left hemispace	96.67	98.73	0.98
Center	99.41	97.41	1.02
Right hemispace	100.28	97.53	1.03
10 N+			
Left hemispace	75.56	79.17	0.95
Center	87.19	76.08	1.15*
Right hemispace	97.51	76.29	1.28*

C, control subjects; N−, neglect absent; N+, neglect present. Asterisks indicate significant differences between LE and RE.
Data from Nico *et al.* (1999).

Table 4 LE and RE as percentages of the extent that subjects were asked to reproduce

	%LE	%RE	LE/RE
Perceived distance reproduction			
8 N+H+	110.00	76.00	1.44*
9 N+H–	89.00	88.00	1.01
5 N–H+	101.00	100.00	1.01
Remembered distance reproduction			
8 N+H+	109.00	78.00	1.40*
9 N+H–	92.00	89.00	1.03
5 N–H+	102.00	99.00	1.03

N+, neglect present; N–, neglect absent; H+, hemianopia present; H–, hemianopia absent.
Asterisks indicate significant differences between LE and RE.
Data from Doricchi and Angelelli (1999).

was executed on the left, on the right, and in a central location with respect to the sagittal midplane of the subject's trunk. In the group of neglect patients significant contralesional over-extension was found in the central location and in right hemispace, but not in left hemispace, where a non-significant contralesional under-extension was observed. The performance of control subjects and right-brain-damaged patients without neglect was fairly accurate in all locations.

The influence of contralesional VFD on the reproduction of horizontal extents was assessed by Doricchi and Angelelli (1999) (see also Chapter 4.5). Two tasks, similar to the task used by Nico *et al.* (1999), were given to eight patients with left neglect and left hemianopia, nine patients with left neglect but without hemianopia, and five patients (four with left and one with right brain damage) with contralesional hemianopia but without neglect. On the first task patients had to reproduce a perceived distance and on the second task they were asked to reproduce a remembered distance. On average, remarkable contralesional over-extension was found on both tasks in patients with neglect and hemianopia but not in patients who showed only neglect or only hemianopia (Table 4).

Complications

The fairly well-defined profile emerging from single-case or small-group studies was somewhat upset by the outcome of a much more extensive investigation on 91 left neglect patients, 43 right-brain-damaged patients without neglect, and 40 age-matched healthy controls (Bisiach *et al.* 1998). Subjects were asked to extend on each side, using a pencil, 75-mm lines to double their original length. Figure 1 shows the distributions of LE/RE for control subjects, patients with neglect, and patients without neglect based on the mean (1.02) and standard deviation (SD) (0.08) of the control group. The first three and the last three columns of each diagram show the number of subjects in whom the ratio LE/RE was above or below two SDs respectively. The proportion of patients with contralesional over-extension was higher in neglect patients (29.67 per cent) than in patients without neglect (20.93 per cent). Ipsilesional over-extension was present in 15.38 per cent of neglect patients and in only one patient without neglect.

At this point, the weaker and stronger implications of the results of experiments on horizontal size reproduction in neglect patients have to be considered. The weaker implication is that these results challenge current interpretations of unilateral neglect (Bisiach *et al.* 1994). Stronger (but much more problematical) implications concern the suitability of these results as a starting point for alternative explanations.

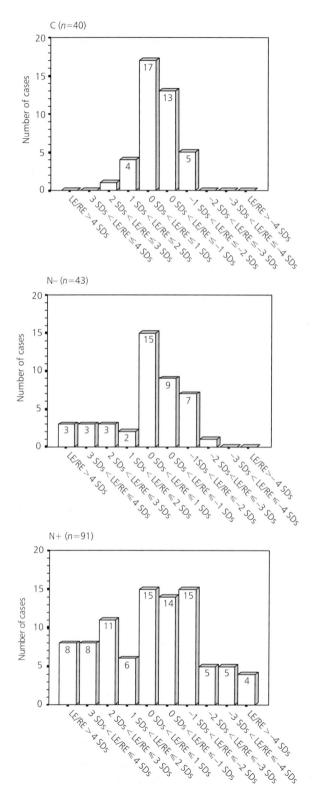

Figure 1 Distribution of LE/RE for control subjects (C), patients with neglect (N+), and patients without neglect (N–) based on the mean and SD of the control group. (Reproduced from Bisiach *et al*. 1998.)

It was suggested that contralesional over-extension could be the consequence of progressive contralesional relaxation of the medium for space representation, such that, for example, two horizontal lines lying side by side are only perceived as equal if the one on the contralesional side is actually longer (Bisiach *et al.* 1998; Bisiach *et al.* 1999 (Fig. 2(a)). This is in agreement with Milner and Harvey's (1995) interpretation of their well-known findings concerning the distortion of horizontal size perception in visuospatial neglect, and militates against an alternative interpretation of those findings in terms of mere imperception of the most contralateral portion of the contralesional stimulus in the visual matching task. The less frequent contralesional under-extension was tentatively interpreted instead as the consequence of contralesional over-relaxation of the representational medium, preventing, beyond a critical point, conscious representation (Fig. 2(b)).

At first sight, this hypothesis may look unfalsifiable. As a matter of fact, it is not. Indeed, it predicts (within certain limits) a higher degree of contralesional over-extension in the reproduction of shorter segments and, in agreement with the results obtained by Nico *et al.* (1999), in the reproduction of more ipsilesionally located segments. It is in fact evident from Fig. 2(b) that if the size of the segment to be extended only stretched, for example, over the two rightmost (arbitrary) units in the grain of the representational medium, left over-extension rather than under-extension would result. On the other hand, left under-extension would be more marked if the segment to be extended shown in Fig. 2(b) were more leftwardly located.

These two predictions were tested by asking 15 left-neglect patients to extend on either side, doubling their original length, 10- or 60-mm horizontal segments located on either side of egocentric space (Bisiach *et al.* 1999). Frontal lobe structures were involved by the lesion in eight patients and spared in seven. In general, both predictions were sustained, but with an unexpected and puzzling discrepancy (Fig. 3). The predicted line-length effect was clearly evident only in neglect patients with frontal lobe damage, while a nonsignificant trend towards an opposite effect was found in patients without frontal damage. In contrast, the predicted hemispace effect was clearly evident only in patients without frontal damage.

Interpretations and puzzles

An *ad interim* interpretation fitting these findings was envisaged. It was suggested that in patients with damage extending to the frontal lobe, neglect might mainly be framed in allocentric coordinates. This would exclude, or minimize, any effect of the working hemispace relative to the sagittal

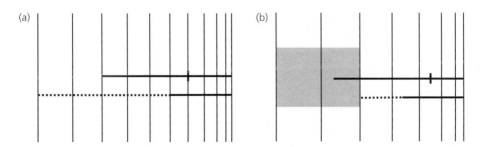

Figure 2 (a) A lower degree of contralesional relaxation of the medium for space representation causing a rightward bisection error (above) and left over-extension (below, dotted line). (b) A higher degree of contralesional relaxation of the medium for space representation causing rightward bisection error and left under-extension. The shading represents the neglected area in which the over-relaxed medium cannot sustain conscious representation. (Reproduced from Bisiach *et al.* 1999.)

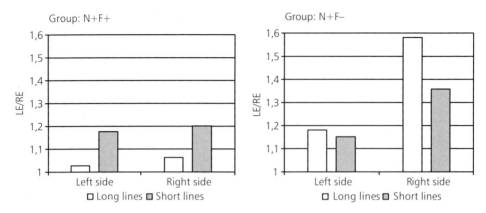

Figure 3 Effects of line length and side of presentation on relative left over-extension by neglect patients on the line extension task. (Reproduced from Bisiach *et al.* 1999.)

midplane of the patient's trunk. In contrast, in patients without frontal damage neglect might mainly be framed in egocentric coordinates, thus giving rise to an apparent hemispace effect. On the other hand, in this group of patients the critical point beyond which the over-relaxation of the medium for space representation can no longer sustain consciousness might be more peripherally located. If this were the case, these patients would, on the contralesional extension task, command a wider space within which (up to a certain limit) contralesional over-extension would actually be more pronounced with longer than with shorter lines.

Of course, this is an entirely *ad hoc* interpretation and must therefore be subjected to independent test. This is a matter for future research, along with other problematical points.

One of these points concerns the role played by contralesional visual field defects. Doricchi and Angelelli (1999) rightly suggested, on the basis of their findings, that concomitant hemianopia could be an important factor underlying contralesional over-extension in neglect patients. On a size-matching task, Ferber and Karnath (2001) found horizontal underestimation of left-sided stimuli in neglect patients with or without hemianopia, as well as in patients with hemianopia but without neglect. However, other findings clearly demonstrate that concomitant hemianopia is neither necessary nor sufficient to give rise to the phenomenon. As mentioned earlier, the two patients examined by Chokron *et al.* (1997) had no visual field defects, and an evident double dissociation between hemianopia and contralesional over-extension was found by Bisiach *et al.* (1998, pp. 343–4). Furthermore, Harvey and Kramer-McCaffery (2001) found horizontal under-estimation of contralesional stimuli in neglect patients, with no difference in performance due to the presence or absence of hemianopia, while right-brain-damaged patients with hemianopia but no neglect showed no left-to-right gradient in line-length estimation.

Another point concerns the negative findings from an experiment by Karnath and Ferber (1999) in which the distance between two points was horizontally reproduced by six neglect patients to the left or right of their subjective 'straight ahead'. There are two possible interpretations for the failure of these authors to demonstrate distortion of represented space. The less interesting interpretation is that their negative conclusion was at least in part based on the acceptance of the null hypothesis in the statistical analysis *vis-à-vis* an evident, albeit nonsignificant, contralesional over-extension. The other interpretation is more interesting and worth further investigation. In their experiment, distance reproduction took place after the disappearance of the model. Therefore shifting the workspace to either side of the subjective 'straight ahead' during reproduction could have correspondingly trailed an allocentric (horizontally anisometric) frame of reference, formerly centered on the model, with it (see also Chapter 4.2). In this case, no left–right change would be expected in length reproduction, contrary to what happens in experiments in which model and reproduction are contemporaneous and are therefore very likely to be included in a single (horizontally anisometric) frame of reference which would entail size distortions if reproduction were to be carried out to the left or to the right of the model.

However, perhaps the most exciting issue is the extent to which horizontal anisometry of space representation is due to perceptual or response bias. Unfortunately, the results of the most extensive study so far conducted (Bisiach *et al.* 1998) in which perceptual and response bias were assessed by means of a variant of the Milner landmark task (Milner *et al.* 1993), were not very demonstrative. Nonetheless, perceptual bias in the manual-response version of the Milner task was found to be significantly higher in patients showing contralesional over-extension. In contrast, response bias was slightly higher in patients with contralesional under-extension in both the verbal-response and manual-response versions of the Milner task. Therefore there is some suggestion that reluctance to orient toward the side of space opposite to the side of the brain lesion could indeed contribute in reducing (or even reversing) the tendency, found in the majority of neglect patients, toward contralesional over-extension in the reproduction of horizontal extents.

To conclude, what we have learned from recent research on horizontal extent reproduction in unilateral neglect urges reconsideration of former theories about a disorder that still remains largely elusive, despite the impressive increase of contributions following the publication of the remark- able volume edited by Weinstein and Friedland in 1977. This is, we believe, axiomatic. Much more problematical is whether theories of neglect based on horizontal anisometry of the medium for space representation will succeed in providing deeper insight into those neural mechanisms whose impairment gives rise to the amazing disorder of conscious perception and representation manifesting itself as unilateral neglect in the full sense of the word.

Acknowledgements

This work is supported by MURST and CNR grants to EB.

References

Bisiach, E., Rusconi, M. L., Peretti, V. A., and Vallar, G. (1994). Challenging current accounts of unilateral neglect. *Neuropsychologia*, **32**, 1431–4.

Bisiach, E., Pizzamiglio, L., Nico, D., and Antonucci, G. (1996). Beyond unilateral neglect. *Brain*, **119**, 851–7.

Bisiach, E., Ricci, R., and Neppi Mòdona, M. (1998). Visual awareness and anisometry of space representation in unilateral neglect: a panoramic investigation by means of a line extension task. *Consciousness and Cognition*, **7**, 327–55.

Bisiach, E., Neppi-Mòdona, M., Genero, R., and Pepi, R. (1999). Anisometry of space representation in unilateral neglect: empirical test of a former hypothesis. *Consciousness and Cognition*, **8**, 577–84.

Chokron, S., Bernard, J. M., and Imbert, M. (1997). Length representation in normal and neglect subjects with opposite reading habits studied through a line extension task. *Cortex*, **33**, 47–64.

Doricchi, F. and Angelelli, P. (1999). Misrepresentation of horizontal space in left unilateral neglect: role of hemianopia. *Neurology*, **52**, 1845–52.

Ferber, S. and Karnath, H.-O. (2001). Size perception in hemianopia and neglect. *Brain*, **124**, 527–36.

Harvey, M. and Kramer-McCaffery, T. (2001). Effects of stimulus size and eccentricity on size distortion in hemispatial neglect. Presented at the 19th European Workshop on Cognitive Neuropsychology, Bressanone, Italy.

Heilman, K. M., Bowers, D., Coslett, H. B., Whelan, H., and Watson, R. T. (1985). Directional hypokinesia: prolonged reaction time for leftward movements in patients with right hemisphere lesions and neglect. *Neurology*, **35**, 855–9.

Karnath, H.-O. and Ferber, S. (1999). Is space representation distorted in neglect? *Neuropsychologia*, **37**, 7–15.

Milner, A. D. and Harvey, M. (1995). Distortion of size perception in visuospatial neglect. *Current Biology*, **5**, 85–9.

Milner, A. D., Harvey, M., Roberts, R. C., and Forster, S. V. (1993). Line bisection errors in visual neglect: misguided action or size distortion? *Neuropsychologia*, **31**, 39–49.

Nico, D., Galati, G., and Incoccia, C. (1999). The endpoints' task: An analysis of length reproduction in unilateral neglect. *Neuropsychologia*, **37**, 1181–8.

Weinstein, E. A., and Friedland, R. P. (Eds) (1977). Hemi-inattention and hemisphere specialization. New York: Raven Press.

4.2 Perceptual and visuomotor processing in spatial neglect

A. David Milner and Rob D. McIntosh

Many of the attempts to tease apart perceptual and motor aspects of neglect have started from a consideration of what might cause the rightward line bisection errors that are typically exhibited by neglect patients. The explanations proposed have tended to fall into two rhetorically opposed camps, emphasizing perceptual and motor factors respectively. The broad concept of directional motor neglect was introduced by Heilman and Valenstein (1979) to explain the salient manifestations of neglect—rather than failing to attend to contralesional stimuli, patients might be unwilling or unable to respond to them. Thus, when attempting to mark the midpoint of a line, the patient's arm movement might be subject to a net rightward vector that induces his or her apparent error of judgment. To test this idea, several studies have employed modified bisection tasks designed to generate different predictions for perceptual and motor impairments (Bisiach *et al.* 1990; Milner *et al.* 1993; Harvey *et al.* 1995). These studies have converged on the conclusion that, while some neglect patients may have a directional motor bias, the majority misbisect for broadly perceptual reasons. Milner and colleagues have explored the perceptual basis of such errors by asking neglect patients to make forced-choice comparisons of the sizes of paired stimuli. These studies have shown that most neglect patients underestimate the horizontal extent of stimuli presented in leftward locations relative to those presented on the right (Milner and Harvey 1995; Milner *et al.* 1998). These original observations have been replicated widely using related techniques (Bisiach *et al.* 1996; Irving-Bell *et al.* 1999; Kerkhoff *et al.* 1999; Kerkhoff 2000). However, although size distortion is reliably observed in tasks where patients compare two simultaneously presented rectangles, some recent data suggest limitations to the phenomenon.

Karnath and Ferber (1999) conducted an experiment designed to characterize the pattern of spatial distortion in neglect. Neglect patients were presented, in otherwise total darkness, with a pair of light-emitting diodes (LEDs), the horizontal separation of which defined a reference distance. Patients were subsequently required to adjust a second pair of LEDs, presented in isolation on their egocentric left or right, to match the remembered reference distance. No perceptual distortions were observed among the seven patients tested. This was interpreted as evidence that the perception of distance might be unimpaired in neglect, despite the well-documented distortions of size perception. This finding has been reassessed by Kerkhoff (2000), who noted that, in addition to the comparison of distances rather than sizes, Karnath and Ferber had employed a sequential comparison procedure rather than presenting paired stimuli simultaneously. Kerkhoff proposed that sequential presentation might have minimized attentional competition between the stimuli and that this factor, rather than the use of 'distance' stimuli, might explain Karnath and Ferber's result.

Kerkhoff (2000) tested neglect patients on a task in which the horizontal extents to be compared were either sizes (of rectangles) or distances (between pairs of small squares), and where the stimuli were presented either simultaneously or sequentially. Perceptual distortions were observed for both size and distance stimuli, but the latter were less severe. This difference was interpreted as a partial dissociation between size and distance processing in neglect. Moreover, perceptual distortions were reduced by sequential presentation, supporting the notion that simultaneous attentional competition contributes to the phenomenon. However, it is notable that significant underscaling of the leftward stimulus occurred in all conditions, even where 'distance' stimuli were presented sequentially. Thus, although this latter condition was designed to parallel the method of Karnath and Ferber (1999), equivalent results were not found. Given that perceptual distortions were observed with sequential presentation, we can perhaps conclude that simultaneous attentional competition is not necessary for the perceptual distortion phenomenon, even if it might be sufficient. In recent studies, we have gathered data that bear on the issues introduced here. The following two sections will focus on these issues.

Perceptual distortions in visual neglect

Distortions of size and distance

Karnath and Ferber (1999) and Kerkhoff (2000) have suggested that perception of inter-object distances in neglect may be less subject to distortion than perception of the sizes of single objects. This proposal is consistent with an earlier report that neglect patients make larger errors when asked to bisect a solid line than when asked to bisect an equivalent distance between two points (Bisiach et al. 1996). However, Bisiach and colleagues did not interpret their result in terms of dissociated processing of size and distance, but offered a more simple explanation. A patient with neglect may fail to look at (or to represent) the true left endpoint of a solid line, but the bisection of an *unfilled distance* demands that both endpoints are seen before the task can be attempted at all. Accordingly, 'the left endpoint of a virtual line constitutes a much more effective attentional cue than the endpoint of a real line' (Bisiach et al. 1996, p. 855).

We decided to address this issue in a straightforward manner. In the first study, a group of right-brain-damaged patients were asked to bisect ten 20-cm black lines and ten 20-cm 'gaps' (between two small black squares). Figure 1 shows that there was a substantial reduction of rightward error amongst neglect patients for gap stimuli as compared to line stimuli. This replicates the observation by Bisiach et al. (1996) and is compatible with either an attentional cueing account or with a partial dissociation between size and distance processing. In order to decide between these explanations, we tested a second series of right-brain-damaged patients on three further bisection tasks. One was a standard line bisection task in which ten 18-cm black horizontal lines were presented. In the other two conditions, an attempt was made to equate the degree of attentional cueing between the line and gap stimuli. In the gap condition, one endpoint was colored red and the other green, with an 18 cm gap between their inner edges. The red stimulus defined the right-hand edge of the gap on five trials and the left-hand edge on five trials, with the configuration alternated between trials. The patient was instructed to look first at the red stimulus and then at the green stimulus, prior to placing the bisection mark, with the examiner pointing to each in turn. The final task was a hybrid of the first two: the red and green gap stimuli abutted the ends of an 18-cm black line and the same cueing procedure was imposed. This constituted a cued line bisection task, with the cueing component matched against the cued gap bisection task. The results obtained are shown in Fig. 2. In the neglect patients, a reduction of rightward bisection error was achieved through the use of gap stimuli, as observed in the first study. However, almost the same

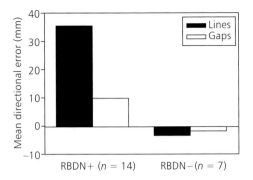

Figure 1 Bisection of lines and gaps in right-brain-damaged (RBD) patients. Positive values indicate rightward errors. Amongst patients displaying neglect for bisection tasks, the severity of impairment is greatly reduced in the gap bisection condition. RBDN+, with neglect; RBDN–, without neglect.

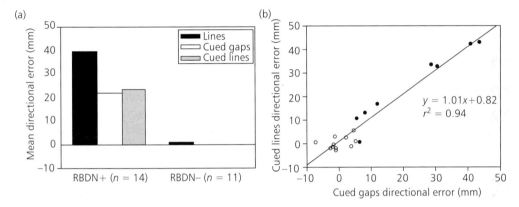

Figure 2 (a) Bisection of lines, cued gaps, and cued lines in right-brain-damaged patients. Positive values indicate rightward errors. When the attentional cueing component is equated between line and gap bisection tasks, equivalent improvements are seen relative to the bisection of uncued lines. (b) Scattergram of mean bisection errors in the cued gap and cued line bisection tasks for all patients (full circles, RBDN+; open circles, RBDN–). The close relationship between the two measures indicates that these tasks depend on common processes.

reduction occurred in the cued line bisection task, suggesting that the reduction of neglect for gap stimuli may have been due entirely to cueing. This interpretation is bolstered by the strong relationship between the patients' performances on the cued gap and cued line bisection tasks. A regression line through the total data set captures 94 per cent of the variability, with a slope of +1.01 and an intercept close to zero (0.82 mm), indicating that the group pattern is representative of the individual patients.

Our findings lead us to concur with the proposal by Bisiach *et al.* (1996) that the improvement of neglect typically observed for gap bisection relates to the attentional cueing inherent in such tasks and does not reflect differential processing of filled and unfilled spatial intervals. Certainly, the study of neglect has provided compelling evidence that the mechanisms underlying the allocation of spatial attention within single objects may be separable from those governing the distribution of attention between discrete objects (Humphreys 1999). However, the study of bisection behavior and size distortion in neglect do not provide any clear reason to believe that a spatial extent, once fully scanned, is judged any differently according to whether it is filled or unfilled.

The role of visual context

We have argued that the apparent distinction between distortions of size and distance in neglect may be an artifact of the different patterns of spatial exploration and attentional allocation that these stimuli elicit. This could explain (in part) why Karnath and Ferber (1999) failed to find any evidence for perceptual distortion in their experiment using sequentially presented gap stimuli. Additionally, Kerkhoff (2000) assessed the role of simultaneous attentional competition in perceptual distortions by comparing performance across conditions in which paired stimuli were presented simultaneously or sequentially. The reduction of size and distance distortions with sequential stimulus presentation led Kerkhoff to conclude that simultaneous attentional competition aggravates the tendency to underestimate leftward extents. As already noted, however, even in the condition designed to replicate Karnath and Ferber's experiment most closely (sequential presentation of gap stimuli), Kerkhoff still observed residual distortion effects, whereas Karnath and Ferber had found no distortion at all. Kerkhoff suggested that this discrepancy might reflect differences in the samples of neglect patients. However, recent data from our laboratory have led us towards a more theoretically motivated account of the differences between these studies.

As part of an investigation into ocular exploration during lateralized size comparisons (see below), we tested three neglect patients on simultaneous and sequential size-matching tasks. The stimuli were solid rectangles, presented on either side of a monitor screen. Paired stimuli appeared together for 6 s (simultaneous condition) or one after the other for 3 s each (sequential condition). The percentages of 'left is smaller' judgments made by each patient in each task condition are shown in Fig. 3, along with data from five age-matched controls. As expected, the neglect patients tended to judge the leftward partner of paired stimuli as smaller. However, there was no reduction of this tendency in the sequential relative to the simultaneous condition (for patient RD, size distortion was actually more severe in the sequential condition). This surprising outcome apparently contradicts the findings of Kerkhoff (2000) and Karnath and Ferber (1999).

In order to make sense of these puzzling results, it may be useful to consider the model of cortical visual processing proposed by Milner and Goodale (1995). These authors have argued for the existence of relatively independent coding systems within the posterior cerebral cortex dedicated to processing visual information for the purposes of perception (the 'ventral stream') and visuomotor control (the 'dorsal stream'). They have proposed that the visual information processed for the purposes of visuomotor control is encoded in an egocentric reference frame in which the absolute sizes of objects are represented. In contrast, the processes giving rise to conscious visual perception are argued to use contextual frames of reference, which represent the spatial relationships between objects in *relative* metrics. In an extension of these ideas, Milner (1997) has argued that perceptual distortions in visuospatial neglect may reflect a breakdown in

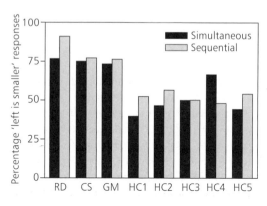

Figure 3 Total percentage of 'left is smaller' judgments in simultaneous and sequential size-matching tasks for three patients with visual neglect (RD, CS, GM) and five age-matched healthy controls (HC1–HC5). The left-sided underestimation exhibited by the patients in the simultaneous presentation condition is not reduced by sequential presentation.

a system for scene representation that puts together visual information received via the ventral stream. Here we would like to propose that a critical factor determining the occurrence of size distortion may be the *relative lateralization of the comparison stimuli in perceptual space*. We assume that whether perceptual space is represented in working memory during a sequential comparison task or is perceived directly during simultaneous presentation, the determinants of stimulus lateralization will be context or scene based rather than being related to egocentric (e.g. body-centered) coordinates. We suggest that this hypothesis could offer a parsimonious account of the discrepancies between our own findings and those of Kerkhoff (2000) and of Karnath and Ferber (1999).

Karnath and Ferber's patients exhibited no perceptual distortions. However, all of their stimuli were presented in isolation, and in otherwise total darkness, so that no external reference frame was available within which to represent the sequentially presented stimuli as lateralized with respect to one another (see also Chapter 4.1). Kerkhoff's subjects were not tested in complete darkness, although the contextual cues available were sparse (the room was darkened and the stimuli were white on a black screen, the borders of which were masked). The degree of perceived lateralization of successive stimuli in this situation will have been greater than in Karnath and Ferber's experiment, perhaps accounting for the modest distortion effects observed in the sequential comparison condition. However, although the contextual cues in Kerkhoff's simultaneous presentation condition would not have been salient, the two stimuli were presented side by side, so that each was lateralized unambiguously by the other's presence. Finally, in our own experiment, all stimuli were black on white, presented on an unmasked monitor in a well-lit room. Under these full contextual cue conditions, stimuli on opposite sides of the screen would have been perceptually lateralized with respect to one another, regardless of whether they were presented simultaneously or sequentially.

We suggest that our provision of salient environmental cues provided equally clear stimulus location information in the simultaneous and sequential conditions, thereby eliciting substantial size distortion in both. In order to test these ideas, we have now developed a sequential size-matching task in which the relative locations of paired stimuli within an environmental frame of reference can be manipulated independently of egocentric coordinates. Our hypothesis predicts that relative lateralization within the environmental frame of reference should be the dominant determinant of size distortion effects. The sole neglect patient so far tested on this task, a 61-year-old man with a right parieto-occipital lesion and complete left hemianopia, has performed in accordance with this prediction.

Perception and visuomotor control in neglect

The application by Milner and Goodale (1995) of their ideas to visuospatial neglect was predicated on the defining fact that visual information on the neglected side has a reduced likelihood of attaining conscious awareness. In Milner and Goodale's model, it is the ventral cortical stream, which passes information to occipitotemporal areas, which furnishes the contents of our visual awareness. In contrast, the dorsal stream is assumed to perform its visuomotor role without the products of its processing entering awareness. Accordingly, Milner and Goodale proposed that many perceptual symptoms of neglect might reflect malfunction in a high-level representational structure where the products of ventral stream processing are integrated and made use of. In other words, it was suggested that visual neglect follows disruption of an elaboration of ventral stream processing (Milner 1997). Consistent with this, the focus for neglect-causing lesions overlaps well into the temporal lobe (Vallar 1993; Karnath *et al.* 2001), while the visuomotor areas lie superiorly in the parietal lobe, in and around the intraparietal sulcus (see Culham and Kanwisher

(2001) for functional MRI evidence). One prediction derived from Milner and Goodale's proposal is that many patients subject to distortions of spatial perception should nevertheless code spatial parameters veridically when programming goal-directed actions. That is, the distortions apparent in the visual perception of the patients should not necessarily affect their visuomotor control, since that would be accomplished by dorsal stream structures unscathed by the brain damage or otherwise refractory to such distortions.

It is important to emphasize the difference between this hypothesis, of dissociated perceptual and visuomotor processing in neglect, and the more familiar notion of a dissociation between perceptual and motor (or 'premotor') contributions to neglect symptoms with which we began this chapter. According to the latter idea, errors (e.g. in line bisection) may result from spatial biases in the processing of sensory inputs, or alternatively from spatial biases in the selection and execution of motor acts (see Mattingley and Driver (1997) for a review). In contrast, the model of cortical processing proposed by Milner and Goodale is concerned with differential processing of visual information for different behavioral purposes, and is orthogonal to the basic distinction between input and output biases. Specifically, Milner and Goodale suggest that the visual processing that gives rise to conscious visual awareness may be largely independent of the neural mechanisms that process the same sensory inputs for the guidance of automatic goal-directed actions. Applied to the neglect syndrome, this model predicts that perceptual biases will not necessarily influence goal-directed actions. In the following two sections, we present preliminary evidence that neglect patients may indeed show preserved visuomotor guidance despite pronounced perceptual biases.

Perception and visuomotor control in gap bisection

In the first study that explicitly contrasted spatial judgments with the visual control of reaching, reduced spatial errors were found when neglect patients were asked to pick up rods centrally rather than to indicate their perceived midpoints (Robertson et al. 1995). We have recently studied several neglect patients in an extension of the pioneering work of Robertson and colleagues. Instead of the bisection of solid rods, we studied the bisection of the space between two stimulus items (i.e. a gap bisection task). Patients were asked to move their hand through the space between two cylinders, one located either 8 cm or 12 cm to the left of midline, and the other 8 cm or 12 cm to the right of midline, under two different task instructions. In the **bisection task**, they were asked to place their right index finger at the exact midpoint of the gap between the two cylinders. In the **reaching task**, they were required to move their finger to any point within a target zone that stretched horizontally across the far edge of the table; the only constraints were that the hand should pass between the two cylinders *en route* and that the movement should be rapid. Our pilot studies had indicated that, for this spatial layout, the optimal hand-path, which minimizes the danger of collision with either cylinder, passes approximately midway between the two cylinders. Therefore our method allows us to compare the spatial analysis that underlies an explicit bisection judgment with that which determines the trajectory of a simple reaching movement made in the presence of potential obstacles. We measured the hand movements of the patients using a magnetic motion analysis system (Minibird, Ascension Technology Ltd). The hypothesis of Milner and Goodale predicts a relative sparing of the latter in many neglect patients, just as has been found in a patient with visual form agnosia resulting from severe bilateral ventral stream damage (McIntosh et al. 2000).

Figure 4 shows the mean transection points, with respect to the center of the gap between the two cylinders, in the bisection and reaching tasks. The mean rightward bisection error of the neglect group was relatively small, and only two patients produced very large rightward errors. This is consistent with the observation that neglect bisection errors tend to be reduced in gap bisection tasks (see above). Nonetheless, the neglect group's mean bisection error was significantly rightward relative to that of the control group. In the reaching task, all subjects reached between

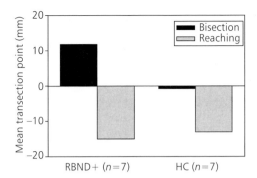

Figure 4 Mean transection point relative to the center of the gap between the two cylinders for neglect patients (RBDN+) and age-matched healthy controls (HC) in bisection and reaching tasks. For the reaching task, the transection point was determined by the lateral position of the right index finger at the point that it crossed the virtual line between the two cylinders. Positive values indicate rightward deviations. The interaction between group and task is significant ($p < 0.05$).

the cylinders at a leftward point with respect to the midpoint of the aperture. This constant bias arises because the marker (the positions of which were used to plot the reaching trajectory) was attached to the right index finger and was therefore leftwardly displaced with respect to the center of the (palm-down) reaching hand. Despite this artifact, it is clear that the characteristic rightward errors of neglect were absent in the reaching task. In fact, the trajectories selected by neglect patients were indistinguishable from those of normal subjects.

This result is suggestive but, by itself, does not establish that the optimal reach trajectory was influenced by the locations of the two cylinders in the workspace. Indeed, the reaching data depicted in Fig. 4 could, in principle, have arisen without subjects having registered the location of either cylinder. In order to quantify the influence that each cylinder exerted upon the reaching response, we calculated the shift in the mean transection point associated with a shift of each cylinder between its two possible locations (averaged across the two locations of the cylinder on the opposite side). The same was done for the responses made in the bisection task. For each cylinder, the distance between the alternative locations (8 and 12 cm from the midline) was 40 mm. Therefore, if a subject bisected perfectly, a 20-mm shift in the bisection response should be induced by shifting either cylinder between its two locations. In the reaching task, it is less easy to predict the change in trajectory that should result from a shift in cylinder location because additional factors are likely to influence the reach (e.g. the movement must be time efficient and easy to execute). However, a comparison of the impact of a shift in the right and the left cylinder should reveal any asymmetry between their respective influences on behavior.

The bisection data gave a very clear result, depicted in Fig. 5(a). As expected, control subjects took precise account of a shift in either cylinder, modifying their bisection responses accordingly. The neglect patients showed a similar response to changes in the position of the right cylinder. However, changes in the position of the left cylinder made very little difference to the bisection responses of the neglect patients, whether this was due to a failure to attend fully to this cylinder or to an inability to code its location accurately. Figure 5(b) shows the data represented in a similar way for the reaching task. The first point to note is that both cylinders were influential in determining the reach trajectories of both subject groups. This confirms that the trajectories selected resulted from the need to avoid collision with either cylinder. Figure 5(b) also shows that, for control subjects, the influence of the two cylinders was approximately equal. For neglect patients, there was a qualitative trend towards a reduced influence of the left-hand cylinder relative to the right-hand cylinder. At present, this trend does not approach significance, but we are continuing to collect data on these tasks. In particular, given a larger patient group, it may be of interest to investigate whether there are differences between patients with and without hemianopia in the relative influences of the two cylinders. At present, we will restrict our conclusions to the broad pattern of the data presented in Figs 4 and 5. In accord with Robertson *et al.* (1995), our results

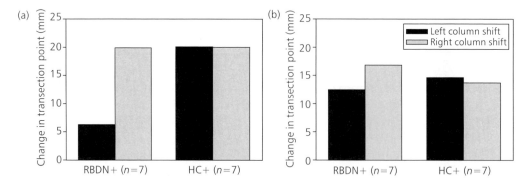

Figure 5 (a) Mean shift of bisection response induced by a 40-mm shift in the location of the left and right cylinders respectively. The interaction between group and side of shift is significant ($p < 0.0005$). (b) Mean shift of reaching response induced by a 40-mm shift in cylinder location. The interaction between task and group and side of shift does not approach significance ($p > 0.3$).

demonstrate that the accuracy of spatial coding (and/or the allocation of spatial attention) can be strongly affected by task demands. In the present study, the crucial difference is between a conscious spatial judgment and a fast automatic reaching response. Our observation that neglect is less evident in the reaching task is fully consistent with the predictions of Milner and Goodale (1995).

Perception and visuomotor control in size processing

In an examination of the visual parameter of size in perception and visuomotor control in neglect, we have tested several patients on a task in which they reach out to grasp one or other of two simultaneously presented cylinders, or instead estimate its diameter. In order to equate roughly the motor requirements between the two tasks, we asked the patients to indicate their perceptual judgments manually, by opening the finger and thumb to match the size of the designated cylinder. The first neglect patient tested on this task (EC) showed clear size distortion when estimating the size of the target objects but not when grasping them (Pritchard *et al.* 1997). As Fig. 6 shows, EC's manual estimations of target diameter were linearly related to target size but her size estimates for targets in left extrapersonal space were systematically smaller than for targets placed on the right. In contrast, in the grasping task EC opened her grip equally wide for objects on either side of space. M.G. Edwards and G.W. Humphreys (personal communication) have recently replicated this pattern of dissociation in a further patient with visual neglect. Moreover, they found that the symmetry of grip scaling to objects on either side of space was maintained even when the grasping task was performed without visual feedback. This indicates that the normality of grip scaling in neglect is not achieved simply by correcting for anticipatory errors on the basis of visual feedback during the reach. These single case studies demonstrate that automatic visuomotor responses (in this case, grip formation) in visual neglect may be unaffected by concurrent misperceptions of object size.

Two recent group studies have provided further evidence that grip formation is symmetrical for objects placed on the neglected and non-neglected sides of space. Harvey *et al.* (2001) found no asymmetry of grip scaling amongst four patients with acute neglect, even under visually open-loop conditions. In our own studies, we applied manual estimation and closed-loop grasping tasks to six further visual neglect patients (McIntosh *et al.* 2001). Again, we confirmed the absence of lateralized abnormalities of grip formation amongst neglect patients. However, none of our patients showed the asymmetric pattern of manual size estimation exhibited by patient

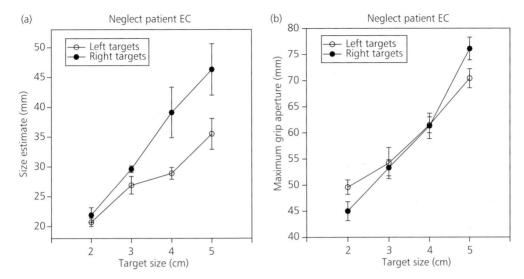

Figure 6 (a) Patient EC's manual size estimates of cylinders presented on the egocentric left or right. The main effect of target side is significant ($p < 0.001$). (b) Patient EC's maximum grip apertures when grasping cylinders on the left or right. Neither the effect of target side nor the interaction of side by size reached significance. (Reproduced from C.L. Pritchard *et al.*, *Neurocase*, **3**, 437–43 (1997).)

EC (Pritchard *et al.* 1997). This null finding was unexpected, especially given the fact that the majority of our patients showed clear leftward size underestimation in pictorial size-matching tasks. This multiple failure to replicate EC's dissociated pattern rather weakens the power of the finding of symmetrical grip formation. It appears that, whilst symmetrical grip scaling may be ubiquitous in neglect, cases of asymmetric manual size estimation may be relatively rare, at least for the manual size estimation task used by Pritchard *et al.*(1997).

However, our observation that asymmetric manual size estimation does not normally accompany size underestimation on standard size-matching tasks may be of some theoretical significance. It implies that the size-underestimation phenomenon is highly sensitive to the structure of the task used to test for it. Standard size-matching tasks always require the size of one stimulus to be judged with respect to that of another. In our manual size estimation task, the target object was always accompanied by a similar object on the other side of space, but this nontarget object was irrelevant to the task. That is, patients were required to estimate the absolute size of the target object without regard to the size of its companion. Our present perspective would suggest that, for the size distortion phenomenon to emerge fully, multiple objects must be represented as occupying relatively lateralized locations within a common environmental frame of reference, so that an element of explicit (or implicit) size comparison can operate (see above). Like many symptoms associated with neglect, size distortion may be a relative and not an absolute phenomenon (Kinsbourne 1987, 1993).

Accordingly, one possible explanation for our null findings in the manual size estimation task is that the separation between objects in left and right space (approximately 21 cm) was too great for any degree of implicit comparison to emerge in the majority of patients. A recent study by Hu and Goodale (2000) may indicate the range over which the estimation of absolute size is liable to be influenced by neighboring objects. In this study, healthy subjects were prone to a size-contrast illusion when making manual width estimates of a cylinder located 2 cm to the left or right of a larger or smaller one (the widths of target cylinders flanked by large distracters were underestimated, and vice versa). However, when reaching to grasp the target cylinder, grip scaling was perfectly accurate. These results fit well with Milner and Goodale's proposal that the perceptual system represents the world in terms of its relative metrics. Furthermore, relative size comparisons may be obligatory when multiple objects occupy the same contextual frame of reference, even when attempting to make absolute size judgments. Accordingly, we would predict that perceptual distortion effects should be observed in the manual size estimates of neglect patients when an arrangement of objects similar to that employed by Hu and Goodale is used. Importantly, of course, we would expect the symmetry of size processing to be preserved for simple grasping responses.

Recent observations on the heterogeneity of subjective size distortion

We have emphasized that the division between perceptual and visuomotor processes proposed by Milner and Goodale (1995) is distinct from the division between perceptual (input) and motor (output) processes that has been more usually addressed in the neglect literature. We have also suggested that the left-sided underestimation of horizontal extents that commonly accompanies neglect may reflect disruption of representational structures linked closely to ventral stream processing. One corollary of this hypothesis is that perceptual distortions should not necessarily affect the spatial processing that underlies the visual guidance of automatic actions in neglect. However, it is important to note that this does not preclude the existence of systematic biases of motor behavior (such as 'directional hypokinesia') in neglect, which might arise from biased motor execution rather than from biased visuomotor processing *per se*. Of special relevance in the present context is the possible role of oculomotor asymmetries in causing apparently 'perceptual' distortions of size.

The first report of size distortion in visual neglect was provided by Gainotti and Tiacci (1971). They reported that neglect was associated with a tendency to overestimate the rightward partner of lateralized pairs of geometrical figures, and they noted that these patients also tended to *fixate* mostly on the rightward figure. Linking these observations, they proposed that 'this asymmetry of visual perception is due to the asymmetric exploration of space shown by patients with unilateral spatial neglect ... the space of visual perception is not homogeneous, but the elements on which gaze is mostly fixed are systematically overvalued' (Gainotti and Tiacci 1971, p. 456). According to this account, the proximal cause of size distortion in neglect is an insufficiency of leftward exploratory eye movements. In order to explore this proposal, we have studied the eye movements made by three neglect patients performing visual size-matching tasks. All three patients underestimated the left partner of paired horizontal rectangles (see Fig. 3). However, their patterns of ocular exploration and verbal responses imply that they may have done so for quite different reasons.

Patient RD, a 50-year-old man with a large right subcortical infarct, exhibited an extreme paucity of leftward ocular exploration. Given his homonymous hemianopia, it would have been impossible for him to see any portion of the left rectangle on the vast majority of trials. However, RD never complained that the discrimination required of him was nonsensical. Instead, in the majority of trials, he chose the left rectangle as the smaller. Moreover, he was no more likely to make 'right is smaller' judgments on trials in which the right rectangle actually was smaller than on any other type of trial, i.e. his verbal responses were random with respect to the stimuli presented but far from random with respect to side of space. These bizarre responses suggest confabulations, with a strong bias to devalue the left side. RD's behavior shows that apparent perceptual size underestimation can result from a high-level response bias. This pattern might be more accurately described as a 'conceptual' undervaluation of leftwardly located stimuli.

Patient CS, a 74-year-old woman with a large right parieto-occipital lesion, did not differ from normal control subjects in terms of the temporal proportions of fixations directed at the left and right paired stimuli. Similarly, the spatial range of her fixations was normal, with the most eccentric fixations landing short of the far end of either rectangle. However, unlike a normal subject, CS had left homonymous hemianopia. Therefore, with the exception of a few trials in which she actually fixated beyond the left-hand edge of the left rectangle, she would have been unable to view its full extent. CS's 'right is smaller' responses were reliably related to stimulus dimensions. Nonetheless, she showed a strong bias to underestimate the left rectangle, choosing the left as the smaller on 76 per cent of trials overall. It seems likely that CS's size underestimation resulted directly from the fact that her leftward scanning was insufficient to compensate for her hemianopia. Thus her behavior is consistent with the proposal by Gainotti and Tiacci (1971) that scanning deficiencies can be sufficient for size underestimation.

A third distinct pattern of behavior was observed in GM, a 53-year-old man with a right inferior posterior parietal infarct. Relative to control subjects, GM's oculomotor exploration was biased *leftwards*, probably as a result of the scanning training that he was receiving from rehabilitation staff. Given his full visual fields, GM would have been able to view the entirety of all presented stimuli. Moreover, 96 per cent of his 'right is smaller' responses were issued on trials in which the right stimulus actually was smaller (with the remaining 4 per cent issued when the paired stimuli were equal), showing that his responses were not random with respect to the stimuli presented. Nevertheless, GM reported that the left stimulus was smaller on 75 per cent of trials overall. This final pattern of behavior shows that scanning deficiencies are not necessary for size underestimation, even if they can be sufficient. This third variety of size underestimation is the only one in which there is strong evidence that the tendency to devalue leftward extents results from a genuine perceptual distortion, in which leftward extents are represented as shorter than equivalent extents viewed in relatively rightward positions.

Our investigations of eye movements in the context of size-matching tasks have so far suggested that the gross symptom of size distortion, as assessed by standard size-matching tasks, may arise at (at least) three levels, which we shall provisionally refer to as conceptual (RD), oculomotor (CS), and perceptual (GM). The heterogeneity revealed by these results is a salutary discovery, which raises a host of issues for future research. For instance, it would be interesting to ascertain what proportion of patients exhibit size distortion for each of the reasons discussed here, whether further 'varieties' of size distortion exist, and whether reliable anatomical correlations can be identified. These findings may also have implications for the hypotheses advanced earlier in this chapter, which we address briefly below.

Concluding comments

We have summarized recent progress on a series of studies in which we are exploring the phenomena of size and distance distortion in neglect patients. We are trying to determine the conditions under which leftward underestimation occurs and to apply the underestimation phenomenon as a tool to explore perceptual and visuomotor factors in neglect. We have used as a heuristic framework the model of Milner and Goodale (1995), according to which perceptual processing is the province of ventral-stream systems in the occipital and temporal lobes. These structures are thought to provide the visual content for representational mechanisms in the right superior temporal and inferior parietal regions, which integrate object information within an appropriate spatial framework. We believe that it is damage to these representational systems that results in the perceptual manifestations of spatial neglect. In contrast, the direct visual control of behavior is thought to be mediated by dorsal-stream networks in the posterior parietal cortex. These are supposed to operate relatively autonomously from perceptual processes, thus retaining immunity from scene-based geometric illusions in healthy observers (Haffenden and Goodale 2000) and (in principle) from lesion-induced perceptual distortions in brain-damaged subjects.

Two major consequences should follow from these ideas. First, what counts as relatively 'leftward' or 'rightward' in creating neglect phenomena should be determined not by the absolute location of the stimuli in egocentric space, but by their location relative to the major visual landmarks that define the environmental frame of reference adopted for the task. Second, there should be some neglect patients who show perceptual changes without concomitant distortions in their visuomotor control. We have presented preliminary evidence supporting both these predictions. However, we have further suggested that the gross symptom of size distortion is not a unitary phenomenon, but may arise in (at least) three distinct ways, which we have provisionally dubbed conceptual, oculomotor and perceptual. That is, patients with neglect may judge leftwardly located stimuli as smaller because of (a) a high-level preference, (b) an incomplete scanning of the left stimulus, or (c) a perception of the left stimulus as smaller despite adequate stimulus exploration. Only the last of these types is fully consistent with the hypothesis that neglect patients represent stimuli presented on the left side of space as compressed relative to equivalent stimuli on the right (Bisiach *et al.* 1996; Milner 1987; Milner *et al.* 1998). Any such case (e.g. our patient GM) also serves as a counter-example to the oculomotor explanation offered by Gainotti and Tiacci (1971). It was of course this kind of 'perceptual' interpretation of the size distortion phenomenon that we attempted to relate to Milner and Goodale's model of cortical visual processing. Therefore, in concluding, it is worthwhile considering briefly how our recent observations on the heterogeneity of size distortion may fit within the general theoretical framework of this chapter.

First, we have provided evidence that leftward size underestimation may result from deficient leftward scanning. This observation is reminiscent of incomplete leftward search amongst neglect patients performing line bisection tasks (see Chapter 4.4) and could potentially provide an explanation for the fact that size distortion phenomena are particularly prevalent and severe amongst neglect patients with hemianopia (see Chapter 4.5). Additionally, the contribution of scanning deficits might also account for the fact that overt cueing or the use of 'gap' stimuli can ameliorate rightward bisection errors (see above) and leftward size underestimation in neglect (Karnath and Ferber 1999; Kerkhoff 2000). Such procedures will generally ensure that the presented stimuli are scanned fully, thereby reducing the influence of uncompensated hemianopia. It should also be noted that incomplete leftward scanning does not exclude the concurrent existence of true perceptual size distortion. Kerkhoff (2000) reported reduced, but still significant, size distortion for gap stimuli as opposed to line stimuli, and we have found similar results for bisection tasks (see above). It is possible that these residual effects reflect true perceptual distortions while the reduction of rightward biases for gap relative to line stimuli represents the contribution of spontaneous scanning deficits under normal circumstances.

A further point to be made with regard to scanning deficits is that, although the proximal cause of leftward size underestimation in a given patient may be oculomotor, the oculomotor bias itself might have an attentional basis. If so, it is possible that scene-based coding is involved in this form of size underestimation as well, in that patterns of exploratory eye movements might well themselves depend on stimulus context and the nature of the response required in the task. Thus, to the extent that the spatial distribution of oculomotor exploration is determined by environmental cues (i.e. by the spatial range of task relevant stimulation), rather than being strictly linked to egocentric coordinates, we would expect size distortion effects to follow the same environmental coordinates. Similarly, it will be of interest to investigate, in neglect patients with scanning deficits, whether patterns of exploratory eye movements are altered when an automatic goal-directed response is required rather than a simple verbal report. These are empirical questions that we are only now beginning to formulate but which we hope soon to address experimentally.

Finally, it is relatively easy to see how Milner and Goodale's model might fit with a high-level response bias such as that observed in RD (see above). Thus, if a patient systematically devalues relatively leftward stimuli, this devaluation should apply to those that he *perceives* as being relatively leftward, and this perception should be determined by environmental context. Moreover, there is no reason to suppose that such a response bias should affect the calibration of movement parameters. However, the model seems unlikely to be especially illuminating with regard to a full understanding of what we have provisionally labelled 'conceptual' distortions. Rather, the bizarre behavior of patient RD presents profound conundrums about the structure of belief systems in neglect and the readiness to confabulate responses in the face of apparently glaring inconsistencies (see also Chapter 1.1). From an experimental standpoint, on the other hand, the more pertinent problem may be that of how to take account of such confabulations when attempting to infer the nature of perception in neglect from a patient's verbal reports.

Acknowledgements

The authors acknowledge the important contributions of Chris Dijkerman, Kevin McClements, and Caroline Tilikete to this research, and are grateful to the Wellcome Trust (Grant 048060) and the Leverhulme Trust (Grant F/268/T) for their financial support.

References

Bisiach, E., Geminiani, G., Berti, A., and Rusconi, M. L. (1990). Perceptual and premotor factors in unilateral neglect. *Neurology*, **40**, 1278–81.

Bisiach, E., Pizzamiglio, L., Nico, D., and Antonucci, G. (1996). Beyond unilateral neglect. *Brain*, **119**, 851–7.

Culham, J. C. and Kanwisher, N. G. (2001). Neuroimaging of cognitive functions in human parietal cortex. *Current Opinion in Neurobiology*, **11**, 157–63.

Gainotti, G. and Tiacci, C. (1971). The relationship between disorders of visual perception and unilateral spatial neglect. *Neuropsychologia*, **9**, 451–8.

Haffenden, A. M and Goodale, M. A. (2000). Independent effects of pictorial displays on perception and action. *Vision Research*, **40**, 1597–607.

Harvey, M., Milner, A. D., and Roberts, R. C. (1995). An investigation of hemispatial neglect using the landmark task. *Brain and Cognition*, **27**, 59–78.

Harvey, M., Jackson, S. R., Newport, R., Krämer, T., Morris, D. L., and Dow, L. (in press). Is grasping impaired in hemispatial neglect? *Behavioural Neurology*.

Heilman, K. M. and Valenstein, E. (1979). Mechanisms underlying hemispatial neglect. *Annals of Neurology*, **5**, 166–70.

Hu, Y. and Goodale, M. A. (2000). Grasping after a delay shifts size-scaling from absolute to relative metrics. *Journal of Cognitive Neuroscience*, **12**, 856–68.

Humphreys, G. W. (1999). Neural representation of objects in space: a dual coding account. *Philosophical Transactions of the Royal Society of London B*, **353**, 1341–51.

Irving-Bell, L., Small, M., and Cowey, A. (1999). A distortion of perceived space in patients with right-hemisphere lesions and visual hemineglect. *Neuropsychologia*, **37**, 919–25.

Karnath, H. -O. and Ferber, S. (1999). Is space representation distorted in neglect? *Neuropsychologia*, **37**, 7–15.

Karnath, H. -O., Ferber, S., and Himmelbach, M. (2001). Spatial awareness is a function of the temporal not the posterior parietal lobe. *Nature*, **411**, 950–3.

Kerkhoff, G. (2000). Multiple perceptual distortions and their modulation in leftsided visual neglect. *Neuropsychologia*, **38**, 1073–86.

Kerkhoff, G., Schindler, I., Keller, I., and Marquardt, C. (1999). Visual background motion reduces size distortion in spatial neglect. *NeuroReport*, **10**, 319–23.

Kinsbourne, M. (1987). Mechanisms of unilateral neglect. In *Neurophysiological and neuropsychological aspects of spatial neglect* (ed. M. Jeannerod), pp. 69–86. Elsevier, Amsterdam.

Kinsbourne, M. (1993). Orientational bias model of unilateral neglect: evidence from attentional gradients within hemispace. In *Unilateral neglect: clinical and experimental studies* (ed. I. H. Robertson and J. C. Marshall), pp. 63–86. Lawrence Erlbaum, Hove.

Mattingley, J. B. and Driver, J. (1997). Distinguishing sensory and motor deficits after parietal damage: an evaluation of response selection biases in unilateral neglect. In *Parietal lobe contributions to orientation in 3D space* (ed. P. Thier and H.-O. Karnath), pp. 309–37. Springer-Verlag, Heidelberg.

McIntosh, R. D., Dijkerman, H. C., Mon-Williams, M., and Milner, A. D. (2000). Visuomotor processing of spatial layout in visual form agnosia. Presented at the Experimental Psychology Society, Cambridge, July 2000.

McIntosh, R. D., Pritchard, C. L., Dijkerman, H. C., Milner, A. D., and Roberts R. C. (in press). Perception and prehension of size in left visual neglect. *Behavioural Neurology*.

Milner, A. D. (1987). Animal models for the syndrome of spatial neglect. In *Neurophysiological and neuropsychological aspects of spatial neglect* (ed. M. Jeannerod), pp. 259–88. Elsevier, Amsterdam.

Milner, A. D. (1997). Neglect, extinction, and the cortical streams of visual processing. In *Parietal lobe contributions to orientation in 3D space* (ed. P. Thier and H.-O. Karnath), pp. 3–22. Springer-Verlag, Heidelberg.

Milner, A. D. and Goodale, M. A. (1995). *The visual brain in action*. Oxford University Press.

Milner, A. D. and Harvey, M. (1995). Distortion of size perception in visuospatial neglect. *Current Biology*, **5**, 85–9.

Milner, A. D., Harvey, M., Roberts, R. C., and Forster, S. V. (1993). Line bisection errors in visual neglect: misguided action or size distortion? *Neuropsychologia*, **31**, 39–49.

Milner, A. D., Harvey, M., and Pritchard, C. L. (1998). Visual size processing in spatial neglect. *Experimental Brain Research*, **123**, 192–200.

Pritchard, C. L., Milner, A. D., Dijkerman, H. C., and MacWalter, R. S. (1997). Visuospatial neglect: veridical coding of size for grasping but not for perception. *Neurocase*, **3**, 437–43.

Robertson, I. H., Nico, D., and Hood, B. (1995). The intention to act improves unilateral left neglect: two demonstrations. *NeuroReport*, **7**, 246–8.

Vallar, G. (1993). The anatomical basis of spatial hemineglect in humans. In *Unilateral neglect: clinical and experimental studies* (ed. I. H. Robertson and J. C. Marshall), pp. 27–59. Lawrence Erlbaum, Hove.

4.3 Spatial anisometry and representational release in neglect

Anjan Chatterjee

Humans can estimate magnitudes of stimuli with considerable consistency. Furthermore, their estimates of magnitude are mathematically lawful. The lawfulness of these estimates suggests that the psychophysical mapping of stimuli to mental representations is shaped by organizational principles of the nervous system. One might anticipate that this mapping would be disrupted by brain damage. In this chapter, we will argue that such disruption occurs in patients with neglect. From casual observation, it is obvious that the world of neglect patients is confined ipsilesionally. It is less obvious that this confinement continues to conform to psychophysical principles.

We start by discussing psychophysical principles in general, and with reference to patients with neglect. We then focus on line bisection tasks, with respect to the graded distortions, or anisometry, of the mental representations of these patients. We then discuss whether the abnormal gradients of attention in neglect are distributed over external space or over internal representations. Finally, we discuss the cross-over phenomenon, which refers to a paradoxical behavior seen when most neglect patients bisect short lines. It is proposed that the cross-over phenomenon follows from a general psychophysical principle and is not confined to visual spatial stimuli. Lastly, we suggest that the cross-over phenomenon points to an underlying instability of mental representations in patients with neglect and to ways in which perceptions are influenced by the context in which stimuli are apprehended.

Quantifying perceptions

Psychophysical relationships

In 1858, Gustav Fechner had a scientific epiphany. He realized that humans quantify their perceptions of stimuli in ways that can be described mathematically. In *The Elements of Psychophysics* (Fechner 1860), he proposed that psychological estimations of stimulus magnitudes were related logarithmically to objective measures of physical stimuli. This relationship

$$y = K \log f,$$

where y represents the subjective psychological estimate and f represents the objective physical measurement, is known as Fechner's law.

Fechner's law held sway for nearly a century until Stevens and colleagues demonstrated that psychophysical relationships are more accurately described by power functions (Stevens and

Galanter 1957; Stevens 1958, 1970). Thus

$$y = Kf^b,$$

which is known as Stevens' law, replaced Fechner's law. Two points about Stevens' law are worth noting. First, power function relationships are found across many perceptual continua, including estimates of brightness, loudness, tactile pressure, length, and area. The generality of this relationship suggests that power laws reflect a fundamental organizational principle by which the human nervous system maps stimuli on to mental representations. Second, the same exponent is found across normal subjects for a given perceptual estimate. The exponents reflect an organizational principle by which specific stimuli are mapped on to mental representations. The constant, by contrast, is sensitive to individual differences and experimental variations.

Neglect and the power law

What happens to lawful psychophysical relationships in neglect when the mapping of stimuli to representation is disrupted? It turns out that neglect patients' awareness of stimuli continues to conform to a power function. However, the exponents of the functions are diminished in comparison with normal (Chatterjee *et al.* 1992*b*, 1994*a,b*; Chatterjee 1995; Chatterjee and Thompson 1998).

Power function relationships in neglect were first observed with cancellation tasks. Chatterjee *et al.* (1992*a*) described a patient with typical left-sided neglect who omitted targets on the left of a cancellation array. On her own, she cancelled targets stereotypically, in that she started at the top right and then moved down vertically in a columnar pattern until she decided that all the targets had been cancelled. When we asked her to cancel targets in an alternating pattern, first on the right and then on the left, she omitted targets in the middle of the array rather than neglecting leftward targets. This observation suggested that her neglect was composed of two components. Firstly, she had an orientation bias toward right space as demonstrated by her performance in the traditional administration of the cancellation tasks. Secondly, she had a pathologically limited capacity to attend to or act on targets regardless of their spatial location. The instruction to alternate the location of targets she cancelled overcame her orientation bias and thereby exposed her capacity limitation.

The capacity limitation to detect targets for this patient was best characterized by a power function. With more targets on stimuli arrays, she cancelled more targets in absolute terms, but fewer targets as a proportion of the array. The relationship of the number of targets on the array to the number she cancelled was described by a power function with an exponent of 0.5. Further experiments demonstrated that the number of targets in the array, and not the density of targets or the time taken on the task, accounted for this relationship (Chatterjee *et al.* 1992*b*).

Psychophysical principles also apply to patients' bisection of horizontal lines. Bisiach *et al.* (1983) reported that neglect patients' bisection of lines was influenced systematically by the length of the target line. Following this initial observation, Halligan and Marshall (1988, 1989) showed that patients consistently made larger errors and were more variable in their transections with longer lines than with shorter lines. They suggested that this error pattern could be viewed psychophysically as evidence for an abnormally large Weber fraction (Marshall and Halligan 1990). (The Weber fraction refers to the magnitude within which one is unable to detect differences between two stimuli.)

To determine whether line bisections can also be described by power functions, we adopted a convention suggested by Bisiach *et al.* (1983). They suggested that a patient's awareness of a line might be considered to be twice the distance from the right end of the line to the point of transection. Using this convention, we studied 16 unselected patients with right brain damage and found that they had an average exponent of 0.80 compared with an average exponent of 0.99 in 16 age-matched normal subjects (Chatterjee *et al*. 1994*a*).

Power function descriptions of neglect performance have been demonstrated in two other tasks. Patients with neglect frequently have an attentional dyslexia in which letters on the left side of words are either neglected or misread. The lengths of the words that patients report seeing are also related to the length of the target words by power functions (Chatterjee 1995). Finally, power function relationships with diminished exponents are also found when patients estimate the magnitudes of stimuli that do not extend in space. Patients' estimates of weights lifted in their left hand are described by power functions with diminished exponents compared with estimates of weights lifted in their right hand (Chatterjee and Thompson 1998).

To summarize, neglect patients' awareness of stimuli is related systematically to the quantity of stimuli with which they are confronted. This systematic relation is described by power functions with exponents that are diminished compared with those of normal subjects. Diminished exponents in these psychophysical power functions suggest that, while patients are aware of incremental changes in stimuli, their awareness of the magnitude of these changes is dampened considerably.

Line bisection and spatial anisometry

Limitations of power function descriptions of line bisection

Line bisection tasks have been used extensively in neglect investigations. The simplicity of the stimuli and the ease of administration of these tasks give them great appeal. As mentioned above, neglect performances across several tasks can be described by power functions. However, in the specific case of line bisections, these descriptions harbor assumptions that limit their interpretation. Figure 1 shows a typical pattern of line bisections by neglect patients showing that greater errors are made with longer lines. Each line is divided into a left segment (l_i) and a right segment (r_i), with i representing different line lengths. As described above, the subjective estimate of any given line was considered to be twice the distance from the right end of the line to the point of

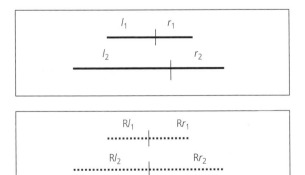

Figure 1 Bisection performances in physical space and its relation to representational space.

transection, or $2r_i$. The right end is used as an anchor because patients orient toward the right end of the line and scan leftward before placing their marks. Power functions were derived from the relationship of different objective line lengths $l_i + r_i$ to the subjective estimates $2r_i$, or

$$2r_i = K(l_i + r_i)^\beta.$$

This method of estimating patients' subjective representations of lines describes the spatial anisometry in neglect to a first approximation. It also raises several questions. How do we know that $2r_i$ is a measure of the patient's representation of the line? $2r_i$ might correlate with the representation of the line in some general way, but the nature of that correlation is not clear. Does it make sense to ascribe specific physical units, such as inches or centimeters, to a linear distance in representational space? Does it seem plausible that a neglect patient's appreciation of linear extent would be characterized by a single power function? If the attentional disturbance is graded along the horizontal axis, might not patients' psychophysics of horizontal linear perception vary over different segments of the line?

An alternative mathematical description of line bisection performance

To address the concerns raised above, we propose an alternative description which focuses on the relationship of the right to the left segments of the transected lines. When subjects bisect lines, they are indicating that their representations of the right and left segments are equal regardless of the objective lengths of these segments. If we label the representation R, then $Rl_i = Rr_i$ by definition, since that is what a bisection task requires of a subject. Importantly, this also means that with longer line lengths, the increase in the left representation is identical to the increase in the right representation. In Fig. 1, $(Rl_2 - Rl_1) = (Rr_2 - Rr_1)$, even though $(l_2 - l_i) \neq (r_2 - r_1)$. These relationships then offer us a link between physical line segments to their mental representations.

The left physical segments are related to the right physical segments by a power function $l = kr^a$. We can then describe the **rate of change** of left-sided physical segments compared with right-sided physical segments over a representational increment that is common to the left and the right sides. The rate of change for the left compared with the right physical segments is described by the first derivative of the function $l = Kr^a$

$$dl/dr = aKr^{(a-1)}.$$

This description incorporates the notion that the spatial anisometry varies dynamically depending on the length of the respective physical segments.

Chatterjee and Thompson (unpublished) investigated 16 patients with right brain damage and five age-matched control subjects to depict these relationships in line bisection performances. Based on their performance on the Behavioural Inattention Test (Wilson *et al.* 1987) and line bisection tasks, seven right-brain-damaged patients had neglect and nine did not. As might be expected, the variability of performance in the neglect subjects was considerably greater than in the brain-damaged control and normal control subjects. For both brain-damaged and normal control populations, the relationship was close to proportional. As the left physical segment increased, so did the right physical segment. Over a common representational increment, the left and the right physical increment increased monotonically. Spatial anisometries of mapping stimuli to representation are not clearly evident. In contrast, in the neglect patients for each increase of the right physical segment, the increase in the left physical segment was disproportionately greater. This relationship can be seen in Fig. 2(a), which shows an average of the group data. For the neglect patients, the left segment increases compared with the right by a power of 1.5. A common representational increment maps onto more physical space on the left as compared with the right. Furthermore, this disparity increases with larger physical segments as shown in Fig. 2(b).

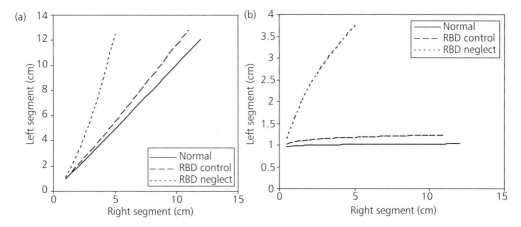

Figure 2 (a) The relationship of left and right segments of bisected lines. The left segment increases with each increment of the right segment. This graph simply demonstrates that in neglect the left segment is longer than the right, and that these patients have left neglect and make larger errors with longer lines. (b) The rate of increase of left versus right physical segments at different lengths of the right physical segment. For the normal control and right-brain-damaged subjects, this increase is proportionate, indicating a lack of anisometry. However, for patients with neglect the curve shows that for each representational increment left-sided space expands compared with right-sided space, and this expansion itself increases with longer segments.

Compression and expansion of space

Discussions of spatial anisometry in neglect often mention compression (Werth and Poppel 1988; Halligan and Marshall 1991) or expansion (Bisiach *et al*. 1996) of space. In these discussions it is important to be explicit about whether one is referring to physical or to representational space. An equivalent segment of representational space maps onto a greater physical distance on the left than on the right. Similarly, an equivalent segment of physical space is compressed further on the left than on the right in representational space. Several findings are consistent with this view. For instance, Milner and colleagues (Milner *et al*. 1993; Milner and Harvey 1995) report that neglect patients perceive left-sided horizontal physical segments as shorter than identical right-sided segments. Similarly, Bisiach *et al*. (1994) reported that neglect patients over-estimate left-sided physical segments when they have to reproduce the horizontal distance described by a right-sided segment. Such overextension of left-sided segments by neglect patients has been reported in several production tasks (Bisiach *et al*. 1996; Chokron *et al*. 1997; Kerkhoff 2000) (but see Bisiach and colleagues (1998) for contrary evidence, and Chapter 4.1 of this book for further discussion).

Viewing the spatial anisometry in neglect as a relative expansion of contralesional physical space and compression of contralesional representational space may also help to explain the counterintuitive findings reported by Karnath and Ferber (1999). They found no distortions of spatial representations in a group of patients with neglect. Their paradigm involved the perception and then reproduction of a horizontal distance. The neglect patients did quite well on this task. However, these data by themselves do not prove that representational anisometry was not present in these patients. In mapping physical space to representational space there may have been a left-sided compression. However, when reproducing this representation onto physical space they would then have expanded the left side. Consequently, relatively normal performance could result from compression in mapping stimuli to representation and then expansion in mapping representation to physical locations in external space.

The distribution of attention and gradients

Attention to external or internal space?

Neglect patients' gradient of attention is clearly tilted toward the right (Kinsbourne 1970, 1987). Could the robust observation that patients' bisections of lines are systematically related to the lengths of objective lines be related simply to the fact that longer lines extend further into ipsilesional space? Perhaps stimuli that extend further in right physical space also attract attention further in that direction and account for the greater deviations of bisection errors with longer lines. We refer to this possibility as the external space hypothesis. Alternatively, patients with neglect may have a pathological limitation of their capacity to sustain an internal representation of the line. This limitation becomes more evident with longer lines. We refer to this possibility as the internal representation hypothesis. These two hypotheses are not mutually exclusive. Typically, longer lines extend further into ipsilesional space and map onto longer representations. Therefore both hypotheses would predict larger errors with longer lines. While not disproving the external space hypothesis, visual illusions provide a test of the internal representation hypothesis.

Testing the internal representation hypothesis

The test of the internal representation hypothesis requires a condition in which patients bisect lines that occupy the same physical extent but different representational extents. Ricci *et al.* (2000) capitalized on the observation that patients with neglect are susceptible to the effects of some visual illusions, such as the Müller-Lyer illusion. Several investigators have reported that neglect patients' bisections are influenced by this illusion such that they bisect lines that appear longer with greater errors than lines that appear shorter (Mattingley *et al.* 1995; Ro and Rafal 1996; Vallar *et al.* 2000) (see also Chapter 4.6). This effect of this illusion is evident even when the patients are unable to report verbally whether the left-sided fins are directed outward or inward. For our purposes, the Müller-Lyer stimuli are not ideal to test the internal representation hypothesis because the 'fins' in the longer-looking lines in the illusion point outward and consequently extend further into ipsilesional external space. Thus Müller-Lyer stimuli extend further ipsilesionally in both external and internal space. To test the internal representation hypothesis, we constructed stimuli adapted from the Oppel–Kundt illusion.

The Oppel–Kundt illusion refers to the phenomenon that horizontal extents are perceived as being longer if they contain more discrete stimuli than if they contain fewer discrete stimuli (see also Chapter 4.6). We showed that lines comprised of fewer segments are perceived as shorter than lines of the same length that are comprised of more horizontal segments (Fig. 3). Ricci *et al.* (2000) reported that three patients with neglect made larger errors on longer-appearing lines despite the fact that these lines occupy the same physical horizontal space. These results support the internal representation hypothesis. They demonstrate that the attentional gradient in neglect which selects rightward stimuli operate on representations that have been processed to some extent.

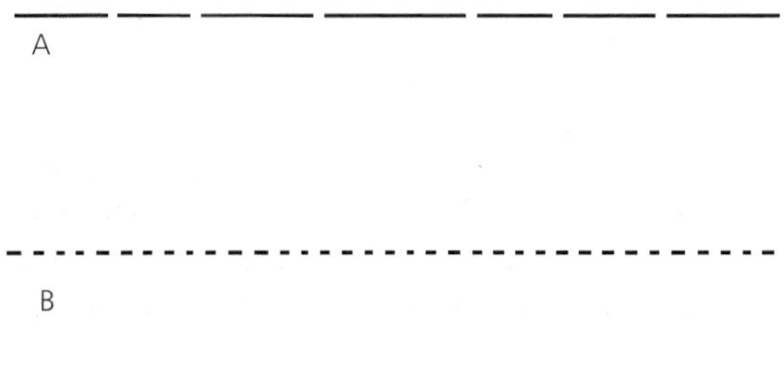

A

B

Figure 3 Examples of stimuli used for the Oppel–Kundt illusion.

Power function descriptions of neglect performance imply that entire magnitudes of stimuli influence performance. Thus, even though patients are 'neglecting' stimuli, something about the overall size of the arrays guides behavior. The pathological selection of stimuli for further processing in neglect must occur after some low-level processing. These relatively low-level processes, such as grouping of visual elements or perception of illusory visual contours, may be selectively damaged with relatively preserved spatial attention (Vecera and Behrmann 1997; Ricci *et al.* 1999). Additionally, as mentioned above, illusory effects may persist despite deficits of spatial attention.

Our suggestion that the anisometry in neglect be viewed as a disordered mapping of stimuli to representation needs to be modified slightly. Neglected stimuli must be processed to some extent, perhaps pre-attentively. The attentional gradient, which is directed ipsilesionally, is distributed over this pre-processed representation. The anisometric mapping of space occurs between this pre-attentively processed initial representation and the attentively processed final representation.

Cross-over, context, and representational release

The cross-over phenomenon

Halligan and Marshall (1988) made a curious discovery, referred to as the cross-over phenomenon, in line bisection tasks. Most patients with left neglect bisect lines to the right of the objective midpoint. However, with short lines (less than 4 cm) they cross over and bisect to the left of the objective midpoint. This cross-over challenges traditional explanations of neglect. Why should an attentional bias to the right shift to the left with short lines? Why should a representational scotoma on the left shift to the right with short lines? Two kinds of explanations (sometimes in combination) have been advanced to explain the cross-over phenomenon. The first invokes something special about the distribution of spatial attention over short lines. The second invokes an exaggeration of a general psychophysical phenomenon.

Attention over short horizontal segments

Marshall and Halligan (1990) initially suggested that patients approach shorter lines differently than they do longer lines. They postulated that the Weber fraction (that segment of line within which one is unable to discriminate between the length of the right and left segments) is larger in patients with neglect than in normal subjects. Their explanation for the cross-over phenomenon was as follows. Patients orient toward the right end of the line (Ishiai *et al.* 1989) and they move their attention leftward till they arrive at the right edge of the Weber fraction at which point they place their mark. Since their Weber fraction is larger than normal and they place their mark at the right edge of this segment, their transections are placed to the right of the line's objective center. However, with shorter lines they traverse the Weber fraction and place their mark at the left edge of this segment. As a result, they transect the line to the left of the line's objective center. The strength of this early hypothesis was that it framed the phenomenon in psychophysical terms. However, the hypothesis was not tested further. The reason why subjects might distribute their attention differently with short than with long lines was not specified.

Anderson offered a theoretical explanation for the cross-over, which proposed an unusual distortion of spatial attention over short lines (Anderson 1996). He started with the general hemispheric organization of spatial attention postulated by Heilman and Van Den Abell (1980) and Mesulam (1981). The right hemisphere is thought to distribute spatial attention widely, encompassing both hemifields, whereas the left hemisphere directs attention more narrowly into the contralateral hemifield. He described these respective attentional fields mathematically as two Gaussian distributions with different parameters (i.e. amplitudes, widths, peak locations) and derived a combined salience function. The function ascribes a variable salience to different sections of the line based on a summation of the two attentional functions. Importantly, when the lesioned right hemisphere is modelled by altering its parameters in specific ways, the saliency function produces an unusual distortion over short horizontal segments close to the midline. In these segments the left side of the line is more salient, whereas with longer lines the right side is more salient. Consequently patients place their transection marks to the left of short lines and to the right of long lines. This theoretical model received some support from eye-movement recording studies. Some patients with neglect tend to dwell on locations slightly to the left of center of horizontal lines, as though these regions were attentionally salient (Barton *et al.* 1998).

Because the cross-over phenomenon is observed with short lines, could the fact that these stimuli lie within an area encompassed by the fovea and can be apprehended without making saccades somehow account for the observation? While this 'foveal' account is not motivated by a clear hypothesis, two lines of evidence suggest that it is unlikely to be relevant to cross-over bisections. First, in some instances patients with left neglect paradoxically hyperorient into left space (Chatterjee, 1998). For example, when asked to point to their body's midsagittal plane while blindfolded most patients with neglect point rightward. However, some patients point into left hemispace (Chokron and Bartolomeo 1998). Similarly, some patients with right hemisphere lesions bisect long lines to the left of true midposition, a phenomenon referred to as ipsilesional neglect (Kwon and Heilman 1991). Adair *et al.* (1998) investigated one patient with such ipsilesional neglect, and found that her bisections were most consistent with an exaggerated cross-over phenomenon (rather than a mirror reversal of contralesional neglect). When presented with longer lines, she continued to place her transection point to the left of the true midpoint. However, the relative location of her transection points shifted rightward as the lines became longer. Thus, in this instance, cross-over bisections occurred with stimuli that could not be apprehended within foveal vision.[1]

The 'foveal account' also assumes that the cross-over phenomenon is specific to idiosyncrasies of visual processing. As we shall discuss later, a cross-over-like phenomenon also occurs when patients make judgments of non-spatial stimuli (Chatterjee *et al.* 2000). From these data we will argue that cross-over bisections are a specific instance of a more general aberration of stimulus processing following right brain damage.

Representational release

Anderson's model predicts that patients have right neglect when they bisect short lines. An alternative hypothesis would be that, rather than neglecting the right side of lines, patients are extending the line leftward in their mind's eye past the line's objective left edge. Because lines are quite featureless, they do not allow one to distinguish easily between these alternatives. In contrast, patients' performances on single-word reading might allow for such a distinction. Similar to lines, words can also be varied in length. In an investigation of patients with neglect dyslexia who omitted or misread leftward letters when reading single words (Chatterjee 1995) it was found that they omitted left-sided letters in long words, but actually confabulated additional letters at the left end of short words. They read two-letter words as having more than two letters. For example, one patient read the word 'my' as 'amy'. By analogy, it was proposed that patients complete or

---

[1] The reasons why in some instances patients show such exaggerated cross-over behavior or why some patients hyperorient into contralesional space is not known, and has not been investigated very much. This behavior may reflect some kind of release phenomenon that remains to be characterized.

confabulate the left end of lines so that they mentally represent these lines as longer than might be done normally. This proposal pointed out that most models of attention incorporate both excitatory and an inhibitory properties. With a left-sided attentional disturbance, one might anticipate both excitatory and inhibitory deficits. Excitatory deficits would result in neglect and inhibitory deficits would result in productive deficits. If the inhibitory deficits occurred at a sufficiently abstract level of representation, the productive errors would be confabulations that were not linked to stimulus properties in any transparent way. A formal test of this representational release hypothesis was provided by Monaghan and Shillcock (1998) who demonstrated its plausibility in a computational model that incorporated both excitatory and inhibitory attentional mechanisms.

Under- and over-estimation of lines

The neglect dyslexia observations suggest that patients with neglect over-estimate the magnitude of small stimuli and under-estimate the magnitude of larger stimuli. This over- and under-estimation of stimuli is a general psychophysical phenomenon that occurs when subjects make magnitude estimates of many different perceptual continua (Laming 1997).

Hollingworth (1909) observed that normal subjects over-estimate the length of small lines and under-estimate the length of longer lines. Mennemeier *et al.* (1998) extended this idea by investigating normal subjects and patients with left brain damage. They found that these subjects also cross over and bisect short lines on the opposite side of where they place their marks with longer lines. Thus the cross-over phenomenon is not unique to neglect, but it seems to be exaggerated in neglect. Mennemeier and colleagues speculated that neglect patients are perceptually anchored to the right end of the line. When they over-estimate short lines, they mentally extend the line past the left end of the objective line and consequently place their transection mark to the left of the objective mid-position.

In a similar vein, Marshall *et al.* (1998) suggested that contextual effects might account for the cross-over effect. They found that the order in which lines of different lengths were presented modified the placement of the transection marks by patients with neglect. Transection marks were placed further leftward when preceded by longer lines, and further rightward when preceded by shorter lines. They suggested that, since the shortest lines are usually preceded by longer lines, these transections end up at the left side of the line's objective mid-point.

Ricci and Chatterjee (2001) investigated contextual effects in line bisection in a series of patients with right brain damage. We replicated the findings of Marshall *et al.* (1998) that lines that precede the target lines modulate the location of the transection on the target line. This modulation occurred with both long and short lines. However, the cross-over was only seen with short lines. Thus, contextual effects contribute to but do not completely account for the cross-over in bisection. Something about the objective size of these lines also seems important, as has also been suggested by Ishiai *et al.* (1997).

Under- and over-estimation of nonspatial stimuli

To test the hypothesis that cross-over bisections represent a specific instance of a more general psychophysical phenomenon, we investigated weight judgments. Chatterjee and Thompson (1998) reported that weight judgments can be described by power functions and that patients with neglect or extinction under-estimate weights on their left side compared with those on their right side. Chatterjee *et al.* (2000) tested two patients with right brain damage. Both markedly under-estimated left-sided weights in general. However, their performance changed with the lightest weight pairs. The first patient was equally likely to judge the lightest left-sided weight as heavier or lighter than the lightest right-sided weight, analogous to the line length at which patients with left neglect are equally likely to place their mark on the left or the right of the line. The second patient reported that that the lightest left-sided weights were heavier than those on the right, analogous to the cross-over phenomenon in line bisections. Based on these data, we proposed that the cross-over phenomenon is a general psychophysical phenomenon not restricted to judgments of visuospatial stimuli. Since the over- and under-estimation of stimuli is a general psychophysical phenomenon, it would apply to weights lifted in both hands. Therefore we reasoned that these contextual effects were exaggerated on the left if the lightest left-sided weights were now judged as heavier than the lightest right-sided weights.

General implications of the cross-over phenomenon

Does the cross-over phenomenon in neglect have any general implications for the mapping of stimuli onto their mental representations? In reviewing the previous accounts of the cross-over in the view of the weight experiments outlined above, Chatterjee *et al.* (2000) proposed the following model for the cross-over effect (Fig. 4). The representation of a stimulus is constrained by at least two factors. The first is the physical characteristics of the stimuli itself. Attention to the stimuli is critical in constraining the representation to the physical features of the stimulus. In addition, memory traces (such as those left from previous stimuli) influence and constrain the representation. Accordingly, contextual effects from the previous stimuli in a series influence the magnitude of the representation. With an attentional impairment, the representation is not tightly linked to the stimuli itself, and as suggested earlier, representational release may occur. In this setting contextual influences modulate representations disproportionately and these contextual effects are exaggerated.

Conclusions and conjectures

The psychophysical range is condensed in neglect

Attentional mechanisms exist in the nervous system because humans are limited in their capacity to process all information at all times, and this capacity is further limited in patients with neglect. Despite their pathological capacity limitation, neglect patients' awareness of stimuli continues to conform to psychophysical power laws. However, their behavior subscribes to power functions with diminished exponents. The diminished exponent means that neglect patients remain sensitive to incremental changes in the magnitudes of stimuli. However, their psychological experience of these changes is dampened compared with normal. Instead of a clean amputation of processing beyond an upper limit, the range of sensory stimuli is compressed into a narrower range of representational space.

The nervous system appears to be designed to appreciate relative rather than absolute changes. With brain damage that produces neglect, the ability to index changes in sensation remains relatively preserved. However, the sensitivity to these changes and an appreciation of absolute magnitudes of sensations are compromised.

In neglect, physical space is expanded and representational space is compressed along the horizontal axis

The preserved effects of visual illusions in neglect suggest that neglect patients process contra-lesional stimuli to some level, perhaps pre-attentively, before the bias to select ipsilesional

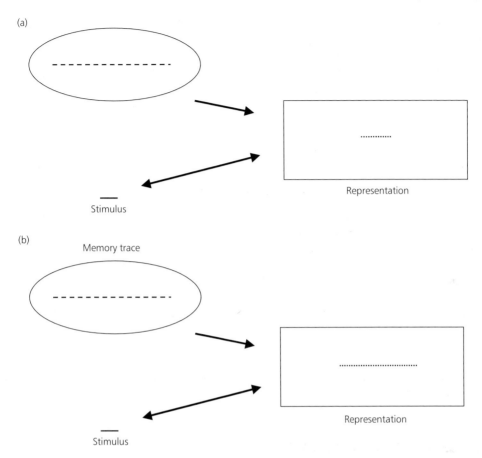

Figure 4 (a) Model of the representation of a stimulus influenced by features of the stimulus itself, as well as the memory trace of similar stimuli encountered previously. Lines are used as an example, but the model applies to words and weights as well. For purposes of the example, the line encountered previously is longer than the stimulus. Therefore the stimulus is pulled to being represented as slightly longer than expected from its objective measure. (b) Model of the representation of the stimulus in a neglect patient. With an attentional deficit, the memory trace has a disproportionate influence, resulting in an exaggerated over-estimation of the representation compared with normal contextual effects. (Reproduced with permission from Chatterjee *et al.* *Neuropsychologia*, **38**, 1390–7 (2000).)

information comes into play. The ipsilesional attentional gradient has specific consequences for the mapping of physical to representational space. Segments of contralesional physical space are compressed in representational space compared with equivalent segments in ipsilesional physical space. This view makes the prediction that on receptive tasks, which map stimuli from physical to representational space, neglect patients will under-estimate left-sided segments. In contrast, on productive tasks, which map representations on to stimuli in physical space, neglect patients will over-estimate left-sided segments. (An exception to this prediction is the situation of a patient with a directional hypokinesia, if the productive task involves a contralesional limb movement.)

The horizontal anisometry in neglect also varies with the size of the stimuli. The relative compression of left-sided representational space increases with longer horizontal stimuli. With short stimuli, the direction of the anisometry reverses.

The cross-over phenomenon in neglect is an exaggeration of a normal psychophysical phenomenon

When humans are confronted with a series of stimuli of varying magnitudes, they tend to over-estimate the stimuli at the lower end of the range and under-estimate stimuli at the upper end of the range. This normal phenomenon is exaggerated in patients with neglect, and underlies the dramatic cross-over bisections often seen in these patients. However, this kind of over- and under-estimation is not confined to stimuli that extend in space. It also occurs with weight estimates. One would predict that a similar phenomenon would be found with magnitude estimates of most stimuli.

Representations in neglect are unstable and at times may be released contralesionally

Representations in neglect are quantitatively and qualitatively unstable. Quantitatively, as mentioned above, neglect patients over-estimate smaller stimuli and under-estimate larger stimuli within a given range. We proposed that memory traces of previously viewed stimuli have a disproportionate influence on the representation. It is possible that previous responses might also have a disproportionate influence on responses,[2] but this possibility has not been investigated. In general, contextual effects of the stimuli on representations and performance in neglect remain under-explored.

Qualitative abnormalities in representational content accompany the quantitative anisometry of the mapping between physical and representational space. The compression of physical space in representational space results in poorer identification or discrimination of contralesional physical stimuli. The expansion of physical stimuli in representational space with small stimuli results in the release of representations and confabulations are more likely. This view predicts that neglect patients are more likely to make contralesional productive errors with small stimuli, when these stimuli are embedded in the context of stimuli covering a range of magnitudes.

Neglect in space, and in time?

Neglect is rightly viewed as a spatial deficit. However, consideration of the cross-over phenomenon leads us to think that temporal in addition to spatial factors influence performance. If Kant was correct in claiming that space and time provide the mental infrastructure for experience, is the spatial distortion in neglect accompanied by distortions of time?

Acknowledgements

The author greatly appreciates the thoughtful comments provided by Lisa Santer, Janice Snyder, and Roberta Daini. This work was supported by the National Institutes on Health (RO1NS37539).

References

Adair, J., Chatterjee, A., Schwartz, R., and Heilman, K. (1998). Ipsilateral neglect: reversal of bias or exaggerated cross-over phenomenon? *Cortex*, **34**, 147–153.

Anderson, B. (1996). A mathematical model of line bisection behaviour in neglect. *Brain*, **119**, 841–50.

Barton, J. J. S., Behrmann, M., and Black, S. (1998). Ocular search during line bisection: the effects of hemi-neglect and hemianopia. *Brain*, **121**, 1117–31.

[2] This possibility was suggested to the author by Mark Mennemeier.

Bisiach, E., Bulgarelli, C., Sterzi, R., and Vallar, G. (1983). Line bisection and cognitive plasticity of unilateral neglect of space. *Brain and Cognition*, **2**, 32–8.

Bisiach, E., Rusconi, M. L., Peretti, V. A., and Vallar, G. (1994). Challenging current accounts of unilateral neglect. *Neuropsychologia*, **32**, 1431–4.

Bisiach, E., Pizzamiglio, L., Nico, D., and Antonucci, G. (1996). Beyond unilateral neglect. *Brain*, **119**, 851–7.

Bisiach, E., Ricci, R., and Modona, M. N. (1998). Visual awareness and anisometry of space representation in unilateral neglect: a panoramic investigation by means of a line extension task. *Consciousness and Cognition*, **7**, 327–55.

Chatterjee, A. (1995). Cross over, completion and confabulation in unilateral spatial neglect. *Brain*, **118**, 455–65.

Chatterjee, A. (1998). Motor minds and mental models in neglect. *Brain and Cognition*, **37**, 339–49.

Chatterjee, A. and Thompson, K. A. (1998). Weigh(t)ing for awareness. *Brain and Cognition*, **37**, 477–90.

Chatterjee, A., Mennemeier, M., and Heilman, K. M. (1992*a*). Search patterns and neglect: a case study. *Neuropsychologia*, **30**, 657–72.

Chatterjee, A., Mennemeier, M., and Heilman, K. M. (1992*b*). A stimulus-response relationship in unilateral neglect: the power function. *Neuropsychologia*, **30**, 1101–8.

Chatterjee, A., Dajani, B. M., and Gage, R. J. (1994*a*). Psychophysical constraints on behavior in unilateral spatial neglect. *Neuropsychiatry, Neuropsychology and Behavioral Neurology*, **7**, 267–74.

Chatterjee, A., Mennemeier, M., and Heilman, K. M. (1994*b*). The psychophysical power law and unilateral spatial neglect. *Brain and Cognition*, **25**, 92–107.

Chatterjee, A., Ricci, R., and Calhoun, J. (2000). Weighing the evidence for cross over in neglect. *Neuropsychologia*, **38**, 1390–7.

Chokron, S. and Bartolomeo, P. (1998). Position of the egocentric reference and directional movements in right brain-damaged patients. *Brain and Cognition*, **37**, 405–18.

Chokron, S., Bernard, J., and Imbert, M. (1997). Length representation in normal and neglect subjects with opposite reading habits studied through a line extension task. *Cortex*, **33**, 47–64.

Fechner, G. (1860/1966). *Elements of psychophysic*. Holt, Rinehart and Winston, New York.

Halligan, P. W. and Marshall, J. C. (1988). How long is a piece of string? A study of line bisection in a case of visual neglect. *Cortex*, **24**, 321–8.

Halligan, P. W. and Marshall, J. C. (1989). Line bisection in visuo-spatial neglect: disproof of a conjecture. *Cortex*, **25**, 517–21.

Halligan, P. W. and Marshall, J. C. (1991). Spatial compression in visual neglect: A case study. *Cortex*, **27**, 623–9.

Heilman, K. M. and Van Den Abell, T. (1980). Right hemisphere dominance for attention: the mechanisms underlying hemispheric assymmetries of inattention (neglect). *Neurology*, **30**, 327–30.

Hollingworth, H. (1909). The inaccuracy of movement. *Archives of Psychology*, **13**, 1–87.

Ishiai, S., Furukawa, T., and Tsukagoshi, H. (1989). Visuospatial processes of line bisection and the mechanisms underlying unilateral spacial neglect. *Brain*, **112**, 1485–1502.

Ishiai, S., Koyama, Y., Seki, K., Sato, S., and Nakayama, T. (1997). Dissociated neglect for objective and subjective sizes. *Journal of Neurology*, **244**, 607–12.

Karnath, H.-O. and Ferber, S. (1999). Is space representation distorted in neglect? *Neuropsychologia*, **37**, 7–15.

Kerkhoff, G. (2000). Multiple perceptual distortions and their modulation in left-sided visual neglect. *Neuropsychologia*, **38**, 1073–86.

Kinsbourne, M. (1970). The cerebral basis of lateral asymmetries in attention. *Acta Psychologica*, **33**, 193–201.

Kinsbourne, M. (1987). Mechanisms of unilateral neglect. In *Neurophysiological and neuropsychological aspects of spatial neglect* (ed. M. Jeannerod), pp. 69–86. Elsevier, Amsterdam.

Kwon, S. E. and Heilman, K. M. (1991). Ipsilateral neglect in a patient following a unilateral frontal lesion. *Neurology*, **41**, 2001–4.

Laming, D. (1997) *The measurement of sensation*. Oxford University Press, New York.

Marshall, J. C. and Halligan, P. W. (1990). Line bisection in a case of visual neglect: psychophysical studies with implications for theory. *Cognitive Neuropsychology*, **7**, 107–30.

Marshall, R. S., Lazar, R. M., Krakauer, J. W., and Sharma, R. (1998). Stimulus context in hemineglect. *Brain*, **121**, 2003–10.

Mattingley, J., Bradshaw, J., and Bradshaw, J. (1995). The effect of unilateral visuospatial neglect on perception of Müller-Lyer illusory figures. *Perception*, **24**, 415–33.

Mennemeier, M., Rapcsak, S. Z., Dillon, M., and Vezey, E. (1998). A search for the optimal stimulus. *Brain and Cognition*, **37**, 439–59.

Mesulam, M.-M. (1981). A cortical network for directed attention and unilateral neglect. *Annals of Neurology*, **10**, 309–25.

Milner, A. D. and Harvey, M. (1995). Distortion of size perception in visuospatial neglect. *Current Biology*, **5**, 85–9.

Milner, A. D., Harvey, M., Roberts, R. C., and Forster, S. V. (1993). Line bisection error in visual neglect: misguided action or size distortion? *Neuropsychologia*, **31**, 39–49.

Monaghan, P. and Shillcock, R. (1998). The cross-over effect in unilateral neglect. Modelling detailed data in the line-bisection task. *Brain*, **121**, 907–21.

Ricci, R. and Chatterjee, A. (2001). Context and crossover in unilateral neglect. *Neuropsychologia*, **39**, 1138–43.

Ricci, R., Vaishnavi, S., and Chatterjee, A. (1999). A deficit of preattentive vision: experimental observations and theoretical implications. *Neurocase*, **5**, 1–12.

Ricci, R., Calhoun, J., and Chatterjee, A. (2000). Orientation bias in unilateral neglect: representational contributions. *Cortex*, **36**, 671–7.

Ro, T. and Rafal, R. (1996). Perception of geometric illusions in hemispatial neglect. *Neuropsychologia*, **34**, 973–8.

Stevens, S. S. (1958). Measurement and man. *Science*, **127**, 383–9.

Stevens, S. S. (1970). Neural events and the psychophysical power law. *Science*, **170**, 1043–50.

Stevens, S. S. and Galanter, E. H. (1957). Ratio scales and category scales for a dozen perceptual continua. *Journal of Experimental Psychology*, **54**, 377–411.

Vallar, G., Daini, R., and Antonucci, G. (2000). Processing of illusion of length in spatial hemineglect: a study of line bisection. *Neuropsychologia*, **38**, 1087–97.

Vecera, S. and Behrmann, M. (1997). Spatial attention does not require preattentive grouping. *Neuropsychology*, **11**, 30–43.

Werth, R. and Poppel, E. (1988). Compression and lateral shift of mental coordinate systems in a line bisection task. *Neuropsychologia*, **26**, 741–5.

Wilson, B., Cockburn, J., and Halligan, P. W. (1987). *Behavioural inattention test*. Thames Valley Test Company, Bury St Edmunds.

4.4 Perceptual and motor interaction in unilateral spatial neglect

Sumio Ishiai

Patients with left unilateral spatial neglect bisect horizontal lines to the right of the true center (Heilman *et al.* 1993). Such errors may reflect a size distortion such that they may perceive linear extents in the left half of egocentric space as shorter than equivalent extents in the right half-space (Milner *et al.* 1993; Milner and Harvey 1995). Studies of eye movements revealed that they hardly ever searched leftward when bisecting lines (Ishiai *et al.* 1989, 1992, 1995, 1996a, 2001). We devised a line extension task (Ishiai *et al.* 1994a,b) to test whether effective orientation to the neglected side would improve left-side underestimation. The patients with neglect following either parietal or frontal lesions extended a horizontal line leftward to double its original length. They executed leftward movements without difficulty, and their line extension performance was nearly accurate compared with the apparent bisection errors. The patients were considered to be able to compare the lengths of the right and left extents because they could attend sufficiently to the left extreme of the extended segment. However, as pointed out by Chokron *et al.* (1997), some patients, especially those with a frontal lesion, tended to show leftward over-extension (Ishiai *et al.* 1994b).

Bisiach *et al.* (1994, 1996) (see also Chapter 4.1) reported a neglect disorder implying a horizontal anisometry of spatial representation. The patients with neglect bisected an actual line and a virtual line between the two points, and then they set the endpoints of the imaginary line on the basis of its printed center. The left endpoint was placed farther from the printed center than the right endpoint. The tendency to left-side over-extension in Bisiach's endpoint task and the line extension task was recently duplicated in a similar task (Doricchi and Angelelli 1999; Nico *et al.* 1999). The central mark and the right or left point are printed on the test sheet. When the right point is printed, the subjects are asked to place the left point so that the left and right points should be equally distant from the central mark. This task is called the 'symmetric positioning task' in this chapter. The left distance was over-extended absolutely compared with the right reference length (Doricchi and Angelelli 1999) or relatively when the performance was compared between the placements of the left and right points (Nico *et al.* 1999).

Patients with neglect show left-side underestimation in the line bisection task and left-side over-extension in the tasks that require leftward extension or localization. We carried out a study to test whether there would be a common mechanism underlying their errors when performing these two types of task. We also intended to answer the question as to why, in the latter tasks, patients with neglect shift attention and execute movements easily to the left side. Many tasks have been devised to investigate the mechanisms of unilateral spatial neglect. Some of them have tried to examine the perceptual and motor aspects separately (see Chapter 4.2). However, unilateral spatial neglect is basically a disorder observed in free viewing conditions. Besides, in clinical manifestation of neglect, the perceptual and motor components are bound tightly together. To clarify the mechanisms of left-side underestimation and over-extension, the present study investigated perceptual and motor interaction, and mental representation, by analyzing movements of the eyes and the hand in unilateral spatial neglect.

Case reports

YH, a 50-year-old right-handed man, was tested 5 months after onset of a middle cerebral artery territory infarction. On CT examination, an extensive lesion involved the frontal, temporal, and parietal lobes. He had left hemiplegia. Left hemianopia was revealed on confrontation testing. His severity of neglect was moderate, and the conventional test score of the Behavioural Inattention Test (BIT) (Wilson *et al.* 1987) was 111 (see Table 1 for scores in the subtests). The scores were abnormal except for the line-crossing subtest.

KO, a 68-year-old right-handed man, was examined 4 months after onset of a middle cerebral artery territory infarction. CT demonstrated an extensive right temporoparietal lesion, and the area of infarction extended into the posterior limb of the internal capsule. He showed left hemiplegia and left homonymous hemianopia. Unilateral spatial neglect was severe, and the BIT conventional test score was 72. The scores in the subtests were all below the cut-off scores (Table 1).

Line bisection and symmetric positioning tasks

Line bisection task

A line 150, 200, or 250 mm long was printed horizontally across the center of a sheet of paper (257 mm × 362 mm). The lines were individually presented to the patients so that the center was located in the sagittal midplane of the trunk. The patients were asked to mark the subjective midpoint on each line with a pencil held in the right hand. They bisected five lines for each length in a randomized order.

We recorded eye-fixation patterns with an eye-camera system (EMR-7, NAC Inc.) (Ishiai *et al.* 1989, 1992, 1995, 1996a, 2001). The head unit of this apparatus, which includes the eye camera and a scene camera, weighs 350 g and is connected to the control unit by flexible cables. The patient could perform the tasks under natural conditions with head movements permitted. The combined picture in which the point of fixation was superimposed on the visual scene was recorded with a videotape recorder. The lateral movements of fixation relative to the presented line were analyzed from the time of line presentation to the time of starting to place the mark.

Table 1 Behavioural Inattention Test: conventional subtest scores

	YH	KO	Cut-off score[a]/full score
Line crossing	36	26	34/36
Letter cancellation	34	29	34/40
Star cancellation	38	16	51/54
Copying	1	0	3/4
Line bisection	0	0	7/9
Drawing	2	1	2/3
Total	111	72	131/146

[a] Cut-off score for Japanese edition of the BIT (Ishiai 1999).

Symmetric positioning task

The patients were presented with a test sheet (257 mm × 362 mm) where a central vertical bar and a right small circle were printed. The right circle was located 75, 100, or 125 mm distant from the central bar. Their task was to mark a left circle at the horizontally symmetric point with a pencil held in the right hand. The examiner demonstrated an ideal performance and asked them to place the left point so that the left and right distances should be equal from the central bar. The patients performed five trials for each distance in a randomized order.

The left distance was measured as a final result. The eye-fixation pattern was recorded throughout the trials with the eye-camera system. Movements of the head were not restricted. The lateral movements of fixation relative to the stimuli were analyzed from the presentation of the test sheet to the time of starting to draw the left circle. The movements of the pencil tip were also recorded after it reached the horizontal level of the central bar and the right circle.

Comparison of left and right distances

Figure 1 shows the overall results for the two patients in the line bisection and symmetric positioning tasks. YH bisected the lines to the right of the true center, and the deviations were greater for the longer lines. In the symmetric positioning task, he over-extended the left distance when reproducing the distance of 75 or 100 mm. The 125-mm trials appeared to be performed almost accurately. As seen in Fig. 1, however, the left points were placed about the same distance to the left of the central bar irrespective of the right distance. KO also showed typical rightward errors in the line bisection task. In the symmetric positioning task, he performed more accurately than YH. However, over-extension on average was observed for the trials of 75- and 100-mm distances.

The right-hand panels of Fig. 1 show the comparison of the results between the two tasks. For the line bisection task, the difference between the left and right extents from the subjective midpoint was calculated. Similarly, for the symmetric positioning task, the difference between the left and right distances was calculated. The analysis of YH's results showed that the left–right difference was greater for the bisections of the longer lines. In contrast, in the symmetric positioning task, the difference became smaller for the longer distances. KO also showed greater left–right differences when bisecting the longer lines. In the symmetric positioning task, the differences were small, reflecting his nearly accurate performance. The left–right difference in the line bisection task was equal to twice the rightward deviation of the subjective midpoint from the actual center. Accordingly, the greater differences for the longer lines are compatible with the typical neglect phenomenon that rightward deviations become greater for longer lines (Halligan and Marshall 1988; Chatterjee 1995). However, the left–right difference in the symmetric positioning task was related inversely, or unrelated, to the distance to be reproduced. These simple comparisons suggest that left-side underestimation in line bisection and over-extension in symmetric positioning resulted from different mechanisms.

Eye movements and line bisection

Eye-fixation pattern

Figure 2 shows the eye-fixation patterns when the two patients bisected the lines. YH made no apparent leftward search in seven of the 15 trials. He placed the subjective midpoint near the left extreme point of fixation on the line (Fig. 2(a)), which corresponds to the eye-fixation pattern characteristic of neglect (Ishiai *et al.* 1989). A month before this study, he always exhibited this

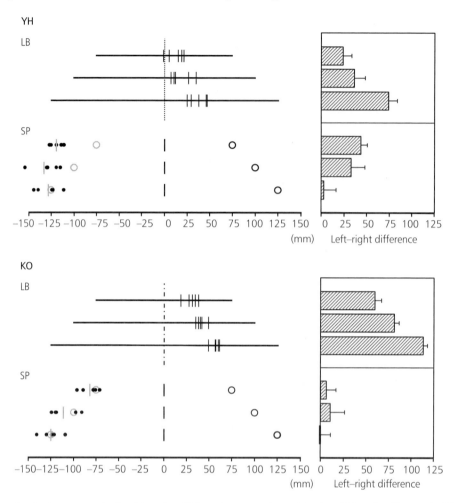

Figure 1 Performances in line bisection (LB) and symmetric positioning (SP) tasks. The vertical bars on the lines show the results for all bisections. In the symmetric positioning task, the black circle and the gray circle represent the right stimulus point and the ideal left point respectively. The subjective left points and their mean position for each distance are shown as the black dots and the gray vertical bars. The right-hand panels show the mean left–right differences with standard deviations for the three length–distance conditions in the two tasks.

typical pattern of neglect without leftward searches. In six of the remaining eight trials, YH showed leftward searches that fell short of the left endpoint. In only two trials, he searched laboriously for the left endpoint (Fig. 2(b)). However, the leftmost fixation was maintained for only about 200 ms, and the gaze returned quickly to the right side. The mark was eventually placed to the right of the actual center.

KO always showed the eye-fixation pattern characteristic of neglect. He persisted in fixating the right-side point at which he later placed the subjective midpoint, and made no leftward search. His eye movements were generally inactive during line bisection, and rightward searches were also infrequent (Fig. 2(c)).

Both patients moved the pencil tip directly to the fixated point on the line. The initiation of hand movements did not affect the gaze direction.

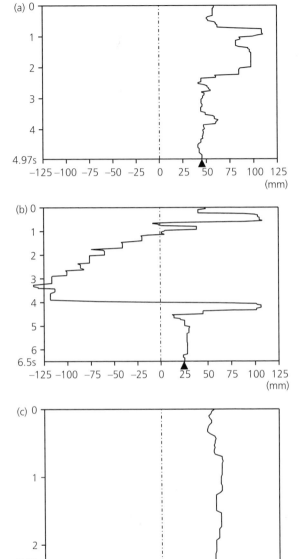

Figure 2 Eye-fixation patterns during line bisection. The horizontal axis indicates the distance from the actual center of the presented line, and the vertical axis indicates the time from the presentation of the line to the placement of the subjective midpoint. The triangle on the horizontal axis shows the location of the subjective midpoint.

Perceived extent and subjective midpoint

Figure 3 shows the relationship between the searched extent and the subjective midpoint for all the bisections of the two patients. The line segment to the right of the left extreme fixation fell in the right visual field at least once during the course of bisection. The perception of the two patients was restricted mostly to this extent, as they had a complete left hemianopia. When YH did not search leftward, the subjective midpoint was placed near the left extreme of the perceived extent. In the eight trials with leftward searches (indicated with asterisks in Fig. 3) he marked to the left of the center of the perceived extent in three trials, to the right side in four trials, and near the center in one trial. In other words, the location of the subjective midpoint relative to the presented line

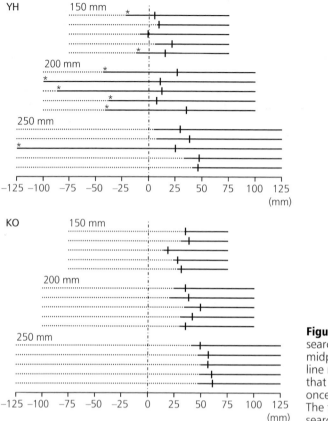

Figure 3 Relationships between searched extent and subjective midpoint for all bisections. The solid line represents the searched extent that fell in the right visual field at least once during the course of bisection. The trials with apparent leftward searches are indicated with asterisks.

was almost unaffected by the size of the leftward searches. This is comparable with the results of previous studies (Ishiai *et al.* 1996*a*; Barton *et al.* 1998). KO made no apparent search to the left side. His subjective midpoint was always placed near the left extreme point of the perceived extent.

Visuospatial processes in line bisection

Patients with typical neglect search to the left side infrequently and insufficiently during line bisection. Their rightward errors of bisection may not be affected by the size of leftward searches or the perceived extents. When patients with left neglect and hemianopia do not search leftward, they place the subjective midpoint near the left extreme of the perceived extent. In this case, the perceived extent does not seem to be 'bisected'. In addition, in bisections with leftward searches, the left side of the perceived segment is not always underestimated. Nevertheless, patients with neglect are considered to understand the task of bisecting a line. Most of them are able to appreciate their rightward errors when forced to fixate the left endpoint after bisection (Ishiai *et al.* 1989, 1995, 1996*a*). The mental representation of a line may be formed on the basis of the attended segment to the right of the fixated point at which the mark is later placed. This may be explained as a completion-like phenomenon (Ishiai *et al.* 1989, 1992; Chatterjee 1995).

The length of a line has been reported to have little true effect on the bisection of patients with severe neglect when their performance is closely examined by controlling line positions relative to the body midline (Koyama *et al.* 1997). In the ordinary midline presentation, the right endpoint of a line is located more to the right side as its length becomes longer. Severe cases may determine their subjective midpoint according to the location of the right endpoint in egocentric space.

After rehabilitation or in the recovery stage, patients with neglect may show some leftward searches during line bisection. However, the searches reach the left endpoint only occasionally, and the duration of the leftmost fixation is very short. Transient attentional shifts to the left side may produce leftward searches, which would not contribute to effective processing of line bisection (Ishiai *et al.* 1996*a*). Significant improvement of bisection seems to require stronger engagement of attention to the left endpoint, as in cueing by letter reporting (Riddoch and Humphreys 1983), forced fixation (Ishiai *et al.* 1995), or pointing to the left endpoint (Ishiai *et al.* 2000).

Patients with neglect fixate the point at which they later place the subjective midpoint. The initiation of hand movements caused no shift of the eyes, although preparation to bisect lines with the right hand might shift overall direction of the gaze to the right side.

Eye and hand movements in the symmetric positioning task

Case YH

Figure 4(a) shows the symmetric positioning performance of YH in the first trial with a 75-mm distance. The fixation gradually shifted to the left side with some rightward searches interspersed.

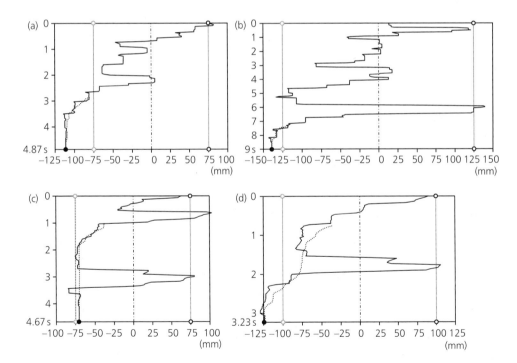

Figure 4 Movements of eyes and hand (pencil tip) during symmetric positioning. The horizontal axis indicates the distance from the central vertical bar, and the vertical axis indicates the time from the presentation of the test sheet to the placement the subjective left point. The black circle, the gray circle, and the black dot on the horizontal axis represent the right stimulus point, the ideal left point, and the subjective left point respectively. The solid line shows the eye movements, and the dotted line shows the movements of the pencil tip after it reached the horizontal level of the central bar and the right point.

He moved the pencil only after his fixation went beyond the ideal left point. After the pencil tip reached the point of fixation, the gaze and the hand moved together further to the left side. In this stage, no rightward search occurred, and over-extension was frequently observed. In the case of the longer 125-mm trials, YH started a reaching movement to the fixation that did not exceed the ideal point (Fig. 4(b)). However, the eyes and the hand moved in coordination to the left side beyond the ideal point. Accordingly, the symmetric point was sometimes misplaced to the left side.

Figure 5 shows analyses for all trials of symmetric positioning. The black crosses in the figure show the points of fixation to which YH initially moved the pencil tip. These points were located nearer to the ideal point (gray circles) than the final left points (black dots). However, in the 75-mm trials the movement of the eyes (black crosses) exceeded the ideal distance. Both the leftward fixation and the additional eye and hand movements resulted in the obvious over-extension. In the 100-mm trials, the pencil tip approached the fixation that fell near the ideal point. The additional movement of the gaze and the hand led to an over-extension of the left distance. In the trials of 125-mm distance, the patient moved the pencil tip to the point of fixation that often undershot the ideal point. The additional movement was also observed, but the left point was placed near the ideal point. The left extreme point of fixation (white crosses) coincided with the subjective left point in most trials for all three distances.

Case KO

KO performed the symmetric positioning task with a different strategy. He shifted his gaze gradually to the left side, and the pencil tip was moved simultaneously (Figs 4(c) and 4(d)) from the central bar or from midway between the central bar and the ideal left point (Fig. 5, leftward

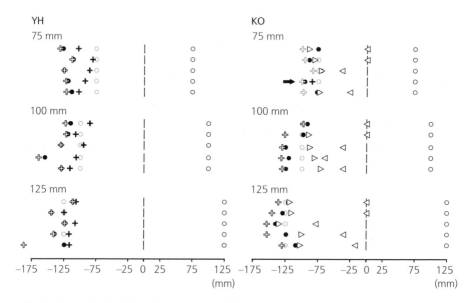

Figure 5 Analyses for all trials of symmetric positioning. The black circle and the gray circle represent the right stimulus point and the ideal left point respectively. The black dot shows the subjective left point, and the white cross shows the leftmost point of fixation. YH moved the pencil directly to the point of fixation (black cross) that went beyond, or fell near, the ideal left point. In contrast, KO started to move the pencil tip from the central bar or from midway between the central bar and the ideal left point (leftward triangle). The rightward triangle shows the location of the pencil tip when the final rightward search started.

triangles). Except in two trials, rightward searching with the eyes occurred before the placement of the left circle. The rightward triangles in Fig. 5 show the locations of the pencil tip when the final rightward search started. When the pencil tip had reached near the ideal point before the rightward search (Fig. 4(c)), the patient made no additional movement and placed the left circle almost accurately (Fig. 5, 75-mm trials 2, 3, and 5, 100-mm trial 2, and 125-mm trials 1–3). In such trials, the returning saccade after the rightward search often overshot the pencil tip, which corresponded to the leftmost fixation (Fig. 5, white crosses). These overshoots resemble those of hemianopic patients who adopt a strategy employing a large saccade to find a target falling in the blind hemifield (Meienberg *et al.* 1981). However, the hypermetric saccades did not result in over-extension of the left distance.

When the point before the rightward search fell short of the ideal point, the patient moved the eyes and the hand further to the left side (Figs 4(d) and 5, 100-mm trials 3–5 and 125-mm trial 4). The additional leftward movement was made without rightward searching and resulted in over-extension in the trials of 100-mm distance. In the fifth trial of 125-mm distance, the rightward search occurred at a point that fell short of the ideal distance, while the patient added no further shift to the left side.

The first trial of the symmetric positioning task, which required the patient to reproduce a 75-mm distance, was unique. The patient started to move the pencil tip from the central bar and exceeded the ideal point. After searching rightward, he moved back to the right side and placed the left circle accurately. Such a rightward movement to correct an over-extension was never found in the other trials of either patient. The lack of corrective rightward movement seems to be a characteristic pattern of neglect in the symmetric positioning task.

The fourth 75-mm trial (Fig. 5, arrow) was exceptionally performed in the same way as YH did; KO moved the pencil only after his fixation went beyond the ideal left point.

Perceptual and motor interaction in symmetric positioning

Activation of a representational map for contralesional space

The symmetric positioning task requires a crossed response to the contralateral imaginary point but not to the visual stimulus itself. When such a response is required into contralesional space, the representational map for that space may be activated in the brain of patients with neglect. A leftward shift of the head and the eyes improved recall for imaginary items in the neglected space, which suggested activation of the engrams for left-sided visuospatial memories (Meador *et al.* 1987). According to the premotor theory (Rizzolatti and Gallese 1988), spatial attention is a correlate of the organization of motor acts. The selection of a motor plan should automatically produce a shift of attention toward the spatial sector where the action will be executed. In the symmetric positioning task, preparation of a leftward response may result in an over-extended representation of the left distance. However, it is possible that the representational map for visual images has a gradual restriction toward the peripheral sector of the left hemispace. The two patients in the present study showed over-extension for the 75- and 100-mm trials but not for the 125-mm trials.

Each hemisphere may be responsible for programming movements of the contralateral hand but also dominant for movement execution within and toward the contralateral hemispace (Heilman *et al.* 1984). The frontal area centered around the frontal eye field may provide a representational map for the distribution of orienting and exploratory movements (Mesulam 1990). Several studies reported that exploratory motor deficits predominate in neglect after lesions that involve the frontal lobe (Bisiach *et al.* 1990; Tegnér and Levander 1991). However, a recent study found that neglect patients with right inferior parietal damage were impaired in making leftward limb movements to targets in left hemispace (Mattingley *et al.* 1998).

The type of response required in the symmetric positioning and line extension tasks appear to induce leftward movements effectively, even when patients with neglect have exploratory deficits in other tasks (Ishiai *et al.* 1994*a*,*b*). The lesion of YH involved the parietal and frontal lobes extensively, and that of KO damaged the parietal but not the frontal lobe. Leftward movements of the right hand may be initiated by activation of the residual function of the right hemisphere or by compensation via left-hemisphere mechanisms or by both. YH directed his gaze to the location that would correspond to the imaginary left point, and KO gradually shifted his gaze to the left side. The resultant perception of the left space probably contributed to a smooth execution of the prepared leftward movement of the hand.

Pathological perceptual and motor interaction

Patients with neglect may have difficulty in dissociating the focus of perception (gaze direction) from the location of motor execution. When they are examined using clinical tests, such difficulty would usually appear in the manifestation of errors on the left side. In free viewing of a flower prepared by the examiner, most patients with neglect were able to discriminate between the presence and absence of the left-side petals (Ishiai *et al.* 1996*b*). However, when copying the flower they left the left side unfinished without noticing the incompleteness. While copying, attention or perception of patients with neglect may be restricted to the right-side petals that they are drawing.

The analyses of their symmetric positioning performances revealed that the patients had difficulty in shifting attention even in the rightward direction from the focus of orientation. They never searched rightward with the eyes when moving the hand to the left extreme distance before placement of the mark. An exaggerated perceptual–motor interaction may also contribute to the leftward over-extension when the response is induced to the left side. Such pathological interaction seems to explain right-sided omissions found in the cancellation tests (Weintraub and Mesulam 1987). When patients with left neglect adopt a compensatory scanning strategy to the left side (Robertson *et al.* 1994), they have difficulty in changing their gaze direction from the left marking point to check omissions on the right side. Prism adaptation (Rossetti *et al.* 1998) (see also Chapter 7.2) produces a discrepancy between the programmed goal of the hand movement and the seen direction of the visual target. This alteration of sensorimotor coordinates may break down the pathological perceptual and motor interaction to improve neglect dramatically.

Impaired disengagement of attention from its current focus seems to be unique to parietal lesions (Posner *et al.* 1984). This deficit of disengagement is reported to be directionally specific to the contralesional side (Posner *et al.* 1987). As the pathological perceptual and motor interaction was also observed in the ipsilesional direction, it is probably not caused by the impaired disengagement of attention. The interaction appeared to be stronger in the patient whose lesion involved the frontal as well as the parietal lobe.

Comparison of two lengths

Patients with neglect often show better performance when judging accuracy of bisection for pre-transected lines than when bisecting lines (Marshall and Halligan 1995; Ishiai *et al.* 1998). The former task requires them to compare two physical lengths, whereas the latter has to be accomplished by estimating the midpoint according to the information provided by a single length. The symmetric positioning task also has to be performed on the basis of a single distance, when the gaze is directed to the imaginary left point in the blank left hemispace. In most trials, however, KO introduced the pencil tip in the visual scene and moved his eyes and hand to the subjective left point. The introduction of the third point enabled the patient to compare the right and left distances. The ability to compare two distances may have compensated for the leftward over-representation which was suggested when KO also determined the left point without moving the pencil tip.

In the line extension task (Ishiai *et al.* 1994*a*,*b*), patients with neglect first placed the pencil tip at the left endpoint of the printed line and then drew an additional line leftward. Recently, we recorded the eye-fixation patterns during line extension in some patients. The movements of the eyes and the hand resembled KO's performance in the symmetric positioning task, especially when he started from the central bar. In the line extension task, the comparison of the left and the right extents is probably easier, as the two line segments are equivalently visible in the course of extension. This is probably why the patients with neglect showed smaller over-extension in our line extension studies.

Use of an egocentric or an allocentric reference frame

In the symmetric positioning task, the imaginary left point may be represented initially in an egocentric reference frame when the central bar is in line with the body midline. YH seemed to perform the task according mainly to this representational process. Patients with neglect may prefer an egocentric or an allocentric reference frame to solve spatial problems, while variable use of either frame may be found in some patients (Chatterjee 1994). Task demands (Behrmann and Tipper 1999) and external cueing (Ishiai *et al.* 2001) may change the selective use of the reference frames. KO probably used an allocentric reference frame additionally to compare the left and right distances at least when he searched rightward before placing the left point. The frontal lobe was involved in the YH's lesion but not in that of KO. Although the allocentric and egocentric functioning of attention may share common mechanisms in the parietal lobe (Fink *et al.* 1997), the frontal lobe might contribute to appropriate and flexible use of the two reference frames. In most trials of symmetric positioning, however, KO showed only one overt search to the right side to compare the two distances on the allocentric frame. Adaptive change of the reference frame appears to be limited in patients with neglect whose perceptual and motor interaction is pathologically exaggerated.

Conclusions

Patients with unilateral spatial neglect adopt different visuospatial processing for the line bisection and the symmetric positioning tasks.

In the line bisection task, leftward searches are absent or are accomplished with marked restriction of size. It is unlikely that the whole extent to the left of the subjective midpoint is perceived but underestimated. The left extent seems to be inferred mainly from the attended right extent, which may be a completion-like phenomenon.

In the symmetric positioning task, when a response is required into the contralesional space, the representational map for that space may be activated in the brain of patients with neglect. Over-extension of the left distance may result partly from over-representation on the left side of the map. However, it is possible that the map has an uncompensated restriction toward the peripheral sector of the left hemispace. An exaggerated 'perceptual–motor interaction' in neglect may also misdirect responses toward the neglected side when the task elicited a leftward orientation. The strategy used to perform a task may be variable among patients as well as trials, which may affect the selective use of the reference frames.

Acknowledgement

This work is supported by a Grant-in-Aid for Scientific Research (C) to Sumio Ishiai from the Ministry of Education, Science, Sports, and Culture, Japan.

References

Barton, J. J. S., Behrmann, M., and Black, S. (1998). Ocular search during line bisection: the effects of hemi-neglect and hemianopia. *Brain*, **121**, 1117–31.

Behrmann, M. and Tipper, S. P. (1999). Attention accesses multiple reference frames: evidence from visual neglect. *Journal of Experimental Psychology: Human Perception and Performance*, **25**, 83–101.

Bisiach, E., Geminiani, G., Berti, A., and Rusconi, M. L. (1990). Perceptual and premotor factors of unilateral neglect. *Neurology*, **40**, 1278–81.

Bisiach, E., Rusconi, M. L., Peretti, V. A., and Vallar, G. (1994). Challenging current accounts of unilateral neglect. *Neuropsychologia*, **32**, 1431–4.

Bisiach, E., Pizzamiglio, L., Nico, D., and Antonucci, G. (1996). Beyond unilateral neglect. *Brain*, **119**, 851–7.

Chatterjee, A. (1994). Picturing unilateral spatial neglect: viewer versus object centred reference frames. *Journal of Neurology, Neurosurgery, and Psychiatry*, **57**, 1236–40.

Chatterjee, A. (1995). Cross-over, completion and confabulation in unilateral spatial neglect. *Brain*, **118**, 455–65.

Chokron, S., Bernard, J.-M., and Imbert, M. (1997). Length representation in normal and neglect subjects with opposite reading habits studied through a line extension task. *Cortex*, **33**, 47–64.

Doricchi, F. and Angelelli, P. (1999). Misrepresentation of horizontal space in left unilateral neglect: role of hemianopia. *Neurology*, **52**, 1845–52.

Fink, G. R., Dolan, R. J., Halligan, P. W., Marshall, J. C., and Frith, C. D. (1997). Space-based and object-based visual attention: shared and specific neural domains. *Brain*, **120**, 2013–28.

Halligan, P. W. and Marshall, J. C. (1988). How long is a piece of string? A study of line bisection in a case of visual neglect. *Cortex*, **24**, 321–8.

Heilman, K. M., Bowers, D., and Watson, R. T. (1984). Pseudoneglect in a patient with partial callosal disconnection. *Brain*, **107**, 519–32.

Heilman, K. M., Watson, R. T., and Valenstein, E. (1993). Neglect and related disorders. In *Clinical neuropsychology* (3rd edn) (ed. K. M. Heilman and E. Valenstein), pp. 279–336. Oxford University Press, New York.

Ishiai, S. (1999). *Behavioural Inattention Test, Japanese edition*. Shinkoh Igaku Shuppan, Tokyo.

Ishiai, S., Furukawa, T., and Tsukagoshi, H. (1989). Visuospatial processes of line bisection and the mechanisms underlying unilateral spatial neglect. *Brain*, **112**, 1485–502.

Ishiai, S., Sugishita, M., Mitani, K., and Ishizawa, M. (1992). Leftward search in left unilateral spatial neglect. *Journal of Neurology, Neurosurgery, and Psychiatry*, **55**, 40–4.

Ishiai, S., Sugishita, M., Watabiki, S., Nakayama, T., Kotera, M., and Gono, S. (1994a). Improvement of left unilateral spatial neglect in a line extension task. *Neurology*, **44**, 294–8.

Ishiai, S., Watabiki, S., Lee, E., Kanouchi, T., and Odajima, N. (1994b). Preserved leftward movement in left unilateral spatial neglect due to frontal lesions. *Journal of Neurology, Neurosurgery, and Psychiatry*, **57**, 1085–90.

Ishiai, S., Seki, K., Koyama, Y., and Okiyama, R. (1995). Effects of cueing on visuospatial processing in unilateral spatial neglect. *Journal of Neurology*, **242**, 367–73.

Ishiai, S., Seki, K., Koyama, Y., and Gono, S. (1996a). Ineffective leftward search in line bisection and mechanisms of left unilateral spatial neglect. *Journal of Neurology*, **243**, 381–7.

Ishiai, S., Seki, K., Koyama, Y., and Yokota, T. (1996b). Mechanisms of unilateral spatial neglect in copying a single object. *Neuropsychologia*, **34**, 965–71.

Ishiai, S., Koyama, Y., and Seki, K. (1998). What is line bisection in unilateral spatial neglect? Analysis of perceptual and motor aspects in line bisection tasks. *Brain and Cognition*, **36**, 239–52.

Ishiai, S., Koyama, Y., Seki, K., and Izawa, M. (2000). Line versus representational bisections in unilateral spatial neglect. *Journal of Neurology, Neurosurgery, and Psychiatry*, **69**, 745–50.

Ishiai, S., Koyama, Y., and Seki, K. (2001). Significance of paradoxical leftward error of line bisection in left unilateral spatial neglect. *Brain and Cognition*, **45**, 238–48.

Koyama, Y., Ishiai, S., Seki, K., and Nakayama, T. (1997). Distinct processes in line bisection according to severity of left unilateral spatial neglect. *Brain and Cognition*, **35**, 271–81.

Marshall, J. C. and Halligan, P. W. (1995). Within- and between-task dissociations in visuo-spatial neglect: a case study. *Cortex*, **31**, 367–76.

Mattingley, J. B., Husain, M., Rorden, C., Kennard, C., and Driver, J. (1998). Motor role of human inferior parietal lobe revealed in unilateral neglect patients. *Nature*, **392**, 179–82.

Meador, K. J., Loring, D. W., Bowers, D., and Heilman, K. M. (1987). Remote memory and neglect syndrome. *Neurology*, **37**, 522–6.

Meienberg, O., Zangemeister, W. H., Rosenberg, M., Hoyt, W. F., and Stark, L. (1981). Saccadic eye movement strategies in patients with homonymous hemianopia. *Annals of Neurology*, **9**, 537–44.

Mesulam, M.-M. (1990). Large-scale neurocognitive networks and distributed processing for attention, language, and memory. *Annals of Neurology*, **28**, 597–613.

Milner, A. D. and Harvey, M. (1995). Distortion of size perception in visuospatial neglect. *Current Biology*, **5**, 85–9.

Milner, A. D., Harvey, M., Roberts, R. C., and Forster, S. V. (1993). Line bisection errors in visual neglect: misguided action or size distortion? *Neuropsychologia*, **31**, 39–49.

Nico, D., Galati, G., and Incoccia, C. (1999). The endpoints' task: an analysis of length reproduction in unilateral neglect. *Neuropsychologia*, **37**, 1181–8.

Posner, M. I., Walker, J. A., Friedrich, F. J., and Rafal, R. D. (1984). Effects of parietal injury on covert orienting of attention. *Journal of Neuroscience*, **4**, 1863–74.

Posner, M. I., Walker, J. A., Friedrich, F. A., and Rafal, R. D. (1987). How do the parietal lobes direct covert attention? *Neuropsychologia*, **25**, 135–45.

Riddoch, M. J. and Humphreys, G. W. (1983). The effect of cueing on unilateral neglect. *Neuropsychologia*, **21**, 589–99.

Rizzolatti, G. and Gallese, V. (1988). Mechanisms and theories of spatial neglect. In *Handbook of neuropsychology*, Vol. 1 (ed. F. Boller and J. Grafman), pp. 223–46. Elsevier, Amsterdam.

Robertson, I. H., Halligan, P. W., Bergego, C., Hömberg, V., Pizzamiglio, L., Weber, E., and Wilson, B. A. (1994). Right neglect following right hemisphere damage? *Cortex*, **30**, 199–213.

Rossetti, Y., Rode, G., Pisella, L., Farné, A., Li, L., Boisson, D., and Perenin M.-T. (1998). Prism adaptation to a rightward optical deviation rehabilitates left hemispatial neglect. *Nature*, **395**, 166–9.

Tegnér, R. and Levander, M. (1991). Through a looking glass: a new technique to demonstrate directional hypokinesia in unilateral neglect. *Brain*, **114**, 1943–51.

Weintraub, S. and Mesulam, M.-M. (1987). Right cerebral dominance in spatial attention: further evidence based on ipsilateral neglect. *Archives of Neurology*, **44**, 621–5.

Wilson, B., Cockburn, J., and Halligan, P. (1987). *Behavioural Inattention Test*. Thames Valley Test Company, Bury St Edmunds.

4.5 The contribution of retinotopic and multimodal coding of space to horizontal space misrepresentation in neglect and hemianopia

Fabrizio Doricchi

The present chapter deals with some apparently paradoxical phenomena concerning horizontal space misperception and misrepresentation in patients with left unilateral neglect. It is not intended to provide a complete review of the issue. Rather, an attempt is made to focus on some empirical findings considered relevant for the understanding of 'misrepresenting behaviors' in neglect patients. A series of studies run by the author with several colleagues are described and the findings are related to those of investigations performed by other researchers in the field.

The problem of space misrepresentation in hemianopia is also considered, and readers are briefly reminded about phenomena of size misperception due to dysmetropsia.

Initial findings

Unilateral neglect is a syndrome characterized by a failure of representing and considering for purposive actions the space contralesional to unilateral brain damage. The syndrome is most frequent after damage of the right hemisphere involving the inferior parietal lobe (Vallar 1998), the frontal lobe, and/or the basal ganglia (Heilman and Valenstein 1972; Husain and Kennard 1996). The double dissociation between unilateral neglect and primary sensory or motor impairments and the reduction of neglect-related visual impairments by means of non-visual proprioceptive or vestibular stimulations have reinforced the conviction that a relevant pathophysiological cause of neglect is the unilateral disruption of neural mechanisms integrating information from different modalities (i.e. visual, proprioceptive, vestibular) (Andersen et al. 1997; Vallar 1998). In the intact organism the hemispherically balanced activity of these mechanisms provides an adaptive representation of extra-personal and personal space maintaining the egocentric spatial frame of reference (i.e. the subjective body midsagittal plane) aligned to the trunk midsagittal plane and ensuring the lateral symmetry of orienting behavior (Ventre et al. 1984).

A few years ago, the idea that unilateral neglect could be simply behaviorally characterized by defective representation and orienting toward contralesional space (or by defective disengagement from the ipsilesional space) (Posner et al. 1984) was seriously challenged by the observation that neglect patients set the contralesional endpoint of a memorized horizontal line (i.e. the 'endpoint task') too far in the neglected hemispace and the ipsilesional endpoint too close in the attended hemispace (Bisiach *et al.* 1994). Just as in the line bisection task, where they typically show ipsilesional deviation of the subjective midpoint, neglect patients seemed to underestimate the contralesional section of the virtual line being reproduced and to overestimate its ipsilesional section. This finding fitted with the results of a series of studies by Milner and coworkers (Milner *et al.* 1993; Harvey *et al.* 1995; Milner and Harvey 1995) demonstrating that neglect patients perceive horizontal line segments positioned in the contralesional egocentric space as being shorter than identical segments positioned in the ipsilesional space. On the basis of these results, Bisiach and coworkers and Milner and coworkers proposed that misperception of horizontal size and distances (possibly linked to an underlying distorted representation of horizontal space) could be a defining feature of the neglect syndrome. Similar interpretative accounts of more specific findings in brain damaged patients and normal subjects can also be found in previous studies (Bisiach *et al.* 1984; Werth and Pöppel 1988; Halligan and Marshall 1991). In particular, Halligan and Marshall (1991) described a patient with left unilateral neglect who, when presented with an arrow positioned below or above an horizontal string of numbers and required to report the number to which the arrow was pointing, showed a systematic ipsilesional deviation in the individuation of the number. The deviation decreased linearly as the position of the arrow shifted toward the ipsilesional section of the string of numbers. This pattern is just as if points in the left hemispace were compressed toward the right, with more contralesional points being more compressed than points near the ipsilesional space.

However, it is important to note that in Halligan and Marshall's case study the patient was not cued or obliged to explore and produce a motor response toward the contralesional space, whereas in the studies by Bisiach *et al.* (1994) and by Milner and coworkers (Milner *et al.* 1993; Harvey *et al.* 1995; Milner and Harvey 1995) patients were explicitly required to evaluate and reproduce a distance or a size in the contralesional space. Also, Halligan and Marshall's study deals with localization in space (i.e. 'where' processing), whereas the studies by Milner and coworkers and by Bisiach and coworkers deal with within- or between-object space (i.e. 'what' processing). These factors potentially indicate that different types or phenomena of horizontal space misrepresentation can be revealed by different behavioral tasks. In the remainder of this chapter, our arguments and conclusions will refer to horizontal space misrepresentation as revealed by distance reproduction tasks explicitly obliging neglect patients to produce ocular and reaching responses toward the contralesional neglected space. As originally suggested by Bisiach *et al.* (1994) (but see also Ishiai *et al.* (1994)), this type of task allows the experimenter to counteract and exclude the influence of factors such as ipsilesional attentional bias, failure of attentional disengagement from ipsilesional space, failure to initiate movements toward contralesional space, or lack of representation of contralesional space. At the same time, these tasks permit us to explore how neglect patients can still represent the contralesional space when obliged to orient and act in that same space. As an example, the findings of Halligan and Marshall (1991) can be entirely interpreted as deriving from ipsilesional attentional and visuomotor bias rather than deriving from a compressed representation of contralesional space (on this point, see also Bisiach *et al.* (1999)). In other words, distance reproduction tasks 'constraining' motor responses toward the neglected space provide a direct measurement of horizontal space misrepresentation, whereas in 'unconstrained' pointing or line bisection tasks, misrepresentation is entirely and indirectly inferred from an ipsilesional bias in performance. In the latter case the 'misrepresentational' interpretation of the performance of neglect patients cannot be operationally disentangled from other interpretations (i.e. ipsilesional attentional bias, defective ipsilesional disengagement, contralesional hypokinesia, contralesional representational scotoma).

These short historical remarks and considerations indicate that the hypothesis viewing horizontal space misrepresentation or misperception as an essential dysfunction of the neglect syndrome can be traced back to the work of Bisiach, Halligan, Harvey, Ishiai, Marshall, Milner, and their coworkers (see also Chapters 4.1 and 4.2).

First study: the influence of concomitant hemianopia and the anatomical correlates of space misrepresentation in unilateral neglect

Looking for an explanation of the paradoxical misrepresenting behaviors of neglect patients and, in particular, of the striking 'far away' endpoint setting in contralesional space observed by Bisiach *et al.* (1994), we noted that the two neglect patients studied by Bisiach and coworkers had complete hemianopia. Also, among the series of seven patients studied by Milner and coworkers, the only patient with negligible misperception of horizontal stimuli was the one with full visual field (patient IH). Furthermore, the neglect patient with representative compression of the contralesional space studied by Halligan and Marshall (1991) also had full hemianopia. With these sparse, although concurrent, findings in mind we further noticed an interesting similarity between the performance of the neglect patients in the endpoint task and the oculomotor behavior documented by Meienberg *et al.* (1986) in hemianopic patients. In this study hemianopics intially performed hypermetric saccades when learning to reach a target in the contralesional blind hemifield (in order to shift away the blind hemifield and bring the lateral target into the seeing hemifield) and hypometric saccades when learning to reach a target in the ipsilesional hemifield (in order not to bring the target into the blind hemifield). After a few trials, hemianopics learned to produce metrically exact seccades.

Based on this evidence, we decided (Doricchi and Angelelli 1999) to investigate the contribution of hemianopia to horizontal space misrepresentation in neglect patients by administering the endpoint task to samples of chronic right-brain-damaged patients with neglect and no hemianopia (N+H−, $n = 9$), to neglect patients with concomitant full hemianopia (N+H+, $n = 8$) and to four left- brain-damaged and one right-brain-damaged patient with contralesional hemianopia and no neglect (N−H+, $n = 5$). In the same study we also first investigated the anatomical correlates of space misperception by superimposing the individual templates of the lesion and by localizing the areas of maximal overlap in each experimental group and in the subgroup of patients showing the highest degree of endpoint-setting asymmetry. All neglect patients showing hemianopia on conventional perimetric testing also had unreliable visually evoked potentials when vertical sinusoidal gratings were displayed at several different temporal frequencies in the contralesional visual field. The main findings of the study were as follows.

- Each of the N+H+ patients had contralesional over-extension and ipsilesional under-extension when reproducing the same (10 cm) horizontal distance (contra minus ipsi asymmetry, 3.25 cm).

- Significant over/under-extension asymmetry was absent in both N+H− (0.2 cm) and N−H+ (0.2 cm).

- In two N+H− patients with selective posterior damage and no hemianopia the degree of over/under-extension was mild and intermediate between that of the N+H+ patients with selective posterior lesions (who had strong asymmetry) and that of the N+H− patients with selective anterior damage (who had no asymmetry).

- The area of maximal lesion overlap in patients with the highest degree of space misperception was centered in the occipital cortical and subcortical structures (BA 17 and 18) (Fig. 1).

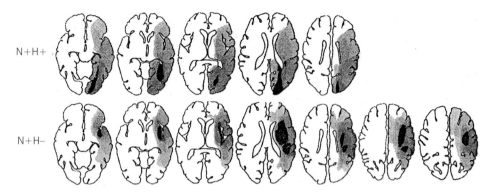

Figure 1   First study: Areas of lesion overlap in patients with neglect and hemianopia (N+H+) and in patients with neglect and no hemianopia (N+H−).

- The ipsilesional deviation of N+H+ (3.6 cm) in the line bisection task (line length, 20 cm) was three to four times higher than in N−H+ (0.87 cm).

- In the overall group of neglect patients there was a significant correlation between the asymmetry of performance in the endpoint-setting task and the ipsilesional deviation in the line bisection task.

- Finally, N+H+ and N+H− had comparable neglect severity in the line and letter cancellation tasks.

    In our view, the main implications of these findings were that distorted representation of horizontal space in neglect patients is not a mere effect of neglect severity and that misrepresentation is due to concomitant unilateral damage of retinotopical representations of space (causing hemianopia) and to damage of higher-order multimodal representations of space (causing neglect). The latter damage would create chronic difficulty in coding spatial positions falling in the retinotopically organized blind field during eye/head gaze shifts. When intact, multimodal representations of space could indeed allow an effective localization of 'blind positions' (through the use of proprioceptive and vestibular cues). As an example, the position of a visual stimulus located in the seeing field before the start of a saccade and in the blind field after the end of the saccade can be still 'held in mind' (Hornak 1995; Gaffan and Hornak 1997) (see also Chapter 6.4) by simply computing the amplitude of the saccade on the basis of the changes in the proprioceptive inputs conveyed by extraocular muscles (assuming, in this example, that head and trunk remain constant). The same reasoning can be applied to head or trunk movements. Therefore, on the basis of the results of this first study, we hypothesized (Doricchi and Angelelli 1999) that misrepresentation of horizontal space in neglect patients depends on the failure or impossibility of compensating for disruption of retinotopic representation of space due to concomitant disruption of neural mechanisms basing the analysis of space on the integration of multimodal cues. The absence of asymmetric performance in N+H− is in keeping with the results of a study by Karnath and Ferber (1999) who found no horizontal space misrepresentation in a task requiring the visual reproduction of horizontal distances (7.5°, 14.7°, or 27.8°) administered to seven patients with neglect but no hemianopia. More recently, Kerkhoff (2000) documented misrepresentation of size and distances (contralesional over-extension and/or ipsilesional under-extension) in a group of 16 neglect patients; 12 of these patients also had concomitant visual field defects (individual data were not reported).

Second study: disentangling visual and proprioceptive-motor influences in visuomotor distance reproduction

Reproducing a distance by setting a pen dot requires eye–hand–arm coordination. In a second study (Doricchi *et al.* 2002*a,b*) we wished to evaluate the visual and proprioceptive-motor components of space misrepresentation by administrating a visuomotor distance reproduction task that had to be performed both with and without visual guidance. Four groups of chronic right-brain-damaged patients (neglect with hemianopia (N+H+, $n = 11$), neglect with inferior quadrantanopia (N+Q+, $n = 5$), neglect without hemianopia (N+H−, $n = 11$), and patients without neglect or hemianopia (N−H−), $n = 9$) and one group of age-matched healthy controls (C, $n = 10$) participated in the study. Subjects reproduced horizontal distances by doubling the length (10 cm) of a line (printed on one lateral side of a paper sheet) toward the contralesional or ipsilesional side of space. The endpoint of the line where the movement started was always located at the center of the sheet. The task was administered in three different conditions: visuomotor (the line is drawn by the patient in free vision), visual (the patient looks and verbally guides the examiner drawing the line), and proprioceptive-motor (the patient is blindfolded and manually explores and doubles the distance subtended by the line). In this way the contribution of visual and hand–arm proprioceptive-motor cues was systematically varied in order to disentangle the role of each of these two factors in visuomotor space misrepresentation. The line bisection and endpoint tasks were also administered. The results showed that relative contralesional over-extension and ipsilesional under-extension of the line was significant only in N+H+ (contra minus ipsi asymmetry, 2.24 cm) and N+Q+ (1.8 cm) when the task was performed under visual guidance (visual line extension). The same lateral asymmetry was significant only in N+H+ (1.76 cm) when distances were reproduced by visually guiding the movement of the limb (visuomotor line extension). No asymmetry was found in any group when the line was doubled without visual guidance (proprioceptive-motor extension). These results indicate that visual input is critical in producing misperception of horizontal space in neglect patients with concomitant visual field defects, whereas the contribution of proprioceptive cues from the arm is negligible.

The results of the line bisection and the endpoint-setting tasks replicated the findings of the first study by Doricchi and Angelelli (1999). N+H+ patients bisected lines (length, 20 cm) with the greatest ipsilesional shift (2.94 cm) from the objective midpoint. This shift was threefold that of N+H− patients (0.82 cm). A similar finding in the line bisection task was first reported by D'Erme *et al.* (1987). N+H+ also had the highest endpoint-setting asymmetry (2.87 cm). In this latter task the asymmetry of N+H− (0.79 cm) was not significantly different from that of C (0.32 cm) or N−H− (0.51 cm). As in the first study, in the overall group of brain damaged patients the asymmetry in the endpoint task was correlated with the ipsilesional deviation in the line bisection task. We also took advantage of the study of samples of C and N−H− to evaluate the consistency of an objection raised by Ferber and Karnath (2001), who argued that in our first study (Doricchi and Angelelli 1999) the performance of N+H− and N−H+ was not compared with that of C or N−H−. According to these authors, these comparisons could demonstrate that N+H− and N−H+ also suffer asymmetry of reproduction in endpoint setting. When we re-analyzed the performance of N+H− and N−H+ from the first study, we observed that the contra minus ipsi asymmetry of N+H− (0.2 cm) and N−H+ (0.2 cm) was not different from that of C (0.3 cm) or N−H− (0.5). These findings contradict the hypothesis advanced by Ferber and Karnath (2001).

Third study: coordinate system of misrepresentation

The aim of this study (Doricchi *et al.* 2002*a,b*) was to try to individuate the spatial coordinate system (or systems) whose disruption is responsible for space misrepresentation in neglect patients. The study of neglect patients with or without hemianopia already allowed us to ascertain the important contribution of the retinotopic space coordinate system to horizontal space misrepresentation. However, adaptive representation of space for action is achieved by integrating retinotopic information with proprioceptive and vestibular cues (Andersen *et al.* 1997). These mechanisms of sensorimotor integration allow the organism to code stimuli impinging on identical retinal positions as being located in different positions of the environment when the position of the eyes in the orbit or of the head over the trunk or of the entire body with respect to the environment changes. Gaze position diffusely modulates the discharge of neurons in occipital (Galletti and Battaglini 1989; Guo and Li 1997), thalamic (Schlag *et al.* 1980; Robinson *et al.* 1990), occipital–temporal (Bremmer 2000), occipital–parietal (Galletti *et al.* 1995), temporal (Bremmer *et al.* 1997), and frontal areas (Boussaud *et al.* 1993, 1998). In the monkey, proprioceptive signals from the neck signalling changes in the relative position of the head over the trunk are integrated in the lateral intraparietal area with visual input and with proprioceptive signals from the eye (Brotchie *et al.* 1995). In nearby area 7a (Snyder *et al.* 1998) and in the parieto-insular cortex (Guldin and Grusser 1998; Faugier-Grimaud *et al.* 1997), vestibular inputs contribute to updating the position of the body after whole-body turns.

In the first experiment of the third study we wished to investigate whether, in neglect patients with or without concomitant hemianopia, changing the position of test stimuli with respect to a patient's body midsagittal plane (i.e. egocentric coordinates) produced any change in the degree of horizontal space misrepresentation. Several authors have already shown that the positioning of stimuli in the ipsilesional body hemispace ameliorates the spatial performance of neglect patients compared with conditions in which stimuli are centered on the body midsagittal plane or are located in the contralesional body hemispace (Vallar 1997). Attending to stimuli on the ipsilesional side of space implies relative ipsilesional eye, head, and trunk rotation; corresponding modifications of proprioceptive input counteract the pathological ipsilesional distortion and rotation of the egocentric frame of spatial reference of neglect patients (Vallar 1997, 1998).

A purely visual task was used. Three colored (green, red, and yellow) unlighted light-emitting diodes (LEDs) placed on a horizontal bar served as test stimuli. The red LED was in a fixed position at the center of the bar, the yellow LED could be moved from the center to the right, and the green LED from the center to the left (patient's viewpoint). At the beginning of a leftward trial, the yellow LED was placed in a fixed position 10 cm (about 10° of the visual angle) to the right of the red LED and the green LED was immediately adjacent to the left of the red one. The reversed arrangement was used in rightward trials. On each trial the experimenter smoothly moved the green LED leftward (or the yellow LED rightward). Patients were required to place the moving LED so as to reproduce, on one side of the bar, the distance between the central red LED and the LED in a fixed position on the other side of the bar. The patient had unlimited time to adjust the LED position. In the first experiment the center of the bar could be aligned to the head–body midsagittal plane of the patient (central position (CP)) or to the head midsagittal plane but presented in the ipsilesional (trunk rotated 30° contralesionally) or contralesional egocentric hemispace (trunk rotated 30° ipsilesionally). Five chronic N+H+ and five chronic N+H− patients participated in the experiment.

In this experiment no effect of trunk turns was observed in either group (Fig. 2). Compared with perfect distance reproduction, N+H+ had significant relative contralesional over-extension (10.3 cm) and ipsilesional under-extension (8.6 cm) whereas N+H− had no asymmetry (contra, 9.6 cm; ipsi, 9.57 cm). Accordingly we concluded that mechanisms concerned with the body-centered coding of space have no role in the genesis of visual space misrepresentation. As pointed out by other authors, who also found no influence of trunk turns on the performance of visual tasks (Vuilleumier *et al.* 1999), the coding of the body-centered position of visual stimuli could be relevant for tasks requiring manual reaching (Nico *et al.* 1999) or the explicit coding of

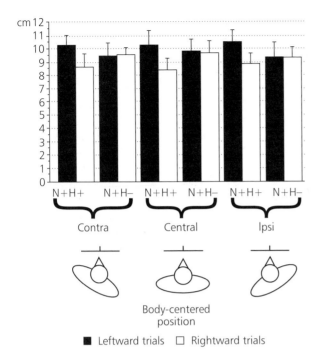

Figure 2 Second study, first experiment: visual horizontal distance reproduction in the contralesional (i.e. leftward trials) and ipsilesional (i.e. rightward trials) head-centered space as function of the body centered position of stimuli. N+H+, patients with neglect and hemianopia; N+H−, patients with neglect and no hemianopia.

extrapersonal positions with respect to the body, but not for pure visual comparison among sizes or distances.

In a second experiment (Doricchi *et al.* 2002*a,b*) we evaluated the effects of separated and combined manipulation of eye and neck position with the aim of defining the influence of eye proprioceptive inputs on the evaluation and reproduction of horizontal distances. For us, it was of particular interest to know that in early retinotopically organized visual areas (V1 and V3a) (Galletti and Battaglini 1989; Guo and Li 1997) lateral gaze deviation determines an increase in the discharge of neurons in the hemisphere contralateral to the direction of gaze shift. Since our first study documented that a relevant anatomical correlate of space misrepresentation in neglect patients was damage of BA 17 and 18 (and of the underlying white matter of the occipital–parietal area), an influence of gaze position on space misrepresentation could have been expected. In the second experiment the same task as used in the first experiment was administered. Here, the center of the bar could be aligned to the head–body midsagittal plane (CP), aligned to the body midsagittal plane but positioned in the contralesional (HC) or ipsilesional head hemispace (HI) (head turn, 30° in each case), or placed in the contralesional (BC) or ipsilesional (BI) head–body hemispace. Ten N+H−, four N+H+, and five N−H+ (three with right and two with left brain damage) patients participated in this second study. All these patients were studied in the chronic phase of the stroke.

The results of this second experiment were more complex (Fig. 3). In the baseline condition (CP) the performance of N+H− was not asymmetric (contra reproduction, 9.8 cm; ipsi, 10 cm). N+H+ and N−H+ had significant and directionally opposed asymmetries of reproduction. N+H+ had relative contralesional over-extension (contra, 11.6 cm; ipsi, 10 cm), and N−H+ had relative contralesional under-extension (contra, 9.7 cm; ipsi, 10.7 cm). In N−H+, relative contralesional under-extension was present in each patient independently of the side of the lesion. The opposed patterns of misrepresentation of N+H+ and N−H+ are

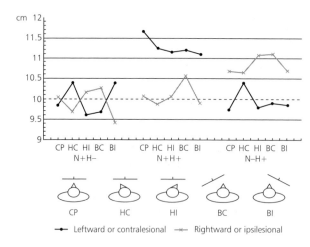

Figure 3 Second study, second experiment: visual horizontal distance reproduction in the leftward (or contralesional) and rightward (or ipsilesional) directions as a function of experimental condition. CP, central position; HC, head turned contralesionally; HI, head turned ipsilesionally; BC, bar in the contralesional head–body hemispace; BI, bar in the ipsilesional head–body hemispace. N+H–, patients with neglect and no hemianopia; N+H+, patients with neglect and hemianopia; N–H+, hemianopic patients without neglect.

congruent with the performance of these patients in the line bisection task. Again, a control group of N+H+ (*n* = 19) had severe ipsilesional deviation (3.26 cm, corresponding to underestimation of the contralesional section of the line), while N−H+ had contralesional deviation (0.49 cm, corresponding to overestimation of the contralesional section of the line). In N+H+ there was no change of the asymmetry across the different experimental conditions. In N+H− the deviation of the eyes toward one side of space (BI or BC conditions), with or without concomitant head deviation in the opposed direction (HI or HC conditions), induced shifting of both endpoints toward the side of space opposite to the direction of gaze shift. In N−H+, the 'reversed' asymmetry was abolished when the head was deviated contralesionally and the center of the bar remained aligned to the body midsagittal line (HC condition, bar positioned in the ipsilesional head hemispace and eyes deviated ipsilesionally, see Fig. 3).

The findings from these two experiments show that horizontal space misrepresentation is not modulated by changes in the body-centered position of stimuli, while it can be modulated by both combined (and directionally opposed) head/eye deviation and by selective eye deviation. These results suggest that space misrepresentation in neglect patients depends on the concomitant disruption of both retinotopic and extra-retinotopic information at a stage of visuospatial processing where the gain of eye-centered retinotopic and head-centered representation of space is not modulated by mechanisms underlying the body centered coding of space. The absence of any modulation from eye or neck proprioception on space misrepresentation in N+H+ confirms that the total unilateral loss of retinotopic representations of space predispose neglect patients to the highest probability of suffering the most severe form of horizontal space misperception. However, is hemianopia a necessary condition for the appearence of space misrepresentation? Retinotopically organized representations are also present outside primary visual cortex in several posterior extrastriate associative visual areas (Galletti and Battaglini 1989) (for a review see Tootell *et al.* (1998)). Also, reaching movements can be coded in eye-centered retinotopic coordinates in the lateral intraparietal area (Batista *et al.* 1999), and the receptive fields of neurons of the ventral section of the same area show 'transitional properties' (Duhamel *et al.* 1997) along a continuum ranging from retinotopic to head-centered coding of space. Therefore the possibility that damage unilaterally disrupting the retinotopic modulation of eye and arm-reaching movements without causing concomitant visual field defects could bring about horizontal space misrepresentation in patients with neglect should be hypothetically acknowledged.

Coda: another new apparent paradox in neglect patients with hemianopia

Finally, we consider an apparent contradiction which seems to be present in the way that N+H+ and N+H− patients perform the line bisection and the 'straight-ahead task'. We repeatedly found that N+H+ patients have a more severe ipsilesional shift when compared with N−H+ (as originally shown by D'Erme *et al.* (1987)). Thus concomitant hemianopia seems to potentiate and worsen contralesional neglect. Ferber and Karnath (1999) found that N+H− patients have a higher ipsilesional shift of the subjective straight ahead than N+H+ patients. These authors interpreted this results by hypothesizing that neglect and hemianopia have opposing lateral biases in the perception of body orientation and that this biases neutralize each other. Thus, according to this view, concomitant hemianopia seems to depotentiate and ameliorate neglect. We have a simpler hypothesis to explain the findings in N+H+ patients in the straight-ahead task and to reconcile them with the opposite findings in the line bisection task. Line bisection depends on the parallel processing and the simultaneous representation of all the spatial points (i.e. positions) constituting the line (Binder *et al.* 1992) . A field cut causes a lateralized reduction of the retinotopic input available for higher-order spatial processing. When performing line bisection, neglect patients with hemianopia fail to compensate for the damaged retinotopic representation of the contralesional half of the line and probably consider only the ipsilesional half for bisection. The straight-ahead task calls into action a completely different way of analyzing space. In this task an LED is moved in darkness from the left to the right or from the right to the left. The subjective straight ahead is calculated by averaging positions set by the patients on rightward and leftward trials (note that in the case of leftward trials the movement of the LED is itself a cue inducing scanning toward the usually neglected side of space). We hypothesize the following.

- In this task hemianopics are aware of their visual field defect and tend to compensate for the defect by setting the straight ahead in the contralesional space independently of the direction of the movement of the LED.
- Patients with neglect and no hemianopia have a rightward bias independently of the direction of the movement of the LED (although this bias could probably be higher on rightward trials); however, the sparing of the retinotopic representation of the contralesional space in these patients smoothens the ipsilesional bias just as in the line bisection task.
- In neglect patients with hemianopia, the slight contralesional shift of the straight ahead is the result of spatial biases alike those found in the endpoint task (see first study) (Doricchi and Angelelli 1999). When the LED moves leftward these patients could perseverate in trying to shift the blind field away in order to maintain the LED in the foveal and parafoveal region of the seeing field, causing relative over-extension in the contralesional field; when the LED moves rightward an opposite tendency could be present (i.e. under-extension) in order not to bring the LED into the blind field moving ipsilesionally. The net average between measurements of the subjective straight ahead on leftward and rightward trials is a subjective straight ahead slightly shifted toward the contralesional side of space.

The findings by Ferber and Karbath could therefore be the result of the specific task adopted to evaluate the straight-ahead position. A study based on a different methodology (e.g. manual pointing to the straight ahead) could lead to different results in N+H+.

Space misrepresentation in hemianopia and dysmetropsia

Hemianopia

When compared with neglect patients, hemianopic patients without neglect have a well-documented opposite bias in the performance of the line bisection task, showing compensatory contralesional deviation toward the blind hemifield (D'Erme *et al.* 1987; Kerkhoff 1993; Barton and Black 1998) (for similar older clinical evidences see the literature briefly reviewed by Ferber and Karnath (1999)). The same deviation is present when setting the subjective straight ahead (Ferber and Karnath 1999) and in pointing tasks (Best 1917). The performance of patients with pure hemianopia in the line bisection task predicts that the same patients should perceive or represent the size of contralesional horizontal stimuli (or an equivalent distance between two stimuli) as being longer than an identical ipsilesional one. The findings in N−H+ in the baseline condition (CP) of the second experiment of the third study fully confirmed this prediction. In the same study we also found that each hemianopic patient, independently of the side of the lesion, consistently judged as 'shorter' the ipsilesional halves of a centrally bisected horizontal bar (Landmark task). Our findings (CP condition) strictly replicate less recent observations by Zihl and von Cramon (1986). These authors asked chronic hemianopic patients (studied 2 months to 7 years after the stroke) to judge whether two visual targets presented along a horizontal perimeter, one in the contralesional and one in the ipsilesional hemifield, were at the same distance with respect to the center of the perimeter. The center of the perimeter was always in line with the head–body midsagittal plane, and in each block of trials the position of one target was maintained fixed whereas that of the target in the opposite hemifield was varied. Exactly as in the baseline condition (CP) of our third study (second experiment), hemianopic patients under-extended distances in the contralesional hemifield and over-extended distances in the ipsilesional hemifield. Also in keeping with these results, one patient with bilateral hemianopia under-extended distances on both sides of space. Therefore the pattern of horizontal space misrepresentation found in hemianopic patients seems opposite to that found in neglect patients with concomitant hemianopia. In our view, this is the probable consequence of the presence, in hemianopics, of spared multimodal coding of spatial positions falling in the retinotopically organized blind field. Multimodal representations of space could promote both awareness (Rizzolatti and Berti 1993) of the retinotopically blind space and the activation of overcompensatory strategies leading to a misrepresention of the space falling in the blind field as being larger than it objectively is. The opposite effects seem to be present in neglect patients with hemianopia.

Opposite to our results and those of Zihl and von Cramon (1986), Ferber and Karnath (2001) recently reported over-extension of size (i.e. horizontal bars) in the contralesional space and under-extension in the ipsilesional space in five hemianopic patients. These authors surprisingly concluded that their findings were compatible with the data of Zihl and von Cramon (their results are opposite to those of Zihl and von Cramon). The interpretation of Ferber and Karnath's findings is made difficult by the influence of some relevant variables that were probably overlooked in their study. First, all patients were examined in the acute phase of the stroke (on average within 20 days of the insult), some of them very early after the stroke (3–10 days). Unawareness of the visual field defect, which can persist well beyond the acute phase in a great proportion of patients (60–70 per cent) (Celesia *et al.* 1997; Zihl 2000) was not assessed. Most unfortunate of all, neglect was evaluated only with a multiple-item cancellation or drawing task and neither line bisection nor straight-ahead tasks were administered. Evaluation of neglect through multi-item tasks (depending on the sequential analysis of an array of spatially distributed items) is insufficient because defective performance of neglect patients in line bisection (requiring the simultaneous and parallel representation of the entire line) can be dissociated from the performance in multiple-item tasks (Binder *et al.* 1992). Therefore, it remains unknown whether Ferber and Karnath's patients had, as documented by all previous investigators, contralesional deviation in line bisection or whether, owing to the recency of the stroke and the unawareness of the visual field defect, they had ineffective compensation of the blind field and ipsilesional deviation. Therefore their results seem rather unusual and not in keeping with all the available evidence in hemianopics (Zihl and von Cramon 1986; D'Erme *et al.* 1987; Kerkhoff 1993; Barton and Black 1998; Kerkhoff 2000; Doricchi *et al.* 2002*a,b*). These studies demonstrate that chronic hemianopics subjectively consider the contralesional part of the horizontal stimuli as being larger than it objectively is, with the consequent tendency to under-extend horizontal size and distances in the contralesional space (and over-extend them in the ipsilesional space) and shift the subjective midpoint of an horizontal line toward the contralesional side.

Dysmetropsia

Dysmetropsia is a disorder of size perception characterized by the apparent modification of the subjectively perceived size of objects which can appear compressed (micropsia) or enlarged (macropsia) compared with their actual size. Micropsia seems more frequent than macropsia and horizontal or vertical size are often independently affected (Frassinetti *et al.* 1999). The disorder can be caused by retinal edema, temporal lobe seizures, migraine, psychoactive drugs (mescaline), and focal brain damage. Some authors (Irving-Bell *et al.* 1999; Karnath and Ferber 1999; Ferber and Karnath 2001) have suggested that manifestation of space misrepresentation in neglect patients with focal brain damage might depend on dysmetropsia (micropsia) affecting the contralesional field. In our opinion, this hypothesis could certainly be applied to specific cases of patients with neglect and no visual field defect (although these type of patients show, as a group, mild or no manifestation of space distortion). Interestingly, in some of these specific cases anosognosia for dysmetropsia could be present because of the frequent association of neglect with unawareness of impaired processing of events in the contralesional personal and extrapersonal space (Vallar 1998). The same hypothesis is less likely to apply to neglect patients with hemi-anopia or to hemianopics. Contralesional dysmetropsia, whether micropsia or macropsia, was reported in patients with unilateral damage of the retrosplenial region (Ebata *et al.* 1991) or of the ventrolateral occipital–temporal extrastriate visual cortex (Cohen *et al.* 1994; Ceriani *et al.* 1998; Frassinetti *et al.* 1999; Safran *et al.* 1999) with no or very limited contralateral visual field defects (i.e. paracentral scotomas). As noted by several authors (Cohen *et al.* 1994; Ceriani *et al.* 1998), complete hemianopia simply prevents the processing of visual stimuli in the extrastriate cortex of the damaged hemisphere and the clinical expression of disorders of size perception. Therefore hypothesizing a role of dymetropsia in the pathogenesis of space misrepresentation in patients with contralateral hemianopia (whether accompanied or unaccompanied by neglect) seems equivalent to formulating the unlikely hypothesis that dysmetropsia is due to some altered functional processing in the intact hemisphere.

Conclusions

On the basis of the empirical findings and the arguments summarized in the present chapter, misperception or misrepresentation of horizontal space, as determined in distance and size repro-duction tasks explicitly requiring orienting toward the contralesional space, cannot be considered as the fundamental dysfunction explaining the rich, varied, and complex symptomatology that can be observed in neglect patients. Rather, horizontal space misrepresentation in neglect patients seems to be the result of concomitant disruption of visual retinotopic and specific multimodal non retinotopic representations of space (probably head centered). Not all neglect patients necessarily suffer misrepresentation, as clearly demonstrated by its absence in the large majority of neglect patients without visual field defects. Therefore neglect can be dissociated from horizontal space misrepresentation. At the same time, and with the exception of cases in which size misperception is due to dysmetropsia, misrepresentation of horizontal space (contra over-extension/ipsi under-extension) is apparently and frequently associated with 'neglect with hemianopia', whereas the 'reversed' form of misrepresentation (contra under-extension/ipsi over-extension) is associated with 'hemianopia without neglect'.

The author is convinced that the initial observations and arguments raised by Bisiach, Halligan, Harvey, Ishiai, Marshall, Milner and their coworkers had the merit of disclosing new clinical phenomena and paradoxes. This drove subsequent investigators (included himself) to reconsider and explore new experimental and theoretical ways of relating the complexity of the clinical expression of the neglect syndrome to the complexity of the neurophysiological mechanisms underlying space computation in the brain. As clearly suggested by Rizzolatti *et al.* (1997), space computation is not a unitary function and different operations of sensorimotor integration are necessary for the spatial organization of the movement of different effectors endowed with different biomechanical properties. It is hoped that the experiments, findings, and arguments reviewed in this chapter will contribute toward the formulation of an articulated taxonomy of neglect-related disorders (Vallar 1998). It is the author's belief that this type of approach has a much higher heuristic value than looking for a fundamental and unique pathophysiological mechanism explaining neglect. At the same time, detailing the links between the disruption of specific representations of space and specific neglect symptoms will provide the basis for developing more effective diagnostic tools and formulating rehabilitative programs meeting the specific needs of each individual patient.

Acknowledgements

The author wishes to thank Professor David Milner for editing the manuscript and Hans-Otto Karnath for providing copies of papers from the less recent German scientific literature.

References

Andersen, R. A., Snyder, L. H., Bradley, D. C., and Xing, J. (1997). Multimodal representations of space in the posterior parietal cortex and its use in planning movements. *Annual Review of Neuroscience*, **20**, 303–30.

Barton, J. J. S. and Black, S. E. (1998). Line bisection in hemianopia. *Journal of Neurology Neurosurgery and Psychiatry*, **64**, 660–2.

Batista, A. P., Buneo, C. A., Snyder, L. H., and Andersen, R. A. (1999). Reach plans in eye centered coordinates. *Science*, **285**, 257–60.

Best, F. (1917). Hemianopsie und Seelenblindheit bei Hirnverlet-zungen. (1917). *Graefes Archiv für Ophthalmologie*, **93**, 49–150.

Binder, J., Marshall, R., Lazar, R., Benjamin, J., and Mohr, J. P. (1992). Distinct syndromes of hemineglect. *Archives of Neurology*, **49**, 1187–93.

Bisiach, E., Cornacchia, L., Sterzi, R., and Vallar, G. (1984). Disorders of perceived auditory lateralization after lesions of the right hemisphere. *Brain*, **107**, 37–52.

Bisiach, E., Rusconi, M. L., Peretti, V. A., and Vallar, G. (1994). Challenging current accounts of unilateral neglect. *Neuropsychologia*, **32**, 1431–4.

Bisiach, E., Ricci, R., Berruti, G., Genero, R., Pepi, R., and Fumelli, T. (1999). Two-dimensional distortion of space representation in unilateral neglect: perceptual and response-related factors. *Neuropsychologia*, **37**, 1491–8.

Boussaud, D., Barth, T. M., and Wise, S. P. (1993). Effects of gaze on apparent visual responses of frontal cortex neurons. *Experimental Brain Research*, **93**, 423–34.

Boussaud, D., Jouffrais, C., and Bremmer, F. (1998). Eye position effects on the neuronal activity of dorsal premotor cortex in the macaque monkey. *Journal of Neuropshysiology*, **80**, 1132–50.

Bremmer, F. (2000). Eye position effects in macaque area V4. *NeuroReport*, **11**, 1277–83.

Bremmer, F., Ilg, U. J., Thiele, A., Distler, C., and Hoffman, K. P. (1997). Eye position effects in monkey cortex. I: Visual and pursuit-related activity in extrastriate areas MT and MST. *Journal of Neurophysiology*, **77**, 944–61.

Brotchie, P. R., Andersen, R. A., Snyder, L. H., and Goodman, S. J. (1995). Head position signals used by parietal neurons to encode locations of visual stimuli. *Nature*, **375**, 232–5.

Celesia, G. G., Brigell, M. M., and Vaphiades, M. S. (1997). Hemianopic anosognosia. *Neurology*, **49**, 88–97.

Ceriani, F., Gentileschi, V., Muggia, S., and Spinnler, H. (1998). Seeing objects smaller than they are: micropsia following right temporo-parietal infarction. *Cortex*, **34**, 131–8.

Cohen, L., Gray, F., Meyrignac, C., Dehaene, S., and Degos, J. D.(1994). Selective deficit of visual size perception: two cases of hemimicropsia. *Journal of Neurology, Neurosurgery, and Psychiatry*, **57**, 73–8.

D'Erme, P., De Bonis, C., and Gainotti, G. (1987). Influenza dell'emi-inattenzione e dell'emianopsia sui compiti di bisezione di linee nei pazienti cerebrolesi. *Archivio di Psicologia, Neurologia e Psichiatria*, **48**, 193–207.

Doricchi, F. and Angelelli, P. (1999). Misrepresentation of horizontal space in left unilateral neglect: role of hemianopia. *Neurology*, **52**, 1845–52.

Doricchi, F., Galati, G., De Luca, L., Nico, D., and D'Olimpio, F. (2002*a*). Horizontal space misrepresentation in unilateral brain damage. I: Visual and proprioceptive-motor influences in left unilateral neglect. *Neuropsychologia*, **40**, 1107–17.

Doricchi, F., Onida, A., and Guariglia, P. (2002*b*). Horizontal space misrepresentation in unilateral brain damage. II: Eye-head centered modulation of visual misrepresentation in hemianopia without neglect. *Neuropsychologia*, **40**, 1118–28.

Duhamel, J. R., Bremmer, F., BenHamed, S., and Graf, W. (1997). Spatial invariance of visual receptive fields in parietal cortex neurons. *Nature*, **389**, 845–8.

Ebata, S., Ogawa, M., Tanaka, Y., Mizuno, Y., and Yoshida, M. (1991). Apparent reduction in the size of one side of the face associated with a small retrosplenial haemorrhage. *Journal of Neurology, Neurosurgery and Psychiatry*, **54**, 68–70.

Faugier-Grimaud, S., Baleydier, C., Magnin, M., and Jeannerod, M. (1997). Direct bilateral cortical projections to the vestibular complex in macaque monkey. In *Parietal lobe contributions to orientation in 3D space* (ed. P. Their and H.-O. Karnath), pp. 57–76. Springer-Verlag, Berlin.

Ferber, S. and Karnath, H.-O. (1999). Parietal and occipital lobe contributions to perception of straight ahead orientation. *Journal of Neurology Neurosurgery and Psychiatry*, **67**, 572–8.

Ferber, S. and Karnath, H.-O. (2001). Size perception in hemianopia and neglect. *Brain*, **124**, 527–36.

Frassinetti, F., Nichelli, P., and di Pellegrino, G. (1999). Selective horizontal dysmetropsia following prestriate lesion. *Brain*, **122**, 339–50.

Galletti, C. and Battaglini, P. P. (1989). Gaze-dependent visual neurons in area V3a of monkey prestriate cortex. *Journal of Neuroscience*, **9**, 1112–25.

Galletti, C., Battaglini, P. P., and Fattori, P. (1995). Eye position influence on the parieto-occipital area PO(V6) of the macaque monkey. *European Journal of Neuroscience*, **7**, 2486–501.

Gaffan, D. and Hornak, J. (1997). Visual neglect in the monkey: representation and disconnection. *Brain*, **120**, 1647–57

Guldin, W. O. and Grusser, O. J. (1998). Is there a vestibular cortex? *Trends in Neuroscience*, **21**, 254–9.

Guo, K. and Li, C. (1997). Eye position-dependent activation of neurones in striate cortex of the macaque. *NeuroReport*, **8**, 1405–9.

Halligan, P. W. and Marshall, J. C. (1991). Spatial compression in visual neglect: a case study. *Cortex*, **27**, 623–9.

Harvey, M., Milner, A. D., and Roberts, R. C. (1995). An investigation of hemispatial neglect using the Landmark task. *Brain and Cognition*, **27**, 59–78.

Heilman, K. M. and Valenstein, E. (1972). Frontal lobe neglect in man. *Neurology*, **22**, 660–4.

Hornak, J. (1995). Perceptual completion in patients with drawing neglect: eye-movement and tachistoscopic investigations. *Neuropsychologia*, **33**, 305–25.

Husain, M. and Kennard, C. (1996). Visual neglect associated with frontal lobe infarction. *Journal of Neurology*, **243**, 652–7.

Irving-Bell, L., Small,M., and Cowey, A. (1999). A distortion of perceived space in patients with right-hemisphere lesions and visual hemineglect. *Neuropsychologia*, **37**, 919–25.

Ishiai, S., Sugishita, M., Watabiki, S., Nakayama, T., Kotera, M., and Gono, S. (1994). Improvement of left unilateral spatial neglect in a line extension task. *Neurology*, **44**, 294–8.

Karnath, H.-O. and Ferber, S. (1999). Is space representation distorted in neglect? *Neuropsychologia*, **37**, 7–15.

Kerkhoff, G. (1993). Displacement of the egocentric visual midline in altitudinal postchiasmatic scotomata. *Neuropsychologia*, **31**, 261–5.

Kerkhoff, G. (2000). Multiple perceptual distortions and their modulation in leftsided visual neglect. *Neuropsychologia*, **38**, 1073–86.

Meienberg, O., Harrer, M., and Wehren, C. (1986). Oculographic diagnosis of hemineglect in patients with homonymous hemianopia. *Journal of Neurology*, **233**, 97–101.

Milner, A. D. and Harvey, M. (1995). Distortion of size perception in visuospatial neglect. *Current Biology*, **5**, 85–9.

Milner, A. D., Harvey, M., Roberts, R. C., and Forster, S. V. (1993). Line bisection errors in visual neglect: misguided action or size distortion? *Neuropsychologia*, **31**, 39–49.

Nico, D., Galati, G., and Incoccia, C. (1999). The endpoints' task: an analysis of length reproduction in unilateral neglect. *Neuropsychologia*, **37**, 1181–8.

Posner, M. I., Walker, J. A., Friedrich, F. J., and Rafal, R. D. (1984). Effects of parietal injury on covert orienting of attention. *Journal of Neuroscience*, **4**, 1863–74.

Rizzolatti, G. and Berti, A. (1993). Neural mechanisms of spatial neglect. (1993). In *Unilateral neglect: clinical and experimental studies* (ed. I. H. Robertson and J. C. Marshall), pp. 87–105. Lawrence Erlbaum, Hove.

Rizzolatti, G., Fogassi, L., and Gallese, V . (1997). Parietal cortex: from sight to action. *Current Opinion in Neurobiology*, **7**, 562–7.

Robinson, D. L., McClurkin, J. W., and Kertzman, C. (1990). Orbital position and eye movement influences on visual responses in the pulvinar nuclei of the behaving macaque. *Experimental Brain Research*, **82**, 235–46.

Safran, A. B., Achard, O., Duret, F., and Landis, T. (1999). The 'thin man' phenomenon: a sign of cortical plasticity following inferior homonymous paracentral scotomas. *British Journal of Ophthalmology*, **83**, 137–42.

Schlag, J., Schlag Rey, M., Peck, C. K., and Joseph, J. P. (1980). Visual responses of thalamic neurons depending on the direction of gaze and the position of targets in space. *Experimental Brain Research*, **40**, 170–84.

Snyder,L. H., Grieve, K. L., Brotchie, P. R., and Andersen, R. A. (1998). Separate body and world-referenced representations of visual space in parietal cortex. *Nature*, **394**, 887–91.

Tootell, B. H., Hadjikani, N. K., Mendola, J. D., Marrett, S., and Dale, A. M. (1998). From retinotopy to recognition: fMRI in human visual cortex. *Trends in Cognitive Science*, **2**, 174–83.

Vallar, G. (1997). Spatial frames of references and somatosensory processing: a neuropsychological perspective. *Philosophical Transactions of the Royal Society of London B*, **352**, 1401–9.

Vallar, G. (1998). Spatial hemineglect in humans. *Trends in Cognitive Science*, **2**, 87–96.

Ventre, J., Flandrin, J. M., and Jeannerod, M. (1984). In search of the egocentric reference: a neurophysiological hypothesis. *Neuropsychologia*, **22**, 797–806.

Vuilleumier, P., Valenza, N., Mayer, E., Perrig, S., and Landis, T. (1999). To see better to the left when looking more to the right: effects of gaze direction and frames of spatial coordinates in unilateral neglect. *Journal of the International Neuropsychological Society*, **5**, 75–82.

Werth, R. and Pöppel, E. (1988). Compression and lateral shift of mental coordinate systems in a line bisection task. *Neuropsychologia*, **26**, 741–5.

Zihl, J. (2000). *Rehabilitation of visual disorders after brain injury*. Psychology Press, Hove.

Zihl, J. and von Cramon, D. (1986). *Zerebrale Sehstörungen*. Kohlhammer, Stuttgart.

4.6 Illusions in neglect, illusions of neglect

Giuseppe Vallar and Roberta Daini

The neurological syndrome of unilateral spatial neglect was definitively conceived by the scientific community as a disorder concerning higher-level cerebral functions, rather than being produced by the derangement of elementary sensory-motor loops, once extensive empirical evidence was provided to the effect that visual, somatosensory, and motor disorders, although frequently associated with neglect, were neither a necessary nor a sufficient condition for neglect to occur. Patients with neglect may show no evidence of visual half-field deficits contralateral to the side of the cerebral lesion (contralesional) (Hécaen 1962; Albert 1973; Bisiach *et al*. 1986; Vallar and Perani 1986), hemiplegia or tactile anaesthesia (Bisiach *et al*. 1986; Vallar *et al*. 1993; Kumral and Evyapan 1999). Conversely, all of these sensory and motor disorders may occur without any detectable evidence of neglect (Bisiach *et al*. 1986), suggesting a double dissociation of function (Vallar 2000).

Converging support for interpretations of neglect as a disorder resulting from the disruption of higher levels of integration came from two sets of observations in the 1970s. Firstly, neglect not only may occur in the absence of elementary sensory and motor disorders, as noted earlier, but is also still present in tactile-proprioceptive exploratory tasks executed without visual control by the unaffected hand ipsilateral to the side of the lesion (ipsilesional) (De Renzi *et al*. 1970; Chedru 1976; Cubelli *et al*. 1991; Vallar *et al*. 1991*a*). Secondly, neglect is not confined to the defective exploration of external (personal or extra-personal) space, but its domain extends to imaginal space (Bisiach and Luzzatti 1978).

A number of comprehensive theoretical accounts incorporate the notion that neglect reflects the disordered function of higher-order processes concerned with spatial cognition. Proposed interpretations include the release of an attentional vector pointing toward the ipsilesional side of space (Kinsbourne 1993), defective attention within the contralesional hemispace (Heilman *et al*. 1993), loss of the neural medium for contralesional space representation (Bisiach and Berti 1987), directional hypokinesia (Heilman *et al*. 1985), and ipsilesional rotation of the spatial frame of reference (Ventre *et al*. 1984). All these general views (Bisiach and Vallar 2000) emphasize the role of the impairment of higher-order spatial systems, with comparatively less attention being paid to the contribution of defective or preserved sensory processing to the shaping of the different manifestations of neglect (Chedru 1976) (see Doricchi and Angelelli, 1999 on the role of left hemianopia, Gentilini *et al*. (1989), and Gilliatt and Pratt (1952) on the role of visual input in neglect) and to the modulatory effects of sensory stimulations (Vallar *et al*. 1997; see also Chapter 7.2). Furthermore, and more importantly, these global accounts fail to appreciate the multicomponent nature of the syndrome of unilateral neglect (Barbieri and De Renzi 1989; Halligan and Marshall 1992; Vallar 1994, 1998).

In the late 1980s, a number of studies concurred in suggesting that one relevant aspect of neglect, shared by its manifold manifestations, is the defective access of otherwise adequately processed information to perceptual awareness. Such preserved nonconscious processing, which may concern both visual and somatosensory stimuli, may include their semantic features (Marshall and Halligan 1988; Bisiach and Rusconi 1990; Vallar *et al.* 1991*b,c*, 1996; Berti and Rizzolatti 1992; Làdavas *et al.* 1993). This dissociation between nonconscious preserved processing and conscious defective processing in neglect may be couched in different theoretical frames. Within an attentional perspective (Umiltà 2001), the nonconscious systems spared in patients with neglect may be conceived as independent of attentional processes which, in turn, support perceptual awareness (Posner 1994). Within a representational account, awareness is an intrinsic feature of the representation of space disrupted in neglect (Bisiach and Vallar 2000).

In this broader context of investigations, aimed at assessing the complete range of preserved perceptual processes in patients with unilateral neglect, **visual illusions** have been used. Visual illusions are a time-honoured tool, long utilized to explore the functional properties of the perceptual system (Coren and Gircus 1978*a,b*; Kanisza 1979). In patients with visual neglect, investigations concerning illusory phenomena have produced three main sets of results. Firstly, there is evidence that processing of visual illusions may be preserved (**illusions *in* neglect**). Secondly, visual illusions of length and position simulate some manifestations of the disorder in normal subjects (**illusions *of* neglect**), thus providing insight into some putative pathological mechanisms such as a distortion of perceptual space (Gainotti and Tiacci 1971; Halligan and Marshall 1991; Milner and Harvey 1995). Thirdly, anatomoclinical correlations in neglect patients, showing preserved versus disrupted illusory effects, provide information concerning their neural basis.

Illusions in neglect

Illusions of length and position

The Müller-Lyer figure (Müller-Lyer 1889; Boring 1942; Porac 1994) and its variants (Coren and Gircus 1978*b*) consists in the phenomenon whereby two identical lines are seen as different in physical length because of the presence of fins with a particular orientation at the line ends. The line with outgoing fins is seen as expanded, and the line with ingoing fins as compressed (Figs 1(b) and 1(c)). Illusory effects are also present when asymmetrical figures are used, and the manual setting of the subjective midpoint of the line is required (Post *et al.* 1998, and references cited therein). A stimulus with a left-sided ingoing fin (Fig. 1(d)) produces an illusory shortening of the left side of the line with a rightward bisection error. A stimulus with a right-sided outgoing fin (Fig. 1(g)) produces a similar effect by an illusory expansion of the right side of the line. A stimulus with a right-sided ingoing fin (Fig. 1(e)) brings about an illusory shortening of the right side of the line, while a stimulus with a left-sided outgoing fin (Fig. 1(f)) induces a lengthening of the left side, both resulting in a leftward bisection error. When fins oriented in the same direction are added to the ends of the line (the Judd or Holding illusion) (Judd 1899; Holding 1970), the stimulus is displaced leftward (Fig. 1(h)), resulting in a leftward transection error, or rightward (Fig. 1(i)), resulting in a rightward error. The Brentano or combined form of the Müller-Lyer figure induces a leftward bisection error when its left side is expanded and its right side compressed (Fig. 1(j)). A Brentano figure with an expanded right side and a compressed left side (Fig. 1(k)) produces a rightward error.

Mattingley *et al.* (1995) investigated the bisection of horizontal lines with unilateral fins and Judd illusion stimuli (Figs 1(d)–1(i)) in seven right-brain-damaged patients. Three line lengths

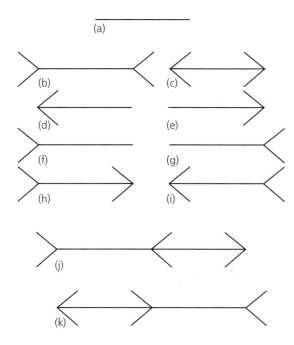

Figure 1 Illusory stimuli used in line bisection: (a) horizontal baseline segment; Müller-Lyer illusion with (b) bilateral outward-projecting fins, (c) bilateral inward-projecting fins, (d) unilateral left-sided inward-projecting fin, (e) unilateral right-sided inward-projecting fin, (f) unilateral left-sided outward-projecting fin, and (g) unilateral right-sided outward-projecting fin; Judd illusion with fins pointing (h) rightward and (i) leftward; (j), (k) Brentano or combined forms resulting from the embedding of two opposite Müller-Lyer illusions ((b), (c)).

(100, 150, and 200 mm) were used, and a group analysis revealed that the patients' subjective midpoint was affected by both right-sided fins (Figs 1(e) and 1(g)) and left-sided fins (Fig. 1(d) and 1(f)), although the latter fell within a putatively neglected region of visual space. Not all patients performed consistently in all conditions, but at least one patient (patient 2) exhibited preserved illusory effects at each line length, with both left-sided and right-sided fins. These largely preserved illusory effects can be contrasted with the patients' inability to report verbally the presence of left-sided fins, regardless of whether they occurred alone (Figs 1(d) and 1(f)) or with right-sided fins (Figs 1(h) and 1(i)).

These results were subsequently confirmed in a single right-brain-damaged patient with left neglect by Ro and Rafal (1996), who used the Judd figure (see Figs 1(h) and 1(i)). The patient exhibited the expected directional effects in a bisection task, although no data from control subjects were provided. Fins pointing rightward (Fig. 1(h)) displaced the patient's subjective midpoint leftward, fins pointing leftward (Fig. 1(i)) had a rightward directional effect. In contrast, in a same–different discrimination task, the patient failed to detect left-sided differences (e.g. Fig. 1(b) versus Fig. 1(i), or Fig. 1(c) versus 1(h)), as patients with left neglect do (Vallar et al. 1994), although stimuli differing in their right side (e.g. Fig. 1(b) versus Fig. 1(h), or Fig. 1(c) versus Fig. 1(i)) were correctly judged as 'different'.

A recent group study by Olk et al. (2001), again using stimuli with unilateral fins and Judd stimuli, confirmed (experiment 1) that right-brain-damaged patients with left neglect may show illusory effects with fins pointing both rightward (Fig. 1(h)) and leftward (Fig. 1(i)), as well as with unilateral fins (Figs 1(d)–1(g)). Five out of the 12 patients were able to report left-sided fins on every trial, four patients on over 80 per cent of the trials, two patients made only a few errors, and one patient (JC) never reported left-sided fins. In most conditions JC showed the expected illusory effects, which, however, proved to be not significant, as analysed in the individual patient. In experiment 2, group analyses revealed illusory effects in the 12 neglect patients, in normal controls, and in right-brain-damaged patients without neglect with both the leftward and the rightward pointing Judd illusion. In this experiment awareness of the left side of the stimulus was assessed by a same–different judgment task similar to the one used by Ro and Rafal (1996). Two of the 12 neglect patients of Olk *et al.* (2001) erroneously judged as 'same' pairs of figures differing in their left side (e.g. Fig. 1(b) versus Fig. 1(i), or Fig. 1(c) versus Fig. 1(h)) on each trial. In line with the earlier findings of Ro and Rafal (1996), one such patient (BM) showed preserved illusory effects, although a statistical analysis was not possible because of the limited number of trials.

Vallar *et al.* (2000), who used the Brentano version of the Müller-Lyer figure, found completely preserved illusory effects in six right-brain-damaged patients with left neglect, both when the left half of the segment was illusorily made longer (Fig. 1(j)), bringing about a leftward directional error, and when it was made shorter (Fig. 1(k)), resulting in a rightward error (Fig. 2). In a second experiment Vallar *et al.* (2000) qualified the dissociation between neglect and the entirely preserved effects of visual illusions, investigating the role of the spatial position of the stimulus. In patients with left neglect a presentation of the stimulus in the left side of space (with respect to the subject's midsagittal plane) increased, as has long been known (Heilman and Valenstein

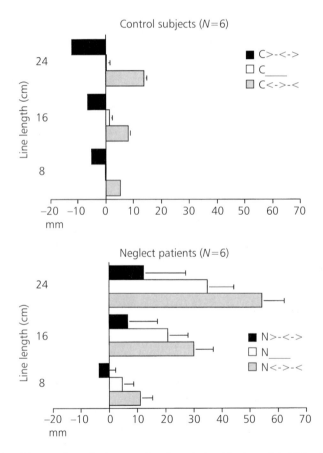

Figure 2 Mean (s.e.) transection displacements of control subjects and right-brain-damaged patients with left visuospatial neglect by line length (8, 16, and 24 cm) and stimulus type (simple line, right-sided outward-projecting fin, left-sided outward-projecting fin). Positive scores denote a rightward displacement of the subjective midpoint with respect to the objective center of the line, and negative scores denote a leftward displacement. (Reproduced with permission from Vallar *et al.*, *Neuropsychologia*, **38**, 1087–97, 2000.)

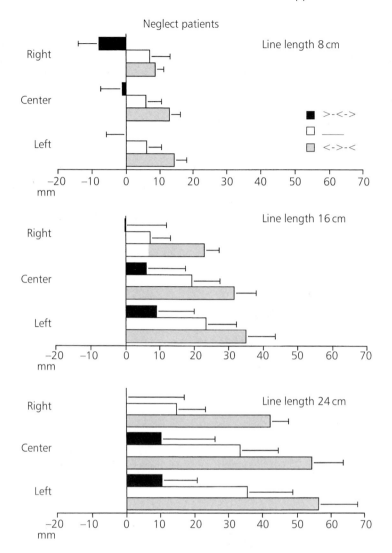

Figure 3   Mean (s.e.) transection displacements of right-brain-damaged patients with left spatial neglect, by line length and stimulus type (see caption to Fig. 2), and spatial position of the stimulus (left, center, and right, with respect to the midsagittal plane of the subject's body). (Reproduced with permission from Vallar *et al.*, *Neuropsychologia*, **38**, 1087–97, 2000.)

1979), the rightward bisection error compared with a center or right-sided position. However, this manipulation did not affect the magnitude of the illusory effects induced by either version of the Brentano–Müller-Lyer illusion (Fig. 3). In contrast, control subjects exhibited the illusory effect, but were not affected by the spatial position of the stimulus (Fig. 4).

The bisection performance of right-brain-damaged patients with left neglect is affected in a similar fashion by the Oppel–Kundt illusion, in which a horizontal line interrupted by vertical cross-bars seems longer as the bars become closer. The configuration which produces an illusory expansion of the left side of the line (Fig. 5(c)) reduces the rightward bisection error; conversely, this is increased by a pattern inducing an illusory lengthening of the right side of the segment (Fig. 5(d)) (Pia and Ricci 2001).

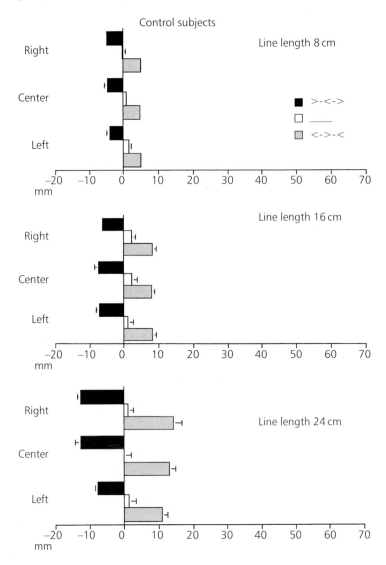

Figure 4 Control subjects: see caption to Fig. 3. (Reproduced with permission from Vallar *et al.*, *Neuropsychologia*, **38**, 1087–97, 2000.)

In two of the studies considered earlier (Ro and Rafal 1996; Olk *et al.* 2001) symmetrical figures were also used (i.e. the Müller-Lyer illusion shown in Figs 1(b) and 1(c)). A consistent finding was that the bilateral outward-projecting fins stimulus (Fig. 1(b)), which is illusorily perceived as longer, brought about a greater rightward error in bisection than the inward-projecting fins stimulus (Fig. 1(c)). Control subjects did not show such an effect (Olk *et al.* 2001). This finding, which may be termed 'illusory line length effect', sheds light on the mechanisms underlying a phenomenon frequently shown by patients with left neglect, namely the disproportionate increase of the ipsilesional error in the bisection of lines of increasing length (Bisiach *et al.* 1983; Vallar *et al.* 2000, and references cited therein). A similar effect of the perceived length of the line on the bisection error of patients with left neglect has recently been found by Ricci *et al.* (2000) using a symmetrical version of the Oppel–Kundt illusion (Figs 5(a) and 5(b)), which, like the Müller-Lyer

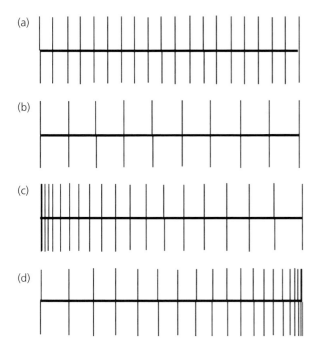

Figure 5 The Oppel–Kundt illusion. Density of the vertical lines: (a), (b) evenly distributed, with different rates; (c) leftward higher density; (d) rightward higher density.

illusion, may increase or reduce the perceived length of the line (see also Chapter 4.3). Taken together, these observations suggest that the pathological bias producing the line-length effect applies not only to physical but also to perceived represented length.

Figures delimited by subjective contours

Mattingley *et al.* (1997) investigated the processing of figures delimited by subjective contours in a patient (VR) with a left-sided visual extinction to double simultaneous stimulation, caused by an extensive lesion in the vascular territory of the middle cerebral artery. VR's left extinction was less severe when the bilateral stimuli formed a subjective figure (Kanisza 1976, 1979) across the visual field than in conditions where such a fill-in did not take place (see earlier evidence that continuous or meaningfully integrated stimuli may overcome neglect (Kartsounis and Warrington 1989)). Processing of these figures was subsequently investigated by Vuilleumier and Landis (1998) in three right-brain-damaged patients with left visual neglect. In a line bisection task, the rightward transection error was comparable across stimulus type (horizontal lines, bars, and rectangles delimited by real or subjective contours, as shown in Fig. 6), with a similar length effect in all stimulus conditions. Vuilleumier and Landis's control condition was a task requiring the bisection of a horizontal empty space, delimited by two dots or vertical segments, with neither real nor subjective contours. Under this condition the three patients did not show any evidence of left neglect in the bisection task, with, if anything, a leftward error. This finding replicates previous observations that the rightward bisection error of patients with left neglect is reduced compared with canonical line bisection when the stimulus is a virtual line, i.e. an empty space between two dots (Bisiach *et al.* 1994, 1996) (although see patient AS, whose rightward error was greater in virtual line bisection). Vuilleumier and Landis (1998) assessed awareness of the presence of the left-sided stimuli used as inducers of the subjective contours by same–different judgments. Patients consistently and erroneously judged configurations which differed in the left-sided inducers, including figures delimited by subjective contours, as 'same'. The patients' performance was

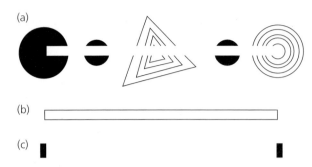

Figure 6 Figures with subjective contours: (a) anomalous surface (horizontal bar) with subjective contours generated by inducers; (b) a surface with real contours; (c) a virtual line, i.e. an empty space between two vertical bars.

errorless both with figures delimited by subjective contours, in which the differences were right-sided, and with similar configurations not inducing subjective contours. In this latter nonillusory condition the patients were able to detect both left- and right-sided differences. This finding shows that bilateral inducers generating subjective contours worsen the patients' ability to detect the left contralesional component stimuli, at least when a same–different judgment response is required. This result differs from the performance of patient VR (Mattingley *et al.* 1997), who showed less left extinction when bilateral stimuli generated a figure with subjective contours across the visual field, compared with sets of similar stimuli which did not induce such an illusory effect. However, no definite conclusions can be drawn; different tasks were used (same–different judgments versus detection), the stimuli were not identical, and Mattingley *et al.*'s patient VR showed no left neglect. This, in turn, was a selection criterion for Vuilleumier and Landis's patients, who also showed left extinction. Nevertheless, these findings suggest that the presence of subjective contours does not systematically facilitate perceptual awareness of left-sided stimuli.

Preserved processing of illusions in neglect

There is converging evidence from a number of different studies that both subjective figures and illusions of length may be adequately processed in patients with left unilateral spatial neglect. Studies investigating the effects of illusions of length (the Müller-Lyer figure and its variants, and the Oppel–Kundt figure) have revealed that, with configurations producing a leftward expansion–rightward compression or a leftward displacement of the line (Figs 1(e), 1(f), 1(h), and 5(c)), the illusory displacement of the subjective center of the line subtracts from the rightward bias which characterizes the bisection performance of patients with left neglect. Conversely, with configurations producing a rightward expansion–leftward compression or a rightward displacement of the line (Figs 1(d), 1(g), 1(i), and 5(d)), the illusory displacement of the subjective center of the line adds to the rightward bias. Figures 2 and 3 illustrate these additive effects in patients with left neglect for the Brentano version of the Müller-Lyer illusion. This preserved processing has been qualified as 'pre-attentive', or not requiring perceptual awareness, on the basis of the observation that, on the one hand, patients show preserved illusory effects on line bisection but, on the other hand, they may fail to detect and report left-sided details of the illusory figures (see patient 2 in Mattingley *et al.* (1995), who never reported left-sided fins but showed complete illusory effects, but see also Ro and Rafal (1996), Vuilleumier and Landis (1998), and Olk *et al.* (2001)). This dissociation in the processing of illusory stimuli can be interpreted in the light of the distinction between 'direct' versus 'indirect' tasks (Palmer 1999, p. 639). A direct task is designed to assess the subject's conscious awareness of a visual presentation (e.g. through detection). An indirect task is designed to assess some process that can be influenced by registered information about the stimulus, even when there is no visual awareness of it. Line bisection can be regarded as a task which taps illusions of length and position in an indirect fashion. In contrast, detection and same–different judgments, concerning the same illusory stimuli or portions of them, can be considered direct tasks. Therefore in patients with left spatial neglect, the level of representation of horizontal extent at which the illusory effects occur appears to be preserved. The indirect–direct task dissociation suggests that this preserved processing may take place without perceptual awareness (see also Chapter 6.1).

This level of visual representation can be qualified as 'nonspatial' and 'retinotopic'. In the study by Vallar *et al.* (2000) the spatial position of the Brentano version of the Müller-Lyer figure affected the bisection error of neglect patients. As found many times before (Heilman and Valenstein 1979), a right-sided position of the stimulus with respect to the midsagittal plane of the subject's trunk reduced the rightward bisection error (Fig. 3). This hemispatial effect, which was not found in normal subjects (Fig. 4), confirms the existence of an egocentric spatial pathological mechanism in the bisection error of patients with left neglect. In contrast, the spatial position of the stimulus did not modulate the extent of the illusory effects shown by either neglect patients or normal subjects (Figs 3 and 4), suggesting that these visual phenomena (preserved in patients with neglect) occur at a nonspatial (retinotopic) level of representation.

Illusions of neglect

As Figs 2 and 4 show, illusions of horizontal extent, such as the asymmetrical versions of the Müller-Lyer figures and the Oppel–Kundt configuration (Figs 1 and 5), induce in normal subjects a rightward or leftward displacement of the subjective midpoint, according to the side of the expansion/compression of the horizontal segment. As noted by Watt (1994), who used the Oppel–Kundt illusion as an illustrative example, these illusory effects mimic the line bisection performance of patients with left unilateral neglect.

Following similar logic, Fleming and Behrmann (1998) used Judd illusion displays (Figs 1(h) and 1(i)) to assess the performance of normal subjects in manual line bisection, and in a task which required them to place the two fins at the ends of an imaginary shaft. This study, in which the illusion-inducing properties of the Judd figures were accurately investigated by varying orthogonally the direction and the angles of the fins, showed that illusory displacements of the shaft induce in normal subjects a directional error similar to the one committed by neglect patients. Such an error is also produced by asymmetrical Müller-Lyer and Brentano configurations (Figs 1(d)–(g), 1(j), 1(k)) (Mattingley *et al.* 1995; Post *et al.* 1998; Vallar *et al.* 2000; Olk *et al.* 2001).

For the Judd figure (an illusion of position, in which the stimulus is displaced), the analogy appears to be consistent with the view that one pathological mechanism underlying contralesional neglect involves the ipsilesional pathological orientation of spatial attention (Kinsbourne 1993; Bisiach and Vallar 2000). The illusory displacement may mimic the ipsilesional shift of lateral spatial attention. For the Müller-Lyer illusion, the analogy is consistent with the view that one pathological mechanism underlying some abnormal behaviors exhibited by right-brain-damaged patients with left neglect is a rightward compression of the internal representation of space at an even rate (Halligan and Marshall 1991), or a shrinkage or compression in size perception confined to, or affecting disproportionately, the left contralesional side of perceived space (see Gainotti and Tiacci (1971) for an early account in terms of over-evaluation of ipsilesional stimuli, and Milner *et al.* (1993), Milner and Harvey (1995), and Karnath and Ferber (1999) for a discussion of these views and empirical data). Alternatively, the spatial medium may be pathologically expanded contralesionally (leftward in patients with left neglect), and compressed ipsilesionally (rightward), making objects in the left side of space, or the left side of objects, disproportionately shorter in their horizontal dimension (Bisiach and Vallar 2000). Distortions of this sort would account for a number of pathological phenomena found in patients with left neglect. These include the patients' rightward error in line bisection, their judging the left half of a horizontal line as shorter than the right (Milner *et al.* 1993), and their underestimation of the horizontal extent of stimuli presented in the left side of egocentric space (Milner and Harvey 1995; Kerkhoff 2000).

However, these simulations of neglect through illusory stimuli are mere analogies, even though they provide suggestions concerning the possible pathological mechanisms producing the ipsilesional displacement of the subjective midpoint in line bisection. As discussed earlier, these illusory effects are preserved in patients with left unilateral neglect. Illusions of length and position, and figures with subjective contours, are likely to arise at a nonspatial retinotopic level of representation (Vallar *et al.* 2000). The anatomical correlates of the preserved illusory effects in right-brain-damaged patients with left unilateral neglect provide converging evidence which supports this conclusion.

The anatomical basis of visual illusions

In recent years, a number of neurophysiological studies in the monkey (von der Heydt *et al.* 1984; von der Heydt and Peterhans 1989; Peterhans and von der Heydt 1991; Grosof *et al.* 1993) and functional imaging experiments in humans (Hirsch *et al.* 1995; Ffytche and Zeki 1996; Larsson *et al.* 1999; Mendola *et al.* 1999) have provided evidence that the neural basis of visual illusions includes the occipital regions (the visual association and the primary visual cortices). These empirical findings, which are not central to the main aim of this chapter and therefore are not reviewed here, concern mainly figures with subjective contours. Based on these suggestions, the anatomical correlates of the processing of visual illusions in patients with left neglect will be considered, focusing on damage versus sparing of the occipital regions and the optic radiations.

Illusions of length and position

In the study by Mattingley *et al.* (1995) a group analysis revealed that right-sided fins induced illusory effects in all conditions, as in control subjects. In contrast, left-sided fins produced only partial effects. This is likely to reflect variability among patients. Mattingley *et al.*'s patient 1, who had severe hypoperfusion in the vascular territory of the right middle cerebral artery, made a systematic left-sided bisection error with left-sided fins, which were presumably treated as visual cues with no illusory effect. In contrast, patient 2, who had a temporoparietal and subcortical stroke lesion, showed completely preserved illusory effects with left-sided fins. The other five patients had lesions involving the frontal, temporal, parietal, or subcortical regions; the occipital lobe was damaged in patient 4. In the recent study by Olk *et al.* (2001), where group analysis showed overall preserved illusory effects, two out of the 12 right-brain-damaged patients with left neglect had lesions extending to the occipital lobe: one patient (KG) showed largely preserved illusory effects, but the other (LC) had a much less consistent performance. In Pia and Ricci's (2001) series of 28 right-brain-damaged neglect patients who showed, as a group, preserved Oppel–Kundt illusory effects, the lesion included the occipital lobe only in four patients (14 per cent).

In two other studies more precise anatomical information was provided, including lesion maps with reference to standard atlases (Damasio and Damasio 1989). The patient of Ro and Rafal (1996) had an extensive temporoparietal lesion which spared the optic radiations and the occipital cortex. In the study by Vallar *et al.* (2000), one patient (GM) showed no illusory effects with left-sided outward-projecting fins (Fig. 1(j)). GM was the only patient in this series with right hemisphere damage extending to the visual association and primary visual cortices. These findings have been replicated and extended in a larger series of right-brain-damaged neglect patients with lesions including the optic radiations, the occipital cortex, or both, and behavioral and electrophysiological evidence of left visual half-field deficits. This group of right-brain-damaged patients with neglect and hemianopia was compared with neglect patients without left visual half-field deficits, and lesions sparing the optic radiations and the occipital cortex. In line with the single-patient observation by Vallar *et al.* (2000), patients with damage extending caudally to the occipital regions showed no illusory effects, which, conversely, were preserved in patients with more anterior damage. This difference was independent of the severity of spatial unilateral neglect, as assessed by cancellation and reading tasks, but, as reported previously (D'Erme *et al.* 1987; Doricchi and Angelelli 1999) (see Binder *et al.* (1992) for related evidence), patients with more posterior damage showed a greater rightward bias in line bisection (Daini *et al.*, 2002).

Figures delimited by subjective contours

The three patients of Vuilleumier and Landis (1998), who showed preserved processing of subjective figures, had cortical or subcortical lesions mapped with reference to a standard atlas (Damasio and Damasio 1989), which spared the primary and secondary visual areas. In a second study, Vuilleumier *et al.* (2001) replicated their earlier findings in a larger series of 12 patients, including the three previously reported cases (Vuilleumier and Landis 1998), with a complete group analysis showing that the rightward bisection error diminished with gap stimuli (an empty space between two dots) compared with horizontal bars formed by either real or illusory contours (Bisiach *et al.* 1996; Bisiach *et al.* 1994). However, after inspection of the individual data, Vuilleumier *et al.* (2001) found that their series separated into two subgroups, differing with respect to their bisection performance with gap stimuli. One subgroup, in which lesions clustered in the inferior-posterior parietal lobule (BA 40), showed the general pattern characterized by a reduction of the rightward bias with gap stimuli. In the other subgroup, in which lesions extended more posteriorly to the lateral occipital lobe (BAs 18 and 19), the bisection error was comparable in all conditions, including gap stimuli. The interpretation of these findings is not straightforward. The average bisection error of subjective versus real figures was similar in both subgroups; the difference concerned a very different stimulus (a gap). However, Vuilleumier *et al.* (2001) also found a significant correlation between the bisection performances of figures with subjective and real contours in the parietal, but not in the parieto-occipital subgroup. With these caveats in mind, their findings suggest, from a neuropsychological perspective, a role of the lateral occipital cortex in the generation of subjective figures.

Conclusions

The available empirical evidence concerning the processing of visual illusions (figures delimited by subjective contours, illusions of length and position) in right-brain-damaged patients with left neglect consistently suggest that the levels of representation where these visual phenomena arise are largely preserved. This behavioral evidence has an anatomical counterpart. Illusory effects are disrupted in patients with left neglect when the lesions extend from the posterior-inferior parietal region, which represents the main anatomical correlate of this disorder (Vallar and Perani 1986; Vallar 2001), more caudally to the occipital regions. Perceptual analysis of visual input, including grouping and figure–ground segmentation (as suggested by experiments using illusory contours), and a relevant part of the multicomponent processes (Coren and Girgus 1978*b*) underpinning estimation of length (as suggested by experiments using variants of the Müller-Lyer and Oppel–Kundt illusions) are likely to take place at a retinotopic level of representation in the visual cortex. These operations are largely independent of the spatial representations, dysfunctional in patients with left neglect, which have more anterior neural correlates in the posterior inferior-parietal and pre-motor frontal regions (Bisiach and Vallar 2000). This functional and anatomical independence is also supported by the finding that the presence or absence of illusory effects in neglect patients is unrelated to the overall severity of neglect itself, as assessed by standard diagnostic test batteries (Vallar *et al.* 2000; Vuilleumier *et al.* 2001; Daini *et al.*, 2002).

In all the studies considered in this review the preserved illusory effects were demonstrated through 'indirect' (Palmer 1999), 'procedural', or 'implicit' tasks (Squire 1992; Roediger and McDermott 1993; Vallar 1999), in which patients were required to communicate that stimulus processing had taken place through a behavioral response (line bisection) rather than by explicitly declaring the detection of the left-sided components of the illusory configurations. A number of studies have emphasized the 'indirect' nature of the preserved illusory effects, showing that patients were unable to process explicitly the left side of the stimulus, as assessed by same–different judgments or detection direct tasks (patient 2 of Mattingley *et al.* (1995); however, see Ro and Rafal (1996), Vuilleumier and Landis (1998), Olk *et al.* (2001), and Vuilleumier *et al.* (2001)). These findings may be taken as evidence that illusory contours and illusions of length and position arise at levels of representation which do not entail perceptual awareness ('pre-attentional' according to some accounts (Mattingley *et al.* 1995; Vuilleumier *et al.* 2001)) but nevertheless may affect the subjects' visuomotor behavior, such as their error in line bisection, with effects adding to or subtracting from the spatial bias brought about by unilateral neglect (Mattingley *et al.* 1995; Ro and Rafal 1996; Vallar *et al.* 2000).

A final issue concerns illusions of length and position as a simulation model of the mechanisms underlying spatial neglect. The simulation appears to include the lateral pathological displacement of spatial attention (the Judd illusion of position) and the relative compression of objects in the left portion of space compared with contralateral objects, or of the left side of objects compared with their right side (the Müller-Lyer figure and its variants, and the Oppel–Kundt figure). On the one hand, data from normal subjects indicate that these illusions provide an effective simulation of one aspect of left spatial neglect, namely the rightward displacement of the subjective midpoint of a horizontal segment. Furthermore, the very nature of illusions of length simulates a horizontal size distortion (Restle and Decker 1977; Cohen *et al.* 1994; Frassinetti *et al.* 1999; Ferber and Karnath 2001), which characterizes some manifestations of unilateral spatial neglect. More specifically, the expansion of the right side of a line and the compression of its left side, induced by appropriately arranged fins, provide an analog of the anisometric distortion of space representation in left neglect. On the other hand, however, the consistent neuropsychological observation of preserved illusory effects of length and position in neglect patients, and of their disruption after damage involving the occipital regions, suggests that such a simulation, plausible as it may be, takes place at a different level of representation and in different regions of the brain.

The view that multiple representations of lateral extension may exist in the brain, within different reference frames, is compatible with the finding that a related perceptual disorder (the underestimation of the horizontal size of contralesional visual objects) has been observed in right-brain-damaged patients with unilateral neglect—a tendency to 'overvalue' the size of ipsilesional drawings (Gainotti and Tiacci 1971) and 'size distortion' (Milner and Harvey 1995). Other empirical data may be found in Kerkhoff (2000) and Ferber and Karnath (2001). These deficits have also been found in patients without neglect ('hemimicropsia' (Cohen *et al.* 1994, case 1; Ferber and Karnath 2001) and 'horizontal dysmetropsia' (Frassinetti *et al.* 1999)), as well as after damage to the left hemisphere (Cohen *et al.* 1994, case 2).It has been suggested that the occipital lobe and, more specifically, the extrastriate visual cortex (Cohen *et al.* 1994; Frassinetti *et al.* 1999) constitute a neural basis for the processing of horizontal length. Consistent with these findings, illusions of length and position are likely, as discussed earlier, to arise in the occipital regions. The precise relationship of these retinotopic representations of horizontal extent, and of their disorders (Frassinetti *et al.* 1999; Vallar *et al.* 2000) (see also Hoff and Pötzl (1938) for an early discussion of the more general concept of anisotropy of visual space), with the 'anisometry' of spatial representation (Bisiach and Vallar 2000), which characterizes some aspects of unilateral neglect, is an issue for future research.

Acknowledgements

This work was supported in part by grants from the Ministero dell'Università e della Ricerca Scientifica e Tecnologica (Cofin99 and Cofin01). We are grateful to Natale Stucchi for a useful discussion about figures with subjective contours.

References

Albert, M. L. (1973). A simple test of visual neglect. *Neurology*, **23**, 658–64.

Barbieri, C. and De Renzi, E. (1989). Patterns of neglect dissociation. *Behavioural Neurology*, **2**, 13–24.

Berti, A. and Rizzolatti, G. (1992). Visual processing without awareness: evidence from unilateral neglect. *Journal of Cognitive Neuroscience*, **4**, 345–51.

Binder, J., Marshall, R., Lazar, R., Benjamin, J., and Mohr, J. P. (1992). Distinct syndromes of hemineglect. *Archives of Neurology*, **49**, 1187–94.

Bisiach, E. and Berti, A. (1987). Dyschiria. An attempt at its systemic explanation. In *Neurophysiological and neuropsychological aspects of spatial neglect* (ed. M. Jeannerod), pp. 183–201. North-Holland, Amsterdam.

Bisiach, E. and Luzzatti, C. (1978). Unilateral neglect of representational space. *Cortex*, **14**, 129–33.

Bisiach, E. and Rusconi, M. L. (1990). Break-down of perceptual awareness in unilateral neglect. *Cortex*, **26**, 643–9.

Bisiach, E. and Vallar, G. (2000). Unilateral neglect in humans. In *Handbook of neuropsychology* (2nd edn), Vol. 1 (ed. F. Boller, J. Grafman, and G. Rizzolatti), pp. 459–502. Elsevier, Amsterdam.

Bisiach, E., Bulgarelli, C., Sterzi, R., and Vallar, G. (1983). Line bisection and cognitive plasticity of unilateral neglect of space. *Brain and Cognition*, **2**, 32–8.

Bisiach, E., Perani, D., Vallar, G., and Berti, A. (1986). Unilateral neglect: personal and extrapersonal. *Neuropsychologia*, **24**, 759–67.

Bisiach, E., Rusconi, M. L., Peretti, V., and Vallar, G. (1994). Challenging current accounts of unilateral neglect. *Neuropsychologia*, **32**, 1431–4.

Bisiach, E., Pizzamiglio, L., Nico, D., and Antonucci, G. (1996). Beyond unilateral neglect. *Brain*, **119**, 851–7.

Boring, E. G. (1942). *Sensation and perception in the history of experimental psychology*, pp. 243 ff. Appleton-Century, New York.

Chedru, F. (1976). Space representation in unilateral spatial neglect. *Journal of Neurology, Neurosurgery, and Psychiatry*, **39**, 1057–61.

Cohen, L., Gray, F., Meyrignac, C., Dehaene, S., and Degos, J. D. (1994). Selective deficit of visual size perception: two cases of hemimicropsia. *Journal of Neurology, Neurosurgery, and Psychiatry*, **57**, 73–8.

Coren, S. and Gircus, J. S. (1978a). *Seeing is deceiving: the psychology of visual illusions*. Lawrence Erlbaum, Hillsdale, NJ.

Coren, S. and Gircus, J. S. (1978b). Visual illusions. In *Handbook of sensory physiology. Perception*, Vol. 8 (ed. R. Held, H. W. Leibowitz, and H.-L. Teuber), pp. 548–68. Springer-Verlag, Heidelberg.

Cubelli, R., Nichelli, P., Bonito, V., De Tanti, A., and Inzaghi, M. G. (1991). Different patterns of dissociation in unilateral spatial neglect. *Brain and Cognition*, **15**, 139–59.

Daini, R., Angelelli, P., Antonucci, G., Cappa, S. F., and Vallar, G. (2002). Exploring the syndrome of spatial unilateral neglect through an illusion of length. *Experimental Brain Research*, **144**, 224–37.

Damasio, H. and Damasio, A. R. (1989). *Lesion analysis in neuropsychology*. Oxford University Press, New York.

De Renzi, E., Faglioni, P., and Scotti, G. (1970). Hemispheric contribution to exploration of space through the visual and tactile modality. *Cortex*, **6**, 191–203.

D'Erme, P., De Bonis, C., and Gainotti, G. (1987). Influenza dell'emi-inattenzione e dell'emianopsia sui compiti di bisezione di linee nei pazienti cerebrolesi. *Archivio di Psicologia, Neurologia e Psichiatria*, **48**, 193–207.

Doricchi, F. and Angelelli, P. (1999). Misrepresentation of horizontal space in left unilateral neglect: role of hemianopia. *Neurology*, **52**, 1845–52.

Ferber, S. and Karnath, H.-O. (2001). Size perception in hemianopia and neglect. *Brain*, **124**, 527–36.

Ffytche, D. H. and Zeki, S. (1996). Brain activity related to the perception of illusory contours. *Neuroimage*, **3**, 104–8.

Fleming, J., and Behrmann, M. (1998). Visuospatial neglect in normal subjects: altered spatial representations induced by a perceptual illusion. *Neuropsychologia*, **36**, 469–75.

Frassinetti, F., Nichelli, P., and di Pellegrino, G. (1999). Selective horizontal dysmetropsia following prestriate lesion. *Brain*, **122**, 339–50.

Gainotti, G. and Tiacci, C. (1971). The relationships between disorders of visual perception and unilateral spatial neglect. *Neuropsychologia*, **9**, 451–8.

Gentilini, M., Barbieri, C., De Renzi, E., and Faglioni, P. (1989). Space exploration with and without the aid of vision in hemisphere-damaged patients. *Cortex*, **25**, 643–51.

Gilliatt, R. W. and Pratt, R. T. C. (1952). Disorders of perception and performance in a case of right-sided cerebral thrombosis. *Journal of Neurology, Neurosurgery, and Psychiatry*, **15**, 264–71.

Grosof, D. H., Shapley, R. M., and Hawken, M. J. (1993). Macaque V1 neurons can signal 'illusory' contours. *Nature*, **365**, 550–2.

Halligan, P. W. and Marshall, J. C. (1991). Spatial compression in visual neglect: a case study. *Cortex*, **27**, 623–9.

Halligan, P. W. and Marshall, J. C. (1992). Left visuo-spatial neglect: a meaningless entity? *Cortex*, **28**, 525–35.

Hécaen, H. (1962). Clinical symptomatology in right and left hemispheric lesions. In *Interhemispheric relations and cerebral dominance* (ed. V. B. Mountcastle), pp. 215–43. Johns Hopkins University Press Baltimore, MD.

Heilman, K. M. and Valenstein, E. (1979). Mechanisms underlying hemispatial neglect. *Annals of Neurology*, **5**, 166–70.

Heilman, K. M., Bowers, D., Coslett, H. B., Whelan, H., and Watson, R. T. (1985). Directional hypokinesia: prolonged reaction times for leftward movements in patients with right hemisphere lesions and neglect. *Neurology*, **35**, 855–9.

Heilman, K. M., Watson, R. T., and Valenstein, E. (1993). Neglect and related disorders. In *Clinical neuropsychology* (3rd edn) (ed. K. M. Heilman and E. Valenstein), pp. 279–336. Oxford University Press, New York.

Hirsch, J., Delapaz, R. L., Relkin, N. R., *et al.* (1995). Illusory contours activate specific regions in human visual cortex: evidence from functional magnetic-resonance-imaging. *Proceedings of the National Academy of Sciences of the United States of America*, **92**, 6469–73.

Hoff, H. and Pötzl, O. (1938). Anisotropie des Sehraums bei occipitaler Herderkrankung. *Deutsche Zeitschrift für Nervenheilkunde*, **145**, 179–217.

Holding, D. H. (1970). A line illusion with irrelevant depth cues. *American Journal of Psychology*, **83**, 280–2.

Judd, C. H. (1899). A study of geometrical illusions. *Psychological Review*, **6**, 241–61.

Kanizsa, G. (1976). Subjective contours. *Scientific American*, **234**, 48–52.

Kanisza, G. (1979). *Organization in vision*. Praeger, New York.

Karnath, H.-O. and Ferber, S. (1999). Is space representation distorted in neglect? *Neuropsychologia*, **37**, 7–15.

Kartsounis, L. D. and Warrington, E. K. (1989). Unilateral visual neglect overcome by cues implicit in stimulus arrays. *Journal of Neurology, Neurosurgery, and Psychiatry*, **52**, 1253–9.

Kerkhoff, G. (2000). Multiple perceptual distortions and their modulation in leftsided visual neglect. *Neuropsychologia*, **38**, 1073–86.

Kinsbourne, M. (1993). Orientational bias model of unilateral neglect: evidence from attentional gradients within hemispace. In *Unilateral neglect: clinical and experimental studies* (ed. I. H. Robertson and J. C. Marshall), pp. 63–86. Lawrence Erlbaum, Hove.

Kumral, E. and Evyapan, D. (1999). Associated exploratory-motor and perceptual-sensory neglect without hemiparesis. *Neurology*, **52**, 199–202.

Làdavas, E., Paladini, R., and Cubelli, R. (1993). Implicit associative priming in a patient with left visual neglect. *Neuropsychologia*, **31**, 1307–20.

Larsson, J., Amunts, K., Gulyas, B., Malikovic, A., Zilles, K., and Roland, P. E. (1999). Neuronal correlates of real and illusory contour perception: functional anatomy with PET. *European Journal of Neuroscience*, **11**, 4024–36.

Marshall, J. C. and Halligan, P. (1988). Blindsight and insight in visuo-spatial neglect. *Nature*, **336**, 766–7.

Mattingley, J. B., Bradshaw, J. L., and Bradshaw, J. A. (1995). The effects of unilateral visuospatial neglect on perception of Müller-Lyer illusory figures. *Perception*, **24**, 415–33.

Mattingley, J. B., Davis, G., and Driver, J. (1997). Preattentive filling-in of visual surfaces in parietal extinction. *Science*, **275**, 671–4.

Mendola, J. D., Dale, A. M., Fischl, B., Liu, A. K., and Tootell, R. B. (1999). The representation of illusory and real contours in human cortical visual areas revealed by functional magnetic resonance imaging. *Journal of Neuroscience*, **19**, 8560–72.

Milner, A. D. and Harvey, M. (1995). Distortion of size perception in visuospatial neglect. *Current Biology*, **5**, 85–9.

Milner, A. D., Harvey, M., Roberts, R. C., and Forster, S. V. (1993). Line bisection errors in visual neglect: misguided action or size distortion? *Neuropsychologia*, **31**, 39–49.

Müller-Lyer, F. C. (1889). Optische Urtheilstäuschungen. *Archiv für Anatomie und Physiologie, Physiologische Abteilung (Supplement-Band)*, **2**, 263–70.

Olk, B., Harvey, M., Dow, L., and Murphy, P. J. S. (2001). Illusion processing in hemispatial neglect. *Neuropsychologia*, **39**, 611–25.

Palmer, S. E. (1999). *Vision science: photons to phenomenology*. MIT Press, Cambridge, MA.

Peterhans, E. and von der Heydt, R. (1991). Subjective contours: bridging the gap between psychophysics and physiology. *Trends in Neurosciences*, **14**, 112–19.

Pia, L. and Ricci, R. (2001). Anisometry of space perception in unilateral neglect. Presented at the Nineteenth European Workshop on Cognitive Neuropsychology, Bressanone, Italy, 21–26 January.

Porac, C. (1994). Comparison of the wings-in, wings-out, and Brentano variants of the Mueller-Lyer illusion. *American Journal of Psychology*, **107**, 69–83.

Posner, M. I. (1994). Attention: the mechanisms of consciousness. *Proceedings of the National Academy of Sciences of the United States of America*, **91**, 7398–403.

Post, R. B., Welch, R. B., and Caufield, K. (1998). Relative spatial expansion and contraction within the Müller-Lyer and Judd illusions. *Perception*, **27**, 827–38.

Restle, F. and Decker, J. (1977). Size of the Mueller-Lyer illusion as a function of its dimensions: theory and data. *Perception and Psychophysics*, **21**, 489–503.

Ricci, R., Calhoun, J., and Chatterjee, A. (2000). Orientation bias in unilateral neglect: Representational contributions. *Cortex*, **36**, 671–7.

Ro, T. and Rafal, R. D. (1996). Perception of geometric illusions in hemispatial neglect. *Neuropsychologia*, **34**, 973–8.

Roediger, H. L. III. and McDermott, K. B. (1993). Implicit memory in normal human subjects. In *Handbook of neuropsychology* Vol. 8 (ed. F. Boller and J. Grafman), pp. 63–131. Elsevier, Amsterdam.

Squire, L. R. (1992). Declarative and nondeclarative memory: multiple brain systems supporting learning and memory. *Journal of Cognitive Neuroscience*, **4**, 232–43.

Umiltà, C. (2001). Mechanisms of attention. In *The handbook of cognitive neuropsychology* (ed. B. Rapp), pp. 135–58. Psychology Press, Philadelphia, PA.

Vallar, G. (1994). Left spatial hemineglect: an unmanageable explosion of dissociations? No. *Neuropsychological Rehabilitation*, **4**, 209–12.

Vallar, G. (1998). Spatial hemineglect in humans. *Trends in Cognitive Sciences*, **2**, 87–97.

Vallar, G. (1999). Neuropsychological disorders of memory. In *Handbook of clinical and experimental neuropsychology* (ed. G. Denes and L. Pizzamiglio), pp. 321–68. Psychology Press, Hove.

Vallar, G. (2000). The methodological foundations of human neuropsychology: studies in brain-damaged patients. In *Handbook of neuropsychology* Vol. 8 (ed. F. Boller and J. Grafman), pp. 305–44. Elsevier, Amsterdam.

Vallar, G. (2001). Extrapersonal visual unilateral spatial neglect and its neuroanatomy. *Neuroimage*, **14**, S52–8.

Vallar, G. and Perani, D. (1986). The anatomy of unilateral neglect after right hemisphere stroke lesions: a clinical CT/Scan correlation study in man. *Neuropsychologia*, **24**, 609–22.

Vallar, G., Rusconi, M. L., Geminiani, G., Berti, A., and Cappa, S. F. (1991*a*). Visual and non-visual neglect after unilateral brain lesions: modulation by visual input. *International Journal of Neuroscience*, **61**, 229–39.

Vallar, G., Bottini, G., Sterzi, R., Passerini, D., and Rusconi, M. L. (1991*b*). Hemianesthesia, sensory neglect and defective access to conscious experience. *Neurology*, **41**, 650–2.

Vallar, G., Sandroni, P., Rusconi, M. L., and Barbieri, S. (1991*c*). Hemianopia, hemianesthesia and spatial neglect: a study with evoked potentials. *Neurology*, **41**, 1918–22.

Vallar, G., Bottini, G., Rusconi, M. L., and Sterzi, R. (1993). Exploring somatosensory hemineglect by vestibular stimulation. *Brain*, **116**, 71–86.

Vallar, G., Rusconi, M. L., and Bisiach, E. (1994). Awareness of contralesional information in unilateral neglect: effects of verbal cueing, tracing and vestibular stimulation. In *Attention and performance. XV: Conscious and nonconscious information processing* (ed. C. Umiltà and M. Moscovitch), pp. 377–91. MIT Press, Cambridge, MA.

Vallar, G., Guariglia, C., Nico, D., and Tabossi, P. (1996). Left neglect dyslexia and the processing of *neglected* information. *Journal of Clinical and Experimental Neuropsychology*, **18**, 733–46.

Vallar, G., Guariglia, C., and Rusconi, M. L. (1997). Modulation of the neglect syndrome by sensory stimulation. In *Parietal lobe contributions to orientation in 3D space* (ed. P. Thier and H.-O. Karnath), pp. 555–78. Springer-Verlag, Heidelberg.

Vallar, G., Daini, R., and Antonucci, G. (2000). Processing of illusion of length in spatial hemineglect: a study of line bisection. *Neuropsychologia*, **38**, 1087–97.

Ventre, J., Flandrin, J. M., and Jeannerod, M. (1984). In search for the egocentric reference: a neurophysiological hypothesis. *Neuropsychologia*, **22**, 797–806.

von der Heydt, R. and Peterhans, E. (1989). Mechanisms of contour perception in monkey visual cortex. I: Lines of pattern discontinuity. *Journal of Neuroscience*, **9**, 1731–48.

von der Heydt, R., Peterhans, E., and Baumgartner, G. (1984). Illusory contours and cortical neuron responses. *Science*, **224**, 1260–2.

Vuilleumier, P. and Landis, T. (1998). Illusory contours and spatial neglect. *NeuroReport*, **9**, 2481–4.

Vuilleumier, P., Valenza, N., and Landis, T. (2001). Explicit and implicit perception of illusory contours in unilateral spatial neglect: behavioural and anatomical correlates of preattentive grouping mechanisms. *Neuropsychologia*, **39**, 597–610.

Watt, R. (1994). Some points about human vision and visual neglect. *Neuropsychological Rehabilitation*, **4**, 213–19.

4.7 Navigation in neglect patients

Luigi Pizzamiglio, Giuseppe Iaria, Alain Berthoz, Gaspare Galati,
and Cecilia Guariglia

Moving into environmental space in everyday living is normally performed under direct visual guidance. Perceived landmarks inform the subject of his or her position while walking from one place to another. However, navigation can be carried out on the basis of internally generated signals, such as somatosensory and vestibular information. These signals update the subject's position and direction with reference to the starting point. This method of navigation is called 'dead reckoning' and does not require vision (Farrell 1996). Another condition consists of moving toward a previously seen target, but without visual feedback (Philbeck et al. 2000). This nonvisual navigation can be effectively calibrated by previous perception of the location and distance of the target (Rieser et al. 1990; Philbeck et al. in press). Performing this method of self-motion requires the integration of visual and nonvisual information. Although the reciprocal influences of visual and nonvisual systems have been increasingly discovered at the psychophysical level, very little is known about the neural substrates involved in this high-level integration in humans.

The study of patients with focal brain damage as they move in the environment with or without vision may provide interesting insights into the role of various cortical areas in controlling different forms of navigation. In this domain, hemispatial neglect is particularly interesting for both clinical and theoretical reasons. One of the main features of hemispatial neglect is the strong anisotropy in processing extrapersonal as well as personal space. Clinical and experimental research documents this asymmetry in spatial processing in a great variety of tasks requiring scanning or different kinds of perceptual evaluation of the environment, or the planning and execution of motor actions (grasping, reaching, throwing, moving the eyes, etc.) (Bisiach 1999).

Very little attention has been given to these patients' potential disorders in navigation in a real environment. Any clinician can provide anecdotal evidence of the difficulty that neglect patients experience in moving in familiar or nonfamiliar environments. However, failure to detect landmarks in the left position of the space would be the obvious interpretation of such a disorder (Bisiach et al. 1993).

Today, knowledge about different navigational systems and about the nature of neglect raises several theoretical issues. The first can be formulated as follows: since hemispatial neglect is a multimodal disorder, does it also produce an anisometry in environmental navigation when using either visual or nonvisual updating?

The second question refers to the integration of visual and nonvisual information. Neuroanatomical data provide a clear picture of frequent impairment of the inferior right parietal lobe in hemispatial neglect (Vallar 1993). On the other side, experimental neurophysiology provides a large body of evidence suggesting high-level integration of different retinal and extraretinal information in the posterior and superior parts of the parietal lobe. Considering the analogy between the cortical areas in monkeys and humans, is it possible that patients with hemispatial neglect show a selective impairment when body movement in space requires integration between visual and nonvisual signals?

Calibration of locomotor control

Two recent studies have dealt directly with the first question. They investigated the capacity of right-brain-damaged patients, with and without neglect, to reproduce perceived distances along linear trajectories by memory. Philbeck *et al.* (2000) studied a group of patients with right posterior parietal lesions and a group of normal controls. Four out of six patients had clinical signs of neglect. The participants were first required to evaluate, either verbally or by walking, the distance between their body and a target perceived either visually or proprioceptively (the participant was passively walked to the target by the experimenter). The target was located 45° to the left or to the right of their midsagittal plane. Right parietal patients perceived egocentric distances and were able to reproduce them similarly to the control group. All participants were able to walk accurately and precisely to the remembered target without vision. The authors concluded that the posterior parietal cortex 'is not critically involved in monitoring and integrating non-visual self motion signals'. Relevant to the present discussion is the fact that the presence of neglect does not impair the ability to update self-location along a straight path, walking toward a target located in the left or the right hemispace.

A study performed in our laboratory addressed similar questions using a different methodology. The aim of the first experiment was to test whether neglect patients reproduce a distance after a whole-body displacement toward both sides of space with the same anisometry observed when they reproduce the length of a line on either side of a horizontal plane. The experiment required the distance replication of rectilinear whole-body translations imposed by a specially designed robot. The participants could replicate a passively imposed whole-body displacement by moving the robot in the same direction (leftward–leftward, rightward–rightward, and forward–forward) or in a different direction (leftward–forward, forward–rightward, etc.) (Fig. 1).

These different conditions allowed us to evaluate whether patients are able to use a 'vestibular memory' for reproducing the distance when the task is to reproduce the passive displacement in the same direction and to generate a representation of the distance when the task is to reproduce the displacement in a different direction. When moving in a different direction, the vestibular and somatosensory information completely changes. In order to replicate the same distance, the passive spatial displacement has to be computed by using some parameters (i.e. velocity profile, time) and comparing them with a successive active displacement based on a different set of sensory information. To prevent the use of the duration of the stimulus to compute the distance, a high proportion of catch trials were introduced in which the time of passive translation was shorter or longer than that in the experimental trials.

Four groups of five participants each were studied: right-brain-damaged patients with neglect (RN+), right-brain-damaged patients without neglect (RN−), left-brain-damaged patients without neglect (LN−), and normal controls (C) of comparable age and education. All patients suffered from unilateral lesions deriving from a single cerebrovascular accident.

The results of the distance replication in the four groups and for the different directions of displacement did not reveal differences in the performances of the four groups. Also, there were no differences between the rightward–leftward direction of movement either when the distance reproduction was performed in the 'same' or in a 'different' direction. None of the interactions between the variables was significant. Considering the velocity profiles produced by the different groups of participants, no clear differences emerged among the three brain-damaged groups;

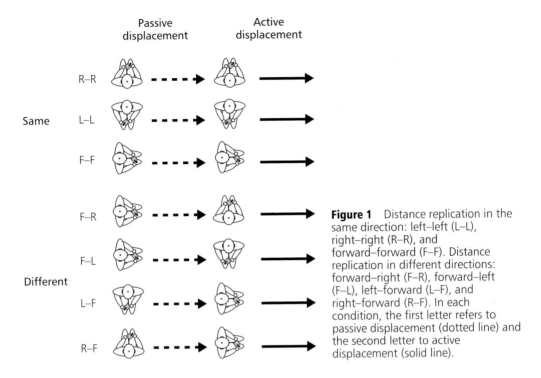

Figure 1 Distance replication in the same direction: left–left (L–L), right–right (R–R), and forward–forward (F–F). Distance replication in different directions: forward–right (F–R), forward–left (F–L), left–forward (L–F), and right–forward (R–F). In each condition, the first letter refers to passive displacement (dotted line) and the second letter to active displacement (solid line).

however, the control group produced a velocity profile that more closely matched the triangular shape of the sample (passive displacement).

The present findings agree with the data obtained by Philbeck *et al.* (2000) in pointing to a lack of asymmetry in processing body displacement in the two levels of the space by using nonvisual signals in both neglect patients and in right and left parietal patients.

A third study is relevant for the potential anisometry of neglect patients when moving in the environment (Bisiach *et al.* 1997). The participants (neglect patients and normal controls) were blindfolded, seated in a wheelchair, and passively pushed along two sides of a rectangular triangle or along three sides of a rectangle. When the wheelchair stopped, while still blindfolded they were asked to indicate the starting point by using a laser pointer. The triangular and rectangular pathways involved either 90° right or 90° left turns. Clearly, the tasks required the participants to build up a spatial representation of the body moving toward the left or the right side of the environmental space by completely relying on vestibular and somatosensory information.

The results of this study did not show any significant difference between neglect or control subjects in indicating the starting point when comparing the rightward and leftward path. Once again, the third study points to a lack of spatial anisometry when the whole body moves in the space and involves the use of nonvisual cues.

Based on these findings, it can be proposed that the integration of nonvisual information in processing a navigational space involves brain structures different from those involved in the interaction between multimodal information and the subjects' segmental responses (movements of the eye, head, trunk, or hand with the subject in a fixed position). Impairments in the latter conditions, which characterize the neglect disorders, do not extend to the processing of moving in environmental space.

Multisensory integration in locomotor control

Regarding the second question posed at the beginning of the chapter, it can be speculated that simple comparisons of body spatial displacements, such as those used in the second and third studies and part of the first study, are so simple that they can be performed at a low level of vestibular processing. The complex integration between visual and nonvisual information, which requires the activity of the parietal cortex, might not be necessary for these kinds of navigational tasks. However, when performing other tasks which require more complex integration of visual and nonvisual information, neglect patients might show the same anisometry, presumably connected with their impairment in integrating multisensory spatial inputs.

A second experiment performed in our laboratory required the participants to perform spatial duplication with or without actual or remembered visual information of spatial location in addition to vestibular inputs. The rationale of the experiment was as follows The participants were passively transported by a robot in either horizontal direction from a visible target to a stop. During the translation they could see several visual landmarks and could code the target position in relation to the landmarks. The task was to return to the target point (Fig. 2). During the 'active return' of the training, all the landmarks and the target were visible. The training did not require any computation or memory of location since the target and the landmarks were visible.

In the first experimental condition, all the landmarks were visible but the target was removed. The participants memorized the position of the target in relation to the visible landmarks. The use of vestibular information may have been marginal.

In the second condition, both landmarks and target were removed. The participants had to combine the vestibular computation of the spatial transportation with the memory of the previous inspected target position by using visual mental imagery and updating the target position in a continuous and dynamic way. The hypothesis was that in patients with spatial anisotropy, such as neglect patients, the condition in which an integration between vestibular and memorized visual spatial location was required would induce a horizontal spatial asymmetry. This experiment was performed with the same four groups of participants and using the same robot as in the

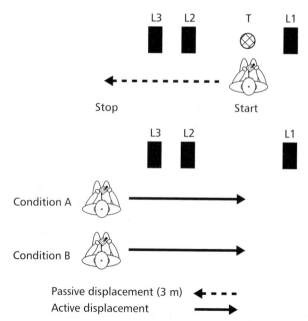

Figure 2 Passive and active conditions: L1, L2, L3, visual landmarks; T, target. The figure shows the case of leftward passive displacement and active returns toward the right side of the space. In the opposite condition landmarks and target were arranged in the mirror image.

study described above. Details relative to the parameters used are described in a separate paper (Pizzamiglio *et al.* in preparation). The results of this study showed that in the first experimental condition the controls and right- and left-brain-damaged patients made undershooting errors in returning to the target location regardless of the direction of the horizontal displacement. In this condition, the need to integrate visual and nonvisual information was marginal, since the available visual inputs could easily be used to solve the problem.

Conversely, in the third condition, which required reliance on vestibular information that provided an estimate of the amount of displacement, together with the memorized position of the previously seen target, neglect patients showed an unequal estimate of their movement toward the left and right side of the space. In particular, neglect patients, as well as other brain-damaged groups, continued to undershoot the target while moving from left to right. However, when the participants moved toward the left side of the space only the neglect group reversed its performance and overshot the target.

General discussion

The studies reviewed so far suggest that brain-damaged patients, including patients with unilateral neglect, can process spatial information as well as normal controls when the entire body is moved. This capacity was observed when they had to reproduce passive translation in the horizontal and spatial plane and even when they had to evaluate a complex passive translation in a wheelchair.

An important point refers to the lack of spatial asymmetry in neglect patients; this is at variance with their anisometric performance when they had to reproduce visually perceived distance on the two sides of a space (Bisiach *et al.* 1996; Chokron *et al.* 1997). One possible explanation is that the comparison between nonvisual inputs (vestibular and somatosensory) required in the task described previously may be performed by neurophysiological structures (i.e. the vestibular nuclei in the brainstem, the thalamus, and different cortical areas) which do not show the same functional asymmetry observed in complex visual processing. The few existing neuroimaging studies on humans, which involved the cortical representation of vestibular information, did not show this asymmetry (Lobel *et al.* 1998).

However, the data from the second experiment did show an anisometry in neglect patients in replicating the distances in the horizontal plane. It must be noted that these results are rather different from those of Philbeck *et al.* (2000). These authors did not find left–right differences in their visually directed walking task. Tentatively, this discrepancy can be attributed to the kind of patients studied (only some patients had neglect and all were capable of walking, indicating less severe lesions) and to a much less complex task. A cognitive analysis of the nonvisual information condition of this experiment requires the computation of the distance to be reproduced on the basis of vestibular and somatosensory inputs and a memory for the location of the previously inspected landmarks and the target. The two categories of information must be integrated in some cortical areas.

On the basis of the work of Grüsser *et al.* (1992), no direct connections are available between the primary visual cortex (V1) and the vestibular cortical areas (PIVC). Therefore, the integration between visual and vestibular inputs must take place on one of the two following pathways: (a) from V1 to V2, MT-MST, parietal area 7, and then to the parieto-insular vestibular cortex (PIVC), or (b) from the superior colliculus, via the pulvinar nucleus of the thalamus, to the PIVC. It can be speculated that asymmetry in evaluating spatial displacement can arise only when there is damage to one or both of these networks connecting visual and vestibular information.

Furthermore, the task used required the subjects to memorize the spatial location of the target, particularly in relation to three visual cues (see the two conditions of the last experiment). In order to respond to this task, the subject had to refer to the relative position in space of both the target and the landmarks. Therefore the subject had to use an object-centered frame of reference. In a recent functional MRI study, Galati *et al.* (2000) showed that when normal subjects respond to a spatial task by using an object-centered frame, there is a strong asymmetric activation of a right parietofrontal system.

It can be suggested that the spatial anisometry in processing movements of the whole body in space, which emerges in neglect patients, can be observed in two conditions.

- Spatial computation must require a multi-sensory integration between vestibular, somato-sensory and visual information.

- Brain lesions most frequently producing such an anisometry are located in the right hemisphere.

More specifically, the lesion may be located either in the parietal lobe, disconnecting the pathway indirectly connecting the striate cortex with the PIVC area, or in areas involved in the connection of the superior colliculus to the PIVC via the pulvinar and the thalamus.

References

Bisiach, E. (1999). Unilateral neglect and related disorders. In *Handbook of clinical and experimental neuropsychology* (ed. G. Denes and L. Pizzamiglio), pp. 479–96. Psychology Press, Hove.

Bisiach, E., Brouchon, L., Poncet, M., and Rusconi, M. L. (1993). Unilateral neglect in route description. *Neuropsychologia*, **31**, 1255–62.

Bisiach, E., Pizzamiglio, L., Nico, D., and Antonucci, G. (1996). Beyond unilateral neglect. *Brain*, **119**, 851–7.

Bisiach, E., Pattini, P., Rusconi, M. L., Ricci, R., and Bernardini, B. (1997). Unilateral neglect and space constancy during passive locomotion. *Cortex*, **33**, 313–22.

Chokron, S., Bernard, J. M., and Imbert, M. (1997). Length representation in normal and neglect subjects with opposite reading habits studied through a line extension task. *Cortex*, **33**, 47–64.

Farrell, M. J. (1996). Topographical disorientation. *Neurocase*, **2**, 509–20.

Galati, G., Lobel, E., Vallar, G., Berthoz, A., Pizzamiglio, L., and Le Bihan, D. (2000). The neural basis of egocentric and allocentric coding of space in humans: a functional magnetic resonance study. *Experimental Brain Research*, **133**, 156–64.

Grüsser, O. J., Guldin, W., Harris, L., Lefebre, J. C., and Pause, M. (1992). Cortical representation of head-in-space movement and some psychophysical experiments on head movement. In *The head–neck sensory motor system* (ed. A. Berthoz, W. Graf, and P. P. Vidal), pp. 497–509. Oxford University Press.

Lobel, E., Kleine, J. F., Le Bihan, D., Leroy-Willig, A., and Berthoz, A. (1998). Functional MRI of galvanic vestibular stimulation. *Journal of Neurophysiology*, **80**, 2699–709.

Philbeck, J. W., Behrmann, M., Black, S. E., and Ebert, P. (2000). Intact spatial updating during locomotion after right posterior parietal lesions. *Neuropsychologia*, **38**, 950–63.

Philbeck, J. W., Behrmann, M., and Loomis, J. M. Updating of locations during whole-body rotations in patients with hemispatial neglect. *Journal of Experimental Psychology: Human Perception and Performance*, in press.

Pizzamiglio, L., *et al.* in preparation.

Rieser, J. J., Ashmead, D. H., Talor, C. R., and Youngquist, G. A. (1990). Visual perception and the guidance of locomotion without vision to previously seen targets. *Perception*, **19**, 675–89.

Vallar, G. (1993). The anatomical basis of spatial hemineglect in humans. In *Unilateral neglect, clinical and experimental studies* (ed. I. H. Robertson and J. C. Marshall), pp. 27–59. Lawrence Erlbaum, Hove.

Section 5 Relation of neglect to attention

5.1 The neurobehavioral analysis of visuospatial attention in the rat

Verity J. Brown

Patients with damage to the right posterior parietal cortex may fail to orient to contralateral stimuli even though there is no evidence of primary sensory or primary motor impairment. In animals, failure to orient to stimuli in different sensory modalities has been reported following unilateral brain damage in a wide range of brain areas, including frontal and parietal cortical lesions, as well as subcortical structures such as superior colliculus, thalamus, and basal ganglia. The term 'sensorimotor neglect' is found frequently in the rat literature to refer to these orientation deficits. It is termed neglect because of the superficial resemblance to the syndrome in human patients. It is not clear, however, whether the 'neglect' in the rat extends to cognitive processes beyond those required for orienting to stimuli, as it does in humans. In this chapter, we will consider ways in which neglect and visuospatial processing are measured in the rat and what can be learned from studies in rats.

Can neglect be studied in a rat?

Some forms of neglect in humans are considered 'representational' (Bisiach and Luzzatti 1978; Bisiach *et al.* 1981); for example, the mind's eye also shows a spatial bias when scanning imagined scenes and the left side is omitted in drawings or copied pictures of objects, even when the paper is placed in the right visual field. Furthermore, the aspect of a stimulus that is neglected depends upon perceptual grouping, with neglect of the left side of multiple objects that are perceived as discrete or the leftmost components when the objects are perceived as a single group. Driver *et al.* (1992) demonstrated that figure–ground resolution of ambiguous stimuli would determine which boundary line was the left side of a 'figure' and hence which line would be neglected.

There is great difficulty in assessing cognitive representational deficits in rats. Not only is it the case that cognitive processes must be inferred from overt behavior, but deficits in response execution must be dissociated from deficits in response selection, which in turn must be distinguished from deficits in perception. For example, when there is disrupted performance in a maze, it may not be possible to dissociate bias in spatial perception from bias in spatial navigation. Spatial biases in posture, position in cage, and hoarding of food have been reported in rats with orientation deficits; although these spatial biases might indicate a distortion of representation of space, it is also possible that the spatial bias, as well as the failure to orient, results from impaired movement. Thus it is not necessary to invoke cognitive mediating factors to account for all spatial biases.

In what sense is the neglect in the rat the same as, or even similar to, the syndrome of neglect in humans? Is there evidence to suggest that what is termed 'neglect' in the rat is homologous, or even analogous, to neglect in primates? As some of the manifestations of neglect in humans might be considered phenomenological, they may not be valuable (indeed, may even be misleading) for understanding the control of spatial attention, and it would not be meaningful to seek the analog of such behaviors in the rat. Demonstrating common features and a shared neural organization would provide evidence that behavior classified as neglect in the rat is homologous to that classified so in humans, but this approach is limited because neither the features of neglect in humans nor the neurological basis of the disorder is understood. Nevertheless, rather than searching for behavior which is analogous to neglect in the rat, an alternative approach is to test the behavioral functions of the area of the rat brain homologous to primate posterior parietal cortex and the circuit of which it is part. If this area has patterns of connectivity in common with areas known to be involved in neglect in primates, this would suggest that it, and the other areas in the network, might also mediate spatial-cognitive behavior.

Functions of rat 'parietal cortex'

The area thought to be equivalent to primate posterior parietal cortex, and therefore most likely to be the place where 'neglect' would be expected following damage, is an anterodorsal part of area Oc2L/Oc2M (Corwin and Reep 1998), which these authors designate PPC. Multimodal 'neglect' has been reported after PPC lesions (King and Corwin 1993; Corwin et al. 1996). Electrophysiological characteristics indicate that this area is involved in spatial processing. For example, Chen and Nakamura (1998) have recorded from 'place cells' that are modulated by the orientation and position of the rat. A consistent feature of PPC lesions in the rat has been the impairment of spatial navigation in maze tasks (Kolb 1990; Crowne et al. 1992; King and Corwin 1992; Spangler et al. 1994; Save and Moghaddam 1996). There is no primary visual impairment or evidence of a learning deficit; rats with PPC lesions are able to solve visual discriminations, even when there is a memory component (see Kolb 1990). The spatial navigation impairment has been attributed to a difficulty in selecting an initial trajectory (Kolb and Walkey 1987; Foreman et al. 1992; Save and Moghaddam 1996). This could be secondary to a failure to use extrapersonal visuospatial cues to orient the head and body before the execution of the motor plan to reach the goal (Kolb 1990). Kolb points out that even when rats are over-trained to the point that the task can be solved, there is still evidence of impaired egocentric spatial navigation. DeCoteau and Kesner (1998) showed that rats with PPC lesions were impaired in detecting spatial displacement of objects, which they suggest possibly indicates an inability to 'switch cognitive strategies', although it could be interpreted as another manifestation of disruption of visuospatial navigation.

The PPC region receives thalamic projections from the lateral posterior nucleus (thought to be equivalent to primate pulvinar) (Chandler et al. 1992), and also projects to medial agranular cortex (AGm) and ventrolateral orbital frontal cortex (Reep et al. 1994). This pattern of connectivity suggests an organization similar to the attentional system of primates (Corwin and Reep 1998). A putative circuit for directing spatial attention has been identified (King and Corwin 1993) which is suggested to be equivalent to the distributed cortical attentional system proposed in primates (Mesulam 1981). The circuit in the rat is thought to involve AGm (King and Corwin 1993), ventrolateral orbital cortex (Corwin et al. 1994), and PPC (Corwin et al. 1996; King and Corwin 1993). Burcham et al. (1997) showed that unilateral disconnection (by knife-cut) of the PPC and AGm produced neglect which was as severe as that following a lesion of either of these areas. They interpret these findings as indicating that AGm and PPC form a cortical attentional system. Although lesions of either PPC or AGm resulted in severe orientation deficits, in PPC lesioned rats the deficits were most severe to visual stimuli, whereas there were no differential deficits across modalities in rats with AGm damage.

Thus, from the above discussion, it is clear that PPC in the rat does have functions—in particular, visuospatial functions—which lend support to the view that the deficits seen following PPC lesions, as well as lesions of the areas with connections to PPC, might be considered as having more than a superficial resemblance to 'neglect' in human patients.

How has neglect been studied in the rat?

Neglect is defined as a failure to respond to contralateral stimuli in the absence of a primary sensory or primary motor deficit. The orientation deficit following unilateral lesions of a variety of structures is often multimodal, suggesting that a primary sensory impairment is unlikely. Recovery may occur at different rates in different modalities, ruling out a primary motor impairment. Thus neglect is inferred specifically if there is a deficit in orienting to stimuli, with no evidence of muscular weakness on the contralateral side. To exclude orientation deficits resulting from hemi-akinesia rather than sensory neglect, rats can be trained to respond away from the side of stimuli; if they are permitted to make a response to the unimpaired side, they would be able to indicate that they have perceived a stimulus on the impaired side. Conversely, if they are required to make a response to the impaired side to indicate detection of a stimulus on the unimpaired side, hemi-akinesia can be excluded. Turner (1973) used this approach to demonstrate that lesions of the lateral hypothalamus (severing the dopaminergic pathway from midbrain to striatum) result in a deficit of sensorimotor integration and not primary sensory or primary motor impairments. Different groups of rats were trained to respond either toward or away from the side of aversive stimuli. The only condition in which the rats were impaired was when they were asked to make contralateral movements toward contralateral stimuli. Nevertheless, Hoyman *et al.* (1979), using tactile stimuli, and Carli *et al.* (1985, 1989), using visual stimuli, demonstrated that rats with striatal dopamine depletion were impaired in responding to the contralateral side, regardless of the side of presentation of stimuli. Although the procedure in these experiments was similar to that used by Turner (1973), it is possible that the conflicting findings are due to the choice of stimuli. The response bias was only seen when the rat had to make the incompatible response of turning toward an aversive stimulus on the contralateral side. The normal reaction of turning away from an aversive stimulus, perhaps coupled with the arousal induced by an impending aversive stimulus, may have enabled Turner's rats to overcome a response bias to turn contralaterally from an ipsilateral stimulus. Both Hoyman *et al.* (1979) and Carli *et al.* (1985) observed impairments in rats making contralateral responses, regardless of the side of presentation of the stimulus. Thus the reliable demonstration of failure to orient to contralesional stimuli seen following depletion of dopamine from the striatum is probably due to hemi-akinesia rather than sensory neglect. It should be noted that this impairment is not purely motoric, but rather is response related in the same sense as used to describe 'frontal neglect' in primates. This raises the obvious question of whether it is possible to identify a neural network subserving attention in the rat similar to that identified in humans (Mesulam 1981).

Schallert *et al.* (1982) developed a test of 'neglect'—the 'patch removal' or 'sticky label' test—which does not involve a lateralized head- or body-orienting response. Adhesive patches are applied to the forepaws of the rats, and the order and latency to contact and remove the patches is recorded. Because there is no requirement to orient the head and body, somatosensory impairments can be distinguished from impairments of spatial orientation. The task has some particular advantages: the test is quick to administer, it can be repeated over days to examine the time course of effects, and no prior operant training is required. Results from this task can also be used to distinguish between the effects of damage to different areas which might have orientation deficits in common. For example, Schallert *et al.* (1982) reported impairments following striatal dopamine depletion using this task, and there are impairments following lesions of AGm (Brown *et al.* 1991) and somatosensory cortex (Barth *et al.* 1990). Lesions of PPC in the rat did not change order or time to contact patches in this task (Ward and Brown 1997).

Another test commonly used in conjunction with orientation tests is paw use in reaching tasks. Posterior parietal cortex in humans and monkeys contributes to reaching accuracy and grasping (Jakobson *et al.* 1991; Nixon *et al.* 1992; Johnson *et al.* 1993; Jeannerod *et al.* 1994), and reaching tasks have the advantage that they may be practically assessed in the rat. Tests of paw reaching have been used to investigate cortical (Castro 1972; Brown *et al.* 1991; Whishaw *et al.* 1986), subcortical (Whishaw *et al.* 1986), and neurochemical (Whishaw *et al.* 1986; Miklyaeva *et al.* 1994) contributions to reaching in the rat. There are grounds on which to suspect that PPC, being mainly concerned with visuospatial processing, would not be important for skilled paw reaching in the rat. For example, Goodale and Carey (1990) have argued that orienting under visual guidance positions the rat toward the target for tactile and olfactory exploration rather than serving to foveate an object for visual identification. Furthermore, it has been argued that paw reaching in the rat is mediated by olfactory rather than visual guidance (Whishaw and Tomie 1989). Therefore visuospatial functions of parietal cortex might only be relevant for paw reaching in mediating the initial orientation to the object to be grasped. On the other hand, spatial deficits akin to the spatial disruption following parietal cortex lesions in humans might be expected to result in generalized deficits in reaching tasks in rats as they do in humans.

In monkeys with posterior parietal damage, reaching deficits are commonly manifested as decreased accuracy of grasping, but there is also evidence of a decrease in attempted reaches with the contralateral limb (Deuel and Farrar 1993). Lesions of rat PPC (Ward and Brown 1997) or AGm (Brown *et al.* 1991) result in a reduction in the use of the contralateral paw to reach for food pellets. In neither case was there evidence of motor deficit; the contralateral paw was used during spontaneous locomotion, for 'bracing' during reaching with the ipsilateral paw, and during pellet manipulation following retrieval with the ipsilateral paw. This implies that sensory processes are not impaired, since successful manipulation of food pellets is dependent on intact sensory feedback (Sabol *et al.* 1985). Perhaps most significantly, the paw preference was not absolute and there was no change in the retrieval success when reaches were made with the contralateral paw. Intriguingly, following either PPC or AGm lesions, the decreased use of the contralateral paw for reaching is accompanied by a reduction in the time spent in the contralateral half of the cage, suggesting an alteration in spatial orientation. This raises the possibility that postural bias might account for the decreased paw use. Video analysis of reaching in the rat has emphasized the importance of posture in reaching (Miklyaeva *et al.* 1994); nevertheless, postural deficits have been shown to impact on reaching ability rather than paw preference. Most importantly, this result is to be compared with that following damage to the forelimb area (FL), which results in reductions in the grasping accuracy of contralateral reaches rather than a decline in contralateral paw use (Whishaw *et al.* 1986; Whishaw and Tomie 1989). Thus the evidence from paw preference further supports the view that *the* PPC–AGm system is involved in the control of spatial orienting, the implication of which might be spatial 'neglect'.

The neural basis of spatial attention in the rat

One of the difficulties of using tests of orientation or paw use is that there are many factors that could result in impairments on such tasks. It becomes necessary to examine the fine points of behavior (e.g. using evidence such as the position in cage) to try to understand complex cognitive processes. The difficulties in the human neglect literature in defining the significance of precise behavioral conditions to tease out features of neglect are magnified in studies with rats. Studies of the psychological processes and neural organization of spatial attention in the rat will result in an increased understanding of the neural basis of attention, which might provide clues about the nature of neglect in humans. Therefore it is important to identify an aspect of either normal or impaired performance that is demonstrably equivalent in rats and primates. It is then possible to study the neural basis of the behavior across species and the circumstances under which it is compromised.

Attention, like any mental process, is necessarily covert and therefore unseen. The challenge that has always faced psychology is to devise tasks that permit measurement of the operation of covert processes. Because attentional selectivity enables the enhanced processing of selected information, it is possible to measure the efficiency of information processing as indicative of the success of attentional selectivity. Using the 'covert orienting' task devised by Posner (1980), covert shifts of attention can be inferred from the reaction time to a visual target. Reaction time is faster when attention has been drawn to the target location by a preceding cue (valid cue) than it is when a cue misdirects attention (invalid cue) away from the subsequent target. The size of the validity effect (the difference between validly and invalidly cued target detection) indicates the strength of the attentional effect. It has been demonstrated that covert shifts of attention are impaired in patients with parietal cortex lesions who also have other classical signs of neglect (e.g. line bisection and cancellation-task deficits) (for a recent review see Losier and Klein (2001)). In particular, patients with lesion damage at the parietal–temporal junction show normal effects of valid cues but are impaired in detecting contralateral targets when their attention is drawn to the ipsilateral side (Posner *et al.* 1984).

Posner *et al.* (1984) have proposed that there are three fundamental components to covert orienting associated with different brain regions. The posterior parietal cortex is thought to be involved in disengagement of attention (Posner *et al.* 1984, 1987; Petersen *et al.* 1989), shifting of attention is thought to be controlled by the superior colliculus (Posner and Driver 1992; Robinson and Kertzman 1995), and engagement of attention at a new location is mediated by the lateral pulvinar of the thalamus (Petersen *et al.* 1987; Posner and Driver 1992). Additional experimental and clinical work has suggested that the anterior cingulate, the lateral frontal cortex, and the basal ganglia are also involved in performance of the task, contributing to target detection and response preparation (Posner and Driver 1992).

The adaptation of this test for animals provides an opportunity to identify an attentional system which is similar across species, for example involving posterior parietal, superior colliculus, and lateral pulvinar (Posner and Petersen 1990). Rats are trained to maintain a nose-poke in a central location while cues and targets are presented in poke-holes to either side of the head. As the head is held still and central and the eyes of a rat are lateral in the head, there can be no overt orienting response to the cue. Reaction time is measured as the time to withdraw from the central location following the peripheral target. In normal rats, the validity effect is about 25 to 50 ms, which is comparable to the effect size seen in humans and monkeys.

There are no deficits of covert orienting following large lesions of frontal cortex (Ward *et al.* 1998). An ischemic lesion of anterolateral cortex (Par1/2 and FL) did result in a transient impairment in movement execution (i.e. movement time) but no impairment of reaction time (Ward *et al.* 1997). As reaction time was not changed in any condition, it follows that this lesion was without effect on the magnitude of the validity effect—by implication, covert orienting (Ward *et al.* 1997). Thus, Par1/2 does not appear to be involved in covert orienting. This result is not very surprising; others have shown that these lesions also do not impair signal detection or vigilance (Muir *et al.* 1996). The effects of a lesion which included PPC were different; although the lesion did not effect the magnitude of the validity effect, reaction time was lengthened to contralateral targets, regardless of the preceding cue (Ward and Brown 1997). There was good evidence that there were no sensory impairments and so they concluded that the reaction time deficits following PPC lesions in the rat were unlikely to reflect an attentional deficit. As there was no differential deficit when targets were invalidly cued, Ward and Brown (1997) suggested that the impairment was 'response related'.

Although the data from the rat would appear to contradict that from patients with parietal lesions, in fact they might be less discrepant than it would appear. In a recent review and meta-analysis, Losier and Klein (2001) note that reaction times to validly cued—as well as invalidly cued—targets are slower contralateral to right parietal lesions. They note that this has been observed many times, although individual studies have perhaps not had the statistical power to establish the conclusion.

It is unlikely that visuospatial orienting of attention is mediated by different neural processes in the rat. For example, manipulations of cholinergic function result in strikingly similar effects across species. There is good evidence that cholinergic systems are involved in covert orienting (Jones *et al.* 1992; Voytko *et al.* 1994; Witte *et al.* 1997; Murphy and Klein 1998; Parasuraman and Greenwood 1998; Davidson *et al.* 1999). Parasuraman *et al.* (1992) reported that patients with Alzheimer's disease have significantly larger validity effects, a consequence of increased costs following invalidly cued targets. Excitotoxic lesions of the basal forebrain in monkeys reveal an analogous selective deficit in covert visuospatial attention orienting (Voytko *et al.* 1994). There are facilitatory effects of cholinergic agonists on covert orienting in primates (Witte *et al.* 1997; Murphy and Klein 1998) and rats (Phillips *et al.* 2000). This is manifest as a reduction in the validity effect, arising from the disproportionate reduction of reaction times to invalidly cued targets, which has been interpreted as enhanced disengagement of attention such that reorientation is more rapid after a distracting invalid cue. Consistent with this, the blockade of cholinergic activity has been associated with deficits in attentional orienting in rats (Phillips *et al.* 2000).

Although the effects of systemic drugs do not indicate which neural structures are involved in covert orienting, the data from rats (Muir *et al.* 1995; Muir *et al.* 1996) and monkeys (Voytko *et al.* 1994) point to the basal forebrain cholinergic cells. These cells project to frontal and parietal cortex and thalamus, including the thalamic reticular nucleus. The thalamic reticular nucleus has been implicated in attentional processes (Guillery *et al.* 1998). Lesions of Rt result in an abolition of the validity effect in the rat (Weese *et al.* 1999) and there is activation of *c-fos* in the thalamic reticular nucleus during visual exploration (Montero 1997) and when rats are attending to cues predictive of reward (McAlonan *et al.* 2000). As both thalamocortical and corticothalamic projections send axon collaterals to the reticular nucleus, the reticular nucleus is in a position to gate the flow of information between thalamus and cortex.

In summary, the orientation of visuospatial attention in the rat is likely to be mediated by similar neural processes as in the primate. Although there are obvious differences in the manifestation of deficits following parietal cortex lesions in different species, focusing on the phenomenology of neglect in humans is likely to be misleading. On the other hand, visuospatial attention can be quantified by measuring the effects of attentional orienting in rats and monkeys. Exploring the neural basis of covert orienting provides clues to understand normal attention as well as manifestations of impaired attention.

References

Barth, T. M., Jones, T. A., and Schallert, T. (1990). Functional subdivisions of the rat somatic sensorimotor cortex. *Behavioural Brain Research*, **39**, 73–95.

Bisiach, E. and Luzzatti, C. (1978). Unilateral neglect of representational space. *Cortex*, **14**, 129–33.

Bisiach, E., Capitani, E., Luzzatti, C., and Perani, D. (1981). Brain and conscious representation of outside reality. *Neuropsychologia*, **19**, 543–51.

Brown, V. J., Bowman, E. M., and Robbins, T. W. (1991). Response-related deficits following unilateral lesions of the medial agranular cortex of the rat. *Behavioral Neuroscience*, **105**, 567–78.

Burcham, K. J., Corwin, J. V., Stoll, M. L., and Reep, R. L. (1997). Disconnection of medial agranular and posterior parietal cortex produces multimodal neglect in rats. *Behavioural Brain Research*, **86**, 41–4.

Carli, M., Evenden, J. L., and Robbins, T. W. (1985). Depletion of unilateral striatal dopamine impairs initiation of contralateral actions and not sensory attention. *Nature*, **313**, 679–82.

Carli, M., Jones, G. H., and Robbins, T. W. (1989). Effects of unilateral dorsal and ventral striatal dopamine depletion on visual 'neglect' in the rat: a neural and behavioural analysis. *Neuroscience*, **29**, 309–27.

Castro, A. J. (1972). The effects of cortical ablations on digital usage in the rat. *Brain Research*, **37**, 173–85.

Chandler, H. C., King, V., Corwin, J. V., and Reep, R. L. (1992). Thalamocortical connections of rat posterior parietal cortex. *Neuroscience Letters*, **143**, 237–42.

Chen, L. L. and Nakamura, K. (1998). Head-centered representation and spatial memory in rat posterior parietal cortex. *Psychobiology*, **26**, 119–27.

Corwin, J. V. and Reep, R. L. (1998). Rodent posterior parietal cortex as a component of a cortical network mediating directed spatial attention. *Psychobiology*, **26**, 87–102.

Corwin, J. V., Fussinger, M., Meyer, R. C., King, V. R., and Reep, R. L. (1994). Bilateral destruction of the ventrolateral orbital cortex produces allocentric but not egocentric spatial deficits in rats. *Behavioural Brain Research*, **61**, 79–86.

Corwin, J. V., Burcham, K. J., and Hix, G. I. (1996). Apomorphine produces an acute dose-dependent therapeutic effect on neglect produced by unilateral destruction of the posterior parietal cortex in rats. *Behavioural Brain Research*, **79**, 41–9.

Crowne, D. P., Novotny, M. F., Maier, S. E., and Vitols, R. (1992). Effects of unilateral parietal lesions on spatial localization in the rat. *Behavioral Neuroscience*, **106**, 808–19.

Davidson, M. C., Cutrell, E. B., and Marrocco, R. T. (1999). Scopolamine slows the orienting of attention in primates to cued visual targets. *Psychopharmacology*, **142**, 1–8.

DeCoteau, W. E. and Kesner, R. P. (1998). Effects of hippocampal and parietal cortex lesions on the processing of multiple-object scenes. *Behavioral Neuroscience*, **112**, 68–82.

Deuel, R. K. and Farrar, C. A. (1993). Stimulus cancellation by macaques with unilateral frontal or parietal lesions. *Neuropsychologia*, **31**, 29–38.

Driver, J., Baylis, G. C., and Rafal, R. D. (1992). Preserved figure–ground segregation and symmetry perception in visual neglect. *Nature*, **360**, 73–5.

Foreman, N., Save, E., Thinus-Blanc, C., and Buhot, M. C. (1992). Visually guided locomotion, distractibility, and the missing-stimulus effect in hooded rats with unilateral or bilateral lesions of parietal cortex. *Behavioral Neuroscience*, **106**, 529–38.

Goodale, M. A. and Carey, D. P. (1990). The role of cerebral cortex in visuomotor control. In *The rat cerebral cortex* (ed. B. Kolb and R. C. Tees), pp. 309–40. MIT Press, Cambridge, MA.

Guillery, R. W., Feig, S. L., and Lozsadi, D. A. (1998). Paying attention to the thalamic reticular nucleus. *Trends in Neurosciences*, **21**, 28–32.

Hoyman, L., Weese, G. D., and Frommer, G. P. (1979). Tactile discrimination deficits following neglect-producing unilateral hypothalamic lesions in the rat. *Physiology and Behaviour*, **22**, 139–47.

Jakobson, L. S., Archibald, Y. M., Carey, D. P., and Goodale, M. A. (1991). A kinematic analysis of reaching and grasping movements in a patient recovering from optic ataxia. *Neuropsychologia*, **29**, 803–9.

Jeannerod, M., Decety, J., and Michel, F. (1994). Impairment of grasping movements following a bilateral posterior parietal lesion. *Neuropsychologia*, **32**, 369–80.

Johnson, P. B., Ferraina, S., and Caminiti, R. (1993). Cortical networks for visual reaching. *Experimental Brain Research*, **97**, 361–5.

Jones, G. M. M., Sahakian, B. J., Levy, R., Warburton, D. M., and Gray, J. A. (1992). Effects of acute subcutaneous nicotine on attention, information processing and short-term memory in Alzheimer's disease. *Psychopharmacology*, **108**, 485–94.

King, V. R. and Corwin, J. V. (1992). Spatial deficits and hemispheric asymmetries in the rat following unilateral and bilateral lesions of posterior parietal or medial agranular cortex. *Behavioural Brain Research*, **50**, 53–68.

King, V. R. and Corwin, J. V. (1993). Comparisons of hemi-inattention produced by unilateral lesions of the posterior parietal cortex or medial agranular prefrontal cortex in rats—neglect, extinction, and the role of stimulus distance. *Behavioural Brain Research*, **54**, 117–31.

Kolb, B. (1990). Posterior Parietal and Temporal Association Cortex. In *The Rat Cerebral Cortex*. (ed. B. Kolb and R. C. Tees), pp. 459–71. MIT Press, Cambridge, MA.

Kolb, B. and Walkey, J. (1987). Behavioural and anatomical studies of the posterior parietal cortex in the rat. *Behavioural Brain Research*, **23**, 127–45.

Losier, B. J. W. and Klein, R. M. (2001). A review of the evidence for a disengage deficit following parietal lobe damage. *Neuroscience and Biobehavioural Reviews*, **25**, 1–13.

McAlonan, K., Brown, V. J., and Bowman, E. M. (2000). Thalamic reticular nucleus activation reflects attentional gating during classical conditioning. *Journal of Neuroscience*, **20**, 8897–901.

Mesulam, M. M. (1981). A cortical network for directed attention and unilateral neglect. *Annals of Neurology*, **10**, 309–25.

Miklyaeva, E. I., Castaneda, E., and Whishaw, I. Q. (1994). Skilled reaching deficits in unilateral dopamine-depleted rats: impairments in movement and posture and compensatory adjustments, *Journal of Neuroscience*, **14**, 7148–58.

Montero, V. M. (1997). C-Fos induction in sensory pathways of rats exploring a novel complex environment: Shifts of active thalamic reticular sectors by predominant sensory cues. *Neuroscience*, **76**, 1069–81.

Muir, J. L., Everitt, B. J., and Robbins, T. W. (1995). Reversal of the visual attentional dysfunction following lesions of the cholinergic basal forebrain by physostigmine and nicotine but not by the 5-HT3 receptor antagonist ondansetron. *Psychopharmacology*, **118**, 82–92.

Muir, J. L., Everitt, B. J., and Robbins, T. W. (1996). The cerebral cortex of the rat and visual attentional function: dissociable effects of mediofrontal, cingulate, anterior dorsolateral, and parietal cortex lesions on a five-choice serial reaction time task. *Cerebral Cortex*, **6**, 470–81.

Murphy, F. C. and Klein, R. M. (1998). The effects of nicotine on spatial and non-spatial expectancies in a covert orienting task. *Neuropsychologia*, **36**, 1103–14.

Nixon, P. D., Burbaud, P., and Passingham, R. E. (1992). Control of arm movement after bilateral lesions of area 5 in the monkey. *Experimental Brain Research*, **90**, 229–32.

Parasuraman, R. and Greenwood, P. M. (1998). Selective attention in aging and dementia. In *The attentive brain* (ed. R. Parasuraman), pp. 461–87. MIT Press, Cambridge, MA.

Parasuraman, R., Greenwood, P. M., Haxby, J. V., and Grady, C. L. (1992). Visuospatial attention in dementia of the Alzheimer type. *Brain*, **115**, 711–33.

Petersen, S. E., Robinson, D. L., and Morris, J. D. (1987). The contribution of the pulvinar to visual spatial attention. *Neuropsychologia*, **25**, 97–105.

Petersen, S. E., Robinson, D. L., and Currie, J. N. (1989). Influences of lesions of parietal cortex on visual spatial attention in humans. *Experimental Brain Research*, **76**, 267–80.

Phillips, J. M., MacAlonan, K., Robb, W. G. K., and Brown, V. J. (2000). Cholinergic neurotransmission influences covert orientation of visuospatial attention in the rat. *Psychopharmacology*, **150**, 112–16.

Posner, M. I. (1980). Orienting of attention. *Quarterly Journal of Experimental Psychology*, **32**, 3–25.

Posner, M. I. and Driver, J. (1992). The neurobiology of selective attention. *Current Opinion in Neurobiology*, **2**, 165–9.

Posner, M. I. and Petersen, S. E. (1990). The attention system of the human brain. *Annual Review of Neuroscience*, **13**, 25–42.

Posner, M. I., Walker, J. A., Friedrich, F. J., and Rafal, R. D. (1984). Effects of parietal injury on covert orienting of attention. *Journal of Neuroscience*, **4**, 1863–74.

Posner, M. I., Walker, J. A., Friedrich, F. J., and Rafal, R. D. (1987). How do the parietal lobes direct covert attention? *Neuropsychologia*, **25**, 135–45.

Reep, R. L., Chandler, H. C., King, V., and Corwin, J. V. (1994). Rat posterior parietal cortex: topography of corticocortical and thalamic connections. *Experimental Brain Research*, **100**, 67–84.

Robinson, D. L. and Kertzman, C. (1995). Covert orienting of attention in macaques. III: Contributions of the superior colliculus. *Journal of Neurophysiology*, **74**, 713–21.

Sabol, K. E., Neill, D. B., Wages, S. A., Church, W. H., and Justice, J. B. (1985). Dopamine depletion in a striatal subregion disrupts performance of a skilled motor task in the rat. *Brain Research*, **335**, 33–43.

Save, E. and Moghaddam, M. (1996). Effects of lesions of the associative parietal cortex on the acquisition and use of spatial memory in egocentric and allocentric navigation tasks in the rat. *Behavioral Neuroscience*, **110**, 74–85.

Schallert, T., Upchurch, M., Lobaugh, N., *et al.* (1982). Tactile extinction: distinguishing between sensorimotor and motor asymmetries in rats with nigrostriatal damage. *Pharmacology, Biochemistry and Behavior*, **16**, 455–62.

Spangler, E. L., Heller, B., Hengemihle, J., *et al.* (1994). Thrombosis of parietal, but not striate, cortex impairs acquisition of a 14-unit T-maze in the rat. *Physiology and Behaviour*, **56**, 95–101.

Turner, B. H. (1973). Sensorimotor syndrome produced by lesions of the amygdala and lateral hypothalamus. *Journal of Comparative and Physiological Psychology*, **82**, 37–47.

Voytko, M. L., Olton, D. S., Richardson, R. T., Gorman, L. K., Tobin, J. R., and Price, D. L. (1994). Basal forebrain lesions in monkeys disrupt attention but not learning and memory. *Journal of Neuroscience*, **14**, 167–80.

Ward, N. and Brown, V. J. (1997). Deficits in response initiation, but not attention, following excitotoxic lesions of posterior parietal cortex in the rat. *Brain Research*, **775**, 81–90.

Ward, N. M., Sharkey, J., and Brown, V. J. (1997). Assessment of sensorimotor neglect after occlusion of the middle cerebral artery of the rat. *Behavioral Neuroscience*, **111**, 1133–45.

Ward, N. M., Marsden, H., Sharkey, J., and Brown, V. J. (1998). Simple and choice reaction time performance following occlusion of the anterior cerebral arteries in the rat. *Experimental Brain Research*, **123**, 269–81.

Weese, D., Phillips, J. M., and Brown, V. J. (1999). Attentional orienting is impaired by unilateral lesions of the thalamic reticular nucleus in the rat. *Journal of Neuroscience*, **19**, 10135–9.

Whishaw, I. Q. and Tomie, J. A. (1989). Olfaction directs skilled forelimb reaching in the rat. *Behavioural Brain Research*, **32**, 11–21.

Whishaw, I. Q., O'Connor, W. T., and Dunnett, S. B. (1986). The contribution of motor cortex, nigrostriatal dopamine and caudate-putamen to skilled motor limb use in the rat. *Brain*, **109**, 805–43.

Witte, E. A., Davidson, M. C., and Marrocco, R. T. (1997). Effects of altering brain cholinergic activity on covert orienting of attention: comparison of monkey and human performance. *Psychopharmacology*, **132**, 324–34.

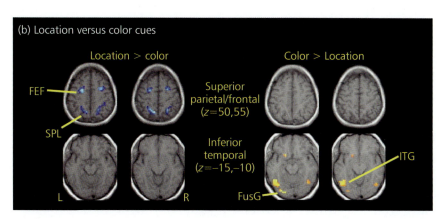

Plate 1 (a) Cue-related activity. Event-related activations to location cues (blue) and color cues (red) are displayed on dorsal and lateral views of a template brain rendered in three dimensions. The areas common to location and color cues are shown in green. (b) Location versus color cues. The results of the direct statistical comparison between location and color cues collapsed across all subjects overlaid onto eight slices of a single subject's normalized anatomical image. The z coordinates for the slices are shown in millimeters in the middle of the panel. Areas more active to location cues than to color cues are shown in blue in the left column; those areas more active to color cues than location cues are shown in red on the right. Abbreviations: PreCG, precentral gyrus; SMA, supplementary motor area; IPS, intraparietal sulcus; SPL, superior parietal lobe; LG, lingual gyrus; FusG, fusiform gyrus; ITG, inferior temporal gyrus; FEF, frontal eye fields.

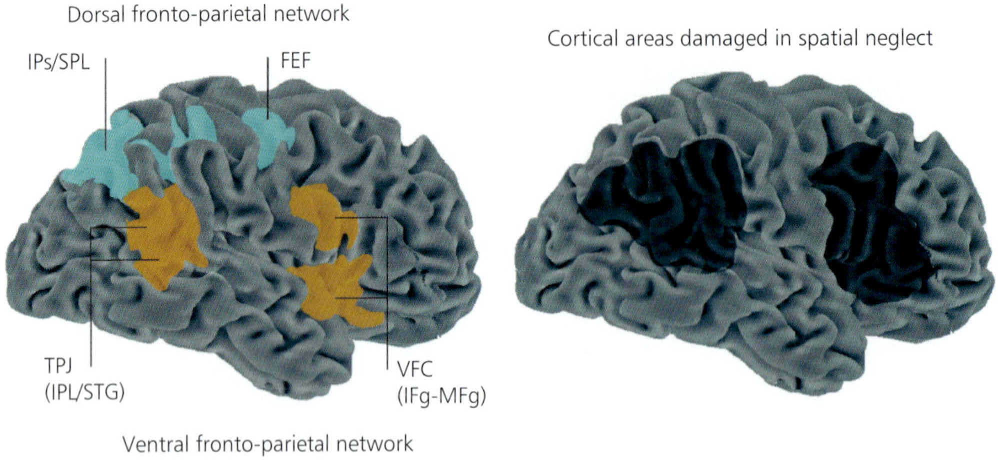

Plate 2 Left: dorsal and ventral fronto-parietal networks as localized in neuroimaging experiments (Corbetta *et al.* 1998; Corbetta and Shulman, 2002). Right: most common regions of damage in spatial neglect.

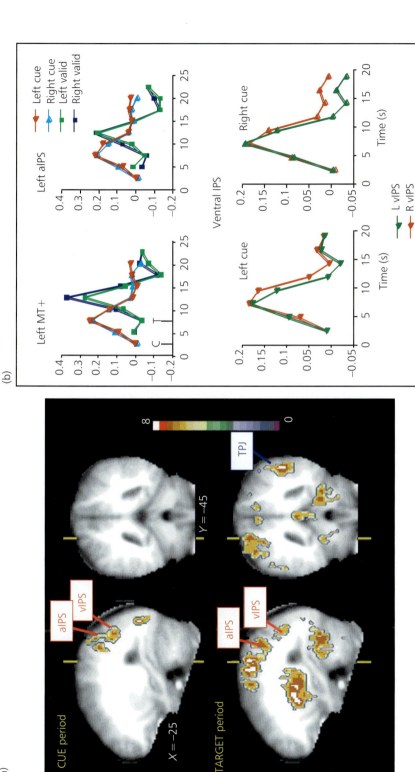

Plate 3 (a) Anova Z-maps of BOLD signal during cue and target periods in left parietal regions (anterior IPS, ventral IPS). Note the absence of significant activation in right TPJ in cue period. Note activation for target detection in both IPS and right TPJ. (b) Upper panels: BOLD signal time courses time-locked to the onset of cue and target stimuli in one occipital (MT+) and one parietal (anterior IPS) region. Note the sustained time course in IPS, but not in MT+, during the cue period, indicating attentional processing of cue location information. Lower panels: signal time course in ventral IPS (left and right hemisphere) in response to leftward and rightward cues. Note the stronger response in right ventral IPS for leftward cues, and no hemispheric difference for rightward cues.

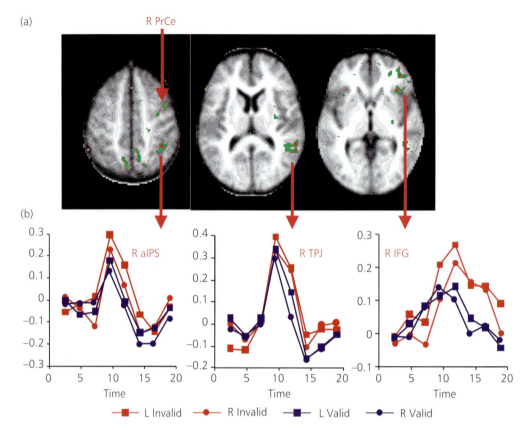

Plate 4 Anova Z-map of the BOLD signal for the effect of target validity. A right-hemisphere lateralized network is revealed when a statistical comparison is made between regions activated for invalid targets and regions activated for valid targets. (b) BOLD signal time courses for the target period demonstrate stronger and slightly more sustained responses for invalidly cued targets than for validly cued targets. Note that the time course for the right IFG peaks slightly later and continues past the end of the trial.

5.2 The neural mechanisms of attentional control

Barry Giesbrecht and George R. Mangun

With the dawn of the cognitive revolution in the late 1950s, psychologists shifted from studying how external forces affected behavioral output to investigating the internal cognitive mechanisms supporting coherent behavior. Since this time, scholars studying attention have explained behavior within the context of dynamic interactions between bottom-up sensory mechanisms and the top-down influences upon them (Fig. 1) (Broadbent 1958). Over the next four decades, another shift has slowly taken place in the psychology of attention aimed at understanding not only the cognitive mechanisms of attention, but also their neural bases. This work, which began in earnest in the 1970s, first focused on the influences of attention on visual sensory processing using physiological measures to quantify changes in visually evoked responses in humans and animals (Eason *et al.* 1969; Van Voorhis and Hillyard 1977; Moran and Desimone 1985). More recent work, which took its lead from studies of deficits in attentional control in neurological patients (Heilman and Valenstein 1979; Mesulam 1981), has turned to investigating the mechanisms of attentional control. This research has implicated a frontoparietal network of brain areas as being involved in attention, particularly visuospatial attention (Mesulam 1990). Over the last decade, the advent of functional neuroimaging has opened up the possibility of investigating in detail the neural mechanisms of attentional control and sensory selection in humans, and a new era of human brain research confronts us (Corbetta *et al.* 2000; Hopfinger *et al.* 2000).

The purpose of this chapter is to provide a snapshot of the current state of the burgeoning literature on the neural mechanisms of top-down attentional control. As an overarching theme, we have focused on visuospatial attention, largely because of its relevance to the issues presented in this book. This chapter is divided into four sections. In the first section, we review three neuroanatomical models of visuospatial attention. Our review of these models is intended to provide an anatomical framework for understanding the empirical research reviewed and presented in later sections. In the second section, we review some of the current literature investigating the neural mechanisms of top-down control. These studies of the top-down control of visuospatial attention can be divided into two categories: those studies aimed at determining *where* control systems are located in cortex, and those that are aimed at determining *how* control is manifest in cortex. The literature review in these first two sections is by no means exhaustive, but rather is intended to provide the reader with a grasp of the main issues in this area. In the third section, we present some of our own work that is aimed at understanding the generality of spatial attentional control mechanisms. Finally, we conclude the chapter by proposing new lines of research that, when combined, will move towards a more complete understanding of top-down attentional control.

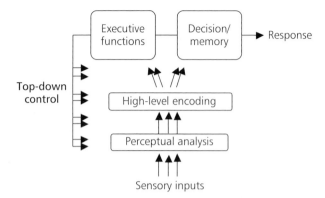

Figure 1 Schematic diagram of the traditional scheme of information processing (Broadbent 1958). In this scheme, sensory stimuli are processed in stages of increasing complexity, from simple features to high-level representations (e.g. categorization and semantics). Although these early processing stages are depicted as being serial, they may not necessarily function in this manner. The information processed by these early stages is then used by executive mechanisms to lead to a decision, internal response, or encoded memory trace as well as to provide top-down influences on the earlier processing stages.

Neuroanatomical models of selective visual attention

As noted above, coherent behavior can be conceptualized as the end result of a dynamic interplay between sensory processing systems and top-down attentional control mechanisms. Disruption of this interplay, as occurs with stroke, leads to severe behavioral deficits. Characterizations of these deficits by neurologists, neuroscientists, and psychologists have furthered our understanding of the cognitive and neural mechanisms of the human attention system. In this section, we review three neuroanatomical models of selective attention, all of which are in large part based on what we know about the impact of brain lesions on behavior. This review will not attempt to delineate between the different models, nor will it include discussions of neurally inspired computational models of selective attention (Laberge 1995; Itti and Koch 2001). Rather, the models we discuss, which span two decades of research, are reviewed because they represent the most common themes present in the cognitive neuroscience of attention.

One of the first comprehensive neuropsychological models of selective attention is Mesulam's model of directed attention (Mesulam 1981, 1990). Mesulam argues that there are four areas that are critical to directed attention: three cortical areas (posterior parietal, cingulate, and frontal cortices), and the subcortical reticular activating system. Based largely on monkey and human lesion work investigating the complex syndrome of unilateral neglect, one cortical region of particular relevance is the posterior parietal cortex (PPC), which among other functions is responsible for maintaining a sensory representation of extrapersonal space. Moreover, Mesulam argues that the posterior parietal cortex, of the right hemisphere in particular, plays an important role in the control of directed attention based on the assumption that it maintains a representation of both contra- and ipsilateral visual space, whereas the left hemisphere only has a representation of the contralateral space. In this model, the cingulate is also thought to be important for control because it is implicated in the maintenance of motivational representations, important for learning and coherent goal-directed behavior. Frontal cortex, with its heavy reciprocal connections with parietal cortex, the superior colliculus, and sensorimotor cortex, is thought to be responsible for storing representations that guide exploratory behaviors such as reaching, scanning, and fixating.

The model posits that the overall efficiency of this frontoparietal attentional network depends on arousal, which is controlled by the reticular activating system.

Another neuroanatomical model of attention is that of Posner and his colleagues (Posner and Petersen 1990; Posner and Rothbart 1991). This model involves the same brain areas as Mesulam's model; however, the models differ in how they are organized into an attentional system. For Posner and colleagues there are three interconnected networks that comprise the attentional system: the anterior network, the posterior network, and the vigilance network. The anterior network is comprised of the cingulate cortex and the supplementary motor area of the frontal cortex. The components of the posterior network are the PPC, the pulvinar, and the superior colliculus. Finally, the vigilance system is made up of the noradrenergic locus coeruleus system. In this framework, both the anterior and posterior networks maintain top-down attentional control. According to the model, the anterior network is responsible for target detection, whereas the posterior network is responsible for orienting to a new location. Orienting is composed of three mechanisms, disengaging attention from its current focus, moving attention to the new location, and re-engaging attention at the new location. In this framework, the disengage and move operations can be thought of as aspects of top-down control, and engaging attention refers to the modulation of incoming information. Based largely on lesion data in neurological patients, the disengage, move, and engage operations are thought to be executed by the PPC (particularly the right hemisphere), superior colliculus, and thalamus respectively (Posner *et al.* 1984, 1985, 1987).

Finally, we consider the biased competition model (Desimone and Duncan 1995). This model provides an account of how visual attention selects objects and/or features of objects in the ventral visual processing stream and locations in the dorsal stream. In this model, selective attention is the result of bottom-up and top-down processes. Bottom-up processes separate stimuli from the background. Top-down processes include biases generated by the application of 'templates' for behaviorally relevant features. For example, when two objects are within a single receptive field, bias may be observed in terms of elevation of maintained activity of cells that code a feature that is behaviorally relevant or expected (Chelazzi *et al.* 1993, 1998). This interaction between top-down and bottom-up processes also includes interplay between working memory and association cortices. As a consequence, top-down control of nonspatial attention is thought to be dependent on the interaction between where templates for objects and object features are generated and maintained in inferior prefrontal cortex and where they are instantiated in temporal cortex. Although their model focuses on selection in the ventral stream, Desimone and Duncan argue that similar principles apply to selection of spatial locations in the dorsal stream. Selection based on spatial position arises from bottom-up and top-down processes, where top-down bias is achieved via templates for a specific location. The difference between attentional control in the dorsal and ventral streams is that, in the former, top-down control is thought to be achieved by an interaction between working memory structures in dorsolateral prefrontal cortex and spatial mechanisms in PPC, paralleling the interaction between inferior frontal and inferior temporal structures in the ventral visual pathway.

Summary

Two points can be made from consideration of these neural models of attention. First, all the models implicate a frontoparietal network of cortical areas in attention, and they also include subcortical structures, particularly the thalamus (Posner and Petersen 1990). Second, not only is there broad anatomical similarity across the models, but there is also a remarkable degree of agreement regarding the areas that are responsible for attentional control. Namely, all models implicate frontal and posterior parietal (especially right-hemisphere) cortices as being involved in the top-down control of spatial attention. The role of frontal areas seems to fall into two classes, working memory in lateral prefrontal areas (Desimone and Duncan 1995), and target detection and motivational aspects of attention in cingulate cortex (Mesulam 1981; Posner and Petersen, 1990). The role of parietal cortex may be considered that of an orienting system (Posner and Petersen 1990), particularly because of its reciprocal connections with lateral prefrontal working memory structures, superior frontal regions (i.e. the frontal eye fields), and retinotopically organized extrastriate regions.

The frontoparietal network and attentional control

Much of what is known about the neural bases of the attentional network has come from neuro-psychological studies of patients with unilateral neglect (Posner *et al.* 1984, 1987; Friedrich *et al.* 1998; Rafal 1998). Although these studies have implicated the frontoparietal network as being involved in attention, precise localization of control functions is difficult because of the poor localization of the sites and extent of lesions from stroke or disease in cortical and subcortical areas. Moreover, a structural lesion in one area may produce functional lesions involving other brain regions via transneuronal degeneration resulting in hypometabolism in those other regions, which may go undetected. However, with the advancement of neuroimaging techniques such as event related potential (ERP), positron emission tomography (PET), and functional MRI (fMRI), we are now able to observe, in high spatial resolution, the frontoparietal network functioning in the healthy human brain.

Early neuroimaging studies converged nicely with previous neuropsychological studies of the attention network. For example, Corbetta *et al.* (1993) compared conditions when subjects shifted attention in the periphery to conditions when attention was maintained foveally. Consistent with the patient literature, Corbetta *et al.* found that, during the attention shifting condition, superior frontal and parietal cortices were activated (relative to passive fixation and foveal conditions). This basic result has been replicated on several occasions, in numerous different laboratories, and has been reviewed extensively elsewhere (Cabeza and Nyberg 1997, 2000; Corbetta 1998; Kanwisher and Wojciulik 2000; Shulman *et al.* 2001). However, two points are worth noting. First, these studies dovetail extremely well with studies of neglect, not only by replicating the general involvement of the frontoparietal network, but also in more precisely locating active structures because of the improved spatial resolution. Second, although these studies afforded greater anatomical specificity because of improved spatial resolution, many do not afford greater functional specificity because of limitations inherent in blocked designs, particularly with PET studies (Corbetta *et al.* 1993). Blocked designs of this sort smear together processing over large periods of time, rendering it difficult to associate a particular activated area with a specific cognitive operation. As a result, many of these studies suffer from inferential limitations pertaining to attentional control because of the inability to decompose top-down mechanisms from bottom-up effects and other processing activity.

More recent event-related designs do not suffer from the same limitations inherent in blocked-design experiments (Buckner *et al.* 1996; McCarthy *et al.* 1997; Burock *et al.* 1998; Rosen *et al.* 1998). In these designs, different trial types are randomly intermixed and, during data analysis, cortical responses time-locked to particular trial types can be averaged. Generally speaking, the responses of these averaged signals can then be compared directly to test specific hypotheses. One of the most notable advantages of the event-related approach is the ability to examine not only the response to particular trials of interest, but also to specific within-trial events. This technique has been employed for many years in human electrophysiology (i.e. electroencephalography (EEG)) and animal neurophysiology (e.g. single-unit recordings) to study the component processes of attentional tasks (Hillyard and Münte 1984; Hillyard *et al.* 1985, 1995; Mangun and Hillyard 1991;

Mangun *et al.* 1993; Yamaguchi *et al.* 1994; Luck *et al.* 1997; Chelazzi *et al.* 1998, 1993). Because fMRI studies of attentional control that are particularly relevant to this chapter apply this 'cue-related' technique, we briefly review two relevant EEG studies before discussing the recent hemodynamic imaging studies.

Harter *et al.* (1989) were the first to decompose the cortical responses to within-trial events in the study of attentional control. They employed a traditional visual cuing paradigm (Posner 1980) to study attentional mechanisms in children, but, unlike many previous EEG experiments of spatial attention which focused on effects of attention on target evoked activity, they investigated the dynamic change in neural activity time-locked to the onset of the cue, but before the target. The inferential logic of this approach is that the cue represents an instruction to direct attention to a particular location in space and, as such, should trigger activity in those areas that are responsible for controlling directed attention. Harter *et al.* reported two ERP effects in response to the attention-directing cues. The first component was a negativity over parietal sites contralateral to the direction indicated by the cue. This response occurred relatively soon after the presentation of the cue, at about 200 ms, and had a duration of about 200 ms. The second component appeared 500 to 700 ms after the cue over occipital sites contralateral to the direction of the cue. Unlike the first component, this deflection was positive relative to the ipsilateral side. Based on the polarity and timing of these components, they were termed the 'early directing attention negativity' (EDAN) and 'late directing attention positivity' (LDAP) respectively. Relating these events to cognitive processes, Harter *et al.* argued that the EDAN component reflected the initiation of control processes, whereas the LDAP component reflected the modulation of retinotopic visual areas corresponding to the location where the target was expected. Consistent with this hypothesis, Hopf and Mangun (2000) recently reported two EDAN-like effects in response to an attention-directing cue: one early over posterior sites (as reported by Harter *et al.* (1989)) and one later over lateral prefrontal sites. These two components are consistent with the notion that top-down control involves parietal cortex mechanisms disengaging attention from its current focus soon after the cue is presented (Posner and Petersen 1990) and maintenance of attention and/or control in lateral prefrontal cortex (Posner and Petersen 1990; Desimone and Duncan 1995). In addition, Hopf and Mangun also observed an LDAP component over occipital–temporal electrodes, which is also consistent with the idea that one of the consequences of attention is the priming of retinotopically organized visual areas (Mangun *et al.* 1993; Hillyard *et al.* 1995, 1998). Together, these studies demonstrate not only the efficacy of using cue-related activity to measure attentional control systems, but, more importantly, the operation of the frontoparietal network well in advance of target presentation.

Two noteworthy event-related fMRI studies have adopted the cue-related approach to isolating brain structures involved in the top-down control of attention (Corbetta *et al.* 2000; Hopfinger *et al.* 2000). These studies are noteworthy for three main reasons. First, they implicate the frontoparietal network in the top-down control of attention. Second, they demonstrate the consequences of attention in two respects: (a) in terms of the impact of control systems on bottom-up sensory processing areas (Hopfinger *et al.* 2000), and (b) the adjustment of the system to breaches of expectation (Corbetta *et al.* 2000). Finally, although they are generally consistent in the patterns of activation, there are also key differences which indicate that the precise functions of the frontoparietal network have yet to be clearly defined. These two studies are reviewed below.

Corbetta *et al.* (2000) tested functional anatomical hypotheses regarding two cognitive operations often assumed to be at work in spatial attention tasks. The first is voluntary orienting to a spatial location, and the second is reorienting to stimuli presented at unattended locations. Based on the models reviewed earlier in this chapter, Corbetta *et al.* hypothesized that voluntary orienting to a location (i.e. directed attention) is mediated by PPC (particularly intraparietal sulcus (IPS)). Reorienting to a new target location, on the other hand, was hypothesized to be mediated by the temporal–parietal junction (TPJ). These complementary hypotheses were tested within the context of a spatial cueing paradigm, in which a central arrow indicated the most likely location of the target. Consistent with the voluntary orienting hypothesis, Corbetta *et al.* found areas of ventral and anterior IPS active during the cue period, but before the target. Interestingly, this activity was protracted in time on a subset of trials in which the cue was followed by a delay and no target, suggesting the maintenance of top-down signals. Similarly, comparison of activations on valid and invalid trials were consistent with the reorienting hypothesis, such that right TPJ exhibited the strongest validity effects in terms of the blood-oxygenation-level-dependent (BOLD) signal and showed very little response to the attention-directing cue (see also Nobre *et al.* (1999) and Arrington *et al.* (2000)). Corbetta *et al.* argued that their results dissociate voluntary orienting mechanisms from target detection mechanisms in parietal cortex, providing evidence converging with the neuropsychological literature implicating posterior parietal cortex as a key attentional control structure (Mesulam 1981; Posner *et al.* 1984, 1987).

Where Corbetta and colleagues focused on parietal involvement in attentional control and breaches of cued expectation, Hopfinger *et al.* (2000) studied control structures and their effect on sensory processing mechanisms. In this study, subjects were presented with an arrow cue at fixation that instructed them to attend to right or left peripheral locations, and then to make a discrimination of a target at that location (i.e. no validity manipulation). Superior frontal, superior and inferior parietal, and superior temporal cortex, were all activated in response to the cues. However, when compared directly with the target activations, only superior frontal cortex, bilateral inferior parietal (IPS), superior temporal, and posterior cingulate areas were more active to the cues than to the targets. Hopfinger *et al.* assessed the impact of the frontoparietal control system on retinotopically organized extrastriate visual areas (identified by retinotopic mapping (Sereno *et al.* 1995)). These researchers found that, in response to the centrally presented cue, there were selective increases in activity in extrastriate areas VP and V4 (representing the peripheral target locations contralateral to the direction of attention) before the target was presented. This result suggests that top-down mechanisms serve to increase the excitability of neurons specialized for processing an upcoming target event (Kastner *et al.* 1999).

Summary

Previous studies of clinical populations, particularly from patients with neglect, provided the first solid evidence identifying the frontoparietal network as being involved in top-down control. The advent of neuroimaging afforded to the opportunity to probe this network *in vivo* in healthy populations. Early studies using blocked PET and fMRI designs provided evidence consistent with the neuropsychological literature that the frontoparietal network is involved in attention. However, owing to the limitations inherent in blocked designs it was not clear which of these areas were involved in control and which were involved in more bottom-up aspects of attentional processing. Event-related methods, like those used in ERP research, allow cortical responses to within trial events to be decomposed. This approach, pioneered by Harter *et al.* (1989), has been adapted to fMRI research with great success. Exploitation of this event-related methodology has allowed researchers to assess the state of the network prior to target presentation and has demonstrated that inferior parietal cortex plays a large role in attentional control.

Mechanisms of attentional control

In the growing literature on attentional control, investigations *localizing* top-down control areas far outnumber attempts at *characterizing* the neural mechanism by which control is achieved. That said, however, there are proposals in the literature purporting to describe how the effects of top-down control are manifest in sensory cortices. Two of these—modulation of baseline activity and modulation of neuronal firing synchrony—are considered in this section.

Baseline modulation

One of the most commonly cited mechanisms of top-down control is a bias in processing before the to-be-attended stimulus is presented. This bias is thought to be manifest in cortex by an increase in baseline firing rates of neurons selective for a behaviorally relevant stimulus. The notion of changes in baseline firing rates acting as a top-down bias mechanism has been incorporated explicitly in the biased-competition model (Desimone and Duncan 1995) as a way of resolving competition among multiple objects in the visual field.

Evidence for baseline shifts in neural firing initially came from monkey neurophysiology (Chelazzi *et al*. 1993, 1998; Luck *et al*. 1997). In one experiment (Chelazzi *et al*. 1993), monkeys performed a delayed match-to-sample task, where each trial began with a brief cue stimulus and after a variable delay (1500–3000 ms) a target display was presented. The monkey's task was to make an eye movement to the object that matched the cue stimulus for a food reward. The critical manipulation was whether the cue was optimal for driving the cells of interest, which were recorded from inferior temporal cortex. The key observation was that, in trials in which the cue was optimal for driving the cell, there was an increase in the spontaneous firing during the delay between the cue and the target. This baseline shift has been replicated in subsequent studies in recordings from earlier ventral visual areas, such as V2 and V4 (Luck *et al*. 1997), as well as in dorsal area LIP (for a review see Colby and Goldberg (1999)).

Recent neuroimaging data with human participants have provided what could be the hemodynamic correlate of baseline shifts in firing rate. For instance, in a study by Kastner *et al*. (1999), subjects were presented with either a sequential display of four complex images in the periphery or a single display of four images in the periphery. These sequential and simultaneous conditions were combined factorially with instructions to attend to one of the peripheral locations or ignore the peripheral stimuli altogether. The instruction to attend was presented 11 s before the stimulus was presented. During this expectation period, when no stimulus was presented, Kastner *et al*. observed increases in baseline activity in retinotopic visual areas representing the location of the to-be-presented target (most notably V4), as well as in the superior parietal lobe (SPL). The results obtained by Hopfinger *et al*. (2000), described in the previous section, also provide converging evidence for baseline modulation of extrastriate visual areas (for other recent examples see Chawla *et al*. (1999) and Martínez *et al*. (1999)).

Although plausible, evidence supporting baseline shifts as a neural mechanism of control is not without ambiguity. For instance, although Luck *et al*. (1997) demonstrated that neurons in V2 and V4 exhibited modulated baseline activity with attention, many of these neurons did not show evidence of an enhanced response to the attended stimuli when they were presented. Similarly, Kastner *et al*. (1999) reported increases in baseline activity not only in V4 and SPL, but also in V1. However, unlike the responses in the later visual areas, the BOLD response in V1 did not exhibit a modulated response when the stimulus was presented. The failure to observe attentional modulations in baseline activity and visually evoked activity in the same neurons suggests that these effects may be the result of different mechanisms (Kastner and Ungerleider 2000).

Neuronal synchrony

Responses of groups of neurons to relevant stimuli are commonly characterized by firing rate changes; however, action potentials from populations can also be characterized in terms of their temporal structure. In particular, the extent to which neurons fire synchronously has been proposed as a computational mechanism by which attentional selection can occur (Niebur and Koch 1994). One hypothesis is that changes in neuronal synchrony reflect an additional, quite different, manifestation of control systems operating in cortex. For example, Steinmetz *et al*. (2000) recently reported an elegant example of the plausibility of neural synchrony as a mechanism of attentional control. In this experiment, monkeys were trained to perform a tactile and a visual task, presented simultaneously. During the testing phase, the monkeys were cued to switch between tasks. The responses of pairs of neurons were recorded from secondary somatosensory cortex contralateral to the tactile stimulation and analyzed for how often they fired at or near the same time when the monkey was attending to the tactile task compared with when it was attending to the visual task. There were two key results. First, almost 66 per cent of the neuron pairs recorded showed synchronous firing during either or both tasks. Second, of those that exhibited synchronous firing, 17 per cent showed changes in synchrony between the visual and tactile tasks, with 80 per cent of these changes being increases in synchrony. The authors argue that such synchronous firing increases synaptic efficiency in the neural representation of the attended location, in much the same way as Desimone and Duncan (1995) argue that shifts in baseline activity resolve competition amongst multiple objects in the visual field.

Consistent with this hypothesis, a very recent study has also reported changes in neural synchrony in extrastriate visual cortex as a function of attention. Fries *et al.* (2001) trained a monkey to perform a visual selective attention task and simultaneously recorded multi-unit activity and local field potentials from sites with overlapping receptive fields in V4. The primary manipulation was whether the monkey's attention was directed, by a visual cue, either inside the receptive field or outside the receptive field. Fries *et al.* reported that during the time between the onset of the cue and the onset of the target display there was a decrease in low-frequency synchronization (e.g. <17 Hz) when attention was directed inside the receptive field. In contrast, they observed an increase in synchronization at higher frequencies with attention (e.g. gamma frequency range, 35–60 Hz). Interestingly, these changes in synchronization were observed in the absence of changes in firing rate as a function of attention. The authors interpret these results within the context of the biased competition model (Desimone and Duncan 1995), in that the changes in synchronization may reflect the resolution of competition between multiple behaviorally relevant stimuli within the visual field by enhancement of these synchronously firing populations in later stages of visual processing.

Summary

In this section we have presented two ways in which top-down control mechanisms can influence neural activity. Although there is substantial evidence supporting baseline shifts in extrastriate cortex, there are ambiguities regarding what the role of these shifts are exactly. This ambiguity is introduced by the fact that some of the neurons showing modulations in prestimulus baseline activity do not show increased response evoked by the presentation of the attended stimulus. An alternative proposal, which is not necessarily mutually exclusive, is that attentional control systems modulate the firing synchrony of populations of neurons. However, as with the baseline shift mechanism, there are also ambiguities regarding the neuronal synchrony proposal, in that only a subset of neurons show modulations of synchrony with attention. Although baseline shifts and neuronal synchrony are plausible control mechanisms, current evidence suggests that, especially in the case of baseline shifts, these patterns of activity likely reflect the *consequences* of top-down attention rather than the control mechanisms themselves.

The generality of the frontoparietal control network

The research reviewed thus far clearly implicates a role for the frontoparietal network in the top-down control of visuospatial attention. One of the issues that we have been studying in our laboratory is the generality of this network. For instance, psychological theory has implicated that not only spatial location as a key dimension on which attentional control systems influence sensory processes (Posner 1980), but also nonspatial attributes such as whole objects, or features such as color or form (Duncan 1984; Hillyard and Münte 1984). Although significant controversy remains concerning the precise relationship between spatial and nonspatial cognitive neural mechanisms, the fact that attending to spatial and nonspatial dimensions results in similar costs and benefits suggests common or, at the very least, interacting control mechanisms (Hillyard and Münte 1984; Kingstone and Klein 1991; Kingstone 1992). In support of this notion, there is emerging neuroimaging evidence, consistent with the behavioral literature, indicating that there may be a great deal of overlap and interaction between the neural systems that mediate spatial and nonspatial attention (McIntosh et al. 1994; Le et al. 1998; Wojciulik and Kanwisher 1999), despite the traditional view that spatial and nonspatial information is processed predominantly by the dorsal and ventral visual streams, respectively (Ungerleider and Mishkin 1982; Milner and Goodale 1993; Haxby et al. 1994). However, not only does the precise relationship between spatial and nonspatial attention remain unclear, it is also unclear how top-down control systems in spatial and nonspatial domains are related. Are they independent, overlapping, or identical? We have recently reported a preliminary experiment that represents an initial step towards understanding this relationship (Giesbrecht et al. 2000).

Method

We asked 10 subjects to participate in a simple cue–target paradigm (Fig. 2). In each trial, subjects were presented a letter at fixation that cued them to attend to the right or left visual field or the color blue or yellow. On location (spatial) trials, the cue was followed by a target display consisting of two green rectangles presented bilaterally in the upper visual field. On color (nonspatial) trials, the target display consisted of blue and yellow rectangles which were overlapped at fixation. Thus,

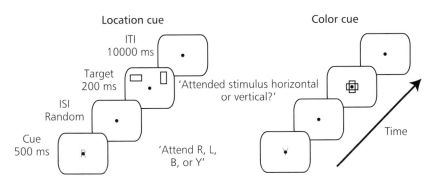

Figure 2 A sample trial sequence from Giesbrecht et al. (2000). At the beginning of each trial a gray cue letter (0.75° × 0.5°) was presented at fixation for 500 ms. On location trials the cue indicated subjects to attend to the right (R) or left (L), and on color trials it indicated subjects to attend to the color blue (B) or yellow (Y). After the cue there was a variable interstimulus interval (ISI) (1000 ms, 8000 ms, or random between 1900 and 7100 ms) during which only the fixation point was visible on the screen. After the ISI, the target display was presented for 200 ms. On location trials, the target display consisted of two green rectangles (1.75° × 1.25°) presented bilaterally in the upper visual field (offset 4° from the horizontal and vertical meridians); on color trials the target display consisted of blue and yellow rectangles (0.875° × 0.625°) which were overlapped at fixation. The task was to indicate the orientation of the relevant rectangle as quickly and accurately as possible. For simplicity, we show here the inverse black–white contrast of the actual stimulus screen and the colors of the target stimuli as black.

spatial and nonspatial tasks were analogous: on location trials subjects were required to orient to one of two locations but not to a color, and on color trials subjects were required to orient to one of two colors but not a location. The interstimulus interval (ISI) between the cue and the target was varied, such that on one-third of the trials it was 1000 ms, on another third it was 8000 ms, and on the final third it was random between 1900 and 7100 ms. The location, color, and ISI trials were randomly mixed. Thus, in each trial subjects did not know whether they would have to orient to a location or to a color, or when the target would be presented after the cue. Subjects were trained extensively before the scanning session and were instructed to maintain fixation at all times, make active use of the information presented in the cue as soon as possible, and to indicate the orientation (horizontal or vertical) of the relevant rectangle quickly and accurately.

Functional images were acquired at 1.5 T and were corrected for asynchronous slice acquisition, motion corrected, spatially normalized to a common stereotactic space (Talairach and Tournoux 1988), and spatially smoothed. The hemodynamic responses to the cues and the targets were modelled separately using the general linear model as implemented in SPM99. The hemodynamic response was modelled as the sum of two gamma functions and its temporal derivative. Statistical significance of our fixed effects analysis was determined using a combined amplitude and extent threshold approach (Forman *et al.* 1995; Xiong *et al.* 1995; Poline *et al.* 1997), as implemented within SPM99.

Results

We measured cue-related brain activity to assess the top-down mechanisms involved in spatial and nonspatial attention. Consequently, in order to obtain maximal separation of the hemodynamic response of attention-directing cues from subsequent visual targets, only data from long ISI trials are reported here. Subjects performed the task well, with no significant differences in response time (location, 860 ms; color, 887 ms; $t(9) = 1.01, p > 0.05$), but a small difference in error rate (location, 10.5 per cent; color, 3.2 per cent; $t(9) = 4.29, p < 0.05$).

Our functional analysis consisted of two steps. First, we identified those areas that were activated in response to location and color cues independently. A statistical threshold of $p < 0.05$, corrected for multiple comparisons, and an extent threshold of eight contiguous voxels were set. The results are shown in Plate 1(a). Areas active only to location and color cues are shown in red and blue respectively. The common areas, i.e. areas activated by both types of cues, are shown in green. These common areas include precentral gyrus, supplementary motor area, parietal cortex (including the superior and inferior parietal lobes, and intraparietal sulcus bilaterally), inferior temporal gyrus, and lingual gyrus. Thus it is clear that there is a great deal of overlap between spatial and nonspatial systems.

To identify those areas that were differentially activated by the two types of cues, the second step of our analysis involved a direct statistical comparison of location and color cues only within those regions that were activated when collapsed across cue type (i.e. the main effect of cue). Because location and color cues were equated for basic sensory processing, those areas involved strictly in the sensory processing of the cue should subtract out, leaving those areas that are preferentially active for either spatial or nonspatial attentional control. The results of this analysis are shown in Plate 1(b) (all clusters shown are significant at $p < 0.05$, extent eight voxels, corrected for multiple comparisons within our region of interest). The group activations overlaid onto four slices of a single subject's anatomical image are shown, starting in superior cortex (e.g. $z = 55$) and moving through to ventral cortex (e.g. $z = -15$). In superior cortex, there were clusters in the superior parietal lobe and the frontal eye fields (both bilateral) that were more active to location cues, whereas there were no dorsal areas more active to color cues. In ventral cortex, on the other hand, there were no areas that were more active to location cues, whereas fusiform, inferior temporal, and lingual gyri were more active to color cues.

Summary

In the preliminary results described above, a frontoparietal network of brain areas became activated in response to attention-directing cues, both spatial and nonspatial. The overlap between spatial and nonspatial cue-related activity probably reflects not only overlap in sensory processing of the cue (e.g. lingual gyrus), but also attentional control mechanisms (e.g. inferior parietal lobe and superior frontal cortex). The direct comparisons between location and color cues revealed that, in these subjects, some of these brain structures were differentially active to the two types of cues, with more dorsal parietal regions supporting spatial orienting and more inferior parietal and ventral cortical areas supporting nonspatial orienting. Overall, these results are consistent with the idea that the cognitive operations involved in attentional control rely on a common network of brain areas, whether the behaviorally relevant dimension is a location or a stimulus feature. However, these results also demonstrate that this general network recruits brain systems selective for control in spatial and nonspatial information.

Concluding remarks

The purpose of this chapter has been to provide a snapshot of the most relevant recent research in the field of the top-down control of attention. Some of this research has identified superior frontal and inferior parietal cortices as key control structures (Corbetta *et al.* 2000; Hopfinger *et al.* 2000). Other research, in monkeys as well as in humans, has suggested that the influence of top-down control mechanisms may be manifest in cortex as modulations in baseline firing rate or firing synchrony in neural populations coding the behaviorally relevant stimuli (Chelazzi *et al.* 1993; Luck *et al.* 1997; Kastner *et al.* 1999; Steinmetz *et al.* 2000; Fries *et al.* 2001). Together, these two lines of investigation have provided important insights into the structure and function of top-down control networks, but these studies represent only the start a growing area of research.

Future directions

A large portion of this chapter has been devoted to what is known about top-down control. As a way of concluding, we would like to look ahead and identify a few of the key issues that need to be addressed in order that we, as a discipline, continue to build on the foundation of these ground-breaking studies. Perhaps the most critical of these questions is the elucidation of the neural mechanism by which control is achieved. Although baseline shifts and neural synchrony are viable proposals, they probably represent the consequences of invoking top-down control systems and not the neural mechanisms by which control is achieved. Another important issue is the generality of the control network. Previous reports indicate that there is overlap in the frontoparietal network in a variety of attention tasks (Wojciulik and Kanwisher 1999). Consistent with these data, the experiment we presented in this chapter provides preliminary evidence that top-down control of attention to different stimulus dimensions also draws on partly overlapping brain areas. The issue of the generality of top-down control mechanisms is being pursued actively in our laboratory and with our collaborators, where studies are addressing whether this network is also responsible for the control of spatial attention in different frames of reference (Wilson and Mangun 2001), to different levels of hierarchical stimuli (Weissman *et al.* 2001), and at short stimulus onset asynchronies (SOAs) and ISIs that are much more similar to those used in behavioral and ERP paradigms (Woldorff *et al.* 2001). Moreover, the relationship between attentional control circuits and other cognitive operations, such as working memory, also need to be addressed in order to achieve a more global understanding of behavior. A few behavioral and neuroimaging studies have attempted to identify the relationship between attention and working memory (Awh and Jonides 1998, 2001; Awh *et al.* 1998, 1999, 2000; de Fockert *et al.* 2001), but none of them have specifically investigated the relationship between attention and working memory control systems. Pursuing these questions fulfils two important obligations of cognitive neuroscience: to formulate a complete understanding of the brain bases of behavior, and to provide clinicians and therapists with information that will help those who have sustained damage to areas that are critical in the top-down control of attention.

Acknowledgements

This research was supported by a training grant from the McDonnell–Pew Foundation's Program in Cognitive Neuroscience and a Postdoctoral Fellowship from the Natural Sciences and Engineering Research Council of Canada, both awarded to BG. Additional support came from a grant from the National Institute of Mental Health awarded to GRM. We thank Gregory McCarthy and Allen Song of the Brain Imaging and Analysis Center, Duke University, for their help with the neuroimaging protocols, and Kevin Wilson and Marty Woldorff for comments on earlier versions of this chapter.

References

Arrington, C. M., Carr, T. H., Mayer, A. R., and Rao, S. M. (2000). Neural mechanisms of visual attention: object-based selection of a region in space. *Journal of Cognitive Neuroscience*, **12** (Supplement 2), 106–17.

Awh, E. and Jonides, J. (1998). Spatial working memory and spatial selective attention. In *The attentive brain* (ed. R. Parasuraman), pp. 353–80. MIT Press, Cambridge, MA.

Awh, E. and Jonides, J. (2001). Overlapping mechanisms of attention and spatial working memory. *Trends in Cognitive Science*, **5**, 119–26.

Awh, E., Jonides, J., and Reuter-Lorenz, P. A. (1998). Rehearsal in spatial working memory. *Journal of Experimental Psychology: Human Perception and Performance*, **24**, 780–90.

Awh, E., Jonides, J., Smith, E. E., *et al.* (1999). Rehearsal in spatial working memory: evidence from neuroimaging. *Psychological Science*, **10**, 433–7.

Awh, E., Anllo-Vento, L., and Hillyard, S. A. (2000). The role of spatial selective attention in working memory for locations: evidence from event-related potentials. *Journal of Cognitive Neuroscience*, **12**, 840–7.

Broadbent, D. E. (1958). *Perception and communication*. Pergamon Press, London.

Buckner, R. L., Bandettini, P. A., O'Craven, K. M., *et al.* (1996). Detection of cortical activation during averaged single trials of a cognitive task using functional magnetic resonance imaging. *Proceedings of the National Academy of Sciences of the United States of America*, **93**, 14878–83.

Burock, M. A., Buckner, R. L., Woldorff, M. G., Rosen, B. R., and Dale, A. M. (1998). Randomized event-related experimental designs allow for extremely rapid presentation rates using functional MRI. *NeuroReport*, **9**, 3735–9.

Cabeza, R. and Nyberg, L. (1997). Imaging cognition: an empirical review of PET studies with normal subjects. *Journal of Cognitive Neuroscience*, **9**, 1–26.

Cabeza, R. and Nyberg, L. (2000). Imaging cognition II: an empirical review of 275 PET and fMRI studies. *Journal of Cognitive Neuroscience*, **12**, 1–47.

Chawla, D., Rees, G., and Friston, K. J. (1999). The physiological basis of attentional modulation in extrastriate visual areas. *Nature Neuroscience*, **2**, 671–6.

Chelazzi, L., Miller, E. K., Duncan, J., and Desimone, R. (1993). A neural basis for visual search in inferior temporal cortex. *Nature*, **363**, 345–7.

Chelazzi, L., Duncan, J., Miller, E. K., and Desimone, R. (1998). Responses of neurons in inferior temporal cortex during memory-guided visual search. *Journal of Neurophysiology*, **80**, 2918–40.

Colby, C. L. and Goldberg, M. E. (1999). Space and attention in parietal cortex. *Annual Review of Neuroscience*, **22**, 319–49.

Corbetta, M. (1998). Frontoparietal cortical networks for directing attention and the eye to visual locations: identical, independent, or overlapping neural systems? *Proceedings of the National Academy of Sciences of the United States of America*, **95**, 831–8.

Corbetta, M., Miezin, F. M., Shulman, G. L., and Petersen, S. E. (1993). A PET study of visuospatial attention. *Journal of Neuroscience*, **13**, 1202–26.

Corbetta, M., Kincade, J. M., Ollinger, J. M., McAvoy, M. P., and Shulman, G. L. (2000). Voluntary orienting is dissociated from target detection in human posterior parietal cortex. *Nature Neuroscience*, **3**, 292–7.

de Fockert, J. W., Rees, G., Frith, C. D., and Lavie, N. (2001). The role of working memory in visual selective attention. *Science*, **291**, 1803–6.

Desimone, R. and Duncan, J. (1995). Neural mechanisms of selective visual attention. *Annual Review of Neuroscience*, **18**, 193–222.

Duncan, J. (1984). Selective attention and the organization of visual information. *Journal of Experimental Psychology: General*, **113**, 501–17.

Eason, R., Harter, M., and White, C. (1969). Effects of attention and arousal on visually evoked potentials and reaction time in man. *Physiology and Behavior*, **4**, 283–9.

Forman, S. D., Cohen, J. D., Fitzgerald, M., Eddy, W. F., Mintun, M. A., and Noll, D. C. (1995). Improved assessment of significant activation in functional magnetic resonance imaging (fMRI): use of a cluster-size threshold. *Magnetic Resonance in Medicine*, **33**, 636–47.

Friedrich, F. J., Egly, R., Rafal, R., and Beck, D. (1998). Spatial attention deficits in humans: a comparison of superior parietal and temporal-parietal junction lesions. *Neuropsychology*, **12**, 193–207.

Fries, P., Reynolds, J. H., Rorie, A. E., and Desimone, R. (2001). Modulation of oscillatory neuronal synchronization by selective visual attention. *Science*, **291**, 1560–3.

Giesbrecht, B., Woldorff, M. G., Fichtenholtz, H. M., and Mangun, G. R. (2000). Isolating the neural mechanisms of spatial and nonspatial attentional control. Presented at the 30th Annual Meeting of the Society for Neuroscience, New Orleans, LA.

Harter, M. R., Miller, S. L., Price, N. J., LaLonde, M. E., and Keyes, A. L. (1989). Neural processes involved in directing attention. *Journal of Cognitive Neuroscience*, **1**, 223–37.

Haxby, J. V., Horwitz, B., Ungerleider, L. G., Maisog, J. M., Pietrini, P., and Grady, C. L. (1994). The functional organization of human extrastriate cortex: a PET-rCBF study of selective attention to faces and locations. *Journal of Neuroscience*, **14**, 6336–53.

Heilman, K. M. and Valenstein, E. (1979). Mechanisms underlying hemispatial neglect. *Annals of Neurology*, **5**, 166–70.

Hillyard, S. A. and Münte, T. F. (1984). Selective attention to color and location: an analysis with event-related brain potentials. *Perception and Psychophysics*, **36**, 185–98.

Hillyard, S. A., Münte, T. F., and Neville, H. J. (1985). Visual-spatial attention, orienting, and brain physiology. In *Attention and performance XI* (ed. M. I. Posner and O. S. M. Marin) pp. 63–84. Lawrence Erlbaum, Hillsdale, NJ.

Hillyard, S. A., Mangun, G. R., Woldorff, M. G., and Luck, S. J. (1995). Neural systems mediating selective attention. In *The cognitive neurosciences* (ed. M. S. Gazzaniga), pp. 665–81. MIT Press, Cambridge, MA.

Hillyard, S. A., Vogel, E. K., and Luck, S. J. (1998). Sensory gain control (amplification) as a mechanism of selective attention: electrophysiological and neuroimaging evidence. *Philosophical Transactions of the Royal Society of London. B. Biological Sciences*, **353**, 1257–70.

Hopf, J. M. and Mangun, G. R. (2000). Shifting visual attention in space: an electrophysiological analysis using high spatial resolution mapping. *Clinical Neurophysiology*, **111**, 1241–57.

Hopfinger, J. B., Buonocore, M. H., and Mangun, G. R. (2000). The neural mechanisms of top-down attentional control. *Nature Neuroscience*, **3**, 284–91.

Itti, L. and Koch, C. (2001). Computational modelling of visual attention. *Nature Reviews Neuroscience*, **2**, 194–203.

Kanwisher, N. and Wojciulik, E. (2000). Visual attention: insights from brain imaging. *Nature Reviews Neuroscience*, **1**, 91–100.

Kastner, S. and Ungerleider, L. G. (2000). Mechanisms of visual attention in the human cortex. *Annual Review of Neuroscience*, **23**, 315–41.

Kastner, S., Pinsk, M. A., De Weerd, P., Desimone, R., and Ungerleider, L. G. (1999). Increased activity in human visual cortex during directed attention in the absence of visual stimulation. *Neuron*, **22**, 751–61.

Kingstone, A. (1992). Combining expectancies. *Quarterly Journal of Experimental Psychology*, **44A**, 69–104.

Kingstone, A. and Klein, R. M. (1991). Combining shape and position expectancies: hierarchical processing and selective inhibition. *Journal of Experimental Psychology: Human Perception and Performance*, **17**, 512–19.

Laberge, D. (1995). Computational and anatomical models of selective attention in object identification. In *The cognitive neurosciences* (ed. M. S. Gazzaniga), pp. 649–63. MIT Press, Cambridge, MA.

Le, T. H., Pardo, J. V., and Hu, X. (1998). 4 T-fMRI study of nonspatial shifting of selective attention: cerebellar and parietal contributions. *Journal of Neurophysiology*, **79**, 1535–48.

Luck, S. J., Chelazzi, L., Hillyard, S. A., and Desimone, R. (1997). Neural mechanisms of spatial selective attention in areas V1, V2, and V4 of macaque visual cortex. *Journal of Neurophysiology*, **77**, 24–42.

McCarthy, G., Luby, M., Gore, J., and Goldman-Rakic, P. (1997). Infrequent events transiently activate human prefrontal and parietal cortex as measured by functional MRI. *Journal of Neurophysiology*, **77**, 1630–4.

McIntosh, A. R., Grady, C. L., Ungerleider, L. G., Haxby, J. V., Rapoport, S. I., and Horwitz, B. (1994). Network analysis of cortical visual pathways mapped with PET. *Journal of Neuroscience*, **14**, 655–66.

Mangun, G. R. and Hillyard, S. A. (1991). Modulation of sensory-evoked brain potentials provide evidence for changes in perceptual processing during visual-spatial priming. *Journal of Experimental Psychology: Human Perception and Performance*, **17**, 1057–74.

Mangun, G. R., Hillyard, S. A., and Luck, S. J. (1993). Electrocortical substrates of visual selective attention. In *Attention and performance XIV: Synergies in experimental psychology, artificial intelligence, and cognitive neuroscience* (ed. D. M. S. Kornblum) pp. 219–43. MIT Press, Cambridge, MA.

Martínez, A., Anllo-Vento, L., Sereno, M. I. *et al.* (1999). Involvement of striate and extrastriate visual cortical areas in spatial attention. *Nature Neuroscience*, **2**, 364–9.

Mesulam, M.-M. (1981). A cortical network for directed attention and unilateral neglect. *Annals of Neurology*, **10**, 309–25.

Mesulam, M.-M. (1990). Large-scale neurocognitive networks and distributed processing for attention, memory, and language. *Annals of Neurology*, **28**, 597–613.

Milner, A. D. and Goodale, M. A. (1993). Visual pathways to perception and action. *Progress in Brain Research*, **95**, 317–37.

Moran, J. and Desimone, R. (1985). Selective attention gates visual processing in extrastriate cortex. *Science*, **229**, 782–3.

Niebur, E. and Koch, C. (1994). A model for the neuronal implementation of selective visual attention based on temporal correlation among neurons. *Journal of Computational Neuroscience*, **1**, 141–58.

Nobre, A. C., Coull, J. T., Frith, C. D., and Mesulam, M.-M. (1999). Orbitofrontal cortex is activated during breaches of expectation in tasks of visual attention. *Nature Neuroscience*, **2**, 11–12.

Poline, J. B., Worsley, K. J., Evans, A. C., and Friston, K. J. (1997). Combining spatial extent and peak intensity to test for activations in functional imaging. *Neuroimage*, **5**, 83–96.

Posner, M. I. (1980). Orienting of attention. *Quarterly Journal of Experimental Psychology*, **32**, 3–25.

Posner, M. I. and Petersen, S. E. (1990). The attention system of the human brain. *Annual Review of Neuroscience*, **13**, 25–42.

Posner, M. I. and Rothbart, M. K. (1991). Attentional mechanisms and conscious experience. In *The neuropsychology of consciousness* (ed. D. M. M. Rugg) pp. 91–111. Academic Press, New York.

Posner, M. I., Walker, J. A., Friedrich, F. A., and Rafal, R. D. (1984). Effects of parietal injury on covert orienting of attention. *Journal of Neuroscience*, **4**, 1863–74.

Posner, M. I., Rafal, R. D., Choate, L. S., and Vaughn, J. (1985). Inhibition of return: neural basis and function. *Cognitive Neuropsychology*, **2**, 211–28.

Posner, M. I., Walker, J. A., Friedrich, F. A., and Rafal, R. D. (1987). How do the parietal lobes direct covert attention? *Neuropsychologia*, **25**, 135–45.

Rafal, R. D. (1998). Neglect. In *The attentive brain* (ed. R. Parasuraman), pp. 489–525. MIT Press, Cambridge, MA.

Rosen, B. R., Buckner, R. L., and Dale, A. M. (1998). Event-related functional MRI: past, present, and future. *Proceedings of the National Academy of Sciences of the United States of America*, **95**, 773–80.

Sereno, M. I., Dale, A. M., Reppas, J. B., *et al.* (1995). Borders of multiple visual areas in humans revealed by functional magnetic resonance imaging. *Science*, **268**, 889–93.

Shulman, G. L., Ollinger, J. M., Linenweber, M., Petersen, S. E., and Corbetta, M. (2001). Multiple neural correlates of detection in the human brain. *Proceedings of the National Academy of Sciences of the United States of America*, **98**, 313–18.

Steinmetz, P. N., Roy, A., Fitzgerald, P. J., Hsiao, S. S., Johnson, K. O., and Niebur, E. (2000). Attention modulates synchronized neuronal firing in primate somatosensory cortex. *Nature*, **404**, 187–90.

Talairach, J. and Tournoux, P. (1988). *Co-planar stereotaxic atlas of the human brain*. Thieme, New York.

Ungerleider, L. G. and Mishkin, M. (1982). Two cortical visual systems. In *Analysis of visual behavior* (ed. D. J. Ingle, M. A. Goodale, and R. J. W. Mansfield), pp. 549–86. MIT Press, Cambridge, MA.

Van Voorhis, S. T. and Hillyard, S. A. (1977). Visual evoked potentials and selective attention to points in space. *Perception and Psychophysics*, **22**, 54–62.

Weissman, D. H., Woldorff, M. G., and Mangun, G. R. (2001). Neural correlates of voluntary orienting for global versus local processing. Presented at the 8th Annual Meeting of the Cognitive Neuroscience Society, New York.

Wilson, K. D. and Mangun, G. R. (2001). Reference frame effects in the top-down control of visual attention: an event-related fMRI investigation. Presented at the 8th Annual Meeting of the Cognitive Neuroscience Society, New York.

Wojciulik, E. and Kanwisher, N. (1999). The generality of parietal involvement in visual attention. *Neuron*, **23**, 747–64.

Woldorff, M. G., Fichtenholtz, H. M., Song, A. W., and Mangun, G. R. (2001). Separation of cue- and target-related processing in a fast-rate visual spatial attention cueing paradigm. Presented at the 8th Annual Meeting of the Cognitive Neuroscience Society, New York.

Xiong, J., Gao, J., Lancaster, J. L., and Fox, P. T. (1995). Clustered pixels analysis for functional MRI activation studies of the human brain. *Human Brain Mapping*, **3**, 287–301.

Yamaguchi, S., Tsuchiya, H., and Kobayashi, S. (1994). Electroencephalographic activity associated with shifts of visuospatial attention. *Brain*, **117**, 553–62.

5.3 Two neural systems for visual orienting and the pathophysiology of unilateral spatial neglect

Maurizio Corbetta, Michelle J. Kincade, and Gordon L. Shulman

Attention defines the ability to select stimuli and actions that are coherent with the behavioral goals of an organism. Attention is not a unitary function since selection problems must be solved at multiple levels of processing, including sensory, cognitive, and motor stages, for behavior to be efficient and goal-directed. Accordingly, current anatomical models of attention propose that different attentional operations, such as selecting a location for an eye movement or detecting a target, are carried out in different brain areas. Similarly, unilateral spatial neglect, the prototypical human model of attentional failure, is no longer considered to be a single impairment, but a heterogeneous constellation of attentional and sensory-motor deficits that are probably mediated by separate neural systems.

In this chapter, we critically evaluate current neurobiological models of attention and unilateral spatial neglect, particularly in relation to neuroimaging results acquired over the last decade. We note that these models do not account for important discrepancies between lesion studies and neuroimaging results. We present a new experiment that clarifies some of these discrepancies, and propose a revision of current models.

Cognitive neuroscience models of attention and neglect

An influential anatomical model of spatial attention and unilateral spatial neglect was proposed by Mesulam (1981, 1999). This model was one of the first to introduce the idea that spatial attention is a distributed function mediated by a 'network' of cortical areas (Heilman and Watson 1977). Prior to this, spatial attention in humans had been widely regarded as a specialized neuropsychological function of the parietal lobes (Critchley 1953). Mesulam suggested that different cortical regions linked within a network perform separate operations of spatial attention. Specifically, posterior parietal, prefrontal, and anterior cingulate cortices would mediate the perceptual, motor–exploratory, and motivational aspects of spatially directed attention.

This model is supported by a wealth of indirect anatomical, physiological, and neuroimaging data as well as some direct observations from lesion studies. Here, we will review some of its key points. Firstly, observations of the effects of lesions that cause unilateral spatial neglect have shown that attention is anatomically distributed in the brain (Heilman and Valenstein 1972; Vallar and Perani 1987; Husain and Kennard 1996; Karnath *et al.* 2001). More recently, brain imaging studies in normal volunteers have consistently localized a network of cortical regions that are active during visual (spatial) attention tasks (Corbetta 1998). These regions include posterior parietal cortex along the intraparietal sulcus (IPS), dorsal frontal cortex near/at the putative human frontal eye field (FEF), and medial frontal cortex near/at anterior cingulate cortex (AC). They are currently considered the core nodes of an attention network whose damage results in unilateral spatial neglect (Mesulam 1999).

Secondly, each node in the network is functionally specialized to implement a different computation related to spatial attention. For example, posterior parietal cortex selects and represents relevant objects, while frontal cortex plans response towards them. This sharp distinction was supported early on by the discovery that neurons in parietal cortex are modulated when attention is covertly or overtly (by eye movements) directed to a visual stimulus, whereas neurons in the frontal eye field are modulated only when the eyes move (Wurtz et al. 1984). However, more recent results support a weaker functional specialization of posterior parietal and frontal regions. Behavioral studies found dissociations between 'perceptual-like' and 'premotor-like' types of neglect (Bisiach et al. 1990; Tegner and Levander 1991), which did not neatly map onto parietal and frontal regions of damage. Single-unit recording studies have reported pure attentional and perceptual modulations in the FEF (Thompson and Schall 1999) and robust planning signals in posterior parietal cortex (Snyder et al. 1997). Finally, imaging studies have not dissociated parietal from frontal activation during perceptual and visuomotor attentional tasks (Corbetta 1998).

Finally, space is asymmetrically represented in posterior parietal and frontal cortex, and this asymmetry explains the higher incidence of left over right space neglect. Right parietal (and frontal) regions direct attention both contralaterally (left space) and ipsilaterally (right space), whereas left parietal (and frontal) regions mainly direct attention contralaterally (right space). This neural asymmetry is suggested by the asymmetric (right greater than left) activation of parietal cortex during some attentional paradigms (see below).

Another influential anatomical model of attention was proposed by Posner and colleagues (Posner and Petersen 1990; Posner and Dehaene 1994). In this model three interacting cortical networks are postulated. A posterior 'orienting' network, centered in posterior parietal cortex and connected subcortical nuclei (superior colliculus and pulvinar), controls 'orienting' of attention. Accordingly, for instance, parietal damage impairs attentional reorienting toward unattended targets in the contralesional field ('disengagement' deficit), while collicular damage slows down movements of attention to a new location of interest. The importance of parietal–collicular–pulvinar networks in orienting is also supported by neuronal and pharmacological studies in primates (Petersen et al. 1987).

A second network, centered in anterior cingulate, is specialized in target detection and operates as a bottleneck regulating the access of targets to working memory/awareness. In recent revisions the anterior cingulate is conceptualized more as a central executive (Norman and Shallice 1985).

The final network is specialized in 'vigilance/alerting' and is centered in the locus ceruleus and ascending projections to the neocortex. Vigilance refers to the ability to monitor the environment for relevant stimuli, particularly under conditions in which very few stimuli are present. Alerting refers to the performance-enhancing effect produced by warning stimuli (Parasuraman et al. 1998). This network is lateralized to the right hemisphere with a core region localized in right frontal lobe, based on positron-emission tomography (PET) studies showing right frontal activation during monitoring of stimuli presented at a very low frequency (Pardo et al. 1991) and reports of vigilance deficits in patients with right frontal damage (Wilkins et al. 1987).

Critique of current anatomical models of attention and unilateral neglect

Discrepancy between functional brain imaging and neuropsychology

Functional brain imaging studies of attention in the last decade have confirmed many of the anatomical predictions of both Mesulam's and Posner's models. Our laboratory initially described a dorsal frontoparietal network which was active when subjects covertly directed attention to peripheral targets (Corbetta *et al.* 1993). Subsequent studies localized these regions more precisely to the IPS–superior parietal lobule (SPL), and to the precentral sulcus and its intersection with the superior frontal sulcus (Corbetta 1998). Later, it was found that the same network is active during the execution of saccadic eye movements to visual stimuli, and that the frontal region may be homologous to monkey FEF (Corbetta *et al.* 1998; Luna *et al.* 1998; Nobre *et al.* 2000). Therefore these regions are not just attentional in nature but part of a circuitry specialized in planning and executing eye movements, and covert attention shifts can be conceptualized as motor plans for an impending eye movement. However, these regions are also modulated by selection for object attributes such as color or shape (Le *et al.* 1998), and this may possibly indicate a more general role of this network in visual, and not just spatial, selection (Wojciulik and Kanwisher 1999).

While this body of work supports the role of IPS–SPL and FEF in visual attention, there is much less support for the notion that these areas are those damaged in patients with unilateral spatial neglect (see Plate 2). Specifically, the parietal region most commonly damaged in patients with unilateral neglect is the inferior parietal lobule (Vallar and Perani 1987). In patients with spatial neglect and no visual field deficit, the superior temporal gyrus is most commonly involved (Karnath *et al.* 2001). Patients with focal injuries involving the superior aspect of the posterior parietal lobes, near the IPS regions active in brain imaging experiments, have deficits in visually guided action known as optic ataxia (Damasio and Benton 1979), but rarely evidence of neglect.

In addition, the 'disengagement' deficit, originally reported by Posner and colleagues, has recently been localized to the temporoparietal junction (TPJ), which includes the inferior parietal lobule and superior temporal gyrus (Friedrich *et al.* 1998). This may explain why the degree of disengagement deficit correlates with the severity of clinical neglect, and why its recovery parallels the clinical recovery of neglect (Morrow and Ratcliff 1988). This localization to TPJ is surprising because many brain imaging experiments adopted variations of Posner's task, yet consistently recruited more dorsal IPS–SPL regions. In contrast, patients with IPS–SPL lesions are impaired in using the probabilistic value of a central (endogenous) cue to predict the location of the target, while patients with TPJ lesions can normally use this form of endogenous expectancy (Friedrich *et al.* 1998).

In summary, these findings emphasize a significant mismatch between the location of parietal areas active during visuospatial attention tasks (IPS–SPL), and the location of lesions that cause neglect and orienting deficits (TPJ). They also suggest that TPJ and SPL may play dissociable roles in orienting, with TPJ being more sensitive to the onset of unattended stimuli, and IPS–SPL more sensitive to the endogenous significance of cues.

A similar mismatch in localization between brain imaging and neuropsychology may exist in the frontal lobe (Plate 2). The putative human FEF region is the frontal core in Mesulam's network based on imaging studies. FEF damage in macaque causes robust neglect (Latto and Cowey 1971). However, the area of frontal damage most commonly involved in cases of neglect in humans includes the lateral and ventral portions of the frontal lobe, and not the more dorsal aspects near/at human FEF (Heilman and Valenstein 1972; Vallar and Perani 1987; Husain and Kennard 1996; Mattingley *et al.* 1998). Patients with frontal lesions including FEF have deficits in voluntary eye movements (Henik *et al.* 1994), but only mild (if any) acute neglect. The more ventral regions of the right frontal lobe have been activated during vigilance tasks in which subjects monitor the environment to detect low-frequency targets (Pardo *et al*. 1991). Vigilance is a major component of the syndrome of unilateral neglect, and right frontal lesions impair vigilance (Wilkins *et al*. 1987).

In summary, it is possible that lesions causing neglect in the frontal lobe do not match with frontal areas of activation during visuospatial attention; rather, they better match the location of regions mediating alerting/vigilance.

Exogenous and endogenous attention

There are two fundamental ways in which we select information in the visual environment: either we pay attention to salient objects or we pay attention to interesting objects. For instance, bright colored objects that stand out from the background, or a sudden flash in the dark, capture our attention immediately and reflexively. At the other extreme, we can search for a familiar face in a crowd. In the latter case, visual perception is guided by internal knowledge or an expectation for a specific visual attribute (e.g. the color of a friend's hat). Most of the time, we operate in environments where sensory saliency and cognitive expectations flexibly interact to generate a coherent and stable visual world.

Psychologists since William James (James 1890) have captured this phenomenological distinction between modes of visual selection in different taxonomies of attention. One distinction is between exogenous and endogenous orienting. These processes were postulated based on the facilitatory effect of simple sensory–exogenous cues (e.g. a peripheral flash) or cognitive–endogenous cues (e.g. an arrow pointing to one location) indicating a likely target location during simple visual detection tasks (Posner 1980). While both types of cues improve performance, the time course of their effect differs substantially. Endogenous cues cause a prolonged facilitation at the attended location, whereas exogenous cues cause a transient facilitation followed by a prolonged inhibition. Therefore it is likely that exogenous and endogenous orienting may be mediated by separate neural systems.

In current models of attention, posterior parietal cortex mediates both forms of orienting. In Mesulam's model, IPS is conceptualized as a 'saliency' map where relevant objects are represented, but there is no clear conceptualization of how these processes may interact in visual perception. In Posner's model, parietal lesions impair both endogenous and exogenous orienting. However, recent work indicates that right parietal patients show a robust orienting deficit only following peripheral cues, and not central cues, and that this deficit is more common in patients with a diagnosis of unilateral neglect (Losier and Klein 2001). These findings suggest the existence of an anatomical separation in posterior parietal cortex between neural systems devoted to endogenous versus exogenous orienting.

A second psychological distinction is the one between orienting and vigilance or alerting (see above for definitions). These two sets of processes are highly interactive under normal conditions. Orienting and target detection increase the level of vigilance, while increased vigilance or arousal facilitates orienting toward novel targets. In pathological conditions like neglect there are also strong interactions between orienting and vigilance/arousal. Robertson and colleagues found that treating vigilance deficits or increasing arousal reduces ipsilesional orienting biases in patients with unilateral neglect (Robertson 1999). This indicates that these two sets of processes are functionally interacting, and based on the location of lesions causing neglect, this interaction may occur in the right TPJ.

At the anatomical level, as discussed earlier, orienting is mediated by parietal and frontal cortex, and vigilance/alerting depend on ascending broad noradrenergic projections from the locus coeruleus to the neocortex. Vigilance/alerting networks are lateralized to the right hemisphere in Posner's model with a core region localized in the right inferior frontal cortex. Therefore neither model explicitly captures the functional interaction that must exist between orienting and vigilance/arousal processes, or points to the parietal cortex as the site of such interaction.

Asymmetric organization of attentional networks

A fundamental issue for research is to explain the clinical lateralization of neglect, and how it might relate to the lateralization of attention networks in the brain. A common current view, mostly based on Mesulam's model, is that frontal and parietal regions in the two hemispheres code asymmetrically for extrapersonal space. Specifically, the right hemisphere controls the allocation of attention to both contralateral and ipsilateral space, while the left hemisphere mainly directs attention to the contralateral (right) space.

This hypothesis is not supported by the available brain imaging evidence. In our initial report, we found that activity in IPS–SPL was stronger contralaterally to the field of attention (Corbetta *et al.* 1993). In addition, left parietal cortex was more active for directing attention to the right field, whereas right parietal cortex was active for attention to both the left and right fields. These findings nicely matched Mesulam's framework. However, more recent studies have reported bilateral parietal activation, with slightly stronger activation in the hemisphere contralateral to the field of attention (Vandenberghe *et al.* 1997, 2000; Corbetta *et al.* 1998). Recent event-related studies have more precisely isolated spatial attentional signals, and still reported largely bilateral IPS activation for directing attention to the left and right fields (Corbetta *et al.* 2000; Hopfinger *et al.* 2000). An important aspect is that attention was always allocated based on endogenous or cognitive cues in all these studies.

In contrast, Nobre *et al.* (1997) have reported strongly right-lateralized IPS–SPL activation during a reflexive covert orienting task. However, when subjects performed the same task under conditions of endogenous cueing, a bilateral activation was recorded. In summary, parietal (IPS) activity may be lateralized to the right hemisphere when subjects orient exogenously, but it is bilateral when they orient based on cognitive cues. This prediction was confirmed in a study by Kim *et al.* (1999).

Anterior cingulate is not involved in stimulus selection, but response evaluation

The anterior cingulate is regarded an important node of attention networks. In Mesulam's model, the cingulate is a motivational center where endogenous expectations (e.g. the intention to attend to the left) are generated. This notion is supported by the traditional role of AC in motivation, cases of patients with neglect after AC damage (Heilman and Valenstein 1972), and anatomical results showing that AC is reciprocally connected with posterior parietal and prefrontal cortex (Mesulam and Mufson 1982). Its role as a central executive is motivated by AC activation in behavioral tasks that require high-level control such as a Stroop task or a divided attention condition for different visual features (Pardo *et al.* 1990; Corbetta *et al.* 1991).

We believe that the inclusion of the anterior cingulate cortex as a critical node in attention networks is not warranted based on either patient studies or more recent neuroimaging work. The majority of patients with anterior cingulate lesions do not have deficits in attentional orienting, but show impairment in response initiation (akinetic mutism) (Laplane *et al.* 1981). Furthermore, cognitive analyses of patients with cingulotomy found limited problems in task switching or selection, but not in orienting (Ochsner *et al.* 2001). Finally, early brain imaging studies averaged attentional control signals with other types of signals (visual, motor, etc.).

More recent functional MRI (fMRI) studies at higher temporal resolution clearly indicate that AC is not recuited during target search or selection, but at or after the time in which a target is detected (Shulman *et al.* 2001). This result is inconsistent with a role of the cingulate in motivation or endogenous expectancy. Other studies have independently supported a role for the AC in response evaluation and monitoring, a late stage process that follows target detection. For example, Carter *et al.* (2000) found high activity in conditions of response conflict independently of task difficulty. Furthermore, primate (Strick 1988) and human (Picard and Strick 1996) studies have identified multiple functional representations in dorsal AC cortex, near the foci active during attention tasks, recruited during high-level motor planning.

In summary, the current evidence supports a role for human AC in response evaluation and monitoring, and not stimulus selection or motivation (see Fig. 1 below).

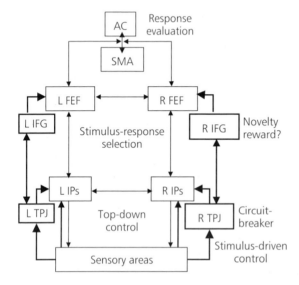

Figure 1 A proposed new model of spatial attention.

Two attentional networks for visual orienting

We have recently identified two regions in human posterior parietal cortex (IPS and TPJ) that are specialized in endogenous orienting and sensory-driven reorienting respectively (Corbetta *et al.* 2000). Here, we show that this distinction extends outside parietal cortex into the frontal lobe, hence identifying two separate attentional networks for visual orienting.

Event-related fMRI evidence for two attentional networks

The paradigm is a modified Posner task. Subjects were shown a small arrow cue at the fovea that predicted the location of a subsequent target with 80 per cent accuracy. A target was then presented at either the cued location (valid target) or the uncued location (invalid target). In some trials, the cue was followed by a 5-s delay and no target was presented. Subjects indicated when they detected a target by pressing a key. The data were analyzed with a linear model that allows the blood-oxygenation-level-dependent (BOLD) signal to be separated for different types of trials and for different intervals within a trial (cue, delay, target detection), while making no a priori assumptions about the shape of the hemodynamic response.

During the cue period (Plate 3(a)), occipital, parietal and frontal regions were active. The signal in IPS (and FEF) was significantly more sustained than in occipital areas (e.g. MT+) (Plate 3(b), upper panel). Therefore, frontal and parietal areas continue to process cue-related information even after the sensory analysis of the stimulus is terminated in the visual system. As subjects direct attention to the target location during the cue period, this sustained signal reflects neural activity for shifting attention. Activity in IPS and FEF was similar in the two hemispheres, independently of the direction of the cue, as expected based on previous studies. However, we also observed evidence of asymmetric spatial coding in the two hemispheres. In the ventral portion of the IPS (near/at V3A/V7), leftward cues produced stronger signals in the right contralateral hemisphere relative to the left ipsilateral hemisphere, whereas rightward cues activated left and right vIPS regions equally (Plate 3(b), lower panel). The same modulation occurred in the dorsal aspect of the FEF cortex. These findings suggest that some regions in IPS and FEF cortex code spatial locations asymmetrically in the two hemispheres. Finally, IPS and FEF were the only brain regions in which the signal remained sustained for the 7-s delay period in which subjects maintained attention onto a peripheral location (not shown). In summary, a striking overlap exists between IPS–FEF areas involved in shifting attention and in maintaining attention onto a location.

Parietal and frontal regions involved in directing attention to a location during the cue period re-activated when a target was detected during the target period (e.g. vIPS, aIPS in lower panel of Plate 3(a)). Therefore these regions are also involved in target and/or response selection. In addition, a novel set of associative parietal, temporal, and frontal regions, which were not active during the cue period, were also recruited (e.g. right TPJ) (Plate 3(a), lower panel).

Some of these regions were selectively modulated when subjects reoriented toward unattended visual targets (Plate 4(a)). Most modulated regions were strongly lateralized to the right hemisphere. Some included regions that were uniquely active during the target period, such as the right TPJ and inferior frontal gyrus (IFG) (Plate 4(a)); others were adjacent to the IPS–FEF system (e.g. right aIPS and PrCes, Plate 4(a)).

In all regions, invalid targets produced a stronger and more sustained signal than valid targets (Plate 4(b)). Since the sensory energy of the target was similar for valid and invalid targets, this modulation cannot be related to sensory differences, but to attentional processes involved in reorienting toward novel sensory events. Interestingly, these reorienting processes were independent of the visual field of the target, because contralateral and ipsilateral targets evoked nonsignificantly different responses (Plate 4(b)). This may indicate that reorienting processes were not spatially selective (see below). Finally, the signal time course in IFG was significantly more prolonged than in other regions, and it was not time-locked to the detection of the target (Plate 4(b)). This may indicate that IFG plays a different role in reorienting than other regions (see below).

In summary, this experiment identifies two separate networks that are differentially modulated during visual orienting. A largely bilateral dorsal frontoparietal network (IPS–FEF network) is recruited during cognitive (endogenous) orienting and during target detection. We propose that this network is involved in stimulus-response selection, both endogenous and exogenous. A second ventral frontoparietal network (TPJ–IFG network), which is strongly right dominant, is predominantly recruited during target detection, particularly when subjects reorient toward unattended visual targets. We propose that this network is involved in reorienting. Finally, reorienting toward unattended stimuli involves the interaction of these two networks in posterior parietal cortex, as illustrated by the recruitment of intraparietal regions (e.g. right aIPS, Plate 4) adjacent to those active during the cue period.

A novel anatomical model of attention

We propose a novel anatomical model of attention that is centered around these two cortical networks (Fig. 1). This model is an evolution of Mesulam's and Posner's models. A dorsal frontoparietal network centered around IPS and FEF mediates stimulus and response selection.

AC is now part of a separate response evaluation system based on its recruitment during response monitoring but not during stimulus or response selection (see above). A separate ventral fronto-parietal network, lateralized to the right hemisphere and centered in TPJ and IFG, mediates alerting a critical component of sensory reorienting. The interaction between IPS and TPJ is critical for explaining the functional interaction between orienting (exogenous, endogenous) and vigilance/arousal. This model provides an anatomical framework to explain some of the inconsistencies between brain imaging and neuropsychology, and a novel interpretation of the hemispheric asymmetries in unilateral spatial neglect.

Functional organization of dorsal frontoparietal network (IPS–FEF)

Stimulus selection

Support for the importance of IPS–FEF in stimulus selection comes from a large number of brain imaging studies (Corbetta and Shulman 1998; Kanwisher and Wojciulik 2000). Specifically, this network is involved in encoding and maintaining cognitive expectations about visual attributes and objects (Kastner *et al.* 1999; Shulman *et al.* 1999*a*). In addition, these areas are involved in visual working memory (rehearsal) (Courtney *et al.* 1996, 1998; Smith *et al.* 1998; Shulman *et al.* 1999*b*) (see also the results of our experiment).

This network is also involved in applying visual expectations to the analysis of incoming stimuli. IPS and FEF are active during visual search and are modulated by target detection (Shulman *et al.* 2001). Interestingly, modulations related to target detection do not occur only in parietal and frontal areas, but also in lower-level visual occipital areas. Since detection requires an interaction between expectation signals and incoming visual information, the IPS–FEF system may be critical for the integration and functional linkage of top-down and bottom-up signals. This linkage may be mediated by feedback projections that reciprocally connect IPS, but not FEF, to multiple visual areas (Lewis and Van Essen 2000) (top-down–bottom-up interaction in Fig. 1). The role of IPS and FEF in the representation of salient sensory stimuli is also strongly supported by single unit studies (Colby and Goldberg 1999; Thompson and Schall 1999). Finally, neural modulation in IPS–FEF during stimulus detection/recognition has been associated to conscious visual processing (Beck *et al.* 2001; Lumer *et al.* 1998).

Response selection

The second important function of the IPS–FEF network is the selection of an appropriate response. This claim is indirectly supported by the strong overlap of areas involved in stimulus selection and those involved in basic sensory–motor transformations like planning and executing an eye or pointing-hand movement to a visual target (Corbetta *et al.* 1998; Connolly *et al.* 2000). Furthermore, neuronal activity in IPS subdivisions has been linked to planning a response by eye or hand movements (Snyder *et al.* 1997). Finally, lesion data support the importance of human parietal cortex in response selection (Goodale *et al.* 1991; Mattingley *et al.* 1998).

Hemispheric organization

The IPS–FEF network is bilaterally active during endogenous orienting toward lateralized stimuli. These findings are inconsistent with its postulated right-hemisphere lateralization during spatial attention (Mesulam 1999). However, in two regions—the ventral sector of IPS (vIPS), corresponding to human V3A/V7, and at the intersection of superior frontal sulcus and precentral sulcus (dorsal FEF)—we clearly see evidence of an asymmetric representation of space, with right-hemisphere regions coding for both contralateral and ipsilateral locations. A similar effect was observed near V3A/V7 in another study (Hopfinger *et al.* 2000). It is possible that these asymmetries may partly contribute to the strong predominance of left hemineglect following right-hemisphere lesions.

A right-hemisphere lateralization may emerge under conditions of exogenous orienting (Nobre *et al.* 1997; Kim *et al.* 1999) or during reorienting toward unattended stimuli (this experiment). This right-hemisphere lateralization may be accounted for by stronger ipsilateral connections between alerting mechanisms in the right TPJ (see below) and ipsilateral IPS (Fig. 1). A predominant right-hemisphere activation of the IPS–FEF network during sensory orienting may explain why normal subjects consistently show a leftward bias in perceptual tasks involving the analysis of sensory stimuli (Reuter-Lorenz *et al.* 1990). It may also explain why maneuvers designed to improve vigilance and alerting (which activate the right inferior parietal cortex) transiently improve leftward orienting in neglect patients (Robertson 1999).

Functional organization of ventral frontoparietal network (right TPJ–IFG)

While selective stimulus processing strongly correlates with activation of the dorsal IPS–FEF system network, reorienting toward novel sensory events engages more ventral parietal and frontal regions, including right TPJ cortex and IFG. We propose that these regions form a network specialized in sensory-driven reorienting. This network has also been identified by Arrington *et al.* (2000) during similar paradigms.

Many putative processes orchestrate the reallocation of attention toward a novel object. Ongoing sensory–motor processes are interrupted, the focus of processing (attention) is disengaged from the current location and redirected toward a new location, and the novel target is identified and its behavioral valence assessed. The main function of this ventral network during orienting is to work as a circuit breaker which interrupts selective processing in the more dorsal IPS–FEF system when a novel relevant stimulus is detected in the visual field. The signal generated in the ventral network reorients the IPS–FEF network to re-map spatially the novel stimulus location. The same network may be important for reallocation of attentional resources after detection of a relevant stimulus.

Right temporoparietal junction

The signal generated in right TPJ may be related to the computation of a novel target location, or it may represent a nonspatial alerting signal informing the dorsal IPS–FEF system of the presence of a novel behaviorally relevant sensory event. Orienting deficits after TPJ damage are directionally selective consistently with the generation of a spatial signal. In fact, right TPJ damage impairs the allocation of attention from the right to the left visual field, while left TPJ damage causes the opposite deficit (Posner *et al.* 1984; Friedrich *et al.* 1998). This directional selectivity was not observed in the BOLD response in right TPJ, which was comparable for targets in left and right visual field. The independence of the BOLD response from target location is more consistent with TPJ generating an alerting signal.

Other results support the notion that right TPJ is more of a 'sentinel' than a spatial processor, and that its activation relates to an alerting signal. Brain imaging studies of vigilance robustly activate the right TPJ (and IFG) (Pardo *et al.* 1991). The detection of oddball targets, which reliably cause vigilance/alerting fluctuations, reliably recruits the right TPJ (and right IFG) (Downar *et al.* 2000). This activity is independent of the location of the target and is time-locked to its detection. Finally, TPJ damage causes the loss of an evoked electrical potential (P300b) that is triggered by the detection of novel stimuli presented at the fovea (Knight and Scabini 1998).

The lateralization of alerting systems to the right TPJ is also supported by anatomical data. Norepinephrine (noradrenaline) terminals from the locus coeruleus (thought to be involved in vigilance) are most densely concentrated in the visual system in the inferior parietal lobule, part of the TPJ region (Aston-Jones *et al.* 1984). Moreover, norepinephrine is more concentrated in the right (than the left) pulvinar of the human brain, a thalamic nucleus that projects to the inferior parietal lobule (Oke *et al.* 1978).

In summary, TPJ plays a critical role in alerting (Fig. 1). We propose that the directional deficit observed after TPJ injury may reflect the loss of facilitatory inputs to neighboring IPS representations, whose imbalance in turn generates a directional spatial bias. This explanation may account for some of the processing deficits observed in neglect (see below).

Inferior frontal gyrus

The other region consistently active during reorienting is the IFG and orbitofrontal cortex. Nobre *et al.* (1999) reported bilateral orbitofrontal activation in blocks of trials containing a high percentage of invalid targets. Arrington *et al.* (2000) recorded higher activity in right IFG during invalid trials than during valid trials. The active region identified by these authors is identical with our IFG response. Finally, right IFG activity has been reported during detection of oddball targets (Downar *et al.* 2000).

Nobre *et al.* (1999) proposed that their modulation reflected either an inhibition to respond in an expected automatic way, or redirection of a response following a violation of expectation. However, motor inhibition or reprogramming would evoke signals that are time-locked to the detection of the unattended target. Instead, IFG manifested a prolonged signal time course that continued after the end of the trial for both valid and invalid targets (Plate 4). Therefore IFG may be involved in more lasting adjustments to a sensory event. We propose that IFG may be involved in reward processes. Reward processes should occur late in the course of a trial. They would not be time-locked to target detection and continue afterwards. Finally, they would be modulated by breaches of expectation (e.g. novelty). This idea is partially supported by the discovery that neurons in orbitofrontal cortex fire at the time of reward and are modulated by reward unpredictability (Tremblay and Schultz 2000). In addition, damage to prefrontal regions abolishes novelty-related evoked potentials (Daffner *et al.* 2000).

Right-hemisphere lateralization

A striking feature of this network is its right-hemisphere lateralization. TPJ was strongly right dominant, and relative lateralization was observed in the insula/IFG during reorienting. As earlier indicated, reorienting also produced right-hemisphere lateralization of more dorsal IPS regions. Other studies support right-hemisphere lateralization of TPJ and IFG during stimulus-driven selection (Arrington *et al.* 2000; Downar *et al.* 2000). This lateralization accounts in large part for the clinical lateralization of neglect (see below).

Functional interactions between right TPJ–IFG and IPS–FEF networks

In healthy individuals, dorsal and ventral orienting systems operate interactively, depending on the mode in which a visual task is performed. Under conditions in which advance information is available, stimulus-response selection is controlled by the dorsal IPS–FEF system. Target detection triggers selective activity in both dorsal and ventral systems. While dorsal signals may be related to conscious processing of the target, activity in the ventral system provides an 'alerting' signal to indicate that the anticipated event has occurred. This may lead to reallocation of attentional resources, and stimulus evaluation in terms of reward processes in the inferior frontal cortex.

However, when a target occurs at an unexpected location, alerting signals in the ventral fronto-parietal system signal to the dorsal system that something worth localizing/detecting has occurred. In order to be informative this signal must contain some spatial information, probably linked to peripheral sensory representation where novel events typically occur. However, the current evidence indicates that spatially selective signals necessary to re-map the new stimulus accurately are hosted in more dorsal IPS–FEF regions.

It is also possible that the ventral TPJ–IFG network is responsible for orienting based on saliency in the visual scene, when we have no specific instruction or current goal requiring attention to a particular object or location. In natural conditions, in the absence of explicit goals or expectations, visual perception is guided by the competitive interaction between low-level features in early visual areas (Desimone and Duncan 1995). It is possible that the TPJ works as a detector of saliency or novelty in the environment.

Two attentional networks and the pathophysiology of neglect

Our model explains some of the discrepancies between neuropsychological studies of neglect and brain imaging studies of visuospatial attention, and provides novel information on the pathophysiology of neglect.

First, the location and hemispheric asymmetry of the exogenous alerting network (particularly the components in TPJ and IFG) nicely matches the location and right-hemisphere dominance of lesions that frequently produce neglect. Therefore neglect must reflect in large part the dysfunction of an alerting mechanism localized in right TPJ. Accordingly, at the acute stage, patients with neglect have problems with vigilance and arousal. As vigilance and arousal improve, deficits in attentional orienting typically become more evident. Another important explanation of the hemispheric asymmetry of neglect is the discovery that some parietal (vIPS) and frontal (dorsal FEF) regions code space asymmetrically in the two hemispheres.

Second, the localization of cognitive-driven orienting mechanisms in IPS explains why patients with SPL/IPS damage cannot properly utilize advance information to select stimulus location. Accordingly, neurons in IPS display not only signals related to endogenous spatial selections, but also signals related to probabilistic reward (Platt and Glimcher 1999).

Third, the proposed interactions between TPJ and IPS may explain why orienting to sensory stimuli is more impaired than voluntary orienting in neglect patients, particularly when competing stimuli are present on the contralesional side. This fact is well known to therapists, who use cognitive cues (e.g. the verbal instruction 'pay attention to the left') to train patients to overcome their neglect of contralesional stimuli. The disruption of exogenous alerting mechanisms in neglect patients with TPJ lesions leads a decreased alerting input to the ipsilateral dorsal IPS–FEF system. This in turn leads to decreased spatial orienting and ineffective selection of left-sided contralesional stimuli. The activation by verbal cues may transiently recruit endogenous orienting mechanisms in the ipsilateral IPS–FEF system, and transiently improve the deficit. However, these voluntary mechanisms are unable to maintain normal attention to the left visual field in the absence of a normally functioning right TPJ, and a potentially disinhibited left TPJ, particularly in the presence of attention-grabbing stimuli in the right visual field.

Fourth, the same functional interaction between TPJ and IPS may also explain why increasing the level of alertness either through sensory cues or self-instructions can improve left-sided attention in neglect patients. Activation of residual alerting mechanisms in right TPJ will increase the drive of ipsilateral IPS–FEF network and thus rebalance the spatial bias.

Finally, neglect patients manifest a characteristic sensory–motor bias toward the right side. Therefore they tend to orient and respond more easily ipsilesionally than contralesionally, particularly when stimuli appear simultaneously in both visual fields. We postulate that this spatiomotor imbalance relates to a functional/anatomical dysfunction of the more dorsal IPS and FEF system. Lesions near/at right TPJ may directly or functionally inactivate the ipsilateral IPS–FEF system. The inactivation of ipsilateral IPS–FEF leads to decreased attention/action to contralateral stimuli. This effect may be compounded by the asymmetric coding of space in vIPS and FEF, as well as by a relative disinhibition of contralateral IPS–FEF with secondary exacerbation of directional biases toward the right space (Kinsbourne 1977).

Conclusions

In summary, the human brain contains two separate neural systems for visual orienting: a 'dorsal' frontoparietal network centered in IPS and FEF responsible for stimulus-response selection, and a more 'ventral' frontoparietal network centered in TPJ and IFG, strongly lateralized to the right hemisphere, which mediates alerting. The two systems interact during normal behavior, and can be selectively damaged by different lesions in the brain. IPS and FEF lesions impair voluntary orienting, whereas TPJ and inferior frontal lesions impair sensory orienting and vigilance. An important issue is how the symptoms of unilateral spatial neglect relate to the dysfunction of these two orienting networks. We suggest that unilateral spatial neglect reflects malfunctioning of both networks through the disruption of the normal interactive processes that regulate the function of these two attentional systems.

References

Arrington, C. M., Carr, T. H., Mayer, A. R., and Rao, S. M. (2000). Neural mechanisms of visual attention, object-based selection of a region in space. *Journal of Cognitive Neuroscience*, **12**, 106–17.

Aston-Jones, G., Foote, S. L., and Bloom, F. E. (1984). Anatomy and physiology of locus ceruleus neurons, functional implications. In *Frontiers of clinical neuroscience*, Vol. 2 (ed. M. G. Ziegler). Williams & Wilkins, Baltimore, MD.

Beck, D. M., Rees, G., Frith, C. D., and Lavie, N. (2001). Neural correlates of change detection and change blindness. *Nature Neuroscience*, **4**, 645–50.

Bisiach, E., Geminiani, G., Berti, A., and Rusconi, M. L. (1990). Perceptual and premotor factors of unilateral neglect. *Neurology*, **40**, 1278–81.

Carter, C. S., Macdonald, A. M., Botvinick, M., *et al.* (2000). Parsing executive processes, strategic vs. evaluative functions of the anterior cingulate cortex. *Proceedings of the National Academy of Sciences of the United States of America*, **97**, 1944–8.

Colby, C. L. and Goldberg, M. E. (1999). Space and attention in parietal cortex. *Annual Review of Neuroscience*, **22**, 319–49.

Connolly, J. D., Goodale, M. A., Desouza, J. F., Menon, R. S., and Vilis, T. (2000). A comparison of frontoparietal fMRI activation during anti-saccades and anti-pointing. *Journal of Neurophysiology*, **84**, 1645–55.

Corbetta, M. (1998). Frontoparietal cortical networks for directing attention and the eye to visual locations, identical, independent, or overlapping neural systems. *Proceedings of the National Academy of Sciences of the United States of America*, **95**, 831–8.

Corbetta, M. and Shulman, G. L. (1998). Human cortical mechanisms of visual attention during orienting and search. *Philosophical Transactions of the Royal Society of London, B 353*, 1353–62.

Corbetta, M., Miezin, F. M., Dobmeyer, S., Shulman, G. L., and Petersen, S. E. (1991). Selective and divided attention during visual discriminations of shape, color, and speed: functional anatomy by positron emission tomography. *Journal of Neuroscience*, **11**, 2383–402.

Corbetta, M., Miezin, F. M., Shulman, G. L., and Petersen, S. E. (1993). A PET study of visuospatial attention. *Journal of Neuroscience*, **13**, 1202–26.

Corbetta, M., Akbudak, E., Conturo, T. E., *et al.* (1998). A common network of functional areas for attention and eye movements. *Neuron*, **21**, 761–73.

Corbetta, M., Kincade, J. M., Ollinger, J. M., McAvoy, M. P., and Shulman, G. L. (2000). Voluntary orienting is dissociated from target detection in human posterior parietal cortex. *Nature Neuroscience*, **3**, 292–7.

Corbetta, M. and Shulman, G. L. (2002). Control of goal-directed and stimulus-driven attention in the brain. *Nature Review Neuroscience*, **3**, 201–15.

Courtney, S. M., Maisog, J. M., Ungerleider, L. G., and Haxby, J. V. (1996). Extrastriate and frontal contribution to face and location working memory, an fMRI study. *Society for Neuroscience* Abstracts, **22**, 968.

Courtney, S. M., Petit, L., Maisog, J. M., Ungerleider, L. G., and Haxby, J. V. (1998). An area specialized for spatial working memory in human frontal cortex. *Science*, **279**, 1347–51.

Critchley, M. (1953). *The parietal lobes*. Edward Arnold, London.

Daffner, K. R., Mesulam, M. M., Scinto, L. F., *et al.* (2000). The central role of the prefrontal cortex in directing attention to novel events. *Brain*, **123**, 927–39.

Damasio, A. R. and Benton, A. L. (1979). Impairment of hand movements under visual guidance. *Neurology*, **29**, 170–8.

Desimone, R. and Duncan, J. (1995). Neural mechanisms of selective visual attention. In Cowan M., editor. *Annual Review of Neuroscience*, **18**, 193–222.

Downar, J., Crawley, A. P., Mikulis, D. J., and Davis, K. D. (2000). A multimodal cortical network for the detection of changes in the sensory environment. *Nature Neuroscience*, **3**, 277–83.

Friedrich, F. J., Egly, R., Rafal, R. D., and Beck, D. (1998). Spatial attention deficits in humans, a comparison of superior parietal and temporal–parietal junction lesions. *Neuropsychology*, **12**, 193–207.

Goodale, M. A., Milner, A. D., Jakobson, L. S., and Carey, D. P. (1991). A neurological dissociation between perceiving objects and grasping them. *Nature*, **349**, 154–6.

Heilman, K. M. and Valenstein, E. (1972). Frontal lobe neglect in man. *Neurology*, **22**, 660–4.

Heilman, K. M. and Watson, R. T. (1977). The neglect syndrome—a unilateral defect of the orienting response. In *Lateralization in the nervous system* (ed. S. Harnad, R. W. Doty, L. Goldstein, J. Jaynes, and G. Krauthamer), pp. 285–302. Academic Press, New York.

Henik, A., Rafal, R., and Rhodes, D. (1994). Endogenously generated and visually guided saccades after lesions of the human frontal eye fields. *Journal of Cognitive Neuroscience*, **6**, 400–11.

Hopfinger, J. B., Buonocore, M. H., and Mangun, G. R. (2000). The neural mechanisms of top-down attentional control. *Nature Neuroscience*, **3**, 284–91.

Husain, M. and Kennard, C. (1996). Visual neglect associated with frontal lobe infarction. *Journal of Neurology*, **243**, 652–7.

James, W. (1890). *Principles of Psychology*, Vol 1. Henry Holt, New York.

Kanwisher, N. and Wojciulik, E. (2000). Visual attention, insights from brain imaging. *Nature Reviews Neuroscience*, **1**, 91–100.

Karnath, H.-O., Ferber, S., and Himmelbach, M. Spatial awareness is a function of the temporal not the posterior parietal lobe. *Nature*, **411**, 950–3.

Kastner, S., Pinsk, M. A., De Weerd, P., Desimone, R., and Ungerleider, L. G. (1999). Increased activity in human visual cortex during directed attention in the absence of visual stimulation. *Neuron*, **22**, 751–61.

Kim, Y. H., Gitelman, D. R., Nobre, A. C., Parrish, T. B., LaBar, K. S., and Mesulam, M. M. (1999). The large-scale neural network for spatial attention displays multifunctional overlap but differential asymmetry. *Neuroimage*, **9**, 269–77.

Kinsbourne, M. (1977). Hemi-neglect and hemisphere rivalry. In *Hemi-inattention and hemispheric specialization*, Vol. 18 (ed. E. A. Weinstein and R. L. Friedland), pp. 41–52. Raven Press, New York.

Knight, R. T. and Scabini, D. (1998). Anatomic bases of event-related potentials and their relationship to novelty and detection in humans. *Journal of Clinical Neurophysiology*, **15**, 3–13.

Laplane, D., Degos, J. D., Baulac, M., and Gray, F. (1981). Bilateral infarction of the anterior cingulate gyri and of the fornices. Report of a case. *Journal of Neurological Science*, **51**, 289–300.

Latto, R. and Cowey, A. (1971). Visual field defects after frontal eye-field lesions in monkeys. *Brain Research*, **30**, 1–24.

Le, T. H., Pardo, J. V., and Hu, X. (1998). 4T-fMRI study of nonspatial shifting of selective attention, cerebellar and parietal contributions. *Journal of Neurophysiology*, **79**, 1535–48.

Lewis, J. W. and Van Essen, D. C. (2000). Corticocortical connections of visual, sensorimotor, and multimodal processing areas in the parietal lobe of the macaque monkey. *Journal of Comparative Neurology*, **428**, 112–37.

Losier, B. J. W. and Klein, R. M. (2001). A review of the evidence for a disengage deficit following parietal lobe damage. *Neuroscience and Biobehavioral Reviews*, **25**, 1–13.

Lumer, E. D., Friston, K. J., and Rees, G. (1998). Neural correlates of perceptual rivalry in the human brain. *Science*, **280**, 1930–4.

Luna, B., Thulborn, K. R., Strojwas, M. H., *et al.* (1998). Dorsal cortical regions subserving visually-guided saccades in humans: an fMRI study. *Cerebral Cortex*, **8**, 40–7.

Mattingley, J. B., Husain, M., Rorden, C., Kennard, C., and Driver J. (1998). Motor role of human inferior parietal lobe revealed in unilateral neglect patients. *Nature*, **392**, 179–82.

Mesulam, M.-M. (1981). A cortical network for directed attention and unilateral neglect. *Annals of Neurology*, **10**, 309–25.

Mesulam, M.-M. (1999). Spatial attention and neglect, parietal, frontal and cingulate contributions to the mental representation and attentional targeting of salient extrapersonal events. *Philosophical Transactions of the Royal Society of London B 354*, 1325–46.

Mesulam, M.-M. and Mufson, E. (1982). Insula of the old world monkey. I: Architectonics in the insulo-orbito-temporal component of the paralimbic brain. *Journal of Comparative Neurology*, **212**, 1–22.

Morrow, L. A. and Ratcliff, G. (1988). The disengagement of covert attention and the neglect syndrome. *Psychobiology*, **16**, 261–9.

Nobre, A. C., Sebestyen, G. N., Gitelman, D. R., Mesulam, M.-M., Frackowiack, R. S. J., and Frith, C. D. (1997). Functional localization of the system for visuospatial attention using positron emission tomography. *Brain*, **120**, 515–33.

Nobre, A. C., Coull, J. T., Frith, C. D., and Mesulam, M.-M. (1999). Orbitofrontal cortex is activated during breaches of expectation in tasks of visual attention. *Nature Neuroscience*, **2**, 11–12.

Nobre, A. C., Gitelman, D. R., Dias, E. C., and Mesulam, M.-M. (2000). Covert visual spatial orienting and saccades: overlapping neural systems. *Neuroimage*, **11**, 210–16.

Norman, D. A. and Shallice, T. (1985). Attention to action: willed and automatic control of behavior. In *Consciousness and self-regulation*, pp. 1–18. Plenum Press, New York.

Ochsner, K. N., Kosslyn, S. M., Cosgrove, G. R., *et al.* (2001). Deficits in visual cognition and attention following bilateral anterior cingulotomy. *Neuropsychologia*, **39**, 219–30.

Oke, A., Keller, R., Mefford, I., and Adams, R. N. (1978). Lateralization of norepinephrine in human thalamus. *Science*, **200**, 1411–13.

Parasuraman, R., Warm, J. S., and See, J. E. (1998). Brain systems of vigilance. In *The attentive brain* (ed. R. Parasuraman), pp. 221–56. MIT Press, Cambridge, MA.

Pardo, J. V., Pardo, P. J., Janer, K. W., and Raichle, M. E. (1990). The anterior cingulate cortex mediates processing selection in the Stroop attentional conflict paradigm. *Proceedings of the National Academy of Sciences of the United States of America*, **87**, 256–9.

Pardo, J. V., Fox, P. T., and Raichle, M. E. (1991). Localization of a human system for sustained attention by positron emission tomography. *Nature*, **349**, 61–4.

Petersen, S. E., Robinson, D. L., and Morris, J. D. (1987). Contributions of the pulvinar to visual spatial attention. *Neuropsychologia* Abstracts, **25**, 97–105.

Picard, N. and Strick, P. L. (1996). Motor areas of the medial wall, a review of their location and functional activation. *Cerebral Cortex*, **6**, 342–53.

Platt, M. L. and Glimcher, P. W. (1999). Neural correlates of decision variables in parietal cortex. *Nature*, **400**, 233–8.

Posner, M. I. (1980). Orienting of attention. *Quarterly Journal of Experimental Psychology*, **32**, 3–25.

Posner, M. I. and Dehaene, S. (1994). Attentional networks. *Trends in Neurosciences*, **17**, 75–9.

Posner, M. I. and Petersen, S. E. (1990). The attention system of the human brain. *Annual Review of Neuroscience*, **13**, 25–42.

Posner, M. I., Walker, J. A., Friedrich, F. J., and Rafal, R. D. (1984). Effects of parietal injury on covert orienting of attention. *Journal of Neuroscience*, **4**, 1863–74.

Reuter-Lorenz, P. A., Kinsbourne, M., and Moscovitch, M. (1990). Hemispheric control of spatial attention. *Brain and Cognition*, **12**, 240–66.

Robertson, I. H. (1999). Cognitive rehabilitation, attention and neglect. *Trends in Cognitive Sciences*, **3**, 385–93.

Shulman, G. L., Ollinger, J. M., Akbudak, E., *et al.* (1999*a*). Areas involved in encoding and applying directional expectations to moving objects. *Journal of Neuroscience*, **19**, 9480–96.

Shulman, G. L., Ollinger, J. M., Petersen, S. E., *et al.* (1999*b*). Effects of cue duration on cued motion detection studied with event-related fMRI. *Society for Neuroscience Abstracts*, **25**, 2.

Shulman, G. L., Ollinger, J. M., Linenweber, M., Petersen, S. E., and Corbetta, M. (2001). Multiple neural correlates of detection in the human brain. *Proceedings of the National Academy of Sciences of the United States of America*, **98**, 313–18.

Smith, E. E., Jonides, J., Marshuetz, C., and Koeppe, R. (1998). Components of verbal working memory: evidence from neuroimaging. *Proceedings of the National Academy of Sciences of the United States of America*, **95**, 876–82.

Snyder, L. H., Batista, A. P., and Andersen, R. A. (1997). Coding of intention in the posterior parietal cortex. *Nature*, **386**, 167–70.

Strick, P. L. (1988). Anatomical organization of multiple motor areas in the frontal lobe: implications for recovery of function. *Advances in Neurology*, **47**, 293–312.

Tegner, R. and Levander, M. (1991). Through a looking glass. A new technique to demonstrate directional hypokinesia in unilateral neglect. *Brain*, **114**, 1943–51.

Thompson, T. G. and Schall, J. D. (1999). The detection of visual signals by macaque frontal eye field during masking. *Nature Neuroscience*, **2**, 283–8.

Tremblay, L. and Schultz, W. (2000). Reward-related neuronal activity during go-nogo task performance in primate orbitofrontal cortex. *Journal of Neurophysiology*, **83**, 1864–76.

Vallar, G. and Perani, D. (1987). The anatomy of spatial neglect in humans. In *Neurophysiological and neuropsychological aspects of spatial neglect* (ed. M. Jeannerod), pp. 235–58. North-Holland, Amsterdam.

Vandenberghe, R., Duncan, J., Dupont, P., *et al.* (1997). Attention to one or two features in left and right visual field, a positron emission tomography study. *Journal of Neuroscience*, **17**, 3739–50.

Vandenberghe, R., Duncan, J., Arnell, K. M., *et al.* (2000). Maintaining and shifting attention within left or right hemifield. *Cerebral Cortex*, **10**, 706–13.

Wilkins, A. J., Shallice, T., and McCarthy, R. (1987). Frontal lesions and sustained attention. *Neuropsychologia*, **25**, 359–65.

Wojciulik, E. and Kanwisher, N. (1999). The generality of parietal involvement in visual attention. *Neuron*, **23**, 747–64.

Wurtz, R. H., Richmond, B. J., and Newsome, W. T. (1984). Modulation of cortical visual processing by attention, perception, and movement. In *Dynamic aspects of neocortical functions* (ed. G. M. Edelman, W. E. Gall, and W. M. Cowan), pp. 195–217. Wiley, New York.

5.4 Mapping spatial attention with reaction time in neglect patients

Carlo A. Marzi, Elina Natale, and Britt Anderson

Patients with hemineglect as a result of a cortical lesion, often centered on the right inferior parietal and the superior temporal lobe (Karnath *et al.* 2001), are characterized by a profound unawareness of the contralesional (left) space. This impairment may concern not only various sensory modalities but also the mental representation of space (Bisiach 1993) and the intention to move in contralesional space (Driver and Mattingley 1998).

Most theories of neglect concur that there is an attentional imbalance favoring the ipsilesional space although the characteristics of such imbalance differ among the various theories (Weintraub and Mesulam 1987; Kinsbourne 1993; Heilman *et al.* 2000). Heilman's and Mesulam's theories can be defined as 'hemispatial' in that they posit that the right, but not the left, hemisphere has a representation of both sides of space and therefore a lesion of the right hemisphere inevitably results in neglect of the left hemispace which remains unrepresented in the brain. The idea of a 'dominance' of the right hemisphere for attention is widely accepted and has recently received support from functional imaging evidence in normal humans. These data show that the right hemisphere is engaged in attentional operations anywhere in the visual field, while the left hemisphere subserves only contralateral attentional operations (Corbetta *et al.* 1993; Nobre *et al.* 1997; Kim *et al.* 1999). Further, Gitelman *et al.* (1999) found that, although their task required attention to be equally shifted to the left and the right hemifields, most of the normal participants employed in the study showed a greater area of activation in the right parietal cortex, consistent with the specialization of the right hemisphere for spatial attention. By the same token, Perry and Zeki (2000) recently found that the right supramarginal gyrus, but not the left, was activated when subjects responded to peripheral stimuli on either side with a saccadic eye movement or a covert attentional shift. Finally, Corbetta *et al.* (2000) have found that the functional MRI (fMRI) response of the right temporal–parietal junction was always stronger than its left counterpart regardless of the hemisphere to which the stimulus was initially presented.

These 'hemispatial' theories of neglect make two predictions as far as distribution of spatial attention in the visual field is concerned.

- There should be a discontinuity at the vertical meridian with attentional deployment sharply decreasing as one moves contralesionally while steadily increasing ipsilesionally.
- There should be an attentional impairment in the ipsilesional field as well given that in this hemifield attentional deployment is now subserved by the left hemisphere only rather than by both hemispheres as in the intact brain.

Furthermore, the left hemisphere has been shown to be less involved in spatial attention than the right hemisphere and this adds to the ipsilesional impairment.

A more detailed version of a hemispatial theory has been provided by Anderson (1996) with a saliency model originally developed to account for the line bisection behavior of neglect patients. According to this model, saliency is mapped to spatial position in the brain and the overall map is the sum of the saliency maps of the two hemispheres. These maps are asymmetric, being magnified in the right hemisphere which is dominant for attentional functions and in which both contra- and ipsilateral hemispaces are represented while only contralateral hemispace is represented in the left hemisphere. A lesion of the right hemisphere modifies the overall saliency map which becomes characterized by two smaller saliency peaks, one corresponding to the center of the visual field and the other an ipsilesional off-center peak corresponding to the saliency peak of the left hemisphere. A neurophysiological counterpart of the hemispatial type of model can be found in recent proposals by Pouget and coworkers (Pouget *et al.* 1999; Pouget and Driver 2000) that the location of the receptive fields of monkey's posterior parietal neurons, which are important for visuospatial behavior, can explain the distribution of attention in hemineglect. These neurons have receptive fields located in both the contra- and ipsilateral visual fields, but the percentage of neurons of a given hemisphere with receptive fields in the ipsilateral hemifield declines as one goes from central to more peripheral field locations. This is true for areas V6A, VIP, and MST, while a more or less strict contralateral representation is present in V1, V2, V3, V3A, MT, LIP, and V6 (C. Galletti, personal communication). Therefore, if this organization can be extended to the human parietal cortex, following lesion of the right hemisphere, the perceptual impairment in the left hemifield should become progressively worse from center to periphery. This is exactly what has been found by Smania *et al.* (1998) in their study using brief visual stimuli presented at various eccentricities across the horizontal meridian of the visual field of neglect patients. They found that the percentage of stimuli that failed to be detected increased sharply in the contralesional field from central to peripheral field locations. In contrast, the percentage of misses was overall smaller in the ipsilesional hemifield and the slope of the eccentricity-detection performance was shallower than in the contralesional field. In addition to a contralesional–ipsilesional gradient in performance, the models of both Anderson (1996) and Pouget *et al.* (1999) predict the presence of an off-center peak of attentional deployment in the ipsilesional hemifield, i.e. in the right hemifield of right-hemisphere-lesioned neglect patients. This is because the saliency peak in the intact left hemisphere in Anderson's model or the most represented portion of the visual field in posterior parietal neurons in Pouget *et al.*'s model do not correspond to the center of the visual field but to an area well within the ipsilesional hemifield. An ipsilesional off-center peak of attentional deployment in the visual field of neglect patients has been found by Karnath (1997), and has been interpreted as related to an ipsilesional shift in the subjective vertical midline which normally coincides with the central vertical meridian. As a consequence, neglect patients tend to explore the visual space more frequently off-center than normal subjects. This result fits with the observation of Barton *et al.* (1998) on ocular search during line bisection and with the off-center ipsilesional peak also found by Smania *et al.* (1998) with manual reaction time (RT). These authors found that in neglect patients RT to lateralized stimuli showed a paradoxical decrease from central to mid-peripheral locations in the ipsilesional hemifield with a peak of faster response around approximately 10° to 20° ipsilesionally. Although the interpretation proposed by the various authors is somewhat different, the consistency of this finding across different studies is remarkable.

In contrast with hemispatial theories, Kinsbourne's theoretical model of neglect (Kinsbourne 1993) proposes that an unopposed vector of the left-hemisphere attentional system drives a subject's attention to the right (Reuter-Lorenz *et al.* 1990). While Kinsbourne did not specify his idea with a mathematical embodiment, others, extrapolating from his theory and their own data, have implied that neglect subjects should show a distortion of spatial attention whereby the processing deficit worsens the more contralesional the target. Bisiach *et al.* (1999*a,b*) have proposed that neglect may involve a Euclidean distortion of space. Further, Bisiach *et al.* (1998) describe a 'relaxation' of space that progressively increases contralaterally to the lesion and contracts ipsilaterally. In another paper by the same group (Bisiach *et al.* 1996), the deficit was predicted to be 'logarithmic.' Milner and colleagues reach a similar conclusion (although intriguingly they describe their postulated deficit as a 'non-Euclidean' distortion), and they conclude that the subjective extent of space is compressed to the left of the lesion, 'the more so in more leftward parts of space' (Harvey *et al.* 1995). Finally, Karnath and Ferber (1999) did not confirm the existence of a subjective space distorsion along the horizontal axis in neglect patients by testing the patients' perception of spatial distance. Regardless of the function that describes the impairment in such models, they predict that there should be no discontinuity at the midline and that subjects with neglect should show a progressive worsening of performance the more leftward one moves, and *they should show a progressive improvement as targets and actions move to the right.* These predictions have not been verified by our RT data (Smania *et al.* 1998), but of course only a formal theory can be verified or disproved by RT data. A competing prediction derived from other computational models of neglect (Anderson 1996) is that the principal focus of attention in neglect subjects should be off-center but should not be monotonically decreasing from right to left.

Here we describe two attempts to cast light on an attentional model of neglect by trying to specify two important aspects. First, we investigate whether the attentional impairment concerns exogenous stimulus-driven attention or endogenous controlled attention. Second, we will try to fit our RT data to the saliency map model of neglect proposed by Anderson (1996), which is a formal model of neglect inspired by clinical data (line bisection).

The overall rationale of our approach depends on the idea that speed of RT (and detection performance) at various locations in the visual field depends on both retinal and attentional factors. In normal subjects the increase in RT with stimulus eccentricity is related to the density distribution of ganglion cells and the cortical magnification factor which decrease on going from central to more peripheral visual field locations (Marzi and Di Stefano 1981; Chelazzi *et al.* 1988). However, it should be noted that the slope of the curve relating RT and eccentricity is strikingly different from the classic acuity curve which depends on the density of cones and as a consequence has a central peak and a sharp fall-off within a few degrees of eccentricity. In contrast, the RT–eccentricity curve does not show a prominent central velocity peak and has a much less abrupt fall-off in speed. This slope fits with the overall density of retinal elements, mainly reflecting the peripheral density distribution of ganglion cells (Marzi and Di Stefano 1981). Therefore it is unlikely that, at least as far as the central portion of visual field is concerned, it reflects the visuotopic organization of primary visual cortex, which has a sharp magnification factor of central vision, but rather reflects the organization of visually responsive posterior parietal and superior temporal areas. In these areas, the magnification of central vision is much less marked than in primary visual cortex. Moreover, the very fact that the slope of the RT–eccentricity function is altered in neglect patients without visual cortical damage (see Smania *et al.* (1998) and the results reported below) supports parietal and temporal areas as substrates for our RT task. On the basis of these considerations, it is reasonable to assume that the pattern of RT responses to stimuli presented along the horizontal meridian reflects the spatial distribution of visual attention, at least as far as stimulus-driven exogenous attention is concerned.

Exogenous versus endogenous attention and neglect

To try and answer the first question we compared detection accuracy and RT for stimuli presented across the visual field in two different attentional conditions: a randomized condition of visual presentation in which brief flashes generated by a light-emitting diode (LED) are presented unpredictably to one of several locations, and a blocked-point condition in which, in a given block of trials, the stimuli are presented to only one location which is always the same. By subtracting RT for a given stimulus location in blocked-point conditions from the RT to the same stimulus under randomized conditions one can ascertain the relative contribution of controlled versus stimulus-driven attention. The assumption is that in the blocked-point condition the subject can focus attention onto the location of the impending stimulus, while in the randomized condition attention is diffuse and is driven onto the correct location by the appearance of the stimulus. If neglect patients are impaired in controlled attention, the difference between the two conditions should be minimal, while if patients are impaired in stimulus-driven attention they should benefit from controlled focused attention.

As a first step, we studied 24 right-handed healthy controls (half females and half males) of comparable age (mean, 58 years; range, 45–78 years) to that of the brain-damaged patients.

The stimuli, consisting of brief LED-generated flashes (10 ms in duration), were presented in one of five positions (5°, 10°, 20°, 30°, and 40°) along the main horizontal meridian in either the left or the right hemifield or in a central position (0°) and in the two conditions of stimulus presentations (blocked-point and randomized). Participants were asked to keep fixation steadily onto a central fixation point and to press a response key with the index finger of the right hand as quickly as possible following stimulus presentation.

Figure 1 shows the mean RT as a function of hemifield, eccentricity of stimulus presentation, and attentional condition. A three-way ANOVA (attentional condition by hemifield by eccentricity) showed a main effect of attentional condition ($F_{(1,23)} = 5.379, p = 0.03$) with the blocked-point condition yielding a faster RT (262 ms) than the randomized condition (274 ms). The main effect of eccentricity was also significant ($F_{(4,92)} = 15.868, p < 0.0001$) with RT increasing as one goes from central to peripheral eccentricities. In contrast, the effect of hemifield was far from significance ($F_{(4,92)} = 108.732, p = 0.677$). No first-order interactions were significant except for attentional condition by eccentricity ($F_{(4,92)} = 2.829, p = 0.029$) with the effect of attentional condition being somewhat larger for peripheral presentations (Fig. 1). It is interesting to note that

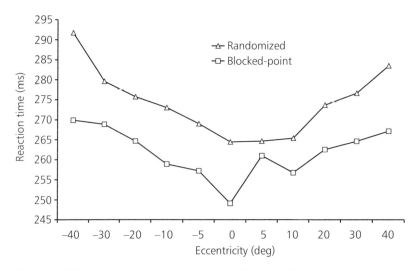

Figure 1 RT under blocked-point and randomized conditions of stimulus presentation at 0°, 5°, 10°, 20°, 30°, and 40° of eccentricity in the left (minus sign on the abscissa) and in the right hemifields of 24 healthy subjects.

the second-order interaction attentional condition by hemifield by eccentricity was not significant ($F_{(4,92)} = 96.263, p = 0.705$), which means that the effect of attentional condition was symmetric across the two hemifields and at the various eccentricities.

As a second step, we studied neglect and control patients (see Table 1 for clinical and demographic details and Table 2 for neuropsychological assessment of neglect) in a task and apparatus similar to that used in the normal subjects. It is important to point out that we selected two neglect patients without hemianopia to avoid the confounding effect of a visual field loss. Controls were two right-brain-damaged patients without neglect or hemianopia and two age-matched healthy controls drawn for comparison purposes from the group of 24 subjects discussed above. Patients used their ipsilesional hand for responding.

We compared both the omission rate (Fig. 2) and the speed of RT (Fig. 3) for the two attentional conditions and the various stimulus locations in either the contra- or the ipsilesional hemifield.

Inspection of Fig. 2, which shows omission rate as a function of hemifield and eccentricity of stimulus presentation, reveals a marked eccentricity-dependent impairment of neglect patients in the contralesional hemifield, while performance is practically faultless in both the brain-damaged and the healthy control groups. Performance in the ipsilesional hemifield (13 per cent of omissions) of neglect patients is better than in the contralesional hemifield (27 per cent of omissions) but is overall worse than in control subjects. More importantly for the present purposes, there is a clear-cut effect of attentional condition with the blocked-point condition yielding a marked improvement of performance in the contralesional hemifield of neglect patients (blocked-point, 20 per cent; randomized, 35 per cent), while there is no effect in the ipsilesional field (blocked-point, 14 per cent; randomized, 12 per cent).

Table 1 Summary of demographic and clinical data for the subject groups

Subject	Age/Sex	Education (years)	Lesion-test (days)	Lesion: side (CT or MRI) and nature
Neglect				
TM	66/F	13	1629	Temporoparietal ischemia
LF	84/M	11	24	Basal ganglia and centrum semiovale ischaemia
Brain-damaged controls				
BC	62/M	5	10	Basal ganglia ischemia
AV	46/M	12	56	Surgical ablation of a ventricular tumor
Healthy controls				
AS	64/F	5		
CM	55/M	19		

Table 2 Patients' performance on neuropsychological assessment of neglect

Patient	Cancellation	Line bisection	Clock dial	Sentence reading	Figure copying
TM	+	NP	NP	–	++
LF	++	+	–	–	–

+, moderate neglect; ++, severe neglect; –, no sign of neglect; NP, not performed.
Test performance used as criterion to classify a patient as suffering from neglect: cancellation, clock dial, sentence reading, and figure copying—at least 15 per cent left-sided targets omitted (++, more than 70 per cent); line bisection—at least 5 per cent of total line lenght leftwards deviated from center (++, more than 20 per cent). To be included in the neglect group a patient had to be impaired in at least two of the above tests.

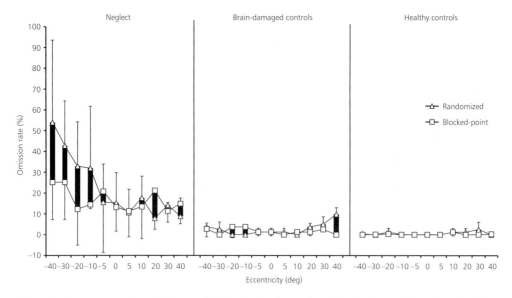

Figure 2   Percentage of omissions under blocked-point and randomized conditions for stimulus presentations at 0°, 5°, 10°, 20°, 30°, and 40° of eccentricity in the left and right hemifields of two neglect patients, two brain-damaged controls, and two healthy controls.

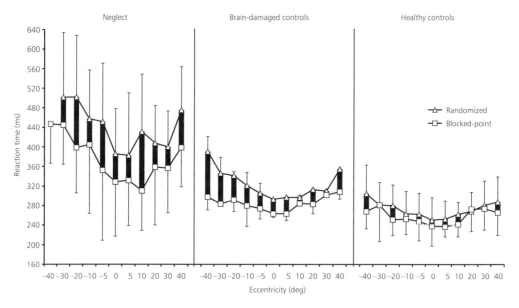

Figure 3   RT under blocked-point and randomized conditions of stimulus presentation at 0°, 5°, 10°, 20°, 30°, and 40° of eccentricity in the left and in the right hemifields of two neglect patients, two brain-damaged controls, and two healthy controls.

   Inspection of Fig. 3, which shows mean RTs for the various stimulus locations, reveals an overall slowing down of neglect patients (406 ms) compared with the other groups (brain-damaged controls, 305 ms; healthy controls, 265 ms). This effect is clearly more pronounced in the contra-lesional hemifield (440 ms) than in the ipsilesional hemifield (385 ms) and is largely eccentricity

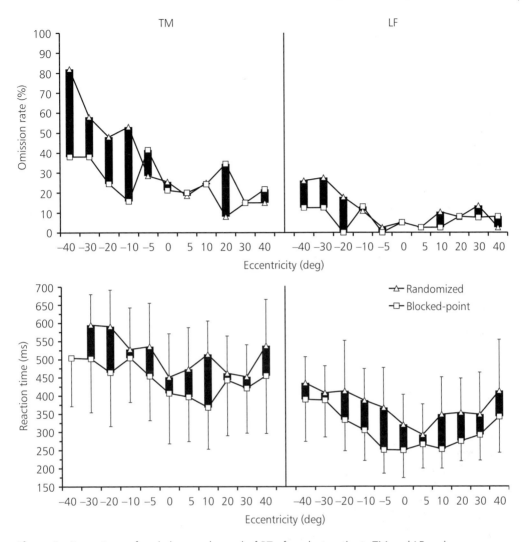

Figure 4 Percentage of omissions and speed of RT of neglect patients TM and LF under blocked-point and randomized conditions of stimulus presentation at 0°, 5°, 10°, 20°, 30°, and 40° of eccentricity in the left and right hemifields.

dependent, becoming increasingly more severe as one goes from central to peripheral locations in the contralesional hemifield. At variance with detection accuracy, the blocked-point condition yielded a similar improvement of performance in both the contralesional and the ipsilesional hemifield. The two neglect patients showed a consistent pattern of results which, despite the small number of patients, reassures on the robustness of the data (Fig. 4).

On the whole, these data confirm previous results (Smania *et al.* 1998) and extend them in two important ways: First, they show that the contralesional impairment in either detection rate or response speed is also present in neglect patients without hemianopia and therefore is likely to be accounted for by attentional rather than by purely sensory factors. Second, neglect patients can benefit from knowing the location of the impending stimuli in the affected hemifield and therefore the bulk of their impairment concerns stimulus-driven rather than controlled attention. This is in keeping with other results showing an impairment of exogenous rather than endogenous attention in neglect patients (Karnath 1988; Làdavas *et al.* 1994; Bartolomeo *et al.* 2001).

Saliency maps and reaction time in neglect

The second question tackled in this chapter is to check the hypothesis of a distortion of the saliency map in neglect patients by using RT as a dependent measure. Various saliency map models of normal visual attention have been proposed (Koch and Ullman 1985; Wolfe 1994; Gottlieb *et al.* 1998; Findlay and Walker 1999; Itti and Koch 2001) but only a few attentional models have been explicitly referred to the behavior of neglect patients (among them, see Pouget and Sejnowski (1997), Mozer (1999), and Chapter 3.2 of this volume). It is important to note that the term 'salience' is operationalized differently in these different models, but they are loosely linked by the idea that there are cognitive maps which influence the allocation of covert attention or eye movements as a prelude to some cognitive operation or behavioral action. Anderson's model has hypothesized a specific functional form for the attentional system: The right-hemisphere salience system is postulated to spread over space bilaterally with the most salient area slightly to the right of body midline. The left-hemisphere salience system is more narrowly focused and centered in contralateral space. Salience can be envisioned as the strength of attraction for the attentional spotlight (Anderson 1999). Because biological distributions often follow a 'bell curve', this functional form, slightly modified, was used as the mathematical instantiation for the salience curves. The presence of the bell-curve form in biological systems is a necessary consequence of the central limit theorem (Hoel *et al.* 1971) and the fact that most complex biological measures reflect the summation of multiple processes with random components. The nomenclature of the salience system (which is used below) can be understood and remembered by considering the 'sf' terms to be scaling factors, the 'sd' terms to be analogous to a standard deviation, and the 'm' terms to represent the means of the distributions. The terms 'r' and 'l' identify the two separate hemispheres. The specific mathematical form of the salience system is the sum of the two separate attentional systems:

$$\text{salience} = \frac{\text{sfl}}{1 + (\text{location} - \text{ml})^2/\text{sdl}^2} + \frac{\text{sfr}}{1 + (\text{location} - \text{mr})^2/\text{sdr}^2}.$$

As part of the evaluation of the present data set, we undertook to fit the subject RT data with a simple linear model, a six-parameter polynomial model, and the salience model. Linear regression is the simplest model and would be the form most consistent with a Euclidean distortion of space. The use of a polynomial regression allows the model to assume a curved shape so that hills of attentional allocation can be detected. It is simply a 'curve-fitting' exercise, but does allow a more direct comparison with the salience model in that both have six free parameters.

All model fitting was done using locally written programs and MATLAB (MathWorks Inc., Natick, MA, USA). Linear, nonlinear, and polynomial regressions followed standard techniques (Graybill and Hariharan 1994). The nonlinear regression was fitted via an iterative Newton–Raphson procedure with initial parameters provided from investigator inspection of the data. In order to be consistent with the underlying theory behind the development of the model, several of the salience model parameters were constrained to positive values (sfl, sfr, sdl, sdr). Additionally, the parameters 'ml' and 'mr' were constrained between −10 and +90 and between −90 and +10 respectively.

Basic regression techniques assume homoscedasticity (equal variance in the dependent measure across all values of the independent measure) and a Gaussian distribution for the dependent variable. It is likely that these assumptions are violated by RT data in general (which often have a skewed distribution) and in neglect subjects in particular (Anderson *et al.* 2000). However, the present data, as the scatter plots demonstrate, did not appear to violate these assumptions seriously and therefore traditional regression techniques, which minimize the squared error of the estimate, were employed. The development of statistical measures for nonlinear regressions are not as fully developed as for linear regression; however, measures of model variance can provide a sense of the relative fitness of one model over another. For comparisons of the different regression fits we used the mean square error as an estimate of variance and its chi-square distribution to calculate 95 per cent confidence intervals. The assumption behind the comparison of model variance is that deviation from a given model can be assessed by the degree to which actual observations differ from the values predicted by the model. The variance of these residual errors is small when the fit is good and larger if the fit is poor. By comparing both the scatter plots and the estimated model variances, a comparison of the different regression models can be made. The RT values have been inverted for model plotting. For each subject, each RT was subtracted from the maximum RT for that subject. This had the effect of making the faster RTs have a greater value on the *y* axis and preserved the ordinal relationships among the RTs. This depiction was felt to be a more natural representation of the salience construct where larger numbers would coincide with greater salience. In the plots, the solid line depicts the salience model, the dotted line shows the linear model, and the broken line shows the polynomial model. Table 3 shows the variance for the linear, fifth-order polynomial, and salience model fits together with the calculated 95 per cent confidence intervals, and Table 4 shows the parameters for the fitting of the salience model.

Table 3 Model variances (with confidence intervals) by subject and condition

Subject	Linear model (95% CI)	Polynomial model (95% CI)	Salience model (95% CI)
Neglect			
TM	124.0 (114.2–135.6)	118.8 (109.4–130.0)	121.1 (111.5–132.5)
LF	114.7 (107.0–123.6)	108.8 (101.4–117.3)	109.9 (102.4–118.4)
Brain-damaged controls			
AV	94.9 (88.9–101.8)	91.6 (85.8–98.3)	92.1 (86.2–98.7)
BC	63.3 (59.4–67.8)	58.7 (55.0–62.9)	59.0 (55.3–63.2)
Healthy controls			
AS	64.7 (60.7–69.4)	61.9 (58.0–66.4)	62.3 (58.4–66.8)
CM	36.9 (34.6–39.6)	35.3 (33.1–37.9)	35.5 (33.3–38.0)

Table 4 Parameters for the fitting of Anderson's salience model by subject

Subject	sfl	ml	sdl	sfr	mr	sdr
Neglect						
TM	329.7	19.6	49.5	25.3	−6.2	10.6
LF	25.6	72.6	6.1	463.2	9.0	74.4
Brain-damaged controls						
AV	144.4	31.8	71.5	343.9	−2.3	91.3
BC	68.1	34.9	1.3	422.2	1.5	92.3
Healthy controls						
AS	459.3	6.3	101.6	85.4	−34.6	2.7
CM	28.5	45.3	13.1	231.4	−2.9	88.0

Subjects TM and LF (left neglect without hemianopia) show the inadequacy of a simple linear model (Fig. 5). Even though the linear regression shows a fit of the proper slope, the scatter plots show that the greatest attentional salience is toward the middle of the spatial field, slightly to the right, and that it decreases in both directions. The linear model cannot capture this behavior, while both the polynomial and salience models do. For both these models, there is 'one hump'. While this could be used as an indictment against the salience model, it may also reflect severe damage to one hemisphere's salience system and the specific focused attentional demands of the RT testing protocol.

The data for AV and BC, the two right-hemisphere-damaged controls, show broad flat curves with peak salience slightly to the right of midline (Fig. 6). In both cases the scaling factors of

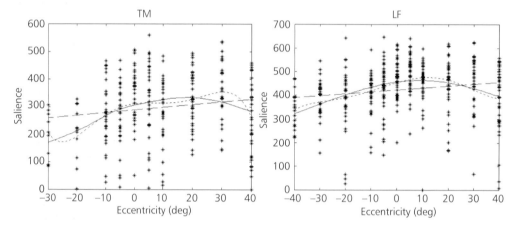

Figure 5 Neglect subjects without hemianopia. This figure shows the fitted curve for the three models in two subjects with neglect. The linear model (dotted line) failed to capture the arched nature of the subjects' salience maps. Both the polynomial model (broken line) and the salience model (solid line) performed better. The plotting conventions are repeated in Figs 6 and 7. The details of converting RT to salience are reported in the text.

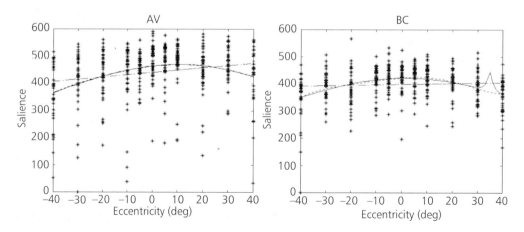

Figure 6 Brain-damaged subjects without neglect or hemianopia. The figure shows the fitted curves and salience data for two subjects without neglect but with right-hemisphere brain damage. Again, the linear model failed to follow the obvious undulating nature of the subjects' salience maps with the downward peripheral curves.

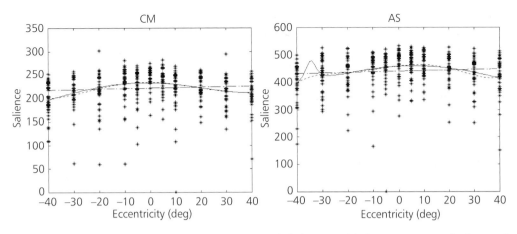

Figure 7 For comparison with Figs 5 and 6 the fits of all three models for two age-matched control subjects are shown. Given the flat salience maps across the visual field tested, all three models provide adequate fits to the data.

the left-hemisphere salience system are less than the right, in accord with theory. Cases CM and AS (normal subjects) are fitted well by all models and do not provide a basis for discriminating among them (Fig. 7).

The RT data from these subjects and the fitted linear, polynomial, and salience models are instructive for evaluating current theories of neglect. First, most theories of neglect, such as those by Bisiach and Milner cited above, explicitly predict that performance worsens the farther to the left the stimulus is presented and improves on going more rightward. This is simply not seen in the current cases and is contradicted by linear models that fit the data from neglect subjects with *negative* slopes, implying less attentional allocation ipsilesionally. Bisiach's expectation of a logarithmic relationship may derive from the power-law-like relationship for the magnitude of errors in line bisection tasks using multiple line lengths. While we did not choose to fit a logarithmic model, the logarithm is a monotonic increasing function so that any fit resulting in poorer allocation of attention to the left would progressively improve to the right. This is not seen in the RT scatter plots or revealed by the polynomial or salience fits. Comparing the parameters of the salience model among the various subjects does not provide a strong case for the specific mathematical form of the salience model, while its ability to capture the general form of subjects' behavior supports the general concepts that underlie the model. Among the cases reported here there is no diagnostic change of parameter values that seems to accompany neglect. The qualitative results from the postulating of two separate salience system and the general characteristics of their spatial distribution are in accord with the behavioral observations. As more empirical data accumulate, it will be necessary to revise the formalism of the model to capture the clinical data better. However, the wide variability of subject RTs in this simple repetitive task suggests an additional challenge. It will also be necessary in future models to include components that can capture the wide variability of neglect subject performance.

These results also show the value of collecting from neglect subjects data of a type and quantity that can be used in the mathematical modelling of neglect behavior. Such collaboration between neglect theory and empirical research will ultimately lead us to a deeper understanding of this important clinical phenomenon. Unfortunately, the analyses so far do not permit a definitive conclusion in favor of any particular theory. They do suggest strongly that a simple linear disturbance of spatial attention is an inadequate model and that using simple curve-fitting programs in the absence of a theoretical rationale is a tenuous practice.

The salience model was a theoretical attempt to account for an unusual behavioral finding, the cross-over effect (Anderson 1997), and it is rewarding that it also seems to be consistent with empirical data derived from other domains and applied to other aspects of neglect behavior. The salience model provided a nice overall fit to the contour of subject data regardless of whether or not the subject had neglect. The fit of the salience model appeared to be as good, on a statistical level, as the more flexible polynomial model. However, the salience model also has problems. It was not consistent in the specifics of its parameters. Considered together, these pros and cons imply that the conceptual details that led to the salience model are probably correct in the outline, and perhaps even in the general shape of the functional form, but that the specific equation chosen is not correct. More importantly, however, the salience model is incomplete as a model of neglect. Neglect occurs across distinct reference frames and there is no mechanism for including this fact in the present model. Further, neglect is notably heterogeneous with severity depending on response mode, near or far space, etc. Again, the salience model is too limited to account for any of these features. Finally, it is very important to distinguish neglect patients with or without hemianopia (Karnath *et al.* 2001) because the presence of a concomitant sensory loss may change the distribution of spatial attention in neglect. In a study currently in progress we are attempting to test specifically the role of hemianopia in the distribution of attention in neglect patients.

Conclusions

In summary, we can draw the following general conclusions. Our RT approach to the study of the distribution of spatial attention across the visual field in neglect patients without hemianopia has provided evidence in broad agreement with hemispatial theories of neglect. Rather than a continuous gradient of increasing attentional deployment from extreme contralesional to extreme ipsilesional visual space, we found a clear-cut hemifield difference in performance. Furthermore, fitting our RT data to the mathematical model of neglect proposed by Anderson (1996) has proved to be a fruitful exercise by allowing rejection of a linear model of attentional distribution and support for a saliency model. Finally, our RT experiments have enabled us to confirm previous evidence of a greater impairment of exogenous rather than endogenous spatial attention in neglect.

Acknowledgements

We wish to thank Dr L. Posteraro, Dr M. Prior, and Dr N. Smania for their invaluable help in recruiting the patients.

References

Anderson, B. (1996). A mathematical model of line bisection behaviour in neglect. *Brain*, **119**, 841–50.
Anderson, B. (1997). Pieces of the true crossover effect in neglect. *Neurology*, **49**, 809–12.
Anderson, B. (1999). A computational model of neglect dyslexia. *Cortex*, **35**, 201–18.
Anderson, B., Mennemeier, M., and Chatterjee, A. (2000). Variability not ability: another basis for performance decrements in neglect. *Neuropsychologia*, **38**, 776–85.
Bartolomeo, P., Sieroff, E., Decaix, C., and Chokron, S. (2001). Modulating the attentional bias in unilateral neglect: The effects of the strategic set. *Experimental Brain Research*, **137**, 432–44.
Barton, J. J., Behrmann, M., and Black, S. (1998). Ocular search during line bisection. The effects of hemi-neglect and hemianopia. *Brain*, **121**, 1117–31.
Bisiach, E. (1993). Mental representation in unilateral neglect and related disorders: the twentieth Bartlett Memorial Lecture. *Quarterly Journal of Experimental Psychology A*, **46**, 435–61.

Bisiach, E., Pizzamielio, L., Nico, D., and Antonucci, E. (1996). Beyond unilateral neglect. *Brain*, **119**, 851–7.

Bisiach, E., Ricci, R., and Modona, M. N. (1998). Visual awareness and anisometry of space representation in unilateral neglect: a panoramic investigation by means of a line extension task. *Consciousness and Cognition*, **7**, 327–55.

Bisiach, E., Neppi-Modona, M., Genero, R., and Pepi, R. (1999*a*). Anisometry of space representation in unilateral neglect: empirical test of a former hypothesis. *Consciousness and Cognition*, **8**, 577–84.

Bisiach, E., Ricci, R., Berruti, G., Genero, R., Pepi, R., and Fumelli, T. (1999b). Two-dimensional distortion of space representation in unilateral neglect: perceptual and response-related factors. *Neuropsychologia*, **37**, 1491–8.

Chelazzi, L., Marzi, C. A., Panozzo, G., Pasqualini, N., Tassinari, G., and Tomazzoli, L. (1988). Hemiretinal differences in speed of light detection in esotropic amblyopes. *Vision Research*, **28**, 95–104.

Corbetta, M., Miezin, F. M., Shulman, G. L., and Petersen, S. E. (1993). A PET study of visuospatial attention. *Journal of Neuroscience*, **13**, 1202–26.

Corbetta, M., Kincade, J. M., Ollinger, J. M., McAvoy, M. P., and Shulman, G. L. (2000). Voluntary orienting is dissociated from target detection in human posterior parietal cortex. *Nature Neuroscience*, **3**, 292–7.

Driver, J. and Mattingley, J. B. (1998). Parietal neglect and visual awareness. *Nature Neuroscience*, **1**, 17–22.

Findlay, J. M. and Walker, R. (1999). A model of saccade generation based on parallel processing and competitive inhibition. *Behavioural and Brain Sciences*, **22**, 661–74.

Gitelman, D. R., Nobre, A. C., Parrish, T. B., *et al.* (1999). A large-scale distributed network for covert spatial attention: further anatomical delineation based on stringent behavioural and cognitive controls. *Brain*, **122**, 1093–106.

Gottlieb, J. P., Kusunoki, M., and Goldberg, M. E. (1998). The representation of visual salience in monkey parietal cortex. *Nature*, **391**, 481–4.

Graybill, F. A. and Hariharan, K. I. (1994). *Regression analysis: concepts and applications*. Duxbury Press, Belmont, CA.

Harvey, M., Milner, A. D., and Roberts, R. C. (1995). An investigation of hemispatial neglect using the Landmark task. *Brain and Cognition*, **27**, 59–78.

Heilman, K. M., Valenstein, E., and Watson, R. T. (2000). Neglect and related disorders. *Seminars in Neurology*, **20**, 463–70.

Hoel, P., Port, S. C., and Stone, C. J. (1971). *Introduction to probability theory.* Houghton Mifflin, Boston, MA.

Itti, L. and Koch, C. (2001). Computational modelling of visual attention. *Nature Reviews Neuroscience*, **2**, 194–203.

Karnath, H.-O. (1988). Deficits of attention in acute and recovered visual hemi-neglect. *Neuropsychologia*, **26**, 27–43.

Karnath, H.-O. (1997). Spatial orientation and the representation of space with parietal lobe lesions. *Philosophical Transactions of the Royal Society of London. B Biological Sciences*, **352**, 1411–19.

Karnath, H.-O. and Ferber, S. (1999). Is space representation distorted in neglect? *Neuropsychologia*, **37**, 7–15.

Karnath, H.-O., Ferber, S., and Himmelbach, M. (2001). Spatial awareness is a function of the temporal not the posterior parietal lobe. *Nature*, **411**, 950–3.

Kim, Y. H., Gitelman, D. R., Nobre, A. C., Parrish, T. B., LaBar, K. S., and Mesulam, M. M. (1999). The large-scale neural network for spatial attention displays multifunctional overlap but differential asymmetry. *Neuroimage*, **9**, 269–77.

Kinsbourne, M. (1993). Orientational bias model of unilateral neglect: evidence from attentional gradients within hemispace. In *Unilateral neglect: clinical and experimental studies* (ed. I. I. Robertson and J. C. Marshall), pp. 63–86. Lawrence Erlbaum, Hillsdale, NJ.

Koch, C. and Ullman, S. (1985). Shifts in selective visual attention: towards the underlying neural circuitry. *Human Neurobiology*, **4**, 219–27.

Làdavas, E., Carletti, M., and Gori, G. (1994). Automatic and voluntary orienting of attention in patients with visual neglect: horizontal and vertical dimensions. *Neuropsychologia*, **32**, 1195–208.

Marzi, C. A. and Di Stefano, M. (1981). Hemiretinal differences in visual perception. *Documenta Ophthalmologica Proceedings Series*, **30**, 273–8.

Mozer, M. C. (1999). Explaining object-based deficits in unilateral neglect without object-based frames of references. *Progress in Brain Research*, **121**, 99–119.

Nobre, A. C., Sebestyen, G. N., Gitelman, D. R., Mesulam, M. M., Frackowiak, R. S., and Frith, C. D. (1997). Functional localization of the system for visuospatial attention using positron emission tomography. *Brain*, **120**, 515–33.

Perry, R. J. and Zeki, S.(2000). The neurology of saccades and covert shifts in spatial attention: an event-related fMRI study. *Brain*, **123**, 2273–88.

Pouget, A. and Driver, J. (2000). Relating unilateral neglect to the neural coding of space. *Current Opinion in Neurobiology*, **10**, 242–9.

Pouget, A. and Sejnowski, T. J. (1997). Lesion in a basis function model of parietal cortex: comparison with hemineglect. In *Parietal lobe contributions to orientation in 3dD space* (ed. P. Thier and H.-O. Karnath), pp. 521–38. Springer, Heidelberg.

Pouget, A., Deneve, S., and Sejnowski, T. J. (1999). Frames of reference in hemineglect: a computational approach. *Progress in Brain Research*, **121**, 81–97.

Reuter-Lorenz, P. A., Kinsbourne, M., and Moscovitch, M. (1990). Hemispheric control of spatial attention. *Brain and Cognition*, **12**, 240–66.

Smania, N., Martini, M. C., Gambina, G., Tomelleri, G., Palamara, A., Natale, E., and Marzi, C. A. (1998). The spatial distribution of visual attention in hemineglect and extinction patients. *Brain*, **121**, 1759–70.

Weintraub, S. and Mesulam, M. M. (1987). Right cerebral dominance in spatial attention. Further evidence based on ipsilateral neglect. *Archives of Neurology*, **44**, 621–5.

Wolfe, J. M. (1994).Visual search in continuous, naturalistic stimuli. *Vision Research*, **34**, 1187–95.

5.5 Spatial extinction and its relation to mechanisms of normal attention

Jason B. Mattingley

It is now widely recognized that spatial neglect following unilateral brain damage is a multifaceted disorder (Driver and Mattingley 1998; Vallar 1998; Driver and Vuilleumier 2001), as illustrated by the broad range of topics covered in this volume. The most salient impairment shown by individuals with neglect is the tendency to ignore otherwise suprathreshold stimuli on the side contralateral to the lesion. This chapter focuses on the phenomenon of **extinction**, which, though apparent in many patients with neglect, can be observed in isolation (Vallar et al. 1994; Driver et al. 1997). For patients with extinction, the problem of detecting contralesional stimuli is exacerbated by the co-occurrence of another stimulus located further toward the ipsilesional side (Bender 1952; di Pellegrino and De Renzi 1995). The phenomenon of extinction suggests a competitive aspect to the spatial bias caused by unilateral brain damage. Indeed, many aspects of spatial neglect seem to be due at least in part to competition from salient stimuli located further toward the ipsilesional side (Mark et al. 1988). The notion of competitive interactions between concurrent stimulus events is a key element of contemporary theories of selective attention (Bundesen 1990; Desimone and Duncan 1995; Duncan 1996); as such, extinction has provided a model example of the effects of attention on perception (Driver et al. 1997; Duncan et al. 1999).

In this chapter we consider the various clinical manifestations of extinction and relate these to relevant data on attentional limits in normal subjects. We then provide an overview of recent findings from studies of extinction that have focused on cross-modal interactions, the effects of temporally asynchronous stimulation, motor competition, and perceptual grouping, and link these results where possible to relevant behavioral, neurophysiological, and brain imaging data. We conclude by considering the possible sites of brain damage that give rise to extinction, and suggest some fruitful avenues for future research.

Clinical manifestations of spatial extinction

Typically, extinction is elicited in the clinic using the 'confrontation' method. The patient is required to detect an examiner's brief finger movements in the visual periphery, whilst fixating the examiner's nose. The basic finding for patients with extinction is that a finger movement occurring in isolation in either hemifield is detected normally, whereas the more contralesional of two simultaneous movements in the two hemifields tends to go unreported (Critchley 1949; Bender 1952). Since the patient is evidently able to detect single contralesional events, it is assumed that afferent processing of contralesional stimuli remains intact, and that it is the presence of the competing ipsilesional stimulus that extinguishes the contralesional event from awareness (Driver *et al.* 1997). Although this interpretation of extinction as a purely competitive deficit is widely accepted, in practice it has proved difficult to demonstrate that extinction does not involve at least some sensory loss for contralesional stimuli. In many right-hemisphere-lesioned patients with neglect, visual evoked potentials are reduced in amplitude and have prolonged latencies for stimuli presented in the contralesional (left) hemifield (Spinelli *et al.* 1994, 1996; Angelelli *et al.* 1996); contrast sensitivity may also be reduced (Angelelli *et al.* 1998). Similar low-level impairments of sensory processing have been revealed in the somatosensory modality for right-hemisphere patients with extinction (Remy *et al.* 1999).

In the typical confrontation test, stimuli are deliberately chosen to be well above threshold, and so estimates of performance for single contralesional events are often at ceiling. Under these circumstances it is difficult to exclude a subtle sensory loss for stimuli on the affected side, which may give rise to a competitive bias favoring ipsilesional events at early stages of sensory processing. Conversely, a patient may detect all contralesional events on bilateral trials, implying that extinction is absent, when the use of briefer or less salient stimuli could potentially have revealed contralesional extinction under similar bilateral presentations (Driver *et al.* 1997). As explained below, recent models of competitive interactions in normal attention have highlighted the interdependency between the **sensory effectiveness** of a stimulus and its **attentional weight** under conditions in which perceptual selectivity is required (Bundesen 1990; Duncan *et al.* 1999). Recent studies of extinction have sought to avoid floor and ceiling effects by using computerized displays that permit more precise control of stimuli, including their duration, size, location, contrast, and so forth.

Despite these caveats, there is little doubt that extinction involves a strong competitive element. Apart from better detection of contralesional events for unilateral versus bilateral trials, extinction patients also report more stimuli on the affected side when instructed to ignore any concurrent ipsilesional events (Karnath 1988). Such strategic control effectively reduces the competitive strength of the ipsilesional stimulus and increases the likelihood that the more contralesional event will reach awareness (Duncan *et al.* 1999). Similarly, having attention cued toward the location of an upcoming contralesional target, either **exogenously** (e.g. by an abrupt peripheral stimulus) or **endogenously** (e.g. by a central symbolic cue), can improve both detection rates and the speed of responses (Posner *et al.* 1984; Morrow and Ratcliff 1988; Friedrich *et al.* 1998). Curiously, there has been relatively little investigation of the role of endogenous control mechanisms in extinction (or neglect), despite extensive evidence that top-down control plays a vital role in perception and action in normal subjects (Monsell and Driver 2000). Kaplan *et al.* (1990) found that right-hemisphere patients were significantly more likely to detect the left visual target in a bilateral trial if it was preceded by several unilateral right-sided trials, compared with just a single unilateral trial on either side or several unilateral *left*-sided trials. This result implies that the competitive advantage for ipsilesional stimuli can be reduced under conditions in which the patient comes to expect a stimulus on the contralesional side. Similar effects have been observed when single- and double-stimulus events are blocked with respect to their hemifield of presentation. Under these conditions right-hemisphere patients improve dramatically when they are able to devote their attention exclusively to a single hemifield (contralesional or ipsilesional) compared with conditions in which they must divide their attention between hemifields (Smania *et al.* 1998; Mattingley *et al.* 2000). These and similar observations suggest that in many cases of extinction top-down control of selective attention is relatively preserved (Làdavas *et al.* 1994; Duncan *et al.* 1999). It would be interesting to test whether this also holds for cases in which the lesion involves areas assumed to be involved in strategic or executive control, such as the prefrontal cortex (Smith and Jonides 1999).

It is often claimed that extinction arises even when both stimuli are presented within the 'intact' (ipsilesional) hemifield, so that the extinguished stimulus is actually closer to the fovea than its ipsilesional competitor (Kinsbourne 1993). In fact, there seems to be little convincing evidence for this claim. In those studies in which right-hemisphere patients showed extinction for concurrent stimuli presented either bilaterally or within the contralesional hemifield, all found that extinction was *absent* for stimuli presented entirely within the ipsilesional hemifield (Rapcsak *et al.* 1987; di Pellegrino and De Renzi 1995; Smania *et al.* 1996; Mattingley *et al.* 2000). di Pellegrino and De Renzi (1995) found that extinction could be elicited for concurrent events within the ipsilesional hemifield if the patient directed attention covertly to a location positioned between the two potential stimulus events, but the presence of extinction in this condition may simply have reflected the difficulty associated with suppressing eye movements toward the attended ipsilesional location (for a related finding in normal subjects, see Mack and Rock (1998)). Although there is reason to be skeptical of claims that visual extinction can occur within the ipsilesional hemifield, this does not exclude the possibility of an abnormal spatial gradient there. Indeed, several studies using reaction time (RT) measures have found that responses to single events can be significantly faster for stimuli located further toward the ipsilesional periphery, relative to more foveal locations on the same side (Ladàvas *et al.* 1990). The apparent discrepancy between detection and RT results may simply reflect the differential sensitivity of these two measures to spatial gradients of attention.

Relation of extinction to normal limits of selective attention

The extinction patient's problem in detecting concurrent sensory events has important parallels with studies showing that even neurologically normal individuals can have problems in detecting simultaneous targets in separate channels of sensory input. Although there are numerous instances of this **dual-target cost**, I shall consider just two examples here. Puleo and Pastore (1978) had participants listen for a low-frequency tone-burst in one ear and a high frequency tone-burst in the other, with all sounds being delivered via headphones. The critical results for present purposes came from a comparison of performance across two conditions: in the **selective-attention** condition, auditory targets could occur in either ear, but participants only had to report those in the monitored ear (left or right, designated in advance); in the **divided-attention** condition, targets could also occur in either ear, but now participants had to report on each ear independently. Performance in the divided-attention condition was as good as in the selective-attention condition, provided that only a single target occurred at a time. In contrast, if in the divided-attention condition targets occurred *simultaneously* in the two ears, there was a significant *decrease* in performance, such that participants failed to report one of the two targets.

Duncan (1980) reported similar results for a visual discrimination task. In his study, participants had to judge whether a digit (the target) appeared in an array of four letters (nontargets). Once again the critical data came from a comparison of performance in two conditions: in the **successive** condition, one pair of characters appeared first, followed half a second later by a second pair; in the **simultaneous** condition, all four characters appeared at once, for the same total duration as those presented in the successive condition. When participants simply had to indicate whether a target digit was present anywhere in the display, performance was equivalent for the successive and simultaneous conditions. Similarly, when they had to determine whether a target was present in each pair of characters independently, performance was roughly equivalent in the successive and simultaneous conditions, provided that only a single target was present. Crucially, however, if two targets appeared, performance declined markedly in the simultaneous versus the successive condition. Thus there was a significant dual-target cost when the relevant visual events were presented simultaneously rather than successively, just as Puleo and Pastore (1978) observed in their auditory task.

These findings suggest that normal subjects are able to monitor multiple potential sources of information provided that only one relevant event (the target) occurs at a time; however, if targets occur concurrently there is a marked cost in performance. This basic limitation is reminiscent of the problem of extinction after unilateral damage (Driver *et al.* 1997). Patients readily detect single-target events on their contralesional side, provided that there is no target on the ipsilesional side to compete for selection. When targets are presented concurrently on the two sides, however, patients detect the ipsilesional item but fail to detect the more contralesional one. In addition to these compelling similarities, there are of course important differences between patients and normal subjects in terms of these dual-target costs. Only unilateral patients exhibit the characteristic **spatially biased** impairment for targets located toward the contralesional side. Moreover, the dual-target decrement in normal subjects only arises for brief masked presentations (Duncan 1980), whereas in patients even suprathreshold targets are missed. This suggests a further deficit in overall attentional **capacity** following unilateral damage, a feature of extinction (and indeed spatial neglect) that has been postulated by several investigators (Karnath 1988; Driver *et al.* 1997; Husain *et al.* 1997; Duncan *et al.* 1999).

Interactions between sense modalities in extinction and normal attention

Extinction has been observed in each of the major sense modalities: vision, touch, audition, and olfaction (Bender 1952; De Renzi *et al.* 1984; Bellas *et al.* 1988). Individual patients may have extinction within just a single modality, or they may show the phenomenon in two or more modalities. Thus, for example, De Renzi *et al.* (1984) observed patients with both visual and auditory extinction. Similarly, Vallar *et al.* (1994) found patients with both visual and tactile extinction. It is not uncommon in clinical practice to find patients with extinction in all three modalities (vision, touch, and audition). On the basis of these findings it is tempting to conclude that the competitive bias that characterizes extinction arises from damage to one or more modality-specific representations (Farah *et al.* 1989; Inhoff *et al.* 1992). It should be noted, however, that most studies that have examined extinction in more than a single modality have used fairly crude clinical measures. These are especially susceptible to floor and ceiling effects, as described above. Several investigators have also failed to equate the salience of stimuli across the different modalities, so that any apparent dissociation in the severity of extinction could be due to baseline differences in the patient's threshold for detecting stimulation in one modality versus the other. In future studies it will be important to ensure that stimuli are scaled to each patient's own threshold for detection, *separately* for each modality.

More recently, the issue of whether extinction can arise for concurrent stimuli in *separate* modalities has generated considerable interest (see Chapter 3.4). This interest has stemmed from two sources. First, single-cell studies in cats and monkeys have revealed that various regions of the brainstem, thalamus, and cerebral cortex contain neurons with bimodal response properties (Graziano and Gross 1995; Stein *et al.* 1995). For instance, in a series of elegant studies in the macaque, Graziano and coworkers have described neurons with spatially overlapping visual and tactile receptive fields (Graziano and Gross 1995, 1998; Graziano *et al.* 1994). The responses of many such neurons are enhanced when temporally coincident tactile and visual stimuli are delivered within their receptive fields, and suppressed when bimodal stimuli are temporally or spatially disparate. Second, there is now a substantial body of evidence to suggest the existence of strong cross-modal links in spatial selective attention (Driver and Spence 1998). Exogenous (nonpredictive) spatial cues have been shown to enhance the speed and accuracy of target discriminations for virtually all combinations of cue and target modality (Spence *et al*. 1998); similar effects have been observed when participants direct their attention endogenously to a particular location in anticipation of targets in a specified modality (Spence *et al*. 2000).

Surprisingly, cross-modal effects in extinction were not investigated systematically until relatively recently. In an early anecdotal account, Bender (1952) observed that unilateral patients would occasionally miss a contralesional visual stimulus if touched simultaneously on the ipsilesional hand, but he presented no data to substantiate his claim. Inhoff *et al*. (1992) failed to find any evidence for visual–tactile cross-modal extinction in a group of right-hemisphere patients, even though each individual exhibited significant extinction for concurrent stimuli in either modality alone. However, numerous recent studies have reported convincing evidence for the existence of cross-modal extinction. Mattingley *et al*. (1997) reported an experiment on three right-hemisphere patients who failed to detect tactile stimuli delivered to the left hand in the presence of a concurrent visual stimulus in the right hemifield; the patients also failed to detect left visual events presented together with a tactile stimulus on the right hand. di Pellegrino *et al*. (1997) reported a right-hemisphere patient with tactile extinction, in whom touches on the left hand were extinguished by concurrent visual events in the right hemifield; crucially, however, this effect was modulated by the position of the ipsilesional hand, with extinction occurring only when the patient's right hand was adjacent to the position of the right-sided visual event, and not when it was located out of view behind the body. This finding fits with neurophysiological data from monkeys (Graziano and Gross 1995, 1998), which show that the visual receptive fields of bimodal neurons move with the hand, thus maintaining spatial coincidence with the tactile receptive fields.

The findings on cross-modal extinction between vision and touch suggest an important role for proprioception in updating the current representation of limb positions, as well as the locations of visual and auditory events with respect to the body. It is well known that rotational deviations of the eyes, head, and trunk can modulate neglect patients' awareness of contralesional visual events (Kooistra and Heilman 1989; Karnath *et al*. 1993; Vuilleumier *et al*. 1999). Similarly in tactile extinction, having patients move their hands to different locations can have a profound impact on the severity of their contralesional impairment. Thus, for example, the proportion of extinguished tactile stimuli is significantly reduced when the arms are crossed and occupy a single hemispace, or when they are crossed so that each hand occupies the opposite hemispace (Smania and Aglioti 1995; Aglioti *et al*. 1999). Even when the hands remain uncrossed, however, we have found that the severity of tactile extinction can be reduced simply by bringing the hands close together within a single hemispace (Driver *et al*. 1996). This latter finding fits with data from normal subjects showing that the ability to ignore tactile distractors delivered to one hand while discriminating a concurrent tactile target on the other is significantly more difficult when the hands are located close together than when they are far apart (Driver and Grossenbacher 1996). Taken together, these results suggest that the competitive interactions that give rise to pathological extinction are played out across multiple brain regions devoted to the processing of inputs from several modalities.

The effects of temporally asynchronous stimuli on extinction

It is typically assumed that extinction is maximal under conditions in which competing stimuli occur simultaneously, in line with work in normal subjects suggesting an attentional limit in reporting concurrent target events (Puleo and Pastore 1978; Duncan 1980). Certainly the standard confrontation technique used to elicit extinction involves delivery of *concurrent* stimulation to different sites on the receptor surface (e.g. the retina or skin). One may ask, however, at what temporal asynchrony the bilateral stimuli delivered in a typical extinction test will be perceived as separate events. As the occurrence of one stimulus becomes further removed in time from the other, contralesional events should presumably begin to be perceived more reliably, since reporting of isolated stimuli on either side is typically close to ceiling in most extinction patients. Recent research has begun to address this question, although there is still some controversy over the interpretation of the results.

di Pellegrino *et al.* (1997) examined a single right-hemisphere extinction patient using asynchronous presentations of left- and right-sided letters. They found that the patient's ability to identify left-sided letters was poorest when a right-sided letter was presented concurrently, and improved steadily as the asynchrony between the two events increased. At stimulus onset asynchronies (SOAs) of ±500 ms, reporting of left stimuli was statistically equivalent for unilateral and bilateral trials. To the extent that they can be generalized, these findings emphasize that, although extinction can occur for asynchronous bilateral events, the contralesional impairment appears maximal under conditions of simultaneity. Intriguingly, however, other experiments using asynchronous presentation of bilateral stimuli suggest that, for the patients, the subjective experience of simultaneous events does *not* correspond to objective simultaneity.

It has long been recognized that the perception of the temporal order of spatially discrete stimuli can be influenced by the direction of spatially selective attention. In his **law of prior entry**, Titchener (1908) stated that 'the stimulus for which we are predisposed requires less time than a like stimulus, for which we are unprepared, to produce its full conscious effect'. In other words, sensory events occurring at a location to which spatial attention is deployed will tend to be perceived prior to physically synchronous events at unattended locations. A common interpretation of the prior entry effect is that the rate of information processing is enhanced at attended relative to unattended locations, so that stimuli occurring at an attended location receive privileged access to awareness (Rorden *et al.* 1997; Stelmach and Herdman 1991; Zackon *et al.* 1999).

The law of prior entry has been examined in several different contexts in normal individuals (Stelmach and Herdman 1991; Zackon *et al.* 1999). In the study by Stelmach and Herdman (1991), observers had their attention directed covertly to one of two placeholders located at an equal eccentricity within the left and right hemifields. Shortly thereafter, two visual targets appeared, one to the left and one to the right. These targets appeared either simultaneously or with a short temporal asynchrony between them. It was found that observers tended to judge the visual target on the attended side as having occurred first, unless the target on the unattended side had a physical lead in time of around 40 ms. In other words, when spatial attention was directed at a particular location, normal observers perceived the target events as asynchronous when they actually occurred concurrently, and as synchronous when the target at the unattended location led physically by 40 ms, as predicted by the law of prior entry. These results reveal the profound impact that selective attention has on the conscious perception of sensory events, a fact that has attracted renewed interest recently in the wake of studies on phenomena such as change blindness (Rensink 1997, 2000; O'Regan *et al.* 1999) and inattentional blindness (Mack and Rock 1998).

If spatial attention is chronically biased toward the ipsilesional side in patients with neglect or extinction, the law of prior entry predicts that ipsilesional events should be perceived earlier than physically synchronous contralesional stimuli. We tested this prediction in two right-hemisphere patients, both of whom extinguished left visual stimuli under bilateral simultaneous stimulation (Rorden *et al.* 1997). Patients were asked to judge the order of onset of two rectangular stimuli presented on the left and right of a central fixation cross. Both stimuli were presented on every trial, either simultaneously or with a temporal gap between them. On asynchronous trials half of the displays involved the stimulus on the left leading in time, and half involved the stimulus on the right leading (Fig. 1(a)). By plotting the proportion of 'right first' responses against the SOA,

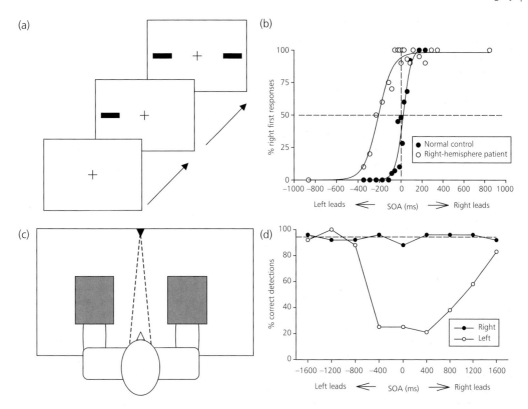

Figure 1 Visual and tactile TOJ tasks used to examine extinction in right-hemisphere patients. (a) Representative display sequence from a single trial in the TOJ task of Rorden *et al.* (1997). Patients maintained fixation on a central cross, which was displayed for 600 ms. Immediately following the offset of the cross, a single bar appeared to the left or right of fixation. This was followed, at a variable SOA (0–864 ms), by a second bar located at an equal eccentricity in the opposite hemifield. Patients were asked to indicate which of the two stimuli appeared first. There were equal numbers of left-first and right-first trials, and these were randomly intermingled. (b) TOJ results for a right-hemisphere patient with left-sided extinction (open circles) and a matched neurologically healthy control (solid circles). The percentage of 'right-first' responses is plotted as a function of SOA. Fitted sigmoid curves are shown separately for each individual. Note the point of subjective simultaneity (50 per cent 'right-first' responses), which is at 0 ms for the control and approximately −200 ms for the patient (adapted from Rorden *et al.* (1997)). (c) Experimental set-up for the tactile TOJ task. The patient fixated a point directly ahead and placed his hands inside occluding cuffs in the left and right hemispace. Brief vibrotactile stimuli were delivered to either hand alone, or to both hands with a variable SOA. The task was to indicate which hand(s) had received a tactile stimulus (left, right or both). (d) Results of the tactile TOJ task, with the percentage of correct detections plotted as a function of SOA. The horizontal broken line shows the mean performance for unilateral trials (pooled across left and right hands). The solid lines show performance on bilateral trials. Note the pronounced decrement in performance for left stimuli on bilateral trials.

we determined the point of subjective simultaneity, i.e. the onset asynchrony at which patients perceived the two events as being simultaneous (Fig. 1(b)). The point of subjective simultaneity in the temporal order judgment (TOJ) task was at an SOA of about zero for neurologically healthy control participants, as would be expected under conditions in which fixation was maintained centrally and attention was distributed equally between the two possible target locations (Stelmach and Herdman 1991). In contrast, both right-hemisphere patients showed a strong prior entry bias in favor of ipsilesional stimuli. They tended to perceive right-sided events as preceding equivalent left-sided ones, unless the left event led physically in time by around 200 ms. For trials in which the left stimulus led by less than 200 ms, the patients tended to perceive the right stimulus as having appeared first.

Following from the early observations of Birch *et al.* (1967), we have also examined prior entry biases in extinction for tactile stimuli. In a collaboration with Kennett, Rorden, and Driver, the author has examined detection of brief vibrotactile events delivered to the left and right hands in a right-hemisphere patient with tactile extinction (Fig. 1(c)). The patient was asked to report the presence of any target event, which could involve a single stimulus to either hand, two stimuli delivered concurrently to both hands, or two stimuli with a variable SOA between them. Each of the patient's hands was located within its own hemispace, and both hands were occluded from view throughout the experiment. As shown in Fig. 1(d), detection of single vibrotactile stimuli on either hand was near ceiling. In contrast, there was a severe decrement in detection of left targets when two stimuli were presented. This impairment for left targets occurred across a range of SOAs, from −400 to +1200 ms, indicating that the occurrence of a right-sided competitor interfered with detection of left targets even when the two events were asynchronous. Preliminary findings have also been reported for an auditory analog of the TOJ paradigm in right-hemisphere patients (Scott *et al.* 1997), suggesting that the ipsilesional attentional bias in extinction can arise in multiple modalities. It seems likely that significant prior entry biases in extinction will also be found for cross-modal designs. Although recent experiments in normal subjects have revealed significant cross-modal prior entry effects (Spence *et al.*, in press), there have been no such investigations in patients to date.

These results suggest that in extinction awareness is severely delayed for contralesional stimulus events, even under conditions in which there is no concurrent ipsilesional competitor. The findings are inconsistent with the popular view that extinction of contralesional stimuli reflects a deficit in disengaging spatial attention from a stimulus on the ipsilesional side (Posner *et al.* 1984), since in the TOJ task the processing of contralesional stimuli is abnormal even for SOAs at which there is no ipsilesional competitor to disengage from. It is currently unclear why extinction is maximal for physically synchronous events (di Pellegrino *et al.* 1997), even though the patients themselves do not experience such events as simultaneous. One possibility is that the tasks used to assess perception of bilateral stimuli rely on different selective mechanisms to those used to assess the perception of temporal order (see Baylis *et al.* (2002) for further discussion). Certainly such task-specific effects have been shown to influence perception of multiple stimuli in other extinction paradigms (Baylis *et al.* 1993; Vuilleumier and Rafal 1999, 2000). Whatever the explanation for this apparent discrepancy, the results from studies of the effects of temporal asynchrony on extinction demonstrate that the processing of contralesional stimuli is impaired even for temporally isolated events. It would seem that the time required to individuate or identify a contralesional target is prolonged relative to an equivalent ipsilesional target in patients with extinction (di Pellegrino *et al.* 1998), consistent with the recent finding of a prolonged attentional blink for foveal stimuli in patients with spatial neglect (Husain *et al.* 1997).

Extinction within the motor domain

Despite the recent surge of interest in the perceptual consequences of unilateral brain damage on perception and awareness, relatively little attention has been devoted to whether aspects of motor control may be similarly affected. One possible reason for this discrepancy is that many unilateral stroke patients have contralesional hemiparesis which may severely restrict their capacity for spontaneous goal-directed actions. However, recent studies of patients with spatial neglect have revealed a variety of deficits involving the preparation and execution of limb movements

(Mattingley and Driver 1997). These deficits range from motor neglect (a failure to use the contralesional limb despite adequate power) to problems in the initiation and execution of movements made with the ipsilesional limb toward contralesional visual targets (Heilman *et al.* 1985; Bisiach *et al.* 1990; Mattingley *et al.* 1992, 1994, 1998; Corben *et al.* 2001). However, there have been few investigations of extinction within the motor domain, despite evidence that execution of bimanual actions requires a fine balance between competition and cooperation of activity within the motor circuits of either hemisphere (Rosenbaum 1994).

In one early study, Valenstein and Heilman (1981) examined a patient with right caudate damage who was asked to raise either hand when it was touched by the examiner. He correctly indicated single touches on either hand, but failed to raise his left hand when touched simultaneously on both. Although this pattern is consistent with left tactile extinction, the patient apparently showed normal detection of the same bilateral tactile stimuli when simply asked to respond verbally to the targets (saying 'left', 'right', or 'both'), suggesting a motoric deficit in responding with the affected limb under conditions in which both hands needed to be moved simultaneously. This clinical result was confirmed empirically by having the patient release a response key with the left or right hand alone, or with both hands simultaneously, depending on the identity of a central symbolic cue. For unimanual responses, the left hand was always slower than the right, but this left-hand cost was especially pronounced when a bimanual response was required. Taken together, these results suggest that actions initiated by the left hand can be disrupted by the simultaneous preparation and execution of movements with the right hand, thus yielding a motor analog of perceptual extinction.

In collaboration with Robertson and Driver, the author has recently tested a number of right-hemisphere patients, all of whom were able to move their left arm, for the presence of motor extinction. Our task involved simple bimanual tapping which was videotaped and scored by independent raters. To establish a baseline level of performance, we initially had participants perform unimanual tapping with either the left (contralesional) or right hand. We then tested their ability to tap *bimanually* for the same duration, either with movements that were in phase (i.e. with both palms raised and lowered together) or out of phase (i.e. with one hand being raised as the other was lowered) (Fig. 2(a)). For some individuals there was either no significant difference between the unimanual and bimanual tapping rates for either hand, or else the tapping rate for each hand was reduced equally in bimanual versus unimanual conditions (i.e. a general decrement for bimanual actions). Crucially, however, there were several patients in whom the rate of left-hand movements was significantly decreased in bimanual versus unilateral conditions, with no such bimanual cost for right-hand movements.

This effect is illustrated for one such patient (JF) in Fig. 2(b). In addition to producing fewer taps with her affected hand in bimanual versus unimanual conditions, JF also stopped moving her left hand altogether in several trials of the bimanual task. She indicated that although she was aware that her left hand had stopped tapping, she was unable to reinstate its movements unless she stopped the right hand and commenced the sequence again. Other patients with motor extinction seemed completely unaware that their left-hand movements had ceased during bimanual activity, and would sometimes continue tapping with the right hand alone until the end of the trial (see Hillis *et al.* (1998) for similar results in patients with thalamic excisions). It is not yet clear whether the phenomena of motor extinction are related to (or caused by) an impairment of proprioception in the affected limb (Vallar *et al.* 1993), a problem in coordinating bimanual actions, or some combination of both. Further experiments will be needed to determine whether such motor deficits can be dissociated from perceptual extinction within the different sense modalities.

A key concept to emerge from recent theories of motor control is that of the **internal model**, in which the motor system generates predictions about the present and future state of the effectors (eyes, hands, legs, etc.) prior to the initiation of an action (Frith *et al.* 2000). A central tenet of

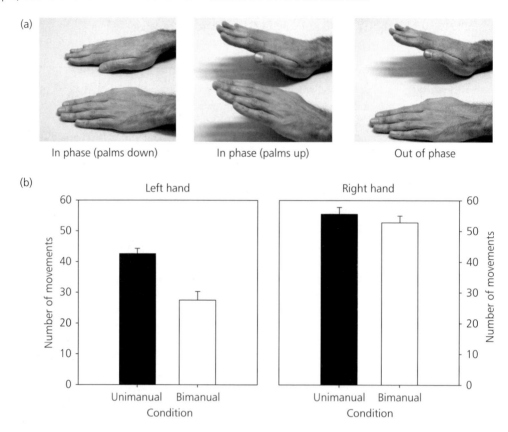

Figure 2 Results of motor extinction experiment. (a) Experimental conditions. Movement sequences were either unimanual (left or right hand alone) or bimanual (in phase or out of phase). Patients maintained central fixation throughout the experiment. (b) Results from a right-hemisphere patient, with separate plots for left (contralesional) and right (ipsilesional) hands. In each plot the number of taps is shown for unimanual versus bimanual conditions (pooled across in-phase and out-of-phase movements, which were equivalent for this patient). Note the significant decrement in left-hand performance in the bimanual condition.

this model is that our conscious experience of voluntary action is derived from the predicted state of the motor system, rather than from its actual state. For the bimanual tapping task described above, right-hemisphere patients with motor extinction may fail to move the left hand not because of a deficit of motor intention *per se*, but because of a failure to monitor the sensory consequences of any left-hand movement under conditions of competition. In the model of Frith *et al.* (2000), unimanual movements of the left hand would be normal since full attention can be devoted to monitoring their sensory consequences. In contrast, when simultaneous movements are made with the right hand, only the sensations associated with its movements are monitored, leaving any sensorimotor discrepancies for the left hand uncorrected. Preservation of the forward model for the appropriate bimanual action would give patients the impression that both hands were moving, but a failure to monitor the sensory consequences of left-hand action would eventually lead to its demise. We are currently conducting further experiments to test this hypothesis, but in the meantime it is clear that unilateral lesions can result in extinction within the motoric as well as the perceptual domain.

Modulating competitive interactions in extinction

As discussed above, extinction may be considered as a pathological exacerbation of the normal limit in attending to multiple concurrent targets, with a characteristic spatial bias induced by the unilateral reduction in competitive strength of sensory inputs. In normal subjects, the multiple-target limit is reduced if competing stimuli form parts of a common object (Duncan 1984; Baylis and Driver 1993) or if they can be grouped together to form a coherent perceptual entity. There is now a wealth of experimental evidence to suggest that normal mechanisms of attention operate on segmented surfaces and objects, rather than on unsegmented regions of visual space (Scholl 2001). This fact has led clinical researchers to investigate the extent to which competitive interactions in extinction might also be reduced under conditions in which bilateral stimulus events, which would otherwise compete for selection, can be linked to form a common object or group. In this section I focus on evidence for the effects of grouping on extinction in vision, since this modality has been studied more intensively than any other.

As we shall see, although extinction can arise after lesions to several different brain areas, it is classically associated with parietal or temporoparietal damage (Posner *et al.* 1984; Friedrich *et al.* 1998). In many cases, therefore, visual processing in preserved regions of the occipital cortex might be expected to provide a neural substrate for early segmentation and grouping of contrale-sional stimuli. Several studies have demonstrated that visual extinction is significantly attenuated when contralesional and ipsilesional events can be grouped together according to principles such as common contrast polarity, colinearity, and connectedness (Ward *et al.* 1994; Gilchrist *et al.* 1996). A recent psychophysical study that employed Gabor patches (sine wave gratings within a Gaussian envelope) as stimuli found that extinction of a patch in the contralesional hemifield was significantly reduced when a simultaneous patch in the ipsilesional hemifield occupied a homologous location and shared the same grating orientation (Pavlavskaya *et al.* 1997). This attenuation was maximal when the two stimuli were within the spatial range normally encom-passed by lateral interactions between neighboring neurons within the primary visual cortex (area V1).

Similar effects of grouping have also been found for visual stimuli whose earliest perceptual processing arises downstream from area V1. Normal processes of visual surface completion, as exemplified by the filling in of illusory figures such as the Kanizsa triangle (Kanizsa 1976), are crucial for providing a three-dimensional representation of the visual world from a two-dimensional retinal image. Such **modal** surface completion is thought to arise 'preattentively' in normal observers, as revealed by extremely rapid ('parallel') processing in visual search experi-ments (Davis and Driver 1994, 1998). Moreover, it is known that single neurons in monkey area V2 respond to illusory contours in much the same way as to conventional luminance-defined edges (von der Heydt *et al.* 1984), and that human extrastriate areas including V2 are activated by Kanizsa illusory figures during functional brain imaging (Ffytche and Zeki 1996).

Mattingley *et al.* (1997) reported on a patient with extensive damage of the right temporoparietal cortex, but with sparing of the mesial occipital lobe, whose extinction of left-sided visual stimuli improved dramatically when these could be completed as part of a common surface with concurrent ipsilesional events. The patient was asked to detect the brief disappearance of quarter-segments from two vertically aligned pairs of black disks located on either side of a central fixation cross (Fig. 3(a)). These segments could disappear from the pair of disks on the left or right (unilateral trials), on both sides simultaneously (bilateral trials), or on neither side (catch trials, as a control for guessing). On bilateral trials, the removal of quarter segments revealed an illusory surface (the white rectangle in Fig. 3(b)) which effectively linked the left and right sides of the display. In control trials, narrow arcs spanned the open segments, preventing any illusory filling in across the two sides of the display on bilateral trials (Fig. 3(a)). Whereas the patient showed severe

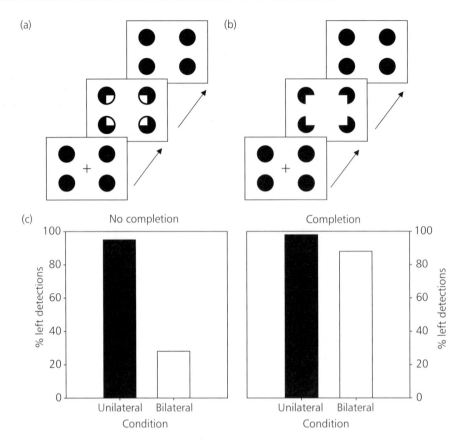

Figure 3 The effects of visual completion on competitive interactions in extinction. (a) Control display with narrow arcs preventing any modal completion across the display. The patient fixated centrally and was asked to report the brief removal of quarter segments from the left or right sides alone, or from both sides (as illustrated). Arrows indicate the temporal sequence of events in each trial. (b) Example display sequence from a bilateral trial of the modal completion experiment, showing a Kanizsa rectangle formed by the removal of quarter segments from each of the circular disks. (c) Graphs showing the percentage of left-sided targets correctly detected for unilateral and bilateral trials, with separate plots for the 'no-completion' and 'completion' conditions illustrated in (a) and (b). Note the significantly greater extinction for bilateral trials in the no-completion displays than in the modal completion displays.

extinction for these control displays, her performance in detecting left-sided events in the displays that yielded an illusory figure was significantly improved (Fig. 3(c)). Indeed, the patient herself often reported the appearance of the illusory rectangle in the experimental condition, providing anecdotal support for our conclusion that bilateral visual events can reach awareness in extinction when they are treated as allies rather than competitors during selection. A similar improvement was observed in the same patient for displays in which two line segments could be perceptually completed by virtue of their apparent occlusion by a central object (**amodal completion** (Michotte et al. 1964)) compared with control displays in which the relevant occlusion cues were removed (Mattingley et al. 1997).

In addition to the effects of early segmentation and grouping processes on extinction, it is clear that numerous other stimulus- and task-specific factors may be important in determining the outcome of the competition between ipsilesional and contralesional events. For instance, line drawings of common objects seem to be stronger competitors for attentional selection than scrambled versions of the same stimuli (Ward and Goodrich 1996), as are faces (Vuilleumier 2000) and stimuli with strong emotional value, such as depictions of faces with fearful expressions and pictures of spiders (Vuilleumier and Schwartz, in press and submitted). Such stimuli may receive priority under conditions of attentional competition because of their biological significance, an observation that has also been made in normal subjects under conditions of inattentional blindness (Mack and Rock 1998). As mentioned earlier, the severity of extinction may also depend on aspects of strategic control, such as the probability of occurrence of lateralized stimuli (Rapcsak et al. 1987), the kind of response to be made (e.g. verbal versus manual (Smania et al. 1996)), or the cognitive set invoked to perform the task (e.g. localization versus enumeration of targets (Vuilleumier and Rafal 1999, 2000)). Empirical investigations of the effects of top-down control on extinction (and spatial neglect) have scarcely begun, but recent findings suggest this is likely to be a focus for future research.

There have also been numerous attempts to reduce the spatially biased competition in extinction by recruiting preserved networks thought to modulate selective attention. At least one influential model of attention, the premotor theory, proposes that selective perception reflects activity in motor circuits responsible for the planning of eye movements to specific locations or objects (Rizzolatti and Camarda 1987). According to this model, covert shifts of spatial attention reflect eye movements that are programmed but not executed. In patients with spatial neglect, the premotor theory assumes that failures to perceive contralesional stimuli reflect an underlying deficit in planning appropriate actions toward the affected side. The pioneering work of Robertson and colleagues (Robertson and North 1992, 1993, 1994; Robertson et al. 1992) has shown that having right-hemisphere patients perform left-hand movements in the contralesional hemispace can significantly reduce their neglect of visual stimuli and can occasionally bring about enduring improvements in activities of daily living.

Such results are often interpreted as providing support for the premotor theory, since the contralesional motor activity required during limb activation improves performance on clinical measures of neglect such as cancellation. However, it seems possible (and perhaps likely) that contralesional limb activation simply increases the frequency and amplitude of contralesional saccades, thus increasing the likelihood that neglected stimuli will be foveated, but without necessarily affecting the distribution of spatial attention. However, in a study of the effects of limb activation on visual extinction, Mattingley et al. (1998) showed that detection of contralesional targets increased significantly when the affected hand (which was hidden from view on the contralesional side of the display) was used to initiate each trial. Crucially, the patient maintained central fixation throughout the experiment, thus permitting any potential effects due to eye movements to be excluded. These findings provide strong evidence that contralesional limb activation actually reduces the competitive advantage for ipsilesional stimuli, and suggests that activity within the motor system can influence perceptual selectivity, as proposed by the premotor theory of attention.

Recall that in addition to their profound spatial bias, many right-hemisphere patients also have a reduced attentional capacity (Driver et al. 1997; Husain et al. 1997; Duncan et al. 1999). This may be related to the impairment of arousal that is common in such patients (Posner and Petersen 1990), and which has been suggested to exacerbate many of the clinical manifestations of spatial neglect (Robertson 1993). A long-standing issue in neurobiological theories of attention (Heilman et al. 1985) has been the extent to which neural systems responsible for mediating arousal are able to influence those concerned with spatial selection. To address this issue, Robertson et al. (1998) examined the effect of providing auditory alerting cues to right-hemisphere patients during a visual TOJ task (see above). The patients, all of whom had neglect and/or extinction, were asked to judge the order of onset of bilateral stimuli that appeared either simultaneously or with a variable SOA between them. In trials without an alerting cue, the patients exhibited a prior entry bias, such that right events were perceived as appearing on average around 500 ms prior to concurrent left events, indicating a spatial bias of attention toward the unaffected side. On the random 25 per cent of trials that were preceded by a salient spatially uninformative alerting cue, this bias was effectively eliminated. These findings provide direct evidence for the interdependency of generalized arousal on the one hand, and spatial selectivity on the other.

Neuroanatomical considerations in spatial extinction

The phenomena of spatial neglect have been variously associated with lesions of the inferior parietal lobule (Vallar and Perani 1986) and superior temporal gyrus (Karnath *et al.* 2001). Relevant anatomoclinical data for extinction are broadly consistent with the patterns observed in neglect, although it has been difficult to draw any firm conclusions. One of the major problems faced by studies seeking to correlate the locus of brain damage with clinical impairments such as neglect has been the difficulty of defining key areas of involvement based upon regions of maximal lesion overlap (Vallar and Perani 1986; Karnath *et al.* 2001). Most patients have large infarctions in the territory of the middle cerebral artery, which has branches that supply most of the lateral convexity of the hemisphere as well as numerous subcortical structures via the lenticulostriate branches (Donnan *et al.* 1991). Moreover, structural imaging can never give the complete picture regarding brain physiology. Functional imaging studies have revealed widespread changes in cerebral blood flow and metabolism even after quite small infarcts (Perani *et al.* 1987), suggesting that the network of brain areas affected in neglect and extinction may be more widespread than commonly assumed.

Early investigators, such as Brain (1941) and Critchley (1949), were amongst the first to suggest a specific relation between the attentional problem of extinction and damage to the association cortex, particularly the parietal lobe. In their classic study of attentional cueing in unilateral lesion patients, Posner *et al.* (1984) described parietal patients as having an 'extinction-like' reaction time pattern, an interpretation that has entrenched the notion of extinction as a distinctly parietal phenomenon. Milner and Goodale (1995) proposed that extinction arises uniquely from damage to the superior parietal lobule, part of the dorsal visual processing stream, whereas spatial neglect arises from damage to the inferior parietal lobule at the interface of the dorsal and ventral streams. Although this separation of lesion sites for extinction and neglect fits with many contemporary accounts of the primate visual system (Milner and Goodale 1995), it is inconsistent with studies showing that extinction can occur after a variety of cortical and subcortical lesions. For instance, of the 46 right-hemisphere-extinction patients examined by Vallar *et al.* (1994), roughly half had circumscribed subcortical lesions, and around a quarter of those with cortical lesions had no damage posterior to the central sulcus. Although this study is somewhat limited by the clinical methods used for assessment, it nevertheless provides some evidence that extinction may not be a strictly parietal phenomenon. Further anatomoclinical correlation studies, using precisely controlled stimulus presentations that avoid floor and ceiling effects, are needed to resolve this issue.

Whether or not it proves possible to 'localize' extinction to a particular brain area, it is nevertheless clear that substantial unconscious processing of extinguished stimuli occurs within undamaged regions of the affected hemisphere. I will not dwell on this issue at length here (although see Chapter 6.1), other than to point out that the nature and extent of any residual processing in extinction will probably be determined by the areas spared by the lesion. As noted elsewhere (Driver and Mattingley 1998; Driver and Vuilleumier 2001), unconscious processing of extinguished objects (McGlinchey-Berroth *et al.* 1993), faces (Rees *et al.* 2000), and words (Schweinberger and Stief 2001) probably arises in most cases from preserved activity within the ventral visual stream (Milner and Goodale 1995). Thus the actual manifestations of unconscious processing, at least for the visual modality, will probably be determined by the extent to which the lesion encroaches on the relevant extrastriate regions within occipital and temporal cortex. It has been suggested that the posterior parietal cortex in primates maintains a 'salience map' of currently relevant spatial locations (Gottlieb *et al.* 1998). If parietal cortex is damaged, there may no longer be a mechanism for binding ventral stream representations to their appropriate locations in space, thus leading to the characteristic loss of awareness for all aspects of contralesional objects (see Driver and Vuilleumier (2001) for a more detailed discussion of this idea).

Two fruitful avenues for future research on the anatomical correlates of extinction are likely to come from the use of functional brain imaging and transcranial magnetic stimulation (TMS). Significant progress has already been made in this direction, and this chapter concludes with a consideration of some recent findings.

Despite the explosion of interest in determining the neural correlates of attention and consciousness in normal subjects (Kanwisher 2001; Kanwisher and Wojciulik 2000), relatively little attention has been devoted to investigating the neural basis of extinction-like phenomena. Fink *et al.* (2000) conducted a positron-emission tomography (PET) study of interhemispheric competition, in which patterns of activation were compared for conditions of partial versus whole reports of letter arrays presented to the left and right hemifields (Sperling 1960; Duncan 1980). For unilateral letter arrays, brain activity was maximal in early visual areas of the contralateral occipital cortex. For bilateral arrays, however, neural activity in early visual areas was significantly reduced relative to that associated with the unilateral arrays, suggesting some degree of neural suppression associated with interhemispheric rivalry. Broadly similar results have been obtained in functional magnetic resonance imaging (fMRI) experiments comparing simultaneous versus successive presentations of visual stimuli in attentional tasks (Kastner *et al.* 1998).

Another approach that has begun to reveal the neurophysiological basis for pathological extinction has come from the use of focal TMS. By delivering a brief high-intensity magnetic pulse to the scalp it is possible to induce a sudden change in electrical current in the underlying cortex, thus producing a reversible 'virtual lesion' in normal subjects (Pascual-Leone *et al.* 2000). By time-locking the TMS pulse to the presentation of lateralized visual or tactile stimuli, several studies have succeeded in producing extinction in normal observers. For example, Pascual-Leone *et al.* (1994) found that repetitive TMS over parietal cortex induced significantly more misses of a contralateral visual target in bilateral than in unilateral presentations. In contrast, similar stimulation of occipital cortex resulted in equivalent misses for both unilateral and bilateral trials. Analogous results have been obtained in the tactile modality, using single-pulse TMS over parietal cortex (Oliveri *et al.* 1999). In a recent series of studies, Oliveri *et al.* (1999, 2000) examined the effects of TMS on the *unaffected* (left) hemisphere of right-brain-damaged patients with tactile extinction. They found that a TMS pulse applied over the left frontal cortex 40 ms after delivery of bimanual tactile stimuli significantly reduced the severity of left-sided extinction in their right-hemisphere patients. These findings are consistent with the notion that pathological extinction involves an interhemispheric competitive bias which favors stimuli transmitted to the intact hemisphere. Presumably the competitive balance is restored by transiently disrupting activity within the intact hemisphere. This is analogous to the effect observed in animal lesion studies, in which a contralesional field defect induced by unilateral occipital ablation is ameliorated by a further lesion of midbrain structures opposite the cortical lesion (Sprague 1966).

Conclusion

An overview of recent clinical and experimental data on pathological extinction following unilateral brain damage has been presented in this chapter. It is clear that this aspect of the broader clinical syndrome of spatial neglect can be traced back to an underlying limit in the normal capacity for attending to multiple target items concurrently, together with a strong spatial gradient in the representation of space arising from unilateral damage of parietal (and possibly other) regions. The studies reviewed here suggest that competitive interactions provide an important mechanism for the selective processing of sensory inputs in the normal brain, and they provide evidence that spatial extinction following unilateral brain damage reflects the outcome of biased competition between simultaneous contralesional and ipsilesional stimuli. The use of fMRI and event-related potentials has already begun to reveal the brain basis for unconscious processing in extinction (Rees *et al.* 2000; Vuilleumier *et al.* 2001). Future studies will no doubt adopt similar approaches to reveal the neural loci for the prior-entry effects, cross-modal interactions, and limb activation and alerting techniques reviewed in this chapter. With further advances in the use of TMS for detecting facilitatory and inhibitory interactions between brain regions (Oliveri *et al.* 2000), it should soon be possible to tease apart the complex dynamics of extinction in normality and pathology.

Acknowledgements

This work was supported by a grant from the Australian Research Council to JBM. The author thanks Nicoletta Beschin, Greg Davis, Jon Driver, Masud Husain, Hans-Otto Karnath, Steffan Kennett, Chris Rorden, and Ian Robertson for their collaborative contributions to the work reviewed here. He also thanks Ada Kritikos for her comments on the manuscript.

References

Aglioti, S., Smania, N., and Peru, A. (1999). Frames of reference for mapping tactile stimuli in brain-damaged patients. *Journal of Cognitive Neuroscience*, **11**, 67–79.

Angelelli, P., De Luca, M., and Spinelli, D. (1996). Early visual processing in neglect patients: a study with steady-state VEPs. *Neuropsychologia*, **34**, 1151–7.

Angelelli, P., De Luca, M., and Spinelli, D. (1998). Contrast sensitivity loss in the neglected hemifield. *Cortex*, **34**, 139–45.

Baylis, G. C. and Driver, J. (1993). Visual attention and objects: Evidence for hierarchical coding of locations. *Journal of Experimental Psychology: Human Perception and Performance*, **19**, 451–70.

Baylis, G. C., Driver, J., and Rafal, R. D. (1993). Visual extinction and stimulus repetition. *Journal of Cognitive Neuroscience*, **5**, 453–66.

Baylis, G. C., Simon, S. L., Baylis, L. L., and Rorden, C. (2002). Visual extinction with double simultaneous stimulation: what is simultaneous? *Neuropsychologia*, **40**, 1027–34.

Bellas, D. N., Novelly, R. A., Eskenazi, B., and Wasserstein, J. (1988). Unilateral displacement in the olfactory sense: a manifestation of the unilateral neglect syndrome. *Cortex*, **24**, 267–75.

Bender, M. B. (1952). *Disorders of perception*. C. C. Thomas, Springfield, IL.

Birch, H. G., Belmont, I., and Karp, E. (1967). Delayed information processing and extinction following cerebral damage. *Brain*, **90**, 113–30.

Bisiach, E., Geminiani, G., Berti, A., and Rusconi, M. L. (1990). Perceptual and premotor factors of unilateral neglect. *Neurology*, **40**, 1278–81.

Brain, W. R. (1941). Visual disorientation with special reference to lesions of the right cerebral hemisphere. *Brain*, **64**, 244–71.

Bundesen, C. (1990). A theory of visual attention. *Psychological Review*, **97**, 523–47.

Corben, L. A., Mattingley, J. B., and Bradshaw, J. L. (2001). A kinematic analysis of distracter interference effects during visually guided action in spatial neglect. *Journal of the International Neuropsychological Society*, **7**, 334–43.

Critchley, M. (1949). The phenomenon of tactile inattention with special reference to parietal lesions. *Brain*, **72**, 538–61.

Davis, G. and Driver, J. (1994). Parallel detection of Kanizsa subjective figures in the human visual system. *Nature*, **371**, 791–3.

Davis, G. and Driver, J. (1998). Kanizsa subjective figures can act as occluding surfaces at parallel stages of visual search. *Journal of Experimental Psychology: Human Perception and Performance*, **24**, 169–84.

De Renzi, E., Gentilini, M., and Pattacini, F. (1984). Auditory extinction following hemisphere damage. *Neuropsychologia*, **22**, 733–44.

Desimone, R. and Duncan, J. (1995). Neural mechanisms of selective visual attention. *Annual Review of Neuroscience*, **18**, 193–222.

di Pellegrino, G. and De Renzi, E. (1995). An experimental investigation on the nature of extinction. *Neuropsychologia*, **33**, 153–70.

di Pellegrino, G., Basso, G., and Frassinetti, F. (1997a). Spatial extinction on double asynchronous stimulation. *Neuropsychologia*, **35**, 1215–23.

di Pellegrino, G., Làdavas, E., and Farnè, A. (1997b). Seeing where your hands are. *Nature*, **388**, 730.

di Pellegrino, G., Basso, G., and Frassinetti, F. (1998). Visual extinction as a spatio-temporal disorder of selective attention. *NeuroReport*, **9**, 835–9.

Donnan, G. A., Bladin, P. F., Berkovic, S. F., Longley, W. A., and Saling, M. M. (1991). The stroke syndrome of striatocapsular infarction. *Brain*, **114**, 51–70.

Driver, J. and Grossenbacher, P. G. (1996). Multimodal contraints on tactile spatial attention. In *Attention and performance XVI* (ed. T. Innui and J. L. McClelland), pp. 209–36. MIT Press, Cambridge, MA.

Driver, J. and Mattingley, J. B. (1998). Parietal neglect and visual awareness. *Nature Neuroscience*, **1**, 17–22.

Driver, J. and Spence, C. (1998). Attention and the crossmodal construction of space. *Trends in Cognitive Sciences*, **2**, 254–62.

Driver, J. and Vuilleumier, P. (2001). Perceptual awareness and its loss in unilateral neglect and extinction. *Cognition*, **79**, 39–88.

Driver, J., Mattingley, J. B., Grossenbacher, P. G., Beschin, N., and Robertson, I. H. (1996). Multimodal attention: interactions between touch, vision and proprioception in spatial selection. Presented at the Third Annual Meeting of the Cognitive Neuroscience Society, San Francisco, CA.

Driver, J., Mattingley, J. B., Rorden, C. R., and Davis, G. (1997). Extinction as a paradigm measure of attentional bias and restricted capacity following brain injury. In *Parietal lobe contributions to orientation in 3D space* (ed. P. Thier and H.-O. Karnath), pp. 401–30. Springer-Verlag, Heidelberg.

Duncan, J. (1980). The locus of interference in the perception of simultaneous stimuli. *Psychological Review*, **87**, 272–300.

Duncan, J. (1984). Selective attention and the organization of visual information. *Journal of Experimental Psychology: General*, **113**, 501–17.

Duncan, J. (1996). Coordinated brain systems in selective perception and action. In *Attention and performance XVI* (ed. T. Innui and J. L. McClelland), pp. 549–78. MIT Press, Cambridge, MA.

Duncan, J., Bundesen, C., Olson, A., Humphreys, G., Chavda, S., and Shibuya, H. (1999). Systematic analysis of deficits in visual attention. *Journal of Experimental Psychology: General*, **128**, 450–78.

Farah, M. J., Wong, A. B., Monheit, M. A., and Morrow, L. A. (1989). Parietal lobe mechanisms of spatial attention: modality-specific or supramodal? *Neuropsychologia*, **27**, 461–70.

Ffytche, D. and Zeki, S. (1996). Brain activity related to the perception of illusory contours. *NeuroImage*, **3**, 104–8.

Fink, G. R., Driver, J., Rorden, C., Baldeweg, T., and Dolan, R. J. (2000). Neural consequences of competing stimuli in both visual hemifields: a physiological basis for visual extinction. *Annals of Neurology*, **47**, 440–6.

Friedrich, F. J., Egly, R., Rafal, R. D., and Beck, D. (1998). Spatial attention deficits in humans: a comparison of superior parietal and temporal-parietal junction lesions. *Neuropsychology*, **12**, 193–207.

Frith, C. D., Blakemore, S. J., and Wolpert, D. M. (2000). Abnormalities in the awareness and control of action. *Philosophical Transactions of the Royal Society of London. Series B, Biological Sciences*, **355**, 1771–88.

Gilchrist, I. D., Humphreys, G. W., and Riddoch, M. J. (1996). Grouping and extinction: evidence for low-level modulation of visual selection. *Cognitive Neuropsychology*, **13**, 1223–49.

Gottlieb, J. P., Kusunoki, M., and Goldberg, M. E. (1998). The representation of visual salience in monkey parietal cortex. *Nature*, **391**, 481–4.

Graziano, M. S. A. and Gross, C. G. (1995). The representation of extrapersonal space: a possible role for bimodal visual-tactile neurons. In *The cognitive neurosciences* (ed. M. S. Gazzaniga), pp. 1021–34. MIT Press, Cambridge, MA.

Graziano, M. and Gross, C. G. (1998). Spatial maps for the control of movement. *Current Opinion in Neurobiology*, **8**, 2195–201.

Graziano, M., Yap, G. and Gross, C. G. (1994). Coding of visual space by premotor neurons. *Science*, **266**, 1054–7.

Heilman, K. M., Bowers, D., Coslett, H. B., Whelan, H., and Watson, R. T. (1985*a*). Directional hypokinesia: Prolonged reaction times for leftward movements in patients with right hemisphere lesions and neglect. *Neurology*, **35**, 855–9.

Heilman, K. M., Watson, R. T., and Valenstein, E. (1985*b*). Neglect and related disorders. In *Clinical neuropsychology* (2nd edn) (ed. K. M. Heilman and E. Valenstein), pp. 243–93. Oxford University Press, New York.

Hillis, A. E., Lenz, F. A., Zirh, T. A., Dougherty, P. M., Eckel, T. S., and Jackson, K. (1998). Hemispatial somatosensory and motor extinction in stereotactic thalamic lesions. *Neurocase*, **4**, 21–34.

Husain, M., Shapiro, K., Martin, J., and Kennard, C. (1997). Abnormal temporal dynamics of visual attention in spatial neglect patients. *Nature*, **385**, 154–6.

Inhoff, A. W., Rafal, R. D., and Posner, M. I. (1992). Bimodal extinction without cross-modal extinction. *Journal of Neurology, Neurosurgery, and Psychiatry*, **55**, 36–9.

Kanizsa, G. (1976). Subjective contours. *Scientific American*, **234**, 48–52.

Kanwisher, N. (2001). Neural events and perceptual awareness. *Cognition*, **79**, 89–113.

Kanwisher, N. and Wojciulik, E. (2000). Visual attention: insights from brain imaging. *Nature Reviews Neuroscience*, **1**, 91–100.

Kaplan, R. F., Verfaellie, M., DeWitt, D., and Caplan, L. R. (1990). Effects of changes in stimulus contingency on visual extinction. *Neurology*, **40**, 1299–1301.

Karnath, H.-O. (1988). Deficits of attention in acute and recovered hemi-neglect. *Neuropsychologia*, **20**, 27–45.

Karnath, H.-O., Christ, K., and Hartje, W. (1993). Decrease of contralateral neglect by neck muscle vibration and spatial orientation of trunk midline. *Brain*, **116**, 383–96.

Karnath, H.-O., Ferber, S., and Himmelbach, M. (2001). Spatial awareness is a function of the temporal not the posterior parietal lobe. *Nature*, **411**, 950–3.

Kastner, S., De Weerd, P., Desimone, R., and Ungerleider, L. G. (1998). Mechanisms of directed attention in the human extrastriate cortex as revealed by functional MRI. *Science*, **282**, 108–11.

Kinsbourne, M. (1993). Orientational bias model of unilateral neglect: evidence from attentional gradients within hemispace. In *Unilateral neglect: clinical and experimental studies* (ed. I. H. Robertson and J. C. Marshall), pp. 63–86. Lawrence Erlbaum, Hove.

Kooistra, C. A. and Heilman, K. M. (1989). Hemispatial visual inattention masquerading as hemianopia. *Neurology*, **39**, 1125–7.

Ladàvas, E., Petronio, A., and Umiltà, C. (1990). The deployment of visual attention in the intact field of hemineglect patients. *Cortex*, **26**, 307–17.

Làdavas, E., Carletti, M., and Gori, G. (1994). Automatic and voluntary orienting of attention in patients with visual neglect—horizontal and vertical dimensions. *Neuropsychologia*, **32**, 1195–1208.

McGlinchey-Berroth, R., Milberg, W. P., Verfaellie, M., Alexander, M. P., and Kilduff, P. T. (1993). Semantic processing in the neglected visual field: evidence from a lexical decision task. *Cognitive Neuropsychology*, **10**, 79–108.

Mack, A. and Rock, I. (1998). *Inattentional blindness*. MIT Press, Cambridge, MA.

Mark, V. W., Kooistra, C. A., and Heilman, K. M. (1988). Hemispatial neglect affected by non-neglected stimuli. *Neurology*, **38**, 1207–11.

Mattingley, J. B. and Driver, J. (1997). Distinguishing sensory and motor deficits after parietal damage: an evaluation of response selection biases in unilateral neglect. In *Parietal lobe contributions to orientation in 3D space* (ed. P. Thier and H.-O. Karnath), pp. 309–37. Springer-Verlag, Berlin.

Mattingley, J. B., Bradshaw, J. L., and Phillips, J. G. (1992). Impairments of movement initiation and execution in unilateral neglect: directional hypokinesia and bradykinesia. *Brain*, **115**, 1849–74.

Mattingley, J. B., Phillips, J. G., and Bradshaw, J. L. (1994). Impairments of movement execution in unilateral neglect: a kinematic analysis of directional bradykinesia. *Neuropsychologia*, **32**, 1111–34.

Mattingley, J. B., Davis, G., and Driver, J. (1997*a*). Preattentive filling-in of visual surfaces in parietal extinction. *Science*, **275**, 671–4.

Mattingley, J. B., Driver, J., Beschin, N., and Robertson, I. H. (1997*b*). Attentional competition between modalities: extinction between touch and vision after right hemisphere damage. *Neuropsychologia*, **35**, 867–80.

Mattingley, J. B., Husain, M., Rorden, C., Kennard, C., and Driver, J. (1998*a*). Motor role of human inferior parietal lobe revealed in unilateral neglect patients. *Nature*, **392**, 179–82.

Mattingley, J. B., Robertson, I. H., and Driver, J. (1998*b*). Modulation of covert visual attention by hand movement: evidence from parietal extinction after right-hemisphere damage. *Neurocase*, **4**, 245–53.

Mattingley, J. B., Pisella, L., Rossetti, Y., Rode, G., Tiliket, C., Boisson, D., and Vighetto, A. (2000). Visual extinction in oculocentric coordinates: a selective bias in dividing attention between hemifields. *Neurocase*, **6**, 465–75.

Michotte, A., Thines, G., and Crabbe, G. (1964). *Les compliments amodaux des structures perceptives*. Publications Universitaires de Louvain.

Milner, A. D. and Goodale, M. A. (1995). *The visual brain in action*. Oxford University Press.

Monsell, S. and Driver, J. (ed.) (2000). *Control of cognitive processes: attention and performance XVIII*. MIT Press, Cambridge, MA.

Morrow, L. A. and Ratcliff, G. (1988). The disengagement of covert attention and the neglect syndrome. *Psychobiology*, **16**, 261–9.

Oliveri, M., Rossini, P. M., Pasqualetti, P., Traversa, R., Cicinelli, P., Palmieri, M. G., Tomaiuolo, F., and Caltagirone, C. (1999*a*). Interhemispheric asymmetries in the perception of unimanual and bimanual cutaneous stimuli: a study using transcranial magnetic stimulation. *Brain*, **122**, 1721–9.

Oliveri, M., Rossini, P. M., Traversa, R., *et al.* (1999*b*). Left frontal transcranial magnetic stimulation reduces contralesional extinction in patients with unilateral right brain damage. *Brain*, **122**, 1731–9.

Oliveri, M., Rossini, P. M., Filippi, M. M., *et al.* (2000). Time-dependent activation of parieto-frontal networks for directing attention to tactile space—a study with paired transcranial magnetic stimulation pulses in right-brain-damaged patients with extinction. *Brain*, **123**, 1939–47.

O'Regan, J. K., Rensink, R. A., and Clark, J. J. (1999). Change-blindness as a result of 'mudsplashes'. *Nature*, **398**, 34.

Pascual-Leone, A., Gomez-Tortosa, E., Grafman, J., Alway, D., Nichelli, P., and Hallett, M. (1994). Induction of visual extinction by rapid-rate transcranial magnetic stimulation of parietal lobe. *Neurology*, **44**, 494–8.

Pascual-Leone, A., Walsh, V., and Rothwell, J. (2000). Transcranial magnetic stimulation in cognitive neuroscience—virtual lesion, chronometry, and functional connectivity. *Current Opinion in Neurobiology*, **10**, 232–7.

Pavlavskaya, M., Sagi, D., Soroker, N., and Ring, H. (1997). Visual extinction and cortical connectivity in human vision. *Cognitive Brain Research*, **6**, 159–62.

Perani, D., Vallar, G., Cappa, S., Messa, C., and Fazio, F. (1987). Aphasia and neglect after subcortical stroke: a clinical/cerebral perfusion correlation study. *Brain*, **110**, 1211–29.

Posner, M. I. and Petersen, S. E. (1990). The attention system of the human brain. *Annual Review of Neuroscience*, **13**, 25–42.

Posner, M. I., Walker, J. A., Friedrich, F. J., and Rafal, R. D. (1984). Effects of parietal injury on covert orienting of attention. *Journal of Neuroscience*, **4**, 1863–74.

Puleo, J. S. and Pastore, R. E. (1978). Critical-band effects in two-channel auditory signal detection. *Journal of Experimental Psychology: Human Perception and Performance*, **4**, 153–63.

Rapcsak, S. Z., Watson, R. T., and Heilman, K. M. (1987). Hemispace-visual field interactions in visual extinction. *Journal of Neurology, Neurosurgery, and Psychiatry*, **50**, 1117–24.

Rees, G., Wojciulik, E., Clarke, K., Husain, M., Frith, C., and Driver, J. (2000). Unconscious activation of visual cortex in the damaged right hemisphere of a parietal patient with extinction. *Brain*, **123**, 1624–33.

Remy, P., Zilbovicius, M., Degos, J.-D., *et al.* (1999). Somatosensory cortical activations are suppressed in patients with tactile extinction: a PET study. *Neurology*, **52**, 571–7.

Rensink, R. A. (2000). The dynamic representation of scenes. *Visual Cognition*, **7**, 17–42.

Rensink, R. A., O'Regan, J. K., and Clark, J. J. (1997). To see or not to see—the need for attention to perceive changes in scenes. *Psychological Science*, **8**, 368–73.

Rizzolatti, G. and Camarda, R. (1987). Neural circuits for spatial attention and unilateral neglect. In *Neurophysiological and neuropsychological aspects of spatial neglect* (ed. M. Jeannerod), pp. 289–313. North-Holland, Amsterdam.

Robertson, I. H. (1993). The relationship between lateralised and non-lateralised attentional deficits in unilateral neglect. In *Unilateral neglect: clinical and experimental studies* (ed. I. H. Robertson and J. C. Marshall), pp. 257–75. Lawrence Erlbaum, Hove.

Robertson, I. H. and North, N. T. (1992). Spatio-motor cueing in unilateral left neglect: the role of hemispace, hand and motor activation. *Neuropsychologia*, **30**, 553–63.

Robertson, I. H. and North, N. T. (1993). Active and passive activation of left limbs: influence on visual and sensory neglect. *Neuropsychologia*, **31**, 293–300.

Robertson, I. H. and North, N. T. (1994). One hand is better than two: motor extinction of left hand advantage in unilateral neglect. *Neuropsychologia*, **32**, 1–11.

Robertson, I. H., North, N. T., and Geggie, C. (1992). Spatiomotor cueing in unilateral left neglect: three case studies of its therapeutic effects. *Journal of Neurology, Neurosurgery, and Psychiatry*, **55**, 799–805.

Robertson, I. H., Mattingley, J. B., Rorden, C., and Driver, J. (1998). Phasic alerting of neglect patients overcomes their spatial deficit in visual awareness. *Nature*, **395**, 169–72.

Rorden, C., Mattingley, J. B., Karnath, H.-O., and Driver, J. (1997). Visual extinction and prior entry: impaired perception of temporal order with intact motion perception after unilateral parietal damage. *Neuropsychologia*, **35**, 421–33.

Rosenbaum, D. A. (1994). *Human motor control*. Academic Press, San Diego, CA.

Scholl, B. J. (2001). Objects and attention: the state of the art. *Cognition*, **80**, 1–46.

Schweinberger, S. R. and Stief, V. (2001). Implicit perception in patients with visual neglect: lexical specificity in repetition priming. *Neuropsychologia*, **39**, 420–9.

Scott, S., Mattingley, J. B., Manly, T., and Wise, R. (1997). Spatial attention deficits and the perception of time. Presented at the Autumn Meeting of the British Neuropsychological Society, London.

Smania, N. and Aglioti, S. (1995). Sensory and spatial components of somaesthetic deficits following right brain damage. *Neurology*, **45**, 1725–30.

Smania, N., Martini, M. C., Prior, M., and Marzi, C. A. (1996). Input and response determinants of visual extinction: a case study. *Cortex*, **32**, 567–91.

Smania, N., Martini, M., Gambina, G., *et al.* (1998). The spatial distribution of visual attention in hemineglect and extinction patients. *Brain*, **121**, 1759–70.

Smith, E. E. and Jonides, J. (1999). Neuroscience—storage and executive processes in the frontal lobes. *Science*, **283**, 1657–61.

Spence, C., Nicholls, M. E. R., Gillespie, N., and Driver, J. (1998). Cross-modal links in exogenous covert spatial orienting between touch, audition, and vision. *Perception and Psychophysics*, **60**, 544–57.

Spence, C., Pavani, F., and Driver, J. (2000). Crossmodal links between vision and touch in covert endogenous spatial attention. *Journal of Experimental Psychology: Human Perception and Performance*, **26**, 1298–1319.

Spence, C., Shore, D. I., and Klein, R. M. Multimodal prior entry. *Journal of Experimental Psychology: General*, in press.

Sperling, G. (1960). The information available in brief visual presentations. *Psychological Monographs: General and Applied*, **74**, 1–29.

Spinelli, D., Burr, D. C., and Morrone, M. C. (1994). Spatial neglect is associated with increased latencies of visual evoked potentials. *Visual Neuroscience*, **11**, 909–18.

Spinelli, D., Angelelli, P., Deluca, M., and Burr, D. C. (1996). VEPs in neglect patients have longer latencies for luminance but not for chromatic patterns. *NeuroReport*, **7**, 815–19.

Sprague, J. M. (1966). Interaction of cortex and superior colliculus in mediation of visually guided behaviour in the cat. *Science*, **153**, 1544–7.

Stein, B. E., Wallace, M. T., and Meredith, M. A. (1995). Neural mechanisms mediating attention and orientation to multisensory cues. In *The cognitive neurosciences* (ed. M. S. Gazzaniga), pp. 683–702. MIT Press, Cambridge, MA.

Stelmach, L. B. and Herdman, C. M. (1991). Directed attention and perception of temporal order. *Journal of Experimental Psychology: Human Perception and Performance*, **17**, 539–50.

Titchener, E. B. (1908). *Lectures on the elementary psychology of feeling and attention*. Macmillan, New York.

Valenstein, E. and Heilman, K. M. (1981). Unilateral hypokinesia and motor extinction. *Neurology*, **31**, 445–8.

Vallar, G. (1998). Spatial hemineglect in humans. *Trends in Cognitive Sciences*, **2**, 87–97.

Vallar, G. and Perani, D. (1986). The anatomy of unilateral neglect after right-hemisphere stroke lesions. A clinical/CT-scan correlation study in man. *Neuropsychologia*, **24**, 609–22.

Vallar, G., Antonucci, G., Guarigha, C., and Pizzamiglio, L. (1993). Deficits of position sense, unilateral neglect and optokinetic stimulation. *Neuropsychologia*, **31**, 1191–200.

Vallar, G., Rusconi, M. L., Bignamini, L., Geminiani, G., and Perani, D. (1994). Anatomical correlates of visual and tactile extinction in humans: a clinical CT scan study. *Journal of Neurology, Neurosurgery, and Psychiatry*, **57**, 464–70.

von der Heydt, R., Peterhans, E., and Baumgartner, G. (1984). Illusory contours and cortical neuron responses. *Science*, **224**, 1260–2.

Vuilleumier, P. (2000). Faces call for attention: evidence from patients with visual extinction. *Neuropsychologia*, **38**, 693–700.

Vuilleumier, P. O. and Rafal, R. D. (1999). 'Both' means more than 'two': localizing and counting in patients with visuospatial neglect. *Nature Neuroscience*, **2**, 783–4.

Vuilleumier, P. O. and Rafal, R. D. (2000). A systematic study of visual extinction: between- and within-field deficits of attention in hemispatial neglect. *Brain*, **123**, 1263–79.

Vuilleumier, P. O. and Schwartz, S. Emotional facial expressions capture attention. *Neurology*, **56**, 153–8.

Vuilleumier, P. O. and Schwartz, S. Spiders, flowers, and other visual things: capture of attention by fear relevant stimuli in patients with unilateral neglect. Submitted for publication.

Vuilleumier, P., Valenza, N., Mayer, E., Perrig, S., and Landis, T. (1999). To see better to the left when looking more to the right: effects of gaze direction and frames of spatial coordinates in unilateral neglect. *Journal of the International Neuropsychological Society*, **5**, 75–82.

Vuilleumier, P., Sagiv, N., Hazeltine, E., *et al.* (2001). Neural fate of seen and unseen faces in visuospatial neglect: a combined event-related functional MRI and event-related potential study. *Proceedings of the National Academy of Sciences of the United States of America*, **98**, 3495–500.

Ward, R. and Goodrich, S. (1996). Differences between objects and nonobjects in visual extinction: a competition for attention. *Psychological Science*, **7**, 177–80.

Ward, R., Goodrich, S., and Driver, J. (1994). Grouping reduces visual extinction: neuropsychological evidence for weight-linkage in visual selection. *Visual Cognition*, **1**, 101–29.

Zackon, D. H., Casson, E. J., Zafar, A., Stelmach, L., and Racette, L. (1999). The temporal order judgement paradigm: subcortical attentional contribution under exogenous and endogenous cueing conditions. *Neuropsychologia*, **37**, 511–20.

Section 6 Cognitive processes in neglect

6.1 Unconscious processing in neglect

Anna Berti

Conscious awareness of sensory events (i.e. conscious recognition and identification of stimuli) allows subjects to comment and act upon the objects of the external world. Its presence is usually inferred from either the subject's overt report of the existence and of the characteristics of the stimulus or by the subject's overt behavior. In unilateral neglect, patients do not report, react, or search for stimuli located in the space contralateral to right-brain damage. When questioned about the presence/absence of contralesional stimuli, they often deny their existence. Even in everyday life they do not use objects which are located in the affected sector of space nor they deploy their attention toward them. Thus they seem to be unaware of contralesional sensory events. The lack of awareness of stimuli coming from the neglected side has often been ascribed to a failure in stimulus processing because of an attentional disorder which prevents any stimulus analysis. However, the view of a complete overlap between stimulus processing and its sensory awareness has been challenged by recent counter-intuitive evidence which has revealed that unperceived stimuli can nonetheless be processed by the nervous system.

In this chapter, we review the evidence demonstrating the existence of unconscious processing of unperceived stimuli in neglect and related disorders, together with the evidence showing how awareness for contralesional stimuli is not an all-or-nothing phenomenon. Implicit processing and modulation of awareness will be discussed with reference to a theory that considers neglect as being due to a disturbance of space awareness.

Unconscious processing in extinction

In the neuropsychological literature, one of the first instances of unconscious processes of unperceived contralateral stimuli has been described in cases of visual extinction. Extinction can either be seen in isolation—and considered a milder form of neglect—or can co-occur with a number of other neglect symptoms. In a classical extinction paradigm the patient is required to detect the presence or report some particular feature of a stimulus presented either alone or paired with another one. Typically, patients do not have problems in single-stimulus trials but miss the leftward stimulus when it is presented together with another stimulus on the right. In a seminal paper, Volpe *et al.* (1979) reported testing four patients with visual extinction on a task in which line drawings of objects or words were presented to the right and the left of a fixation point. The patients had to judge whether the two stimuli were the same or different. Two of the patients denied the presence of any stimulus on the left side and claimed that the test was silly because, they argued, it is not possible to say whether two stimuli are the same or different when only one is presented in the visual field. Nonetheless when the patients were forced to guess, they gave correct same–different judgments. This outcome suggested a dissociation between phenomenal experience of the visual stimuli (absent) and their neural processing (present). Indeed, correct above-chance same–different judgments can only be achieved if somewhere in the brain a (putative nonconscious) representation of the stimuli is available. According to Volpe and collaborators, the brain damage prevents the access to consciousness of the representation that, nonetheless, guided the patients' behavior.

One problem raised by this study is that of the cognitive level of processing that the unseen stimulus can reach. One possibility is that only low-level sensory processing can be carried out nonconsciously by the damaged brain. Another possibility is that the extinguished information can be analyzed even semantically without becoming conscious. Volpe and coworkers favored the second hypothesis and proposed that full—sensory and semantic—processing of the extinguished stimuli was responsible for the patients' correct discrimination. However, in the study just described, it is difficult to draw firm conclusions about the level of processing reached by the unperceived stimulus because low- and high-level processes were confounded in the design. Indeed, when the stimuli were the 'same' they not only belonged to a given object category but were also physically identical, and when they were 'different' they were both physically different and belonged to different semantic categories. Therefore the correctness of patients' responses might have been based only on intact sensory processing that sorted the category on the basis of visual similarity.

The problem of the level of processing that unperceived visual stimuli can reach has been further investigated by Berti *et al.* (1992) in a study of a single patient (EM). This patient, who was affected by left visual field extinction, was tested using a paradigm similar to that used by Volpe *et al.* (1979). The stimuli were photographs of real objects briefly presented to the right, to the left, or on both sides of a fixation point. In single-stimulation trials the patient was able to identify and name the objects depicted in the photographs.

In conditions of double simultaneous stimulation two photographs were presented, one to the right and one to the left of the fixation point. The objects could belong to either the 'same' category or to 'different' categories; when they were the 'same' they could be either physically identical or physically different (i.e. two different exemplars of a watch), whereas when they were 'different' they could be either physically very similar or physically dissimilar (Fig. 1).

In *double-stimulation* conditions, the patient was sometimes aware that 'something' was presented in the affected field, but she could only say that this 'something' was a sort of light. Although she was never aware of the identity of left-side stimuli, she could judge whether they belonged to the same or different categories. Moreover, she also gave correct same–different judgments when the stimuli were physically different but belonged to the 'same' category, and when they were physically similar but belonged to the 'different' category. Therefore it was concluded that EM was able to process not only the physical features of the unperceived stimulus, but also their semantic relation.

It is worth noting that extinction has been usually studied using simple and briefly presented visual events. Therefore it has generally been mainly characterized as a two-dimensional phenomenon, affecting meaningless visual stimuli (Marzi *et al.* 1996), letters (di Pellegrino and DeRenzi 1995), line drawings of objects (Volpe *et al.* 1979), or photographs of real objects (Berti *et al.* 1992). In most of these cases unconscious processing has been demonstrated. An interesting question is whether extinction (and nonconscious representations of the extinguished stimuli) can also be found for real three-dimensional objects, or whether extinguished, but still processed, information can enter awareness once that three-dimensional object representation is activated. Recently, Maravita (1997) has described, in the somatosensory domain, extinction for both dimension and recognition of three-dimensional geometric shapes. A patient with light touch extinction

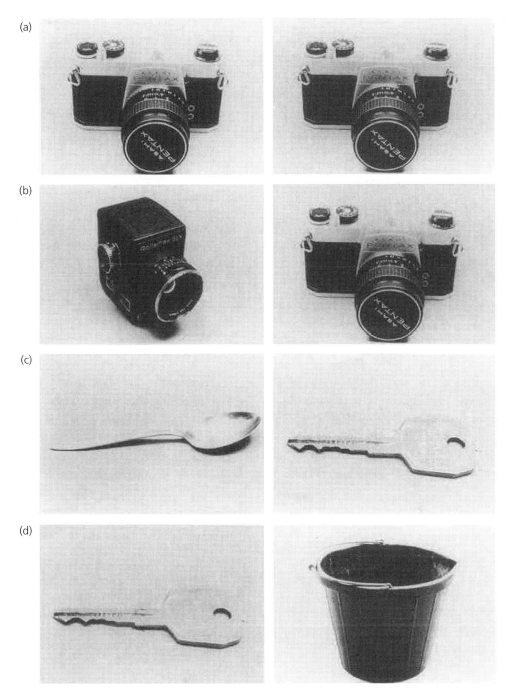

Figure 1 Examples of the stimuli used in the visual same–different task: (a) same–identical condition (stimuli have physical and categorical similarity); (b) same–different condition (stimuli have only categorical similarity); (c) different–similar condition (stimuli have only physical similarity); (d) different–dissimilar condition (stimuli had no similarity). See text for explanation. (Adapted from Berti *et al.*, *Neuropsychologia*, **30**, 403–15 (1992).)

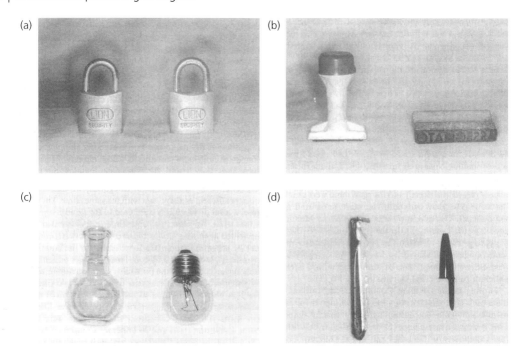

Figure 2 Examples of the stimuli used in the tactile same–different task: (a) same–identical condition (stimuli have physical and categorical similarity); (b) same–different condition (stimuli have only categorical similarity); (c) different–similar condition (stimuli have only physical similarity); (d) different–dissimilar condition (stimuli have no similarity). See text for explanation. (Adapted from Berti *et al.*, *Neuropsychologia*, **37**, 333–43 (1999).)

was unable to say which of two different spheres, placed simultaneously in the two hands, was the larger. Sometimes he was not even able to say that the left-hand object was a sphere; nonetheless, he presented with a tactile illusion that could only be obtained if normal processing of the shape of the left-hand object was carried out.

Berti *et al.* (1999) also found categorical processing of the extinguished stimulus in the tactile–haptic domain. A paradigm similar to that used in the previous study (Berti *et al.* 1992) (Fig. 2) was employed, but this time the patient was asked to judge real three-dimensional objects placed in the right and left hands. The patient (ENM) showed extinction of left-side objects similar to that shown by EM. He claimed that he felt that something was placed in his left hand, but he had no idea of what it was, not even whether it was a real object. Nevertheless, he was able to make correct same–different judgments on the stimuli when they were categorically the same but physically different, and when they were categorically different but physically similar.

These data show that the extraction of three-dimensional information from a real object is not sufficient to trigger a conscious representation of it.

Unconscious processing in neglect

In the neglect domain, the first instance of nonconscious processing of the left-side stimuli can be found in a study conducted by Halligan and Marshall (1988). They described a neglect patient who resolutely denied any differences between line drawings of two houses, identical on the right side, but with bright red flames coming out from the left window of one of them. Despite this explicit denial of any difference between the two stimuli, when asked in which of the two houses she would have preferred to live in, the patient consistently chose the nonburning house. This behavior suggested that the patient covertly recognized the semantic content of the stimuli so that its *unconscious* representation influenced the conscious patient's choice. However, a subsequent study by Bisiach and Rusconi (1990) showed that results like those described by Halligan and Marshall (1988) do not necessarily imply unconscious *semantic* processing of the unperceived stimuli. Using stimuli similar to the 'burning house', Bisiach and Rusconi (1990) described two patients who consistently made a 'nonsemantic' choice, for instance the burning house. This means that the patients' responses, although related to an implicit processes of the neglected stimuli, could be perceptually, and not semantically, based.

Conceptually similar findings were later reported by Vallar *et al.* (1994). They asked five neglect patients to give same–different judgments on pairs of line drawings of animals. The pairs were composed of two pictures shown one above the other. Same pairs were composed of two identical drawings. Different pairs consisted of a drawing of an animal and a drawing in which the left half of that animal had been substituted by the left half of a different animal. All patients misjudged the different pairs as 'same'. However, when asked which of the two drawings more appropriately corresponded to the name of the animal depicted in the nonchimeric picture, three patients made the correct choice and noticed the presence of the chimeric picture, whereas one patient made the correct choice without noticing the presence of the different left half of the animal. Another patient gave paradoxical responses, choosing the chimeric figure instead of the picture depicting the full animal. The consistent choice of one of the two pictures in this case indicates that the patient's responses were not at chance and therefore that, at some stage of the visual information processing, some aspects of the unreported stimulus had influenced the patient's behavior. However, one cannot conclude that the choice was made on semantic grounds.

Nonconscious perception up to the level of meaning extraction was demonstrated in neglect patients by Berti and Rizzolatti (1992). They used a priming paradigm in which line drawings of objects were tachistoscopically presented to the right and left of a fixation point. Presentation of left-side prime stimuli was always followed by right-side target stimuli. The target could be categorically related to the prime (congruent conditions) or unrelated (noncongruent condition). In the congruent condition the stimuli could be perceptually identical (highly congruent condition) or dissimilar (congruent condition). Patients were instructed to press one or the other of two keys depending on whether the right-side figure was an animal or a fruit. Five patients always denied the occurrence of left visual stimuli. Nonetheless, they showed significantly shorter reaction times to the right-side stimuli in the highly congruent and congruent conditions (743 and 750 ms respectively) than in the noncongruent condition (855 ms). These data showed that stimuli from the neglected side can be processed by the visual system and that this process can reach a categorical level of representation. Berti and Rizzolatti (1992) also ran a control condition in which the primes were shapes physically similar to the drawings used as stimuli, but not recognizable as animals or fruit (Fig. 3). In the congruent condition with meaningless shapes they did not obtain a priming effect, showing that the facilitation in reaction time in the congruent condition with meaningful drawings was not due to putative physical similarity amongst exemplars within a category. Implicit categorical processing for symmetric–asymmetric line drawings of objects has recently been reported by Doricchi and Galati (2000).

Nonconscious processing of neglected information has also been demonstrated for verbal material, i.e. for words or parts of words that are not explicitly reported by neglect patients. Instances of low-level implicit analysis of meaningful letter strings can be found in those cases of neglect where the lexical status of a word influences the patient's reading. Indeed, it has often been observed that patients with neglect dyslexia are better at reading real meaningful words than meaningless string of letters (Behrmann *et al.* 1990). An opposite dissociation was described by Bisiach *et al.* (1990).

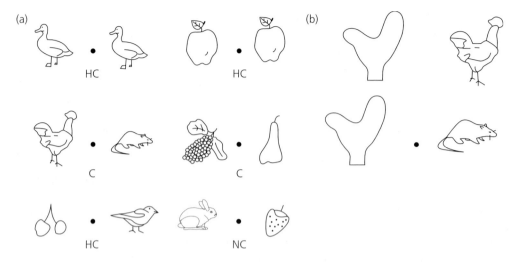

Figure 3 Examples of the stimuli used in the priming experiment: (a) combination of stimuli used for the highly congruent (HC), congruent (C) and noncongruent (NC) conditions; (b) example of how meaningless shapes have been derived from meaningful line drawings (upper pair) and of the control condition corresponding to a congruent trial (lower pair). See text for explanation. (Reproduced from Berti and Rizzolatti, *Journal of Cognitive Neuroscience*, **4**, 345–51 (1992).)

They reported the case of patient EB who neglected or miscompleted the left side of 10-letter meaningful words and pronounceable nonwords. However, this patient was able to report correctly all letters from stimuli in which the left part of the words had been substituted by a string of consonants. In this case, despite the severity of neglect shown in reading conventional words, either the physical (word form) or the lexical status of the left part of the letter string affected patients' awareness of the left part of the stimulus. In any case (both when patients read words better than nonwords and vice versa), in order to affect the patient's performance *differently* the left part of the letter string must have been processed *always*, and not just when a correct reading was achieved.

The word-form and the lexical effects described above do not necessarily imply that semantic processing can be carried out on the unperceived verbal stimuli. However, subsequent research has shown that the meaning of the unperceived words could also be processed implicitly. Làdavas *et al.* (1993) demonstrated nonconsious semantic priming during a lexical decision test. They asked a neglect patient to press a bar as soon as possible at the presentation of real words projected in the good ipsilesional field; no response was required if nonwords were presented. In go trials, before the presentation of the right visual field word (target), another word, which could be either semantically related or unrelated to the target word, was presented to the left visual field (prime). Responses to right target words preceded by semantically related prime words were faster than responses to trial when a semantically unrelated words was presented as prime. In a forced choice detection task with a yes–no response, the patient was at chance in detecting left visual field words, showing no awareness of the stimuli that caused the priming effect. Similar priming effects of left-sided stimuli were also shown by McGlinchey-Berroth *et al.* (1993) in four patients with visual neglect.

Berti *et al.* (1994) have demonstrated semantic processes for the *left* neglected part of content words. They described patient MD, affected by neglect dyslexia, who made omission errors in reading common words and words that indicated colors. For instance, when asked to read the Italian word *marrone*, which means 'brown', he read *one*, which does not mean anything in

Italian. When forced to say what word it might have been, he still did not read the left part of it, but claimed that the meaning could be related to something that had to do with nuclear power such as 'neutron' or 'proton'. A Stroop color task (Stroop 1935) was carried out on this patient. He was asked to name the color in which words were written as quickly as possible. The color could be congruent with the meaning of the word (the word 'red' written in red ink) or incongruent (the word 'red' written in green). Lists of congruent and incongruent words were presented. Patient MD showed longer naming times for the list of words whose meaning did not correspond to the color in which were written. In other words, although he was not able to read explicitly the left part of words, the meaning of those words strongly influenced the color-naming task. This showed that the left neglected part of words was implicitly processed up to the level at which the reading process is completed, i.e. up to the level of meaning extraction. Indeed the interference effect in the Stroop test is due to the competition for the output buffer between the two color words that became activated in the incongruent condition of the task, i.e. the word that is actually written and the word depicting the color of the written word. More recently, Berti *et al.* (2000) have shown an influence of the meaning of the unreported left side of words, embedded in string of nonreadable consonants, on the position of the neglect point in reading a complex string of letters. The word could be in the center, on the right, or on the left of the meaningless string (e.g. for the word MATITA (pencil) the stimuli could be ZFGMATITARBD, MATITAZFGRBD, or ZFGRBDMATITA). The patients were simply requested to read the stimulus. It was found that in some patients with neglect dyslexia the neglect point was influenced by the position of the real word in the string, and in particular that the neglect point was moved to the left when the meaningful word was on the left. This was interpreted as an implicit effect of the semantic aspect of the stimulus on the patient's reading performance. Interestingly, when the neglect point was moved to the left by the presence of the meaningful stimuli, the words was almost always read again with neglect errors. For instance, a patient could read the 12-letter string ZFGRBDMATITA as $------$ TITA (omitting the first eight letters) and the string MATITAZFGRBD as $--$ TITAZFGRBD (this time omitting only two left letters). This showed that the pre-attentive effect of the meaning did not trigger any conscious experience of the left-side part of the stimulus.

In summary, the study of both extinction and neglect patients has demonstrated that the fate of the unreported stimuli is not necessarily that of being completely lost by the nervous system. The level at which unperceived stimuli are processed can be very high, although some experiments used tasks and paradigms that did not allow unconscious processing based on physical/pictorial characteristics to be disentangled from unconscious processing also involving the semantic attributes of the stimulus. The experiments that used categorization tasks and purely verbal material are the most convincing examples of processing without awareness of the semantic content of neglected information.

A tentative explanation of processing without awareness in neglect

Understanding of the phenomenon of unconscious processing in neglect may be improved if one considers the similarities and differences with respect to blindsight, another syndrome characterized by unawareness for contralesional stimuli. Blindsight is a neurological condition in which a visual field deficit is consequent upon damage to the primary visual occipital areas. Patients with either syndrome are not *aware* of the stimuli presented contralateral to the brain damage, but in both cases it is possible to demonstrate unconscious processing of unperceived stimuli. However, there are important differences between the two syndromes. Behaviorally, although both kinds of patients deny the existence of contralesional stimuli, a subject with blindsight acknowledges being blind, whereas a neglect patient does not report any problem with his or her vision; in other words, while blindsight patients complain of losing information from one side of the world, neglect patients usually do not report such a lack of experience. From a physiological point of view, in blindsight subjects the brain damage which prevents an overt detection and recognition of stimuli is located in an area (the striate cortex) that has always been related to primary visual processes and where neurons code visual information in retinal coordinate. As a consequence, blindsight manifests itself in retinal coordinates. In contrast, the brain areas whose damage is responsible for neglect are not primary sensory areas, but associative areas not responsible of the visual processes *per se*. Neurons in these areas code visual information in a system of nonretinal coordinates. Therefore neglect manifests itself in nonretinal coordinate. As pointed out by different authors, while the challenge in blindsight is that of explaining the possibility of processing (unconsciously) visual stimuli despite the well-documented visual field defect, in neglect the question is why patients do not report stimuli that can be physiologically processed, at least by visual occipital areas. Indeed, Berti and Rizzolatti (1992) (see also Làdavas *et al.* (2000) and Driver and Vuilleumier (2001) for similar considerations) claimed that the demonstration that neglect patients can process visual shape presented to the neglected side to a very high level of elaboration is not surprising when one considers the functional–anatomical organization of the visual cortical system. It is generally accepted that there is a segregation between centers for space representation (dorsal stream) and centers for stimulus perception (ventral stream) (Ungerleider and Mishkin 1982). The parietal areas whose damage usually produces neglect are part of the dorsal stream and are mostly involved in space analysis and in the control of visually guided movement. In contrast, perception of form depends mostly on the activity of inferotemporal areas of the ventral stream. As a consequence, the capacity of shape analysis and categorization shown by neglect patients is exactly what one would expect from the functional–anatomical properties of the intact ventral chains of visual centers. Also, the fact that neglect patients can be implicitly affected by illusory stimuli even when they do not perceive the left part of the illusory configuration has been ascribed to the normal functioning of intact occipital extrastriate areas (see Chapter 4.6). A similar interpretation can be proposed for explaining priming and related effects obtained in neglect patients using verbal material. The areas primarily involved in reading and more generally in language processes are intact in neglect patients. Thus, what we have to explain is why, despite the integrity of the cognitive systems underlying the various implicit processes found in neglect, patients are unaware of the product of the processing carried out on the stimuli falling in the affected sector of space. To explain this apparent paradox, Berti and Rizzolatti (1992) proposed that the encoding of space is a necessary prerequisite for the conscious perception of sensory events. If spatial encoding is prevented or impaired, as it is in neglect, stimuli do not reach consciousness even when processed up to a semantic level. Therefore, if our brain cannot locate a stimulus in space, the presence and the identity of the stimulus does not enter consciousness. In this view awareness depends on the normal functioning of space representations i.e., the 'where' enables the 'what'.

Rizzolatti and Berti (1993) advanced a theory that considers neglect as being mainly due to a disorder of space awareness. According to this theory, based on the neurophysiological characteristics of the brain centers devoted to space representation (Rizzolatti *et al.* 2000), space awareness would depend upon the joint activity of several perceptuomotor cortical and subcortical pragmatic maps that are part of the dorsal stream of visual information processing (see also Chapter 3.3). The synergic activity of all these different maps is responsible for the emergence of awareness for the stimuli presented in different sectors of space and of the execution of the correct action in that space. Thus the functioning of a composite multicomponential structure, distributed in discrete brain areas, represents the necessary condition for gaining a conscious experience of the stimuli of the external world onto which actions have to be executed. A lesion of one or more of the dorsal stream maps induces a decrement of the total activity of the system; the activity produced by the other intact or quasi-intact maps is not sufficient for generating normal awareness in the space sector affected by the brain lesion. In other words, the dorsal stream has a crucial role in the activation of the visual representation of the ventral stream (Doricchi and Galati 2000). The decrement of the neural activity consequent on brain damage is also tuned by the competition that arises between the right damaged and left intact, hemisphere space representations, so that the representation that depends upon the affected hemisphere becomes weaker. Nonetheless, stimuli are processed by the intact brain regions devoted to specific cognitive elaboration. It is worth noting that what is weaker is the representation of space and not that of the stimuli *per se*. As already said, they may receive a full cognitive analysis (e.g. a semantic representation of a word) without this reaching consciousness. Thus a weaker space representation interferes with the chain of events that is crucial for attaining stimulus awareness and therefore for accomplishing the correct motor act.

Modulation of awareness

Position in space

The theory of a multicomponent network for space awareness not only accounts for nonconscious processing of neglected stimuli, but also predicts the possibility that space awareness can be modulated by factors that selectively activate the maps for spatial representation. One important component in the differential activation of space awareness is the position of the object with the respect to its distance from the patient's body and its relative position with respect to different systems of body coordinates.

A discrete brain lesion can affect only the part of the circuit that preferentially codes the space outside hand-reaching distance; in this case awareness will be affected mainly in the nonreachable space, whereas a stimulus presented in near space, coded by the map that has not been damaged, can be detected (Cowey *et al.* 1994; Vuilleumier *et al.* 1998). In contrast, brain damage affecting mainly the representation of the space surrounding the body would cause a lack of awareness for stimuli presented in near space (Halligan and Marshall 1991; Berti and Frassinetti 2000). Animal studies have shown that areas that are specialized for coding near space can also contain a small percentage of neurons that represent far space and vice versa. Therefore damage of a given brain area, although affecting mainly the representation of one space sector, may also impair, although less severely, another sector of space. As a consequence, the double dissociations between far- and near-space neglect found in humans are never of the strong type (see also Chapter 3.3), i.e. neglect is also present in the space sector that is not directly affected by the brain lesion, whereas awareness for the stimuli located in the affected space may fluctuate and not be completely lost because of the small percentage of neurons in the unaffected brain map which can still represent, although in a weaker way, that sector of space.

Awareness can also be influenced by the relation between the current posture of the patient with respect to the spatial position of the stimulus. An amelioration of the sensory awareness for visual events is usually observed when the visual stimulus is delivered to the right of the trunk midline (Bisiach *et al.* 1985*b*) irrespective of its position on the retina (Kooistra and Heilman 1989; Karnath *et al.* 1991). In the tactile–haptic domain, stimulus awareness depends upon the spatial location of the hand in space. Smania and Aglioti (1995) have shown that a tactile stimulus delivered to the left hand of patients with tactile extinction had better chance of being experienced and reported if the left hand was positioned in the right space. Berti *et al.* (1999) found that even tactile identification and recognition of meaningful object was influenced by the position of the hands. In patient ENM (who had tactile extinction for meaningful objects) they observed that there was a tendency for an amelioration of awareness for stimuli manipulated by the left hand when the left hand was positioned in the right hemispace. Interestingly, stimulus awareness for the right unaffected hand was impaired when the right hand was located in the left space. These results demonstrate that the lack of awareness for contralesional stimuli in neglect and extinction is not related to damage to primary sensory cortices, and therefore endowed in a system of retinal and somatotopic coordinates, but instead to a system for the representation of spatially determined events that code space in nonretinal coordinates. Awareness in neglect is not an all-or-nothing phenomenon but depends on the stimuli being within the shadow of a weaker representation of space. Manipulation that would change the relationship between the impaired space and the position of the stimuli affects awareness.

Physiological and behavioral manipulations

If space awareness depends on the normal activity of a multiplicity of brain maps for space representations, the activity of a partially damaged circuit should be increased when specific physiological or behavioral manipulations determine the activation of neural pathways that encroach upon and project to the damaged brain regions devoted to spatial representations. The temporary increase in neural activity may re-equilibrate the imbalance between right and left representations and lead to transient emergence of stimulus awareness. This can be observed when particular kinds of physiological or behavioral maneuvers are applied. For instance, caloric stimulation with cold water in the left ear may induce a temporary remission of the left-side symptomatology in neglect patients (Cappa *et al.* 1987). Awareness for contralesional sensory events emerges and remains present while the physiological effect of stimulation (e.g. saccades toward the affected side) lasts, so that neglect patients who were not able to search for and detect stimuli on the left side become able to carry out many different perceptual and motor tasks in the affected space. A possible interpretation of this effect is that the caloric manipulation, which impinges on the vestibular–proprioceptive paths projecting to the cortex (Bottini *et al.* 1994; Bottini *et al.* 2001), directly modulates the spatial maps whose level of activation was diminished by the brain damage. The possibility of reacting to neglected stimuli under certain physiological conditions clearly demonstrates that inputs from the left affected side can be processed, but that their detection becomes part of the patient's conscious experience only when the rivalry between the two hemispheres, caused by the brain damage, is diminished by the activation induced with the physiological stimulation.

Other authors obtained improvement in left-side processing with task manipulation that combined the differential effect of action performed in the left space with the hand performing the action (Halligan *et al.* 1991; Robertson and North 1992). In particular, the influence of proprioceptive activation on the emergence of awareness in the neglected sector of space has been shown by Làdavas *et al.* (1997) in a study where the task manipulation consisted of passively moving the patient's hand in either ipsilesional or contralesional space. The authors found that neglect patients were more accurate in naming objects projected onto the left side of a 90° mirror which inverted left and right space (Tegner and Levander 1991) when the left hand was passively moved in the left contralesional space than when it was moved in the right space. Since the stimuli and the hands were reflected in a mirror that inverted right and left space, and a direct view of the stimuli and of the stimulated hand was prevented by a board, the better performance was clearly due to the proprioceptive information related to the limb position and not to visual cueing. This study clearly showed that the activation of intact proprioceptive path caused by the stimulation of the hand located in a specific position in space was able to modulate, by projecting to areas that are part of complex circuit for space representation partially damaged by the brain lesion, the impaired representation related to extrapersonal space.

Spatial transpositon

Patients with unilateral brain lesion may be able to report the presence and/or the identity of a stimulus presented to the contralesional side of the body or of the space only if they refer it to the ipsilesional side (allochiria) (Obersteiner 1882). Although this phenomenon has usually been described for elementary stimuli, recent neuropsychological evidence of allochiric transposition for complex meaningful percepts has been obtained in patients with unilateral neglect. Halligan et al. (1992) described a patient who, in copying a butterfly, omitted the left-side wing. However, he drew some of the left-side details on the right wing. Vallar et al. (1994) reported a patient who, when asked to described the picture of a chimera constituted by a deer on the left and a kangaroo on the right, traced the contour of the head of the kangaroo and said: 'Here one could draw a deer'. Similarly, tracing the head of a swan on a shark left–swan right chimera he said: 'Here one could draw a shark'. Interestingly the patient had no apparent conscious experience of the chimeric nature of the configuration. The allochirich behavior is obviously related to the capacity of processing left-side-neglected stimuli up to the semantic level of analysis discussed in the previous sections. What is striking is the dissociation between the 'what' (object recognition) and the 'where' (space localization) of the patient's conscious experience. However, if we assume that space enables awareness for sensory events, allochiria seem to further confirm this hypothesis. The transposition of left-side content to the right space suggests that a necessary condition for gaining access to conscious experience of a sensory events is the possibility of locating it in space, whatever space representation is available.

Input–output component of space awareness

The brain areas devoted to space representation have neurons that are specialized for programming motor acts toward specific space sector. Therefore brain damage to these areas impairs not only the sensory aspect of space coding but also the programming of action directed in the affected space sector. Patients may have problem in initiating movements with the ipsilesional unaffected hand toward contralesional space (directional hypochinesia) (Heilman et al. 1985). This impairment of the motor component of the space representation has been found to influence awareness not only for stimuli presented in the affected side of space, but even for stimuli presented in the good visual field. Patients in whom the input and output components of the task have been disentangled by stimulus manipulation (e.g. a mirror that causes a left–right inverted image of the display) may not be aware of stimuli which, although appearing on the right side of the space visible on the mirror, have to be reached by a motor act toward the affected sector of space (Tegner and Levander 1991). Bisiach et al. (1985a) studied neglect patients using a panel with two rows of light-emitting diodes (LEDs), one green and one red. The LEDs were on both the right and the left of a central fixation point. Four response keys were present below the LEDs, two on the right side of the panel and two on the left. Patients were asked to name either the color of the light that was flashed (first experiment) or to press a response key that was lighted in each trial either on the side of the flashing LED or on the opposite side (second experiment). In the first experiment, when color naming was requested, patients were always fully aware of right-side stimuli and almost never aware of the left. However, in the second experiment, when a motor response was required, awareness was strongly influenced by the side where the motor response had to be given. It was found that awareness for left-side stimuli ameliorated when the response key to left-side stimuli was lighted on the right side. Even awareness for *right*-side stimuli was influenced by the side of the motor response because, when the response key was lighted on the left (neglected) side, patients often showed incorrect reactions—pressing either the key of the right side, which was unlit but of the corresponding color, or the lighted key of the wrong color—or no response at all, as if they had not seen anything on the right good space. One patient (FS) spontaneously denied that any stimulus had occurred in the ipsilesional (unaffected) visual field. In this experiment the temporal sequence of the events is such that the side of the motor response has to be decided *after* the occurrence of the visual stimulus on the good or the affected space. Therefore it is the possibility of gaining access to the motor response, and not only the impaired input procesess, which gates the 'normal' sensory information (coming from the right side of space) out of consciousness and sometimes leads the 'affected' left-side stimulus to be normally perceived and responded to. These results show that consciousness of a sensory event can be precluded when the motor component within a sensory–motor cycle is impaired, whereas awareness for a contralesional visual event can be reached if the sensory–motor cycle is not blocked at the level of the output processes.

Conclusion

Neglect studies have shown that information which has been fully processed in all its features may not be consciously acknowledged, when its spatial location is not analyzed. In other words, brain damage can cause a spatially constrained disorder of awareness. The deficit observed is a disorder of awareness because the processing of a specific kind of stimulus can still be possible while the consciousness for the product of that process is impaired (Umiltà 2000). Moreover, the disturbance is spatially constrained because the processing *and* the conscious experience for information coming from space sectors not affected by the brain damage remain possible.

As we have seen, an interesting property of the network for space awareness is that, since it is distributed anatomically and differentiated physiologically, it can be damaged in only one, or a few, of its components, so that there is the possibility of modulating awareness by task manipulation that impinges upon the spared neurons of the multiple pragmatic maps for space representation. This shows that awareness is not an all-or-nothing phenomenon but can appear to be dissociated depending upon the relation between stimulus and space processing.

These observations not only call into question important psychological assumptions about the correspondence between stimulus processing and its conscious experience, but also threaten the concept of the structural unity of consciousness (Bisiach and Berti 1995). Phenomenal experience, as it is inferred from the behaviour of normal subjects and from our own experience, has the quality of unity. However, data like those coming from the research on nonconscious processes in neglect, showing that brain damage can selectively affect a single stream of consciousness and that the differential activation of distributed space representations can recalibrate a spatially constrained disorder of awareness, suggest that the structure of conscious processes is not unitary and monolithic, but is multicomponential and dynamic (Berti, 2000). Whatever proposal turns out to be adequate for explaining the details of the structure of conscious processes, it is clear that, on the basis of neuropsychological observations, consciousness cannot be considered an indivisible and *heirarchically* superimposed component of the mind. In contrast, consciousness should be considered as a property emerging from a composite and modular organization of the cognitive system, where the coding of the stimulus in space play a crucial role.

Acknowledgement

This work was supported by a MURST-PRIN grant to AB.

References

Behrmann, M., Moscovitch, M., Black, S. E., and Mozer, M. (1990). Perceptual and conceptual mechanisms in neglect dyslexia. Two contrasting case studies. *Brain*, **113**, 1163–83.

Berti, A. Neuropsychological syndromes and the structure of conscious processes. In *The Emergence of the Mind: Proceedings of the 9th International Conference*. Fondazione Carlo Erba, Milan, 2000.

Berti, A. and Rizzolatti, G. (1992) Visual processing without awareness: evidence from unilateral neglect. *Journal of Cognitive Neuroscience*, **4**, 345–51.

Berti, A. and Frassinetti, F. (2000). When far becomes near: re-mapping of space by tool use. *Journal of Cognitive Neuroscience*, **12**, 415–20.

Berti, A., Allport, A., Driver, J., Dienes, Z., Obury, J., and Oxbury, S. (1992) Levels of processing for visual stimuli in an 'extinguished' field. *Neuropsychologia*, **30**, 403–15.

Berti, A., Frassinetti, F., and Umiltà, C. (1994). Nonconscious reading? Evidence from neglect dyslexia, *Cortex*, **30**, 181–97.

Berti, A., Oxbury, S., Oxbury, J., Affanni, P., Umiltà, C., and Orlandi, L. (1999) Somatosensory extinction for meaningful objects in a patient with right hemisphere stroke. *Neuropsychologia*, **37**, 333–43.

Berti, A., Plazzi, S., Maravita, A., and Stracciari, A. (2000). Object and space coding in neglect dyslexia. Presented at the 18th European Workshop on Cognitive Neuropsychology, Bressanone, 24–29 January 2000.

Bisiach, E. and Berti, A. (1995) Consciousness in dyschiria. In *The cognitive neurosciences* (ed. M. S. Gazzaniga), pp. 1331–40, MIT Press, Cambridge, MA.

Bisiach, E. and Rusconi, M. L. (1990) Break-down of perceptual awareness in unilateral neglect. *Cortex*, **26**, 643–9.

Bisiach, E., Berti, A., and Vallar, G. (1985*a*). Analogical and logical disorders underlying unilateral neglect of space. In *Attention and performance XI* (ed. M. I. Posner and O. S. Marin), pp. 239–49. Lawrence Erlbaum, Hillsdale, NJ.

Bisiach, E., Capitani, P., and Porta, E. (1985*b*) Two basic properties of space representation in the brain: evidence from unilateral neglect. *Journal of Neurology, Neurosurgery, and Psychiatry*, **48**, 141–4.

Bisiach, E., Meregalli, S., and Berti, A. (1990). Mechanisms of production control and belief fixation in human visuospatial processing: clinical evidence from unilateral neglect and misrepresentation. In *Quantitative analysis of behavior*. Vol. IX:*Computational and clinical approach to pattern recognition and concept formation* (ed. M. L. Commons, R. J. Herrnstein, S. M. Kosslyn, and D. B. Mumford), pp. 3–21. Lawrence Erlbaum, Hillsdale, NJ.

Bottini, G., Sterzi, R., Paulesu, E., *et al.* (1994) Identification of the cerebral vestibular projection in man: a positron emission tomography activation study. *Experimental Brain Research*, **99**, 164–9.

Bottini, G., Karnath, H. O., Vallar, G., *et al.* (2001). Cerebral representation for egocentric space: functional-anatomical evidence from caloric vestibular stimulation and neck vibration. *Brain*, **124**, 1182–96.

Cappa, S., Sterzi, R., Vallar, G., and Bisiach, E. (1987) Remission of hemineglect and anosognosia during vestibular stimulation. *Neuropsychologia* **25**, 775–82.

Cowey, A., Small, M., and Ellis, S.(1994). Left visuo-spatial neglect can be worse in far than in near space. *Neuropsychologia*, **32**, 1059–66.

di Pellegrino, G. and DeRenzi, E. (1995) An experimental investigation on the nature of extinction. *Neuropsychologia*, **33**, 153–70.

Doricchi and Galati (2000). Implicit semantic evaluation of object symmetry and contralesional visual denial in a case of left unilateral neglect with damage of the dorsal paraventricular white motter. *Cortex*, **36**, 337–50.

Driver, J. and Vuilleumier, P. (2001) Perceptual awareness and its loss in unilateral neglect and extinction. *Cognition*, **79**, 39–88.

Halligan, P. W. and Marshall, J. C. (1988) Blindsight and insight in visuo-spatial neglect. *Nature*, **336**, 766–7.

Halligan, P. and Marshall, J. M. (1991) Left neglect for near but not for far space in man. *Nature*, **350**, 498–500.

Halligan, P. W., Manning, L., and Marshall, J. C. (1991) Hemispheric activation vs spatio-motor cueing in visual neglect: a case study. *Neuropsychologia*, **29**, 165–76.

Halligan, P. W., Marshall, J. C., and Wade, D. T. (1992) Left on the right: allochiria in a case of left visuo-spatial neglect. *Journal of Neurology, Neurosurgery, and Psychiatry*, **55**, 717–19.

Heilman , K. M., Bowers, D., Coslett, H. B., Whelan, H., and Watson, R. T. (1985). Directional hypokinesia. *Neurology*, **35**, 855–9.

Karnath, H. O., Schenkel, P., and Fischer, B. (1991). Trunk orientation as the determining factor of the 'contralateral' deficit in the neglect syndrome and as the physical anchor of the internal representation of body orientation in space. *Brain*, **114**, 1997–2014.

Kooistra, C. A. and Heilman, K. M. (1989). Hemispatial visual inattention masquerading as hemianopia. *Neurology*, **39**, 1125–7.

Làdavas, E., Paladini, R., and Cubelli, R. (1993). Implicit associative priming in a patient with left unilateral neglect. *Neuropsychologia*, **31**, 1307–20.

Làdavas, E., Berti, A., Ruozzi, E., and Barboni, F. (1997). Neglect as a deficit determined by an imbalance between multiple spatial representations. *Experimental Brain Research*, **116**, 493–500.

Làdavas, E., Berti, A., and Farnè, A. (2000). Dissociation between conscious and non-conscious processing in neglect. In *Beyond dissociation: interaction between dissociated implicit and explicit processing* (ed. Y. Rossetti and R. Revounsuo), pp. 175–193. J. Benjamins, Philadelphia, PA.

McGlinchey-Berroth, R., Milberg, W. P. Verfaellie, M., Alexander, M., and Kilduff., P. T. (1993). Semantic processing in the neglected field: Evidence from a lexical decision task. *Cognitive Neuropsychology*, **10**, 79–108.

Maravita, A. (1997) Implicit processing of somatosensory stimuli disclosed by a perceptual after-effect. *NeuroReport*, **8**, 1671–4.

Marzi, C. A., Smania, N., Martini, M. C., *et al.* (1996). Implicit redundant-target effect in visual extinction. *Neuropsychologia*, **34**, 9–22.

Obersteiner, H. (1882). On allochiria: a peculiar sensory disorder. *Brain*, **4**, 153–63.

Rizzolatti, G. and Berti, A. (1993). Neural mechanisms of spatial neglect. In *Unilateral neglect: clinical and experimental studies* (ed. I. H. Robertson and J. C. Marshall), pp. 87–105. Taylor & Francis, London.

Rizzolatti, G., Berti, A., and Gallese, V. (2000). Spatial neglect: neurophysiological bases, cortical circuit and theories. In *Handbook of neuropsychology*, Vol. 1 (ed. F. Boller, J. Grafman, and G. Rizzolatti), pp. 503–37. Elsevier, Amsterdam.

Robertson, I. H. and North, N. (1992). Spatio-motor cueing in unilateral neglect: the role of hemispace, hand and motor activation. *Neuropsychologia*, **30**, 553–63.

Smania, N. and Aglioti, S. (1995). Sensory and spatial component of somaesthetic deficit following right brain damage. *Neurology*, **45**, 1725–30.

Stroop, J. R. (1935). Studies of interference in serial verbal reactions. *Journal of Experimental Psychology*, **18**, 643–62.

Tegner, R. and Levander, M. (1991). Through a looking glass: a new technique to demonstrate directional hypochinesia in unilateral neglect. *Brain*, **114**, 1943–51.

Umiltà, C. (2000). Conscious experience depends on multiple brain systems. *European Psychologist*, **5**, 3–11.

Ungerleider and Mishkin (1982). Two cortical visual systems. In *The analysis of visual behavior* (ed. D. J. Ingle, M. A. Goodale, and R. J. Mansfield). MIT Press, Cambridge, MA.

Vallar, G., Rusconi, M. L., and Bisiach, E. (1994). Awareness of contralesional information in unilateral neglect. In *Attention and performance XV* (ed. M. Moscovitch and C. A. Umiltà), Cambridge, MA, MIT Press.

Vuilleumier, P., Valenza, N., Mayer, E., Reverdin, A., and Landis, T. (1998). Near and far visual space in unilateral neglect. *Annals of Neurology*, **43**, 406–10.

Volpe, B. T., Ledoux, and Gazzaniga, M. S. (1979). Information processing in an 'extinguished' visual field. *Nature*, **282**, 722–4.

6.2 Primary sensory deficits after right brain damage—an attentional disorder by any other name?

Peter W. Halligan and John C. Marshall

The clinical presentation of patients who 'ignore' objects, events, or people on the side of space opposite their brain damage (clinically termed visual–spatial neglect (VSN)) has been described in the medical literature for well over a century. Although there were comparatively few studies of VSN prior to the 1970s, the last 25 years has spawned a proliferation of research from the related fields of clinical neuropsychology (Bisiach and Vallar 1988; Heilman *et al.* 1993), cognitive neuropsychology (McCarthy and Warrington 1990; Robertson and Marshall 1993), cognitive neuroscience (Jeannerod 1987; Thier and Karnath 1997), and neuro-rehabilitation (Robertson and Halligan 1999).

Recent findings have had important consequences for neuropsychological theory and clinical practice, while also questioning many strongly held beliefs in a conceptually and clinically unified syndrome of VSN (Heilman and Valenstein 1979; Vallar 1994). Most manifestations of the 'neglect syndrome' have been shown to dissociate across patients (Barbieri and DeRenzi 1989; Stone *et al.* 1998; Vallar 1998). Even within such relatively simple tasks as copying or spontaneous drawing there are many qualitatively distinct patterns of impairment that could each be called lateralized 'neglect' (Marshall and Halligan 1993; Halligan and Marshall 2001).

The original account of the syndrome has become so fragmented in the last decade (Halligan and Marshall 1994; Stone *et al.* 1998) that even its original architects were forced to concede the need for revision:

> Although at one time we thought that the variety of neglect subtypes could be explained by variations in severity and in means of elicitation, we currently believe that neglect is not a unitary disorder. There is increasing evidence that neglect can be subdivided by the presumed underlying mechanisms: inattention (sensory neglect), disorders of action and intention (motor neglect), and representational disorders. (Heilman *et al.* 1994)

Despite the growing number of studies that have questioned the integrity of a unified construct, the clinical definition and the traditional methods used to assess VSN and to distinguish the condition from other sensory and cognitive disorders has survived remarkably intact. A standard textbook description of visual neglect defines the condition as '... the failure to report, respond, or orient to novel or meaningful stimuli presented to the side opposite a brain lesion, when this failure cannot be attributed to either sensory or motor defects' (Heilman *et al.* 1993).

Since the 1970s, VSN has been conceptualized (almost exclusively) in terms of higher-level cognitive deficits using for the most part behavioral measures derived from clinical neuropsychology.

This proclivity for 'cognitive' explanations (attentional, intentional, and/or representational) over the past 30 years assumed that a firm line could be drawn between behavioral symptoms due to sensory–motor deficits (e.g. hemianopia or hemiparesis) and those due to higher-level processes (e.g. VSN). Most contemporary accounts of VSN employ the above clinical definition and the more widespread distinction between 'primary' (low-level, sensory–motor) and 'cognitive' (high-level) deficits. Such a distinction is not specific to the study of neglect (see Bay (1953) and Bender and Feldman (1972) for analogous arguments about agnosia), although the assumption that the behavioral manifestations of neglect performance are not due to 'primary' sensory–motor deficits has rarely been questioned since the 1970s (but see Marshall *et al.* (1993)).

Since the definition of neglect provided by Heilman and colleagues does not in itself specify how the condition should be assessed or how it should be distinguished from the effects of primary deficits, the presenting symptoms of VSN have tended to be 'defined' ostensibly by the clinical bedside tasks used to reveal them rather than by any principled understanding of their nature (Milner 1997). As such, selective (impaired) lateralized performances are described as instances of 'perceptual', 'representational', 'attentional', 'intentional', or 'motor' neglect on the basis of a superficial characterization of the eliciting task conditions. This approach is problematic, since it reserves higher-level cognitive explanations for a limited range of lateralized symptoms whose main justification is that they were derived from measures other than those used by neurologists/neuro-ophthalmologists to assess 'primary sensory deficits'. It was not always so.

As Cohen (1993, p. 194) writes:

> Many neurologists prior to 1950 did not distinguish disorders of neglect from other unilateral sensory disturbances. The neglect of one side of the body or environment that some patients with contralateral brain lesions exhibited was considered to result from deafferentation of sensory pathways and or sensory cortex. This position was supported by the high incidence of primary sensory disturbances in these patients ... therefore the unilateral quality of neglect seems to fit with the unilateral nature of the many sensory disturbances, in which the ascending sensory pathways are disturbed unilaterally.

In the absence of a principled rationale for the selection of the behavioral tests employed to diagnose VSN (many of which predate the formal emergence of neglect as a clinical entity), it is timely to (1) review the conceptual distinction drawn between primary and **high-level** deficits insofar as they relate to current accounts of VSN, (2) critically examine whether the behavioral measures currently employed are capable of distinguishing between the two levels of deficit, and (3) consider whether it remains theoretically or clinically useful to retain a strong conceptual distinction between different levels of impairment within functionally specific but nevertheless integrated visual information processing systems.

We do not suggest that some (or all) of the many heterogeneous clinical forms of VSN can or should be explained by primary sensory disorders (e.g. visual field deficits), or that all forms of supposedly primary sensory deficits originate from higher-level deficits. Rather, we will argue that the traditional conceptual divide between the former and the latter is predicated upon differential task demands and criterion measures that are currently justified by little more than tradition. Thus the distinction may need to be revised for the benefit of understanding both types of deficit (Halligan, Marshall, and Wade, 1990).

The historical basis for the conceptual divide between 'primary' and 'high-level' deficits

The historical origins of the hierarchical view of visual processing ('low-level' versus 'high-level' vision) which subsequently dominated much of experimental neurobiology and clinical neuropsychology over the last century, have been comprehensively reviewed by Zeki (1993).

Zeki traces this distinction back to a conceptual (rather than empirical) parcelling of 'seeing' into a sensory experience followed by subsequent high-level 'interpretations'. Consequently,

> there has been a tendency, dictated partly by philosophical speculation and partly by neurological speculation to separate the problem of sensing from that of understanding . . . Central to these concepts, and the first among them, was the neurologists' philosophical view of vision and, indeed of the brain, the supposition that cortical vision was a dual [hierarchical] process consisting, first, of the reception and analysis of visual 'impressions'—the process which led to 'seeing'—and, next of their 'association' with previous impressions—a process which led to 'understanding' what was seen, each process having a separate and anatomically distinct cortical seat.

This in turn assumed that

> . . . a distinctive cortical function such as 'seeing' should be reflected in a distinctive cortical architecture, while a function such as 'association' should be reflected in a different cortical architecture. (Zeki 1993, p. 48)

In addition to providing a heuristic framework for understanding the effects of brain damage, this division legitimated the pursuit of independent methods which, over time, became characteristic of different clinical specialities (e.g. neuro-optometry and neuropsychology), each pursuing independent lines of research. The consequences of this division were to be long lasting. The development of cognitive accounts of agnosia and VSN was delayed by the notion that they were due to primary sensory disorders (either bilateral or unilateral).

> In accepting this doctrine neurologists had come, by the turn of the century, to develop a deeply philosophical attitude about the brain, usually without realising it. . . . it would be no exaggeration to say that adherence to this doctrine retarded our present notion of the organization of the visual cortex and of brain function by well over a century. Until the last two decades and possibly even today, most visual neurobiology was concerned with relatively low levels of vision and in particular with the retina. (Zeki 1993, pp. 3–4)

More importantly, this 'philosophical speculation' was instrumental in suggesting which functions should be attributed to the different anatomical brain areas and the interpretation of the behavioral consequences that followed relatively discrete pathology to different brain areas. The initial clinical evidence was derived from a purported distinction between visual field deficits (VFDs) and agnosia, where '. . . lesions in one part of the visual cortex led to blindness, lesions in another part led to a condition in which patients could see but could not understand what had been seen' (Zeki 1993).

The fact that many patients with lateralized neurological symptoms apparently failed to show evidence of 'primary deficits' using conventional neuro-optometry and neurological methods explains why in the 1970s neuropsychologists confidently asserted that VSN was a 'higher-level' disorder' that could not (by definition) be attributed to the effects of 'primary deficits'.

The late development of VSN as a 'high-level' cognitive deficit

Before VSN became a household name in behavioral neurology and cognitive neuropsychology in the 1980s, the term was often used to describe a subset of clinical behaviors not explicitly distinguished from those attributed to unilateral sensory disturbances (Bender 1952; Battersby *et al.* 1956; Eidelberg and Schwartz 1971; Weinstein and Friedland 1977). This failure to discriminate is not too surprising given the strong association between what is now regarded as VSN and other neurological and neuropsychological deficits following large lesions of the right hemisphere. This point is illustrated in Fig. 1, which shows that many right-brain-damaged patients

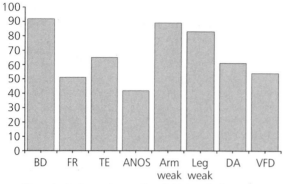

Figure 1 Frequency of perceptual and motor problems in a sample of patients with unilateral neglect (Hier *et al.* 1983): BD, block design; FR, face recognition; TE, tactile extinction; ANOS, anosognosia; DA, dressing apraxia; VFD, visual field deficit.

with visual neglect also suffer face recognition disorders, constructional impairments, extinction, arm and leg paralysis, dressing apraxia, and visual field deficits.

Consequently, the classical description that emerged after the Second World War defined neglect rather loosely as a variable disturbance of visuospatial functions commonly found within a larger constellation of sensory, motor, and other spatial disorders. Informal observation of patient behavior provided the initial basis and ultimately the face validity for both the pathological construct and the development of quantitative diagnostic tests. These included the following:

- failure to notice people approaching from the left
- failure to eat food from the left side of the plate
- failure to dress or groom the left side
- omission of letters, numbers, and/or words on one side of the page when reading
- omission of one side of the contents of a picture during verbal description or drawing
- failure to pick up coins or cards on the affected side
- omission, distortions, and asymmetries in spontaneous drawing and writing.

Although initially a descriptive clinical label derived from countless clinical observations of the behavior of right-brain-damaged patients, VSN made a clean break with its sensory-related past in the early 1970s. This conceptual transformation resulted in more elaborate neuropsychological and neurophysiological attempts to explain the unilateral deficits in terms of impairments to hemispherically lateralized cognitive systems. One potential problem (often overlooked) was that the clinical features and criterion tasks remained unchanged. Researchers continued to employ many of the same clinical methods to diagnose VSN that were in use before the condition was formally recognized as an autonomous clinical entity (Zingerle 1913; Pineas 1931; Brain 1941). Unlike optometry, which developed technically sophisticated means of refining the diagnosis of visual problems, simple bedside tests continued to be used to provide an objective and quantifiable indication of the underlying deficit in neglect. On cancellation, line bisection, and figure copying, patients would be classified as showing VSN if they failed to cancel items located on the left side of the page, bisected lines to the right of true center, and/or omitted or distorted the left side of their drawings.

Since the 1950s, over 50 different tests have been used to provide a quantifiable index of VSN, in the belief that all were somehow capable of tapping the largely unspecified cognitive or high-level disturbances assumed to be implicated in the disorder. In most cases, clinical experience rather than theory provided the justification for particular tasks. Furthermore, few studies attempted to relate the selection of these tests to their ability to predict the functional behavioral characteristics that clinically gave rise to the underlying construct in the first place (Halligan *et al.* 1991). Furthermore, researchers tacitly assumed that the tasks employed were collectively capable of detecting 'high-level' cognitive pathology over and above those effects due to co-occurring primary sensory–motor deficits.

Since the formal diagnosis of primary (e.g. VFD) and higher-level (VSN) disorders ultimately relies upon performance on behavioral tests and since both require simple verbal or motor responses, differential diagnosis of VSN from sensory and/or motor symptoms (e.g. VFD/plegia) was always difficult even after the widespread availability of CT and, more recently, MRI lesion localization (Heilman *et al.* 1993). Precise lesion localization (where available) is not sufficient to distinguish between sensory and high-level disorders in the absence of precise evidence establishing reliable associations between a damaged brain region (derived from structural radiological scans) and selective behavioral performance. Localized (mal)functions are open to different functional interpretations: the behavioral effects of the brain damage could be the product of a disconnection between two relatively intact centers or the result of damage to an area not itself directly responsible for the lost or impaired capacity but nevertheless involved in mediating the response.

Accordingly, the problem of deciding which lateralized symptoms should be attributed to VSN rather than VFD was decided largely by fiat. Given that the standardized neurological and opthalmological measures for 'primary sensory deficits' (e.g. visual field deficit) had been established long before the first published reports of neglect as a formal medical construct, clinical measures used to define VSN were not (by definition) considered to result from primary sensory deficits.

Can clinical measures currently employed to detect 'primary sensory deficits' truly exclude higher-level cognitive deficits?

It is generally accepted that VFD and VSN represent functionally unrelated disorders that differ in terms of lesion location, eye movements, and prognosis (Halligan 1999). A visual field cut (hemianopia or scotoma) is assumed to result from damage to the 'sensory pathways' which transmit visual information from the retina to visual cortex or to occipital cortex itself. Eye-movement recordings have clearly shown that hemianopic patients employ a series of stepwise saccadic eye movements which permit them to find and fixate objects initially located in the blind hemifield (Meienberg *et al.* 1981, 1986). Conversely, patients with neglect make fewer fixations and spend a shorter time exploring the contralesional side (Behrman *et al.* 1997). There is also considerable evidence that many patients with homonymous hemianopia develop over time a consistent set of compensatory eye and head movements directed to the affected side (Ishiai *et al.* 1987; Meienberg *et al.* 1983). In patients where performance on formal perimetry or, more commonly, the less reliable confrontation tests (Trobe *et al.* 1981)) indicates that visual stimuli falling on a particular area of the retina cannot be reliably reported, the assumption is that the 'primary' processing necessary (but not sufficient) for higher-level visual functions has been selectively disconnected or impaired.

Although such deficits undoubtedly exist, distinguishing their effects from 'attentional disorder' after right-hemisphere damage is not straightforward; in both cases, assessments ultimately rely on the patient's ability to report or otherwise respond to specific targets located on the affected side. The problem arises when one patient purportedly shows neglect but not a visual field deficit and another patient purportedly has a visual field deficit but no neglect. Since neglect implies a failure in perceptual awareness in the left field (e.g. a failure to detect targets on the left side of a cancellation or copying task), how is it possible for such a patient to report reliably stimuli located in the left visual field when responding to confrontational visual field testing?

To address these issues it is necessary to consider briefly the history of the methods employed to assess the visual fields. Unlike the assessment of visual neglect, formal visual field assessment began early in the nineteenth century; the first perimeter was designed by Purkinje in 1825 (Grüsser and Landis 1991). Thirty years later, in 1856, von Graefe introduced the first systematic assessment in ophthalmology. The aim of perimetry was to provide a quantifiable indication of 'simple sensations'(e.g. those provoked by static or moving point sources of white or colored light) detected by the subjects within their visual field. Assuming that primary visual cortex was specialized for 'basic' sensory or 'low-level' visual functions, disorders of visual detection ('blindness') were commonly attributed to damage to primary visual cortex and the optic radiations (and hence termed 'primary deficits').

Visual field testing charts the relationship between the known spatial location of objects presented during steady fixation of gaze and the subject's ability to detect or describe them. Visual fields testing involves charting the 200° arc of vision and can assess color vision, flicker sensitivity, contrast sensitivity, pupillary responses, and motion detection. There are several ways of testing a patient's visual fields, but the most common clinical method involves confrontational testing whereby the examiner moves a target inward from different locations in the periphery of the subject's visual field. On the basis of normative findings, different patterns of visual loss have been associated with particular diseases of the eye, optic nerves, and central nervous system (Hensen 1993).

Given the apparently simple nature of the task demands, failure to provide a correct verbal report could be construed as a qualitatively elemental or low-level form of visual processing deficit by comparison with the 'higher levels' of visual processing involving perceptual judgments, complex discriminations, or attentional orientation. It was widely assumed that appropriate activation of primary visual (striate) cortex in these tasks was sufficient for the conscious detection of the object in the visual field. However, formal perimetry and indeed clinical confrontation testing depends upon '. . . the co-operation of the patient, on his general attentiveness and on his ability to restrict eye movements, concentrating on a small fixation target throughout' (Grüsser and Landis 1991, p.138). Although traditional methods of visual field assessment have clearly been successful in demonstrating the topography of the afferent visual pathways and considerable inter-individual consistency of correspondence between the retina and striate cortex, the apparent simplicity of the subject's response (consciously to detect and report a spot of light) conceals the many different cognitive processes necessary to perform the task adequately. It is easy to assume that relatively simple tasks (e.g. detection of simple stimuli) do not require the involvement of high-level cognitive processes such as attention. But response to visual field assessment requires cognitive processes similar to those involved in tests of VSN (e.g. vigilance, selective attention, verbal/motor processing of response, working memory, etc). Consequently, it is unclear (other than in terms of task complexity) why failure consciously to detect and register the location of a simple stimulus should not be considered to involve deficits in some of the cognitive processes needed to perform visual neglect tasks.

Furthermore, the extrapolation that impaired performance on simple detection tasks is equivalent to the clinical term 'blindness' was originally based on Lissauer's anatomical distinction between cortical blindness and psychic blindness (agnosia) (Lissauer 1890). Despite the fact that Lissauer's distinction was based on animal experiments, cortical (or cerebral) blindness was assumed to be a total loss within a particular region of the visual field 'of all conscious vision due to lesions of the visual radiations or visual cortex representing that region' (Grüsser and Landis 1991, p. 147). In contrast, 'Poppelreuter (1917) claimed that some rudimentary vision was always present in the blind field' (Heywood 1996, p. 756). Subsequent reports of 'blindsight' (using forced choice discrimination tasks) by Weiskrantz (1986) provided convincing experimental evidence that visual information could be processed in those parts of the visual field considered on perimetry to be 'blind'. Moreover, Kentridge *et al.* (1999) showed that the attentional selection of spatial information can be relatively intact in patients with a visual field deficit who show blindsight. In these experiments, attention was directed by symbolic cues in the subject's spared field of vision or by cues presented in his blind field. Cues in the blind field were effective in directing attention to a second location remote from that at which the cue was presented. In such cases, it is known that a variety of residual and alternative visual pathways systems can arise from thalamic nuclei and bypass V1 (Weiskrantz 1986).

Comparing measures of VFD and VSN

A brief comparison of the two forms of assessment respectively employed to elicit VFD and VSN demonstrates some of their shared cognitive demands (and differences therein):

(1) Visual field testing crucially involves gaze fixation, which makes considerable demands on endogenously controlled visual attention. The extent to which this methodological control involves attention during visual field assessment was eloquently demonstrated by Walker *et al.* (1991). The patient in question had severe left-sided neglect and had been diagnosed by her neuro-ophthalmologist, using standard perimetry, as suffering from a left homonymous hemianopia. Walker and colleagues showed, using a computer set-up similar to standard VFD testing, that the woman did not report stimuli in particular locations. In both experimental procedures, the woman was required to stare at a central fixation point while waiting to detect stimuli on either side of the screen. By switching off the central fixation point a sixth of a second before presenting the lateralized test stimuli, Walker *et al.* (1991) showed that the patient was better able to detect and report the stimuli on the left. The improved results were interpreted as eliminating the attentional demands of having to maintain central fixation as required by traditional VFD testing. In other words, the requirements of gaze fixation acted as a form of cueing of the patient's attention to a central point with the resultant extinction of objects to the left of fixation and hence the apparent hemianopia. This study by Walker *et al.* (1991) strongly suggests that the procedures of maintaining central fixation involved in standard field plotting (e.g. perimetry or confrontation) can introduce attentional factors into visual field testing and hence mislead the examiner's interpretation of the deficit.

(2) Throughout visual field assessment the subject must also maintain vigilance (i.e. sustained attention) so as to detect when and where the light stimulus is introduced into the visual fields.

(3) Furthermore, the subject has to divide his or her attention between the fixation point and the peripheral object (physical extent, color, and shape) introduced by the examiner.

By convention, visual field performance is assessed in terms of a unified frame of reference where the orientation of head, trunk, and eye fixation are all congruent. In contrast, neglect is usually assessed in free vision without explicit control over head or eye movements and analyzed by reference to the patient's midsagittal plane. While fixation ensures that the visual field examined can be brought into correspondence with the retinal field projected onto V1, the diagnosis of VSN does not operate solely within this restricted frame of reference. However, the fact that assessing VFDs makes explicit use of the known connections between retina and striate cortex does not imply that VFDs originate entirely within this primary anatomical system.

Using standard confrontational testing techniques, but employing different lateralized positions of gaze, Nadeau and Heilman (1991) reported a patient (without evidence of visual neglect) who showed a 'gaze-dependent hemianopia'. When the patient directed his gaze 30° to the right (such that the left retinotopic field was now in right hemispace *vis-à-vis* the midsagittal plane) he showed a marked improvement in movement detection, object naming, shape identification, and color naming over the standard condition with 'straight-ahead' fixation. The authors suggest

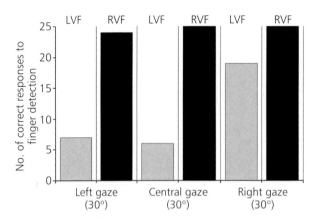

Figure 2 Performance of a patient with an apparent hemianopia which varies depending on where the eyes are pointing. When gazing centrally (central gaze), detections in the left visual field (LVF) were less than in the right visual field (RVF). This was also the case when gazing to the left (left gaze). With right gaze, on the other hand, the number of left-sided detections increased dramatically. In other words, an attentional disorder was masquerading as a peripheral visual disorder. (Adapted from Kooistra and Heilman (1989).)

that the results from the standard confrontation condition in this case represent more than just primary visual dysfunction and that the gaze-direction effects arise from the influence of attentional or intentional factors. This speculation is supported by an earlier case study of a neglect patient by Kooistra and Heilman (1989). Using confrontation assessment, Kooistra and Heilman described a patient with a right thalamic and temporo-occipital lesion who demonstrated a left visual field defect, in addition to neglect on standard tasks such as line cancellation and line bisection. In an attempt to disentangle the effects of neglect and visual field deficit, the patient was instructed to look to the left or the right while engaged in the same visual field assessment. When confrontation testing took place with the patient's eyes directed either straight ahead (as in traditional testing) or 30° towards the left, the patient failed to report stimuli presented in the relative left visual field. However, with her eyes directed 30° towards right hemispace, the visual field defect appeared to resolve. These results suggest that the patient had visual neglect which, upon conventional confrontation testing, was masquerading as a visual field defect. The findings in this patient are summarized diagramatically in Fig. 2. A similar effect with respect to hemianesthesia was reported by Smania and Aglioti (1995); detection of left-sided tactile stimuli after right brain damage improved when the left hand was located in right hemispace.

The effects of VFD on traditional tests of VSN

Since VFD and VSN assessments ultimately require conscious visual processing, presumably mediated in part at least by similar cognitive processes, it is instructive to know how patients with visual field deficits (with and without visual neglect, however defined) perform on traditional 'neglect tests' such as line bisection. The answer was originally raised in early German clinical reports (Axenfeld 1894; Liepmann and Kalmus 1900) and recently investigated by several groups (D'Erme *et al.* 1987; Kerkhoff 1993). Barton and Black (1998) reported that right-brain-damaged patients with left visual field defects but without neglect (measured on a variety of traditional bedside tasks) showed reliable contralesional displacement to the left on line bisection, whereas right-brain-damaged patients with neglect (but without VFD) showed ipsilesional displacement to the right. Hence, if lateral displacement *per se* (as opposed to contralesional versus ipsilateral displacement) were the defining factor, there would be no firm basis for distinguishing (at a behavioral level) between a cognitive or a low-level ('sensory') account of task performance. What might produce such a contralateral bisection bias in hemianopia? One factor suggested by Barton and Black (1998) that could generate an abnormal bias is:

> a change in attentional distribution ... space on their blind side acquires greater salience, leading to an attentional gradient that is strategically adaptive for their disability. Whether the altered gradient is pathological (in neglect) or adaptive (in hemianopia), the result may be a bias in perceptual judgment in the direction of the gradient, causing ipsilateral bisection bias in hemineglect and contralateral bisection bias in hemianopia.

Interactions between hemianopia and neglect on line bisection are also of interest. However, the evidence here is divided. Several studies (D'Erme *et al.* 1987; Doricchi and Angelelli 1999; Daini *et al.*, in press) have shown that neglect patients with homonymous hemianopia make greater ipsilesional bisection errors. In contrast, Ferber and Karnath (1999) showed that the presence of a visual field defect in some patients with left visual neglect could interact to effectively reduce or even cancel the traditional rightward deviation on bisection. The assumption here was that a directionally orthogonal deviation produced by a low-level sensory deficit could modulate a high-level (attentional) deviation. The reports of directional differences when the effects of both visual field deficits and visual neglect interact (i.e. are found to be co-present) might be explained by the differential sensitivity and task demands of the measures used and/or the possibility that, in some cases, VFD performance resulted from attentional rather than sensory deficits.

The situation is different with respect to other operational measures of VSN. It is no surprise that some patients with 'hemianopia' perform within normal limits on such traditional paper-and-pencil tests of visual neglect as cancellation. Without the constraint of fixation, the ability to direct eye movements and attention into the blind field will typically compensate for the sensory loss. Finally, double dissociations between VFD and VSN (Halligan *et al.* 1991) may be taken as strong evidence for the historical distinction between the two types of visual deficits, but the validity of this conclusion does not require that the dissociated deficits are not in themselves attentional! Therefore this contrast between VFD and VSN is qualitatively no different from the finding that all the major clinical tests of visual neglect have also been found to doubly dissociate.

Can (some) 'visual sensory deficits' be explained in terms of damage to high-level processes?

Is there evidence, then, for extending the domain of disorders of attention to include what were once considered low-level sensory deficits? A number of converging studies have shown that impairments such as visual field deficits, somatosensory disorders, and motor disorders, traditionally conceived as primary deficits, involve impairments of higher-order cognitive processes.

Preserved physiological processing of somatosensory stimuli without awareness

Studies by Vallar *et al.* (1991*a,b*) found normal sensory or visually evoked potentials when stimuli were delivered to the left side in patients diagnosed with somatosensory and low-level visual deficits in addition to their neglect. The findings were considered to be evidence that brain areas other than primary visual or somatosensory cortex contribute to perceptual awareness. Although not clinically practical in all cases, such neurophysiological techniques remain the gold standard for distinguishing between the behavioral effects of lateralized primary sensory deficits and attentional deficits where clinical measures are insufficient.

Relative incidence of left and right sided primary sensory deficits

It is generally assumed that basic motor and sensory pathways are equivalently connected to both hemispheres. Yet only recently have studies formally examined the relative incidence of 'primary' neurological disorders (visual field defects, motor loss, and proprioceptive loss) after unilateral stroke. In a landmark study, Sterzi *et al.* (1993) showed that the incidence of 'primary' deficits in a large community-based epidemiological study was reliably greater following right brain damage (after controlling for any selection bias due to patient exclusion). The results were summarized as follows:

> The incidence of deficits of sense of pain was 57 per cent in right and 45 per cent in left brain damaged patients. Similarly, the incidence of contralesional visual half field deficits was 18 per cent in right brain damaged patients and 7 per cent in left brain damaged patients. Finally 95 per cent of right brain damaged patients exhibited motor deficits, which were found in only 85 per cent of left brain damaged patients (Vallar 1997, p. 1402).

Sterzi *et al.* (1993) explain their findings in terms of attentional deficits that were not detected by conventional neurological assessment. The results confirm that traditional neurological measures may elicit behavioral deficits other than those arising from purely 'primary' sensory loss.

Modification of primary sensory–motor deficits

It has been known for many years that caloric stimulation of the vestibular system can produce a dramatic but short-lived improvement in visual neglect. However, such short-term beneficial effects have also been found to extend to basic sensory–motor deficits after right brain damage. In a review of caloric stimulation and other sensory techniques (vestibular and optokinetic), Vallar *et al.* (1997) showed that these procedures could improve (albeit temporarily) somatosensory function and motor performance on the affected side of the body. This suggests that the original anesthesia/paresis may not have been caused entirely by primary damage, but by attentional/intentional factors which could be briefly but strikingly modified by caloric stimulation. Vestibular stimulation improves not only extra-personal visuospatial neglect (Rubens 1985), but also neglect for internally generated images (Geminiani and Bottini 1992), hemianesthesia (Vallar *et al.* 1990, 1993), hemiplegia (Rode *et al.* 1992), anosognosia (Cappa *et al.* 1987), and somatoparaphrenia (Bisiach *et al.* 1991). These positive effects occur even though clear instances of double dissociations among all these disorders have been documented. Similarly, optokinetic stimulation in right-brain-damaged patients may improve (or worsen) extra-personal visuospatial neglect (Pizzamiglio *et al.* 1990), deficits of position sense (Vallar *et al.* 1993), and left motor deficits in right-brain-damaged neglect patients (Vallar *et al.* 1997).

Attentional modification for treating VFD

Zihl (1995) and Kasten *et al.* (1998) have shown that attentional training can attenuate the physical boundaries of a VFD. Trexler (1998) reported a 52-year-old woman who, having suffered a posterior left hemisphere infarction and right homonymous hemianopia, showed volitional attentional control over the size of her scotoma. An independent examiner performed visual field mapping using Goldmann perimetry in three different conditions: without volitional effort, with volitional effort, and with distraction. On standard examination, the patient demonstrated a dense right homonymous hemianopia, regardless of stimulus parameters, except for preservation of a small island in the right inferior quadrant. When asked to concentrate on perceiving the right visual field, she demonstrated a full right lower quadrant and a normal sensitivity gradient for smaller and dimmer stimuli. Having to perform a competing cognitive task (counting backwards from 100 by sevens) while concentrating on perceiving right visual field stimulation eliminated this perceptual advantage and her dense right homonymous hemianopia returned without the preserved island of vision in the right lower quadrant. A positron-emission tomography study of the patient showed that significant increases in cerebral blood flow in contralateral medial prefrontal cortex, and in ipsilateral dorsolateral frontal, temporoparietal, and insular cortex, were associated with volitional control of the visual field defect.

Conclusion

At the very beginning of cognitive science, it was thought that information flow through the 'mind' started with elementary 'sensations' which were successively elaborated by more 'cognitive' functions until the now more complex representations could access memory traces (Clarke and Dewhurst 1972; Marshall 1982). Anatomically, the neural substrate that supported this flow of information was initially conjectured to be the ventricular system: All the senses projected to the first ventricle (the 'sensus communis') in (what are now) the frontal lobes; further processing culminated in access to memory in the fourth (or sometimes fifth) ventricle in (what is now) occipital cortex. Somewhat later, equivalent psychological theories had the neural substrates of sensation located in primary occipital cortex (vision), primary temporal cortex (hearing), and primary parietal cortex (somatosensory processing). The representations in these areas were then further elaborated in secondary and tertiary 'association' cortices, before transfer to memory, now located in the hippocampus (Clarke and Dewhurst 1972).

In modern terminology, these theories postulated that all information processing was 'bottom-up', in terms of both cognitive and neuroanatomical 'flow'. Currently, however, 'top-down' flow from high-level functions that is capable of modulating sensory input is regarded as of equal importance to 'bottom-up' processing. Indeed, for the visual system (and perhaps for all systems), top-down modulation seems to reach back to the initial cortical stages of bottom-up processing. There is now considerable psychophysical and physiological evidence to show that activation in early visual areas can be modulated by attentional systems located in parietal association and frontal cortex. The results of both neuroimaging (Chawla *et al.* 1999) and single-cell neurophysiology (Desimone 1998) show that top-down influences can modulate neural activity in extrastriate and striate cortex (Somers *et al.* 1999). Directed attention can increase activity in human visual cortex even in the absence of visual stimulation (Kastner *et al.* 1999). Even more striking are the related findings from functional imaging that reveal preparatory 'baseline attentional shifts' in brain activity that can modulate activity in sensory brain areas *before* stimulus onset, i.e. while the subject prepares to process the anticipated stimulus. (Driver and Frith 2000). Findings of this nature clearly make the clean separation of 'primary' deficits, such as a visual field cut, and high-level deficits, such as neglect, difficult to sustain.

The mere clinical fact that some patients show deficits on one set of tasks whereas others show deficits on other tasks does not in itself provide sufficient reason to justify a qualitative distinction between VFD and VSN. Can 'sensation' in such cases be meaningfully dissociated or decoupled from cognitive processing during visual field testing? Is it reasonable to claim that the different consciously mediated processes of selective, divided, and sustained attention involved in VSN testing are not involved in more 'basic' tasks? The pertinence of these questions is demonstrated by the fact that there are now several attested cases of attentionally modulated performance in supposedly primary sensory deficits. Whether it is useful to retain the conceptual distinction between different levels of impairment (as assessed by conventional measures) within functionally specific but nevertheless integrated visual information processing systems remains to be seen.

References

Axenfeld, D. (1894) Eine eifnache, Methode, Hemianopie zu zu diagnotiziren Neurologisches Zentralblatt, 437.

Axenfeld, T. (1915). Hemianopische Gesichtsfeldstörungen nach Schädelschüssen. *Klinische Monatsblatter für Augenheilkunde*, **55**, 126–43.

Barbieri, C. and DeRenzi, E. (1989). Patterns of neglect dissociation. *Behavioural Neurology*, **2**, 13–24.

Barton, J. J. and Black, S. E. (1998). Line bisection in hemianopia. *Journal of Neurology, Neurosurgery, and Psychiatry*, **64**, 660–2.

Battersby, W. S., Bender, M. B., Pollack, M., and Kahn, R. L. (1956). Unilateral 'spatial agnosia' ('inattention') in patients with cerebral lesions. *Brain*, **79**, 68–93.

Bay, E. (1953). Disturbances of visual perception and their examination. *Brain*, **109**, 99–14.

Behrmann, M., Watt, S., Black, S. E., and Barton, J. J. (1997). Impaired visual search in patients with unilateral neglect: an oculographic analysis. *Neuropsychologia*, **35**, 1445–58.

Bender, M. B. (1952). *Disorders in perception*. C. C. Thomas, Springfield, IL.

Bender, M. B. and Feldman, M. (1972). The so-called 'visual agnosias'. *Brain*, **95**, 173–86.

Bisiach, E. and Vallar, G. (1988). Hemineglect in humans. In *Handbook of neuropsychology* (ed. F. Boller and J. Grafman), pp. 195–222. Elsevier, Amsterdam.

Bisiach, E., Rusconi, M. L., and Vallar, G. (1991). Remission of somatoparaphrenic delusion through vestibular stimulation. *Neuropsychologia*, **29**, 1029–31.

Brain, R. (1941). Visual disorientation with special reference to lesions of the right cerebral hemisphere. *Brain*, **64**, 244–72.

Cappa, S. F., Sterzi, R., Vallar, G., and Bisiach, E. (1987). Remission of hemineglect and anosognosia during vestibular stimulation. *Neuropsychologia*, **25**, 775–82.

Chawla, D., Rees, G., and Friston, K. J. (1999). The physiological basis of attentional modulation in extrastriate visual areas. *Nature Neuroscience*, **2**, 671–6.

Clarke, E. and Dewhurst, K. (1972). *An illustrated history of brain function*. Sandford Publications, Oxford.

Cohen, R. A. (1993). *The neuropsychology of attention*. Plenum, New York.

Daini, R., Angelelli, P., Antonucci, G., Cappa, S. F., and Vallar, G. (2001). Exploring the syndrome of spatial unilateral neglect through an illusion of length. *Cortex*, **37**, 710–4.

D'Erme, P., De Bonis, C., and Gainotti, G. (1987). Influenza dell'emi-inattenzione e dell'emianopsia sui compiti di bisezione di linee nei pazienti cerebrolesi. *Archivio di Psicologia, Neurologia e Psichiatria*, **48**, 193–207.

Desimone, R. (1998). Visual attention mediated by biased competition in extrastriate visual cortex. *Philosophical Transactions of the Royal Society of London. Series B, Biological Sciences*, **353**, 1245–55.

Doricchi, F. and Angelelli, P. (1999). Misrepresentation of horizontal space in left unilateral neglect: role of hemianopia. *Neurology*, **52**, 1845–52.

Driver, J. and Frith, C. (2000). Shifting baselines in attention research. *Nature Reviews Neuroscience*, **1**, 147–8.

Eidelberg, E. and Schwartz, A. S. (1971). Experimental analysis of the extinction phenomenon in monkeys. *Brain*, **94**, 91–108.

Ferber, S. and Karnath, H.-O. (1999). Parietal and occipital lobe contributions to perception of straight ahead orientation. *Journal of Neurology, Neurosurgery, and Psychiatry*, **67**, 572–8.

Geminiani, G. and Bottini, G. (1992). Mental representation and temporary recovery from unilateral neglect after vestibular stimulation. *Journal of Neurology, Neurosurgery, and Psychiatry*, **55**, 332–3.

Grüsser, O. J. and Landis, T. (1991). *Visual agnosias and other disturbances of visual perception and cognition*. Macmillan, London.

Halligan, P. W. (1999). Hemianopia and visual neglect: a question of balance? *Journal of Neurology, Neurosurgery, and Psychiatry*, **67**, 565–6.

Halligan, P. W. and Marshall, J. C. (Eds.) (1994). *Spatial Neglect: Position Papers on Theory and Practice*. Lawrence Erlbaum Associates, Hove, East Sussex.

Halligan, P. W. and Marshall, J. C. (1994).

Halligan, P. W. and Marshall, J. C. (2001). Graphic neglect—more than the sum of the parts. *NeuroImage*, **14**, S91–7.

Halligan, P. W., Marshall, J. C., and Wade, D. T. (1990). Do visual field deficits exacerbate visuo-spatial neglect? *Journal of Neurology, Neurosurgery, and Psychiatry*, **53**, 487–91.

Halligan, P. W., Cockburn, J., and Wilson, B. A. (1991). The behavioural assessment of visual neglect. *Neuropsychological Rehabilitation*, **1**, 5–32.

Heilman, K. M. and Valenstein, E. (1979). Mechanisms underlying hemispatial neglect. *Annals of Neurology*, **5**, 166–70.

Heilman, K. M., Watson, R. T., and Valenstein, E. (1993). Neglect and related disorders. In *Clinical neuropsychology* (ed. K. M. Heilman and E. Valenstein), pp. 279–336. Oxford University Press, New York.

Heilman, K. M., Valenstein, E., and Watson, R. T. (1994). The what and the how of neglect. *Neuropsychological Rehabilitation*, **4**, 133–9.

Hensen, D. B. (1993). *Visual fields*. Oxford Medical Publications, Oxford.

Heywood, C. A. (1996). Visual field deficits. In *The Blackwell dictionary of neuropsychology* (ed. J. G. Beaumont, P. M. Kenealy, and M. J. C. Rogers), pp. 755–9. Blackwell, Oxford.

Hier, D. B., Mondlock, J., and Caplan, L. R. (1983). Behavioural abnormalities after right hemisphere stroke. *Neurology*, **33**, 337–44.

Ishiai, S., Furukawa, T., and Tsukagoshi, H. (1987). Eye-fixation patterns in homonymous hemianopia and unilateral spatial neglect. *Neuropsychologia*, **25**, 675–9.

Jeannerod, M. (ed.) (1987). *Neurophysiological and neuropsychological aspects of spatial neglect*. North-Holland, Amsterdam.

Kasten, E., Wust, S., Behrens-Baumann, W., and Sabel, B. A. (1998). Computer-based training for the treatment of partial blindness. *National Medicine*, **4**, 1083–7.

Kastner, S., Pinsk, M. A., De Weerd, P., Desimone, R., and Ungerleider, L. G. (1999). Increased activity in human visual cortex during directed attention in the absence of visual stimulation. *Neuron*, **22**, 751–61.

Kentridge, R. W., Heywood, C. A., and Weiskrantz, L. (1999). Attention without awareness in blindsight. *Proceedings of the Royal Society of London. Series B, Biological Sciences*, **266**, 1805–11.

Kerkhoff, G. (1993). Displacement of the egocentric visual midline in altitudinal postchiasmatic scotomata. *Neuropsychologia*, **31**, 261–5.

Kooistra, C. A. and Heilman, K. M. (1989). Hemispatial visual inattention masquerading as hemianopia. *Neurology*, **39**, 1125–7.

Liepmann, H. and Kalmus, E. (1900). Über einer Augenmastörung beu Hemianopikern. *Berliner Klinische Wochenschrift*, **38**, 838–42.

Lissauer, H. (1890). Ein Fall von Seelenblindheit nebst einem Beitrage zur Theorie derselben. *Archiv für Psychiatrie und Nervenkrankheiten*, **21**, 222–70.

McCarthy, R. A. and Warrington, E. K. (1990). *Cognitive neuropsychology: a clinical introduction*. Academic Press, New York.

Marshall, J. C. (1982). Models of the mind in health and disease. In *Normality and pathology in cognitive functions* (ed. A. W. Ellis), pp. 1–18, Academic Press, London.

Marshall, J. C. and Halligan, P. W. (1993). Visuo-spatial neglect: a new copying test to assess perceptual parsing. *Journal of Neurology*, **240**, 37–40.

Marshall, J. C., Halligan, P. W., and Robertson, I. H. (1993). A critical review of contemporary theories of unilateral neglect. In *Unilateral neglect: clinical and experimental studies* (ed. I. H. Robertson and J. C. Marshall), pp. 311–29. Lawrence Erlbaum, Hove.

Meienberg, O. (1983). Clinical examination of saccadic eye movements in hemianopia. *Neurology*, **33**, 1311–15.

Meienberg, O., Zangemeister, W. H., Rosenberg, M., Hoyt, W. F., and Stark, L. (1981). Saccadic eye movement strategies in patients with homonymous hemianopia. *Annals of Neurology*, **9**, 537–44.

Meienberg, O., Harrer, M., and Wehren, C. (1986). Oculographic diagnosis of hemineglect in patients with homonymous hemianopia. *Journal of Neurology*, **233**, 97–101.

Milner, A. D. (1997). Neglect, extinction, and the cortical streams of visual processing. In *Parietal lobe contributions to orientation in 3D space* (ed. P. Their and H.-O. Karnath), pp. 3–22. Springer-Verlag, Berlin.

Nadeau, S. E. and Heilman, K. M. (1991). Gaze-dependent hemianopia without hemispatial neglect. *Neurology*, **41**, 1244–50.

Pineas, H. (1931). Ein Fall non Raumlicher Orientierungs-stroung mit Dyschirie. *Zeitschrift für die Gesamte Neurologie und Psychiatrie*, **133**, 180–95.

Pizzamiglio, L., Frasca, R., Guariglia, C., Incoccia, C., and Antonucci, G. (1990). Effect of optokinetic stimulation in patients with visual neglect. *Cortex*, **26**, 535–40.

Robertson, I. H., and Halligan, P. W. (1999). *Spatial neglect: a clinical handbook for diagnosis and treatment*. Lawrence Erlbaum, Hove.

Robertson, I. H. and Marshall, J. C. (ed.) (1993). *Unilateral neglect: clinical and experimental studies*. Lawrence Erlbaum, Hove.

Rode, G., Charles, N., Perenin, M. T., Vighetto, A., Trillet, M., and Aimard, C. (1992). Partial remission of hemiplegia and somatoparaphrenia through vestibular stimulation in a case of unilateral neglect. *Cortex*, **28**, 203–8.

Rubens, A. (1985). Caloric stimulation and unilateral visual neglect. *Neurology*, **35**, 1019–24.

Smania, N. and Aglioti, S. (1995). Sensory and spatial components of somaesthetic deficits following right brain damage. *Neurology*, **45**, 1725–30.

Somers, D. C., Dale, A. M., Seiffert, A. E., and Tootell, R. B. (1999). Functional MRI reveals spatially specific attentional modulation in human primary visual cortex. *Proceedings of the National Academy of Sciences of the United States of America*, **96**, 1663–8.

Sterzi, R., Bottini, G., Celani, M. G., *et al*. (1993). Hemianopia, hemianaesthesia and hemiplegia after right and left hemisphere damage: a hemispheric difference. *Journal of Neurology, Neurosurgery and Psychiatry*, **56**, 308–10.

Stone, S. P., Halligan, P. W., Marshall, J. C., and Greenwood, R. J. (1998). Unilateral neglect: a common but heterogeneous syndrome. *Neurology*, **50**, 1902–5.

Thier, P. and Karnath, H.-O. (ed.) (1997). *Parietal lobe contributions to orientation in 3D space*. Springer-Verlag, Berlin.

Trexler, L. E. (1998). Volitional control of homonymous hemianopia: a single case study. *Neuropsychologia*, **36**, 573–80.

Trobe, J. D., Acosta, P. C., Krischer, J. P., and Trick, G. L. (1981). Confrontation visual field techniques in the detection of anterior visual pathway lesions. *Annals of Neurology*, **10**, 28–34.

Vallar, G. (1994). Left spatial hemineglect: an unmanageable explosion of dissociations? No. *Neuropsychological Rehabilitation*, **4**, 209–12.

Vallar, G. (1997). Spatial frames of reference and somatosensory processing: a neuropsychological perspective. *Philosophical Transactions of the Royal Society of London. Series B, Biological Sciences*, **352**, 1401–9.

Vallar, G. (1998). Spatial hemineglect in humans. *Trends in Cognitive Sciences*, **2**, 87–97.

Vallar, G., Sterzi, R., Bottini, G., Cappa, S., and Rusconi, M. L. (1990). Temporary remission of left hemianesthesia after vestibular stimulation: a sensory neglect phenomenon. *Cortex*, **26**, 123–31.

Vallar, G., Sandroni, P., Rusconi, M. L., and Barbierie, S. (1991*a*). Hemianopia, hemianaesthesia and spatial neglect: a study with evoked potentials. *Neurology*, **41**, 1918–22.

Vallar, G., Bottini, G., Sterzi, R., Passerini, D., and Rusconi, M. L. (1991*b*) Hemianesthesia, sensory neglect, and defective access to conscious experience. *Neurology*, **41**, 650–2.

Vallar, G., Antonucci, G., Guariglia, C., and Pizzamiglio, L. (1993). Deficits of position sense, unilateral neglect and optokinetic stimulation. *Neuropsychologia*, **31**, 1191–1200.

Vallar, G., Guariglia, C., Nico, D., and Pizzamiglio, L. (1997). Motor deficits and optokinetic stimulation in patients with left hemineglect. *Neurology*, **49**, 1364–70.

Walker, R., Findlay, J. M., Young, A. W., and Welch, J. (1991). Disentangling neglect and hemianopia. *Neuropsychologia*, **29**, 1019–27.

Weinstein, E. and Friedman, R. (ed.) (1977). *Hemi-inattention and hemispheric specialisation*. Raven Press, New York.

Weiskrantz, L. (1986). *Blindsight*. Oxford University Press.

Zeki, S. (1993). *A vision of the brain*. Blackwell Scientific, Oxford.

Zihl, J. (1995) Visual scanning behavior in patients with homonymous hemianopia. *Neuropsychologia*, **33**, 287–303.

Zingerle, H. (1913). Ueber Storrungen der Wahrnemung des eigenen Koerper Gehirnerkrankungen. *Monatschift für Psychiatrie und Neurologie*, **34**, 13–36.

6.3 Spatial, temporal, and form-binding effects in vision: the contribution from extinction

M. Jane Riddoch and Glyn W. Humphreys

Initial visual processing is thought to involve a number of separable dimensions, with these dimensions being processed to some degree in different neural areas. Evidence to support this line of reasoning comes from a number of different methodologies including neurophysiological studies of single cell activity (Desimone and Ungeleider 1989), functional brain imaging (Watson *et al.* 1993; Tootell *et al.* 1995), and neuropsychological studies of patients with isolated perceptual deficits (Humphreys 1999). For example, the different neural areas may be separately impaired as a result of brain damage resulting in selective impairments such as the visual perception of form (Milner *et al.* 1991), color (Heywood *et al.* 1991), and motion (Zihl *et al.* 1983). However, we normally perceive a coherent world in which colors are *integrated* with shape and movement. Therefore integration or binding processes represent a fundamental aspect of visual processing. The focus of this chapter is on the nature of the processes which allow form elements to be bound into contours, contours to be bound into shapes, and the conjunctions of surface features such as color and form to be bound together (e.g. a red apple in a blue bowl, rather than a blue apple in a red bowl). We present the case for several different forms of binding in visual processing; some are the function of the ventral visual system (e.g. the binding of elements into contours and the binding of contours into shapes), while others may come about through the involvement of the dorsal visual pathway (mediating the binding of surface features and shapes). Thus, damage to early visual processing within the ventral visual stream can disrupt the binding of contours into shapes, although the binding of form elements into contours can still operate (as in integrative visual agnosia discussed below). Binding of form elements into contours may also be disrupted as a result of damage to the ventral stream; thus, patients with shape agnosia are unable to recognize or discriminate between even simple geometric forms (Milner *et al.* 1991).[1] In some circumstances patients with damage to the dorsal stream (resulting in visual extinction) can show benefits in performance as a result of processing via the ventral stream. Preserved form binding can operate implicitly in such patients. For example, Humphreys *et al.* (2000) examined the report of shape and surface detail in a patient (GK) with Bálint's syndrome. GK demonstrated left-side visual extinction in perceptual report tasks, failing to report the left member of a pair of stimuli. However, extinction was reduced when stimuli grouped (according to collinearity, connectedness, or shape similarity for example) (Fig. 1) (Ward *et al.* 1994; Gilchrist *et al.* 1996; Mattingley *et al.* 1997).

---

[1] Although binding of elements into contours and binding of contours into shapes are both functions of the ventral visual pathway, they may be separately impaired as a result of brain damage. Patient HJA was able to bind elements into contours, but impaired in the binding of contours into shapes (see below).

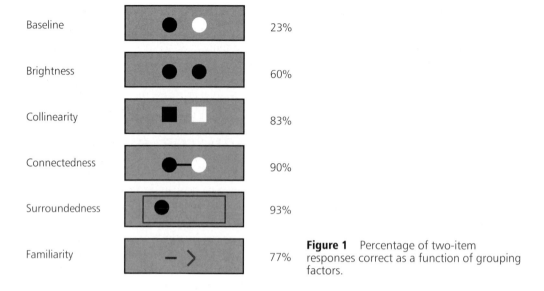

Baseline		23%
Brightness		60%
Collinearity		83%
Connectedness		90%
Surroundedness		93%
Familiarity		77%

Figure 1 Percentage of two-item responses correct as a function of grouping factors.

In contrast, evidence indicates that the binding of shape to surface information about objects is disrupted after damage to the dorsal visual pathway (e.g. to the parietal lobe) even when the binding of elements into contours, and contours into shapes, is relatively preserved (see below).

The distinction between the proposed different forms of visual processing in the dorsal and ventral streams maps well with a theoretical account of object recognition put forward by Grossberg and colleagues (Grossberg and Mingolla 1985; Grossberg and Pessoa 1998), who were amongst the first to propose that the perception of surface properties of objects depends on two operations: first, a process of boundary formation performed by a boundary contour system (BCS) which uses grouping processes such as collinearity and good continuation to form bounded contours of shapes; second, a process of 'filling in', within the bounded regions, performed by a feature contour system (FCS). Activation within the FCS generates the surface properties of objects. We present neuropsychological evidence consistent with these ideas in the following two sections.

Temporal factors may also influence binding. Neurophysiological data on synchronized firing of neurons suggests that different features of an object may be bound by time (Eckhorn 1999). Thus, cells responding to features from one object are synchronized and fire at a different time from cells responding to other objects. Later in the chapter we present neuropsychological data suggesting that binding may be based on the common temporal onset of visual stimuli. The evidence that we have in this regard suggests that such binding is relatively transient, and it is not maintained when stimuli are presented for longer durations. Transient binding by common onset may provide one way in which visual information is provisionally organized until more sustained binding processes generate stable perceptual representations.

Binding elements into contours, and binding contours into shapes

Brain damage may impair the ability to bind features into shapes, particularly under conditions in which multiple items are present in the field when there may be competition in assigning elements between shapes (Humphreys *et al.* 1992). In a detailed study of an agnosic patient (HJA), Humphreys *et al.* have shown the contrast between relatively good assignment of elements into shapes when only one item is present, and poor assignment of elements to multiple shapes. HJA was profoundly agnosic and particularly impaired at recognizing line drawings. Despite this, he performed well on the Efron shape-matching task (Humphreys *et al.* 1992). However, he was impaired at search tasks that required that visual elements bind together in a spatially parallel manner across a field containing multiple stimuli. HJA took part in a number of experiments where targets were defined on the basis of a particular conjunction of form features (e.g. a horizontal and vertical line combining to form an inverted T) relative to homogeneous distractors containing the same features but in a different arrangement (e.g. upright Ts). Normal subjects can detect such targets efficiently by binding elements in targets and distractors in parallel and then grouping and rejecting distractors on the basis of their 'bound' feature conjunctions (Duncan and Humphreys 1989; Humphreys *et al.* 1989). HJA was unable to do this and was significantly impaired relative to age-matched controls. Nevertheless, he could detect targets in parallel when they were differentiated by a salient feature from distractors (e.g. a T having a contrasting orientation to distractors), and so he was capable of processing elements in parallel when the binding of form elements together was not crucial. He could also conduct efficient serial search for form-conjunction targets amongst heterogeneous distractors (e.g. upright and 90° rotated Ts). For normal subjects, segmentation of targets and distractors by similarity at the level of feature conjunctions is disrupted when heterogeneous stimuli are presented, and subjects then adopt a serial search strategy. HJA's deficit was not apparent under these circumstances, although it appeared when parallel binding of form elements was necessary.

The distinction between intact coding of basic form features (e.g. oriented edge elements), and impaired binding into shape has been further illustrated in more recent experiments with HJA, using simple shape-matching tasks. Giersch *et al.* (2000) presented line drawings of three geometric shapes which could be spatially separated, superimposed, or occluding (Fig. 2). Subsequently, target and distractor arrays were presented (with the relative locations of the shapes being altered in distractor arrays). HJA performed relatively well on this task with separated shapes, but performed poorly with superimposed and occluding shapes. Interestingly, the deficit with occluding shapes was most pronounced when the length of the occluded edge was small—the condition when the

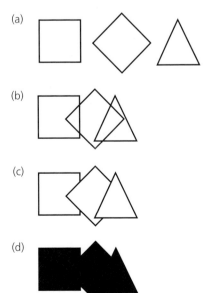

Figure 2 Examples of the stimuli used by Giersch *et al.* (2000): (a) spatially separated; (b) superimposed; (c) occluding; (d) occluding silhouettes.

missing fragment should be easiest to compute based on collinearity between the nonoccluded edges (Fig. 2(c)). Other data showed that HJA sometimes used the occluded edge to segment the occluder, and sometimes assigned the edge to the shapes as if it were visible. These results suggest that HJA could compute the occluded edge (using collinearity), but he was then impaired at assigning it to the correct shape and using it in the process of segmenting the multiple shapes. Feature coding, including edge grouping by collinearity, precedes feature binding into shapes and multiple shape segmentation. HJA also performed this shape-matching task reasonably well with silhouettes. This is of additional interest. Normal subjects tend to find silhouettes more difficult to match than line drawings, presumably because local details that facilitate segmentation of shapes are lacking and hence performance relies on more global descriptions of the overall configuration (Giersch et al. 2000). HJA seemed able to use these global descriptions reasonably well, given his relatively good matching of silhouettes. However, the local detail present in line drawings (e.g. the occluded edges) disrupted his performance, because of his impaired binding and segmentation of the shapes.

The contrast between HJA's good performance with silhouettes and his poor performance with line drawings extended beyond simple shape-matching tasks. Riddoch and Humphreys (1987) first reported this tendency in an object decision task with HJA (see also Lawson and Humphreys (1999) for further recent evidence). With complex stimuli, the problem with line drawings can be demonstrated even with single items. The problem was even greater with limited presentation times, and it was also exacerbated by overlapping figures (Riddoch and Humphreys 1987). A similar pattern of performance, with strong effects of figural overlap and better performance with silhouettes, has been reported by Butter and Trobe (1994) with their agnosic patient. Patients described by DeRenzi and Lucchelli (1994) and Kartsounis and Warrington (1991) have also shown poor performance with overlapping figures despite good discrimination of simple Efron shapes. In more complex line drawings, edges provide cues for segmentation of objects into parts and they must also be bound correctly to yield appropriate object descriptions. Thus, in some patients with agnosia there seems to be an impairment in the interplay between grouping and segmentation, which leads to an incorrect parsing of perceptual wholes. This incorrect parsing can come about because grouping of part-to-wholes is relatively weak when compared with segmentation operations between parts. The deficits in agnosic patients suggest that object recognition in complex images depends on processes that bind edge contours into their correct spatial relations, and that support appropriate segmentation between 'figural' elements and elements occupying the perceptual 'ground'. Agnosic patients, such as HJA, typically have lesions of the ventral visual system (for example, in HJA's case there are bilateral lesions involving the lingual and fusiform gyri (see Riddoch et al. (1999) for an MRI scan)), suggesting that the grouping of parts into objects and the segmentation of figural objects from the perceptual ground depend on an intact ventral visual system. It is interesting that HJA remained able to group local form elements based on collinearity (even though these elements need not then be represented in the correct figure–ground relations in an image). This suggests that the grouping of local form elements may take place in areas of primary visual cortex that are preserved. Neurophysiological evidence is consistent with this, with local grouping contingent on horizontal connections between cells in regions as early as V1 (Gilbert and Wiesel 1989; Gilbert 1992).

Binding surface information to shape

Neuropsychological evidence for deficits in the binding of form and surface detail has come from patients with parietal lesions. For instance, Friedman-Hill and coworkers (Friedman-Hill et al. 1995; Robertson et al. 1997) reported data on a patient (RM) with Bálint's syndrome following bilateral parietal lesions. Although able to detect targets defined by the difference in a single feature relative to the distractors, RM was severely impaired at search for a target defined by conjunctions of form and surface detail (Humphreys and Price 1994). In addition, even under free viewing conditions, RM generated illusory conjunction errors by failing to combine the colors and shapes of the stimuli correctly. Thus, given a red X and a green O, RM was likely to report the presence of a green X and a red O. Friedman-Hill and coworkers argue that the parietal lesions suffered by their patient had the effect of disrupting attention to the spatial locations of stimuli, in turn causing an impairment in the binding process. On this view, attention to the location of a target is required to raise the activation for the features of that stimulus relative to the features of other (distractor) stimuli in the field; this enables the activated (attended) features to be bound whilst distractor features are filtered out (Treisman 1998). Attention may be necessary for binding. Alternatively, the parietal lobe may contain a spatial map that aligns attributes from the same object that are computed in separate neural areas (e.g. color and form).

One interesting aspect of patients with this deficit in binding form to surface detail is that the binding of form information itself may be relatively spared. For example, illusory conjunctions are typically based on the migrations of color between whole letters, and patients with Bálint's syndrome usually have relatively good object and word recognition (see Baylis *et al.* (1994) for evidence on RM's word recognition). As we have indicated earlier, preserved form binding can operate implicitly in such patients. Humphreys *et al.* (2000) have demonstrated that extinction can be reduced in patient GK when stimuli group (according to collinearity, connectedness, or shape similarity, for example) (Fig. 1). This grouping seemed to occur preattentively since detection was contingent on a stable group being formed between the ipsi- and contralesional items. In addition to this, GK made many illusory conjunction errors in which the surface properties of the grouped shapes could be exchanged. Binding of the forms did not guarantee correct binding of form to surface detail. Humphreys *et al.* (2000) argue that the results support a two-stage account of visual binding: initially, form elements are bound together on the basis of *Gestalt* properties (intact in GK), prior to the form information being integrated with surface details (impaired in GK, and indicated by the illusory conjunctions of surface detail and form). Humphreys *et al.* (2000) suggest that the assignment of surface properties to forms requires an interaction between ventral and dorsal (parietal) brain areas which link object and surface properties, possibly on the basis of their common location. GK's parietal lesions disrupted the linkage process. In addition, Humphreys *et al.* showed that, whilst extinction was influenced by the relative spatial locations of shapes (left-side shapes being extinguished), illusory conjunctions were not. Humphreys *et al.* account for these contrasting effects of visual field in terms of the integrated competition hypothesis (Duncan *et al.* 1997). According to this hypothesis, perceptual report is contingent on competition between separate objects. This competition can become unbalanced after a spatially selective lesion, so that a stimulus in one location consistently loses the competition for selection; there is spatial extinction. This competition can be reduced if visual elements group, with the elements within a perceptual group being selected together. This can include selection of spatial detail as well as shape information. However, if there is a misalignment of elements within the parietal lobe, the surface information may be miscombined to generate illusory conjunctions. These miscombinations may be equally frequent from the ipsi- and contralesional fields, since they arise on occasions when the attributes of stimuli have been recovered.

These results on the effects of grouping on extinction again indicate that some forms of binding can be effected in neural areas unaffected by parietal damage. Interestingly, grouping between parts of shapes can be demonstrated even in patients who find it extremely difficult to attend to spatial locations. For example, even when he is able to report visual stimuli, GK is very impaired at judging whether stimuli appeared at fixation or up to 3° away (Humphreys *et al.* 1994). It is difficult to attribute any binding in this case to attention to the spatial location occupied by the reported stimulus, contrary to views that attention plays a causal role in this binding process (Treisman 1998).

Temporal binding

Binding contingent on synchronized neural activity has been proposed as one alternative to binding resulting from attention to a spatial location. Physiological studies have shown that there can be stimulus-dependent synchrony of firing between widely separated brain areas (Gray *et al*. 1989; Singer and Gray 1995; Eckhorn 1999). For instance, neurons responding to bars that are collinear and move together will fire in a time-locked manner, whereas neural firing is not synchronized if the bars move in an uncorrelated manner. Thus, binding may result from cells firing in synchrony, and temporal synchrony may be imposed by connections between cells that respond to elements that co-occur in perceptual groups (see Hummel and Biederman (1992) for one implementation of this idea in a computational model). Such connections may allow coalitions of features to be bound rapidly and in a spatially parallel manner, although attention may subsequently be needed to form stable representations based on such coalitions. There is also some behavioral evidence for temporal synchronization in the input being important for feature binding in humans (Fahle 1993; Elliott and Müller 1998). For instance, detection of a target formed by grouped elements is facilitated when the elements are pre-cued by features that appear synchronously, relative to when the pre-cued features appear asynchronously (this facilitation occurs even when observers cannot detect temporal asynchrony in the pre-cues, providing another piece of evidence for implicit binding in vision). Further data on time-based binding comes from neuropsychology and is based on the phenomenon of 'anti-extinction'.

As we have indicated above, extinction reflects poor report of a contralesional stimulus when it is placed in competition for selection with an ipsilesional item. This has been reported after a number of different brain lesions, including frontal and temporal lesions, and damage to the basal ganglia, white matter, thalamus, and internal capsule (Vallar *et al*. 1994). To date, the opposite phenomenon (anti-extinction) has only been reported twice. This term can be used to describe circumstances in which there is *better* detection of a contralesional stimulus when it occurs with an ipsilesional item than when the contralesional stimulus appears alone (Goodrich and Ward 1997; Vaishnavi *et al*. 2000). Recently we have demonstrated anti-extinction effects in patient GK in tasks requiring the identification of bilaterally presented letters (Humphreys *et al*., 2002). The anti-extinction effects only occurred with short stimulus presentations. At these durations there was poor identification of single letters presented in GK's left field, and improved identification of letters presented simultaneously with a letter in the right field. With longer exposures, there was improved report of single left letters whilst, if anything, report of the stimulus decreased on two-item trials. These data are shown in Fig. 3.

In contrast with these results, when the stimuli were defined by common onset, there was no evidence for anti-extinction when letters were defined by offsets of contours in masks. Consequently, Humphreys *et al*. proposed that a possible mechanism for the improved report of two items may have been the grouping of the stimuli by common onset, with the effects of grouping by common onset dissipating over time (even though the stimuli remain in the field with prolonged exposure durations). An alternative account is that the onsets of stimuli in the left and right fields briefly cue attention to the spatial region where the stimuli fall, enabling left as well as right letters to be reported. Single left letters, briefly presented, may not serve as such good attentional cues; hence there is poor identification on single left trials. To test between these accounts, Humphreys *et al*. examined the effects of having flanking stimuli onset around a central letter defined by an offset. The display conditions were as illustrated in Fig. 4. If the onsets cue

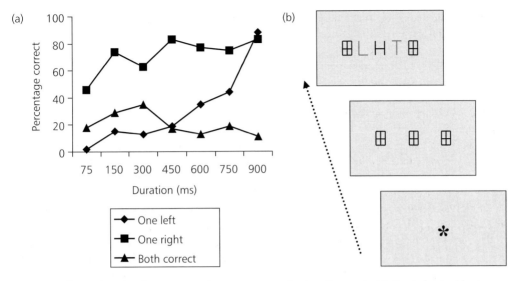

Figure 3 Illustrating the time course of events on a trail when the central letter is flanked by two letters.

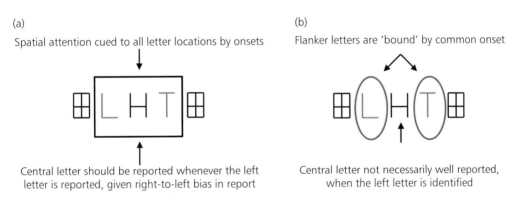

Figure 4 Illustrating the spatial attention and common onset accounts.

attention around a spatial area, the central letter (falling within this area) should be relatively easy to report when the left letters are identified through anti-extinction. On the other hand, if anti-extinction is based on grouping by common onset, then the central letter need not be well identified since, being defined by an offset, it should not group strongly with the flanking letters.

The results showed that report of the central letter in anti-extinction trials actually decreased when the left letter was identified. In contrast, in trials where there was only a single left flanker letter, report of the central letter was significantly better when the left letter was identified than when it was not. The data do not fit with the idea that the flanking letters cued attention. Instead, the results are consistent with a grouping account since when onset letters group they are reported together and prior to the central (offset) letter being identified. On trials with just a left flanker, the central (offset) letter was typically identified first, as it was in a preferred (central) location. This bias was overridden by grouping on trials with two letter onsets. Owing to grouping, the right onset letter supports report of the left onset letter, but this benefit (the source of the anti-extinction effect) lasts only as long as the grouping signal persists. If the grouping signal is transient, report of the left letter may decrease on two-item trials as GK then responds with a general bias to select right-side items first. Anti-extinction changes to extinction as the stimulus duration increases. Why do the onsets still not lead to good report of left-side items with longer stimulus durations? There are several possibilities here. One is that offsets, occurring briefly after onsets, help to support temporal grouping (with brief stimulus durations). Another is that development of a sustained response to the stimuli (with prolonged exposures) reinforces the bias to the right, thus generating extinction effects. We may further speculate that the transient binding by common onset, revealed in anti-extinction effects, provides the visual system with a 'quick but dirty' representation of the world. To provide a more accurate veridical representation there may need to be a more sustained binding process sensitive to properties such as collinearity, shape similarity, connectedness, etc.—the factors found to reduce extinction with more prolonged stimulus exposures in patient GK.

Conclusions

We have considered evidence suggesting that there can be several kinds of binding in vision. Damage to early visual processing within the ventral visual stream can disrupt the binding of contours into shapes, although the binding of form elements into contours can still operate. This suggests that the process of binding elements into contour is distinct from the process of binding contours into shapes. The latter form of binding seems to operate within the ventral visual system. On the other hand, damage to the parietal lobe can disrupt the binding of shape to surface information about objects, even when the binding of elements into contours, and contours into shapes, seems to be relatively preserved. These findings are consistent with a multistage account of binding in vision, which distinguishes between the processes involved in binding shape information (in the ventral visual stream) and the processes involved in binding shape and surface detail (involving interactions between the ventral and dorsal streams). In addition, it appears that a further transient form of binding can take place, based on stimuli having common visual onsets. The function of transient binding may be to provide the visual system with a rapid representation of the world. However, transient binding may be of little use for functions such as object recognition which may require the appropriate binding of form and surface information and which may result from a later and more sustained binding process.

Acknowledgements

This work is supported by the Medical Research Council.

References

Baylis, G. C., Driver, J., Baylis, L. L., and Rafal, R. D. (1994). Reading of letters and words in a patient with Balint's syndrome. *Neuropsychologia*, **32**, 1273–86.

Butter, C. M. and Trobe, J. D. (1994). Integrative agnosia following progressive multifocal leuko-encephalopathy. *Cortex*, **30**, 145–58.

DeRenzi, E. and Lucchelli, F. (1994). Are semantic systems separately represented in the brain? The case of living category impairment. *Cortex*, **30**, 3–25.

Desimone, R. and Ungeleider, L. G. (1989). Neural mechanisms of visual processing in monkeys. In *Handbook of neurophysiology*, Vol. 2 (ed. F. Boller and J. Grafman), pp. 267–99. Elsevier Science, New York.

Duncan, J. and Humphreys, G. W. (1989). Visual search and visual similarity. *Psychological Review*, **96**, 433–58.

Duncan, J., Humphreys, G. W., and Ward, R. (1997). Competitive brain activity in visual attention. *Current Opinion in Neurobiology*, **7**, 255–61.

Eckhorn, R. (1999). Neural mechanisms of visual feature binding investigated with microelectrodes and models. *Visual Cognition*, **6**, 231–66.

Elliott, M. A. and Müller, H. M. (1998). Synchronous information presented in 40 Hz flicker enhances visual feature binding. *Psychological Science*, **9**, 277–83.

Fahle, M. (1993). Figure–ground discrimination from temporal information. *Proceedings of the Royal Society of London. Series B, Biological Sciences*, **254**, 199–203.

Friedman-Hill, S., Robertson, L. C., and Treisman, A. (1995). Parietal contributions to visual feature binding: Evidence from a patient with bilateral lesions. *Science*, **269**, 853–5.

Giersch, A., Humphreys, G. W., Boucart, M., and Kovi ́aks, I. (2000). The computation of occluded contours in visual agnosia: Evidence of early computation prior to shape binding and figure–ground coding. *Cognitive Neuropsychology*, **17**, 731–59.

Gilbert, C. D. (1992). Horizontal integration and cortical dynamics. *Neuron*, **9**, 1–13.

Gilbert, C. D. and Wiesel, T. N. (1989). Columnar specificity of intrinsic horizontal and corticocortical connections in cat visual cortex. *Journal of Neuroscience*, **9**, 2432–42.

Gilchrist, D., Humphreys, G. W., and Riddoch, M. J. (1996). Grouping and extinction: evidence for low-level modulation of visual selection. *Cognitive Neuropsychology*, **13**, 1223–49.

Goodrich, S. J. and Ward, R. (1997). Anti-extinction following unilateral parietal damage. *Cognitive Neuropsychology*, **14**, 595–612.

Gray, C. M., Konig, P., Engel, A., and Singer, W. (1989). Oscillatory responses in cat visual cortex exhibit inter-columnar synchronisation which reflects global stimulus properties. *Nature*, **359**, 231–3.

Grossberg, S. and Mingolla, E. (1985). Neural dynamics of form perception: boundary completion, illusory figures, and neon color spreading. *Psychological Review*, **92**, 173–21.

Grossberg, S. and Pessoa, L. (1998). Texture segregation, surface representation and figure–ground separation. *Vision Research*, **38**, 2657–84.

Heywood, C., Cowey, A., and Newcombe, F. (1991). Chromatic discrimination in a cortically blind observor. *European Journal of Neuroscience*, **3**, 802–12.

Hummel, J. and Biederman, I. (1992). Dynamic binding in a neural network for shape recognition. *Psychological Review*, **99**, 480–517.

Humphreys, G. W. (1999). Integrative agnosia. In *Case studies in the cognitive neuropsychology of vision* (ed. G. W. Humphreys), pp 41–55. Psychology Press, London.

Humphreys, G. W., Cinel, C., Wolfe, J., Olson, A., and Klempen, N. (2000). Fractionating the binding process: neuropsychological evidence distinguishing binding of form from binding of surface features. *Vision Research*, **40**, 1569–96.

Humphreys, G. W. and Price, C. J. (1994). Visual feature discrimination in simultanagnosia: a study of two cases. *Cognitive Neuropsychology*, **11**, 393–434.

Humphreys, G. W., Quinlan, P. T., and Riddoch, M. J. (1989). Grouping effects in visual search: effects with single- and combined-feature targets. *Journal of Experimental Psychology: General*, **118**, 258–79.

Humphreys, G. W., Riddoch, M. J., Quinlan, P. T., Donnelly, N., and Price, C. A. (1992). Parallel pattern processing and visual agnosia. *Canadian Journal of Psychology*, **46**, 377–416.

Humphreys, G. W., Romani, C., Olson, A., Riddoch, M. J., and Duncan, J. (1994). Non-spatial extinction following lesions of the parietal lobe in humans. *Nature*, **372**, 357–9.

Humphreys, G. W., Riddoch, M. J., Nys, G., and Heinke, D. (2002) Unconcious temporal binding: neuropsychological evidence from antiextinction. *Cognitive Neuropsychology*, **19**, 361–80.

Kartsounis, L. D. and Warrington, E. K. (1991). Failure of object recognition due to a breakdown of figure–ground discrimination in a patient with normal acuity. *Neuropsychologia*, **29**, 969–80.

Lawson, R. and Humphreys, G. W. (1999). The effects of view in depth on the identification of line drawings and silhouettes of familiar objects: normality and pathology. *Visual Cognition*, **6**, 165–96.

Mattingley, J. B., Davis, G., and Driver, J. (1997). Pre-attentive filling in of visual surfaces in parietal extinction. *Science*, **275**, 671–4.

Milner, A. D., Perrett, D. I., Johnston, R. S., *et al.* (1991) Perception and action in 'visual form agnosia'. *Brain*, **114**, 405–28.

Riddoch, M. J. and Humphreys, G. W. (1987). A case of integrative agnosia. *Brain*, **110**, 1431–62.

Riddoch, M. J., Humphreys, G. W., Gannon, T., Blott, W., and Jones, V. (1999). Memories are made of this: the effects of time on stored visual knowledge in a case of visual agnosia. *Brain*, **122**, 537–59.

Robertson, L. C., Treisman, A., Friedman-Hill, S., and Grabowecky, M. (1997). A possible connection between spatial deficits and feature binding in a patient with parietal damage. *Journal of Cognitive Neuroscience*, **9**, 295–317.

Singer, W. and Gray, C. M. (1995). Visual feature integration and the temporal correlation hypothesis. *Annual Review of Neuroscience*, **18**, 555–86.

Tootell, R. B. H., Reppas, J. B., Kwong, K., *et al*. (1995). Functonal analysis of human MT and related visual cortical areas using magnetic resonance imaging. *Journal of Neuroscience*, **15**, 3215–30.

Treisman, A. (1998). Feature binding, attention and object perception. *Philosophical Transactions of the Royal Society*, **353**, 1295–306.

Vaishnavi, S., Calhoun, J., Southwood, M. H., and Chatterjee, A. (2000). Sensory and response interference by ipsilesional stimuli in tactile extinction. *Cortex*, **36**, 81–92.

Vallar, G., Rusconi, M. L., Bignamini, L., Geminiani, G., and Pizzamiglio, D. (1994). Anatomical correlates of visual and tactile extinction in humans: a clinical CT scan study. *Journal of Neurology, Neurosurgery, and Psychiatry*, **57**, 464–570.

Ward, R., Goodrich, S. J., and Driver, J. (1994). Grouping reduces visual extinction. *Visual Cognition*, **1**, 101–9.

Watson, J. D. D., Myers, G. R., Frackowiak, R. S. J., *et al*. (1993). Area V5 of the human brain: evidence from a combined study using positron emission tomography and magnetic resonance imaging. *Cerebral Cortex*, **3**, 79–84.

Zihl, J., von Cramon, D., and Mai, N. (1983). Selective disturbance of movement vision after bilateral brain damage. *Brain*, **106**, 313–40.

6.4 The role of spatial working memory deficits in pathological search by neglect patients

Jon Driver and Masud Husain

Recent research has suggested that neglect consists of a number of dissociable components, with different patients demonstrating somewhat different types of impairment (Robertson and Marshall 1993; Vallar 1998; Mesulam 1999; Driver and Vuilleumier 2001). Our view is that most neglect patients may actually suffer from *combinations* of component deficits, with each component exacerbating the others to produce the florid symptoms seen in the clinic and in daily life. For example, a visual attentional bias may combine with impairments of motor planning or execution in many patients (Heilman *et al.* 1985a; Mattingley *et al.* 1998; Husain *et al.* 2000).

A multicomponent nature for neglect is perhaps unsurprising when one considers the very large lesions that are commonly involved in severe cases. Such lesions can affect many different brain regions, encompassing areas not just within the parietal lobe but also in frontal and/or superior temporal cortex, plus subcortical nuclei (such as the basal ganglia and thalamus) as well as white-matter tracts, thereby leading to disruption in many other remote areas (Vallar and Perani 1986). Viewed from this anatomical perspective, it is perhaps inevitable that patients with diffuse and variable lesions will suffer disruption to more than one function, and that different combinations of deficit might exist in different patients.

Of course, quite severe neglect can sometimes be seen in patients with more focal lesions, particularly when the right inferior parietal lobe is involved. However, even such cases, we suggest, will typically have damage to several different functional areas. We note, for example, that recent neurophysiological work on the posterior parietal lobe in monkeys has already revealed important differences in function between closely neighboring areas in and around the intraparietal sulcus (Andersen *et al.* 1997; Rizzolatti *et al.* 1997; Snyder 2000). Thus, even damage confined to the parietal lobe may result in various combinations of deficit, depending upon exactly which areas and/or connections are disrupted.

However, such considerations should not lead to the conclusion that there are no common principles in neglect. For example, an attentional bias to the ipsilesional side may be present in many neglect patients, perhaps all. Nor does a multicomponent perspective entail that the only possible approach in research is to fractionate the syndrome into innumerable different varieties (Halligan and Marshall 1992). Instead, one can seek to identify the component deficits which are common in neglect (bearing in mind the typical lesions) and study how these influence each other when combined, jointly producing the pathological behaviors which typify the syndrome.

Here we focus on one possible contributing component to the neglect syndrome that has received relatively little attention to date, namely deficits in **spatial working memory**. Although others have considered the possible role of impaired spatial working memory in representational (or 'imaginal') aspects of neglect (Ellis *et al.* 1996; Beschin *et al.* 1997) our concern here is specifically with the role of spatial working memory deficits in visual search. We should emphasize from the outset that we are *not* suggesting that spatial working memory deficits provide the sole explanation for neglect in any individual case. Instead, we are proposing that when *combined* with other deficits that are common in the syndrome (e.g. attentional biases towards the ipsilesional side), deficits in spatial working memory may contribute substantially to the pathological behaviors that are typically observed.

In particular, we propose that impaired spatial working memory may contribute to recursive examination of ipsilesional locations in many visual tasks. Such re-examination of ipsilesional space may account for an important aspect of the search behavior of neglect patients observed in everyday life as well as in clinical tests of neglect such as cancellation. Typically, patients with neglect fail to search contralesional locations when viewing a cluttered scene (such as the room around them or a cancellation sheet), exploring mainly ipsilesional locations. Strikingly, they continue to do this even when given *unlimited* time. Yet the same individuals may be capable of perceiving contralesional stimuli in less cluttered displays, and may demonstrably be able to saccade to extreme contralesional locations when requested.

One possible explanation for some patients' failure to explore contralesional locations in cluttered environments is that, in addition to their bias in attention towards the ipsilesional side, they may fail to keep track of which locations they have already searched. The *combination* of such deficits, we suggest, would lead to recursive examination of ipsilesional locations. Neglect patients may look back repeatedly to their favored side partly because they do not retain the fact that they have already explored locations there.

Why might spatial working memory deficits be expected in neglect patients?

There are several grounds for suspecting that spatial working memory might often be affected in neglect. First, recent functional imaging studies of normal volunteers (Jonides *et al.* 1993; D'Esposito *et al.* 1998) have shown that a variety of spatial working memory tasks activate a network that is strikingly similar to the network of areas implicated in typical neglect lesions (i.e. a predominantly right-lateralized network involving parietal and frontal areas, plus subcortical structures such as the basal ganglia). Second, single-cell recording studies in monkeys demonstrate that neurons in related parietal and frontal areas play a role in maintaining spatial information over delay periods for various spatial working memory tasks (e.g. delayed saccades) (Mazzoni *et al.* 1996; Colby and Goldberg 1999). Third, patients with lesions involving the parietal lobe exhibit deficits in saccadic tasks that require location information to be maintained and/or updated across eye-movements (Duhamel *et al.* 1992; Heide *et al.* 1995). Fourth, recent functional imaging studies demonstrate parietal activation, predominantly in the right hemisphere, when healthy subjects perform tasks which place demands on remembering spatial location across saccades (Heide *et al.* 2001; Tobler *et al.* 2001). Fifth, behavioral and evoked reaction potential studies in normal volunteers suggest that processes of spatial attention and of spatial working memory are closely related (Awh and Jonides 2001), such that deficits in the former (as commonly proposed for neglect) might also be expected to be associated with deficits in the latter.

Finally, many standard tests for neglect may involve an overlooked spatial working memory component. For instance, in search tasks, patients are required to find multiple targets arrayed across a cancellation sheet or a display screen, sometimes in the presence of multiple intermingled nontargets. Efficient search behavior in such tasks may require that previously inspected locations are not revisited (Klein 2000). This may involve spatial working memory for those locations that have already been searched.

How spatial working memory deficits might contribute to pathological search

Neglect patients typically show pathological visual search behavior (Eglin *et al.* 1989; Karnath and Fetter 1995; Behrmann *et al.* 1997; Niemeier and Karnath 2000) which has several characteristics. They often begin by inspecting items towards the ipsilesional edge of the display. Although they will typically move on to examine some further items, spontaneous search rarely proceeds fully to the contralesional side (even when the patient is demonstrably capable of perceiving items there in isolation, and of saccading there when requested). Instead, search typically goes back to those ipsilesional items that have already been examined (and often moves on again, only to return again recursively). Figure 1 shows an example of such behavior in the eye-movement pattern of one neglect patient when searching for multiple Ts among Ls (Husain *et al.* 2001). Similarly recursive searching can be seen in several other studies of neglect patients (Chedru *et al.* 1973, Fig. 2(f); Behrmann *et al.* 2000, Fig. 7), although this aspect was not always emphasized in the reports.

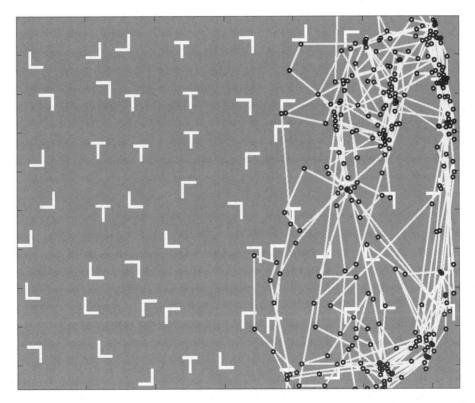

Figure 1 Example record of eye movements and fixations in a right-parietal neglect patient, when searching for multiple Ts among Ls. Note the neglect of left locations, and the repeated returns to rightward locations (after several intervening saccades). Note also that leftward saccades were as common as rightward saccades overall in this patient's search. When refixating previously inspected and detected targets on the right, the patient often indicated (incorrectly) that he had found them for the very first time. (Adapted with permission from Husain *et al.*, *Brain*, **124**, 941–52 (2001).)

Most existing accounts of neglect can readily explain why search typically *begins* on the ipsilesional side—this is due to a lateral bias in attention and/or exploration following the lesion which favors stimuli on the ipsilesional side. However, it is perhaps less obvious why search then fails to proceed fully in the contralesional direction, even given unlimited time, especially since neglect patients can be observed to make as many saccades in the contralesional as in the ipsilesional direction within the region that they do search (Niemeier and Karnath 2000; Husain *et al.* 2001).

We propose that a deficit in spatial working memory (specifically, in retaining the locations of items already searched, across saccades), when *combined* with the attentional bias to the ipsilesional side that is conventionally proposed, might explain such pathological search. The attentional bias to one side would lead search to start with ipsilesional items. Although search might then start to proceed elsewhere, a deficit in keeping track of previously searched locations would lead patients to return to those locations most favored by their attentional bias. These would appear to them to be 'new' locations still to explored, owing to the proposed spatial working memory deficit. This would substantially exacerbate the impact of the attentional bias. If the patients cannot retain which locations have been already searched, they would be under the erroneous impression that their search is proceeding to new unexplored locations, when in fact old ground is being covered over and over again. This could explain why patients typically fail to explore contralesional locations, even when given unlimited time, in both clinical tests and daily life.

Eye-movements and reports during multi-target search

We recently tested these ideas in a single case with enduring left visual neglect (but intact visual fields) after focal right inferior-parietal damage (Husain *et al.* 2001). We measured his eye movements while requiring him to search for Ts among Ls, as for the display shown in Fig. 1. With the displays used, this task required each item to be fixated in turn, even in normal volunteers. Critically, we also tested spatial working memory during the search process by requiring the patient (and age-matched normal volunteers) to indicate whether each particular T was being fixated for the first time (and thus was a new discovery), or whether it had already been fixated earlier during the search. This decision was indicated by making a button-press while fixating a particular T. Note that this button-press response did *not* change the visual display (unlike cancellation marks in standard cancellation tests for neglect, but like visual search in daily life where inspected locations receive no visible mark). Hence there was nothing in the display itself to tell viewers whether they had already inspected any particular item; only memory for previously searched locations could convey this.

Normal subjects rarely refixated previously searched items. Moreover, when doing so they misjudged the item to be a new discovery even more rarely. This suggests that normal subjects retain which locations they have already searched in their working memory, contrary to some recent proposals that even normal visual search may show little or no short-term memory (Horowitz and Wolfe 1999) (for an opposing view see Klein (2000) and Kristjansson (2000)). The parietal neglect patient's behavior was strikingly abnormal in several respects. First, as would be expected, he neglected many left targets, rarely fixating items on the contralesional side of the display (Fig. 1). This arose even though he made as many saccades in the contralesional direction as in the ipsilesional direction, within the ipsilesional region that was searched (Niemeier and Karnath 2000). Second, the patient *re*fixated previously inspected targets (which were mainly on the right) at a highly abnormal rate (Fig. 1). His refixation rate (i.e. number of refixations on targets divided by the number of individual targets fixated) was 4.1 for displays like Fig. 1, more than 13 times the mean rate of 0.3 for normal subjects searching the same displays.

The third observation to such proposals in this patient provides the crucial new finding as regards possible deficits in spatial working memory. When refixating previously inspected items, unlike normal individuals, the patient often judged (as indicated by his button-press responses) that he was fixating them *for the first time*, erroneously treating them as new discoveries. This suggests a spatial working memory deficit in keeping track of locations already searched across saccades. Such a deficit may be consistent with other demonstrations that parietal patients are impaired in retaining location information across saccades in simpler eye-movement tasks (e.g. double-step saccades) (Duhamel *et al.* 1982; Heide *et al.* 1985).

The parietal patient who showed spatial working memory deficits in our search tasks also showed deficits on conventional measures of spatial working memory. Specifically, he had a Corsi block span of only 3 on both conventional clinical testing and on computerized CANTAB measures (Owen *et al.* 1990). He was also impaired on the CANTAB battery's version of Petrides' self-ordered pointing task (Petrides and Milner 1982). It is possible that perceptual neglect could have made some contribution to scores on these conventional measures (as any contralesional locations that are perceptually neglected would presumably not be remembered). However, his Corsi deficit remained even when all tested locations were in the ipsilesional hemifield. Likewise the self-ordered pointing task still showed a deficit when only locations in the ipsilesional third of the display were analyzed. In any case, note that the spatial working memory deficit observed in our novel search tasks (i.e. via the button-presses which indicated that previously searched locations were mistaken by the patient for new discoveries) did *not* concern neglected locations; rather, this deficit was found precisely for those locations which had already been searched (any memory deficit could not be tested for unexplored locations).

One might suggest that the spatial working memory deficit in such a patient could bear no relation to his neglect, but simply be present in addition, owing to the substantial lesion. In contrast, we would propose that the spatial working memory deficit may contribute to the neglect for contralesional locations, exacerbating such neglect substantially. We suggest that the spatial working memory deficit, when combined with an ipsilesional attentional bias, would lead the patient to visit recursively ipsilesional locations that had already been examined, which he evidently considered as potentially new target locations. Such recursive search of the locations favored by his attentional bias would prevent search from ever proceeding to the less favored locations. In contrast, search in a person with intact spatial working memory would naturally proceed to less salient locations after initial examination of those which appear most salient, because such an individual would remember that these salient locations had already been examined.

In support of our proposal of a relation between the spatial working memory deficit, and the severity of contralesional neglect. We found that the patient's neglect increased as the load on his limited spatial working memory was increased (Husain *et al.* 2001). For example, as the number of items in the display was increased (so that the number of visited locations to be remembered also increased), his neglect and his mistaken treatment of previously searched locations as new discoveries both rose in a tightly correlated manner (Fig. 2). This finding is consistent with our proposal that as spatial working memory increasingly fails (leading to more recursive search of ipsilesional locations), so neglect of contralesional locations should also increase in severity. An increased tendency to treat previously searched items on the right as new discoveries was associated with stronger left neglect.

Spatial working memory deficits versus deficits in disengaging or perseveration

Many investigators (Heilman *et al.* 1985b; Kinsbourne 1987; Bisiach and Vallar 1988; Robertson and Marshall 1993; Mesulam 1999) have previously commented on the fact that neglect patients appear to become 'locked' onto the ipsilesional side of displays. Some authors have proposed

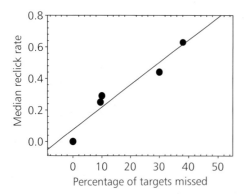

Figure 2 Plot showing that the degree of neglect (percentage of targets missed) was strongly correlated with the rate of reclicking for previously detected targets when later refixating them. Each point concerns a different condition of spatial working memory load, for the patient studied by Husain *et al.* (2001). (Adapted with permission from Husain *et al.*, *Brain*, **124**, 941–52 (2001).)

that this may reflect a specific difficulty in 'disengaging' attention from ipsilesional locations (Posner *et al.* 1984). We would not disagree that such deficits may contribute to neglect, but it is important to note that they differ from the present proposals and findings. The parietal patient in our search study (Husain *et al.* 2001) actually made as many saccades in the contralesional as in the ipsilesional direction within the region searched, demonstrating that he was in fact able to disengage from particular ipsilesional locations to shift his search in a more contralesional direction (Niemeier and Karnath 2000). Moreover, when he refixated ipsilesional locations, this was typically after numerous intervening saccades, again indicating that his refixations did not simply reflect a total inability to disengage from any particular fixated location on the ipsilesional side. Finally, note that our critical observation was *not* simply the high rate of refixations on ipsilesional items (such refixations have in fact also been observed in several previous studies (Chedru *et al.* 1973; Behrmann *et al.* 1997)). Instead, the critical new result was that the patient explicitly indicated that he (mistakenly) thought that he was fixating particular targets on the ipsilesional side *for the very first time*, when in fact he was actually refixating them. It is this aspect of our results which indicates a spatial working memory deficit, and which was associated with stronger contralesional neglect in those conditions where it became more pronounced.

Note that our proposals and findings also differ from previous observations concerning 'perseverative' behavior during cancellation tasks. It is a common clinical observation that some neglect patients may make multiple visual marks on individual items during standard paper-and-pencil cancellation tasks (Na *et al.* 1999; Rusconi *et al.* in press). Such behavior cannot be due to deficient memory for which locations have already been examined, since a visible mark is present at each visited location to indicate the previous visit(s) directly when any further mark is made (we return to this point later when introducing revised cancellation tasks which can assess spatial working memory). Rather than reflecting impaired spatial working memory, perseverative re-cancellations with visible marks may instead just reflect the compulsive perseverative tendencies classically associated with frontal damage. Indeed, two recent studies have found that re-marking in standard cancellation tasks is indeed linked to frontal damage in particular (Na *et al.* 1999; Rusconi *et al.*, in press). It should also be noted that the parietal patient studied in our search tasks (Husain *et al.* 2001) *never* made such visible recancellation marks throughout many sessions of standard cancellation tests over several years of examination. Moreover, his tendency to mistake previously fixated targets for new discoveries in our search tasks (which did not involve any visible marks) cannot be attributed to perseverative tendencies (see Husain *et al.* (2001) for further discussion of this).

Group study of eye-movements and reports during multitarget search

The patient studied in detail with our search tasks (Husain *et al.* 2001) is only a single case. One might reasonably ask how common such spatial working memory deficits are in neglect patients, and whether they are typically associated with more severe neglect, as predicted if such deficits exacerbate neglect as we propose. Together with our collaborators (Mannan, Mort, Hodgson, and Kennard) we have recently studied a larger group of 16 patients with various lesions. As in our single-case study, we measured eye-movement patterns while each patient searched for multiple Ts among Ls, while also measuring with button-presses (which leave no visible mark) whether the patient judged that he or she was fixating any particular target for the first time, or instead judged that he or she had already examined it. Analysis of the group dataset is ongoing, but several preliminary conclusions can already be drawn. First, the pattern showed by the parietal case of Husain *et al.* (2001) is by no means unique. Neglect patients with lesions to specific regions of the intraparietal sulcus or inferior parietal lobe show a similar impairment. Second, neglect patients without damage to these areas do not appear to show this deficit. Third, the degree of neglect across patients correlated with the severity of the trans-saccadic spatial working memory impairment, suggesting that a failure to retain searched locations does indeed exacerbate spatial neglect.

Spatial working memory in cancellation tasks

In the remainder of this chapter, we consider how possible spatial working memory deficits might affect performance on a standard diagnostic test for neglect, namely cancellation tasks. In doing so, we describe a new variant of the cancellation task ('invisible' cancellation) which provides a clin-ically applicable method for investigating the role of spatial working memory at the bedside. This new task turns out to provide a more sensitive measure for neglect than standard cancellation tasks.

   In the usual paper-and-pencil procedure for cancellation, the task is highly analogous to visual search (i.e. look for multiple targets, sometimes among intermingled nontargets), except that each target found should now receive a visible mark with the pencil. As noted above, these visible marks mean that (in principle at least) working memory may no longer be needed to register which targets have already been examined, as each of these should have a permanent mark on them. However, pencil-marks made in cancellation procedures are often not easily resolvable from unmarked targets and distractors *within peripheral vision*. Therefore patients may have to fixate each individual item to determine whether it has already been marked. Thus, even when previously found targets are cancelled, patients may nevertheless demonstrate pathological recursive search through ipsilesional locations if they cannot resolve their cancellation marks in peripheral vision and are also unable to retain which locations they have already searched.

   To examine this issue, we have introduced an extreme manipulation of mark visibility into cancellation tasks (Wojciulik *et al.* 2001). In one condition, marks are made with a thick red pen, so that they are now highly visible even in peripheral vision. In the other critical new condition, marks are made *invisibly* from the patients' perspective (i.e. marks are made with the other end of the pen, which has no ink, using carbon-paper beneath the cancellation sheet so that marks can be registered for later scoring). According to our proposals concerning the role of spatial working memory deficits in pathological search by neglect patients, we should expect the invisible-mark condition to produce stronger neglect (i.e. more failures to mark contralesional targets) than the condition with highly visible marks. The latter should provide a clearly visible reminder of which locations have already been searched, whereas this must be retained in spatial working memory for the invisible-mark condition. Hence spatial working memory deficits should lead to recursive search of ipsilesional locations, and thus stronger neglect of contralesional locations, in the invisible-mark condition.

The reverse prediction (i.e. more neglect with highly visible than with invisible marks during cancellation) can also be motivated. For instance, highly visible and salient marks made initially for targets on the ipsilesional side might lock the patients' attention onto that side, making it even harder for them to disengage their attention (Posner *et al.* 1984) to shift towards more contralesional targets. In one well-known study, Mark *et al.* (1988) compared standard cancellation (i.e. with pencil-marks) with a new condition in which targets were rubbed out with an eraser rather than cancelled. They found less neglect in the new condition. This might be intepreted as the eraser facilitating disengagement from ipsilesional items (as Mark *et al.* suggested) by making these invisible. Such a perspective would presumably predict more neglect with highly visible than with invisible marks for our own cancellation studies. On the other hand, it may be possible to reinterpret Mark *et al.*'s eraser study in terms of spatial working memory contributions to neglect. Once an item has been erased, it may no longer have to be retained in working memory as already examined, in order to prevent revisits there, since search rarely goes to empty locations.

In our first 'invisible' cancellation study (Wojciulik *et al.* 2001), we compared highly visible marks versus invisible marks in a single case (who had frontal and subcortical damage in the right hemisphere). The results were clear, revealing that neglect in cancellation was more severe with invisible marks than with highly visible marks. This accords with our prediction based on the suggested role of spatial working memory deficits in exacerbating neglect. The highly visible red marks would provide an aid to any patient with such a deficit, by clearly indicating which target locations have already been examined, to prevent the recursive search through them that might otherwise have been caused by poor retention of their locations.

Of course, in daily life people do *not* usually make highly visible marks on each location that they examine when searching through a natural scene. Hence the invisible-mark condition may better capture the pathologically recursive search patterns that can be seen in daily-life settings for the patients. Note also that the invisible-mark cancellation test in effect provides a low-tech clinically applicable version of the search paradigm in which we used computerized measures of eye position combined with computerized button-presses as described earlier (Husain *et al.* 2001). Because of its low-tech nature, the 'invisible' cancellation test (which requires only paper, pen, and carbon-paper) can be more readily applied in clinical settings at the bedside.

Group study of cancellation with invisible versus highly visible marks

We have recently applied the new 'invisible' cancellation test to a heterogenous group of 23 right-hemisphere stroke patients, selected as neglect suspects on the basis either of their lesions (which were typically large right middle cerebral artery infarctions), or on the basis of clinical reports (indicating the presence of neglect in daily life or on standard tests) (Wojciulik *et al.*, in preparation). As in the single-case study by Wojciulik *et al.* (2001), we again compared cancellation with invisible marks (recorded on carbon paper) with cancellation of the same search sheets with highly visible thick red marks. The group data on all 23 patients confirmed that more severe neglect (i.e. more failures to mark contralesional targets) was found overall in the *invisible-mark* condition. Moreover, this pattern was particularly evident in those patients who showed only mild neglect when cancelling with highly visible marks (Fig. 3). Finally, among the latter cases, neglect of contralesional targets during the invisible-mark condition was stronger for those patients who revisited ipsilesional targets (to make another invisible mark there) at a higher rate. This is consistent with our proposal that recursive search through ipsilesional targets (caused by a failure to retain which locations have already been searched) can exacerbate neglect of contralesional targets.

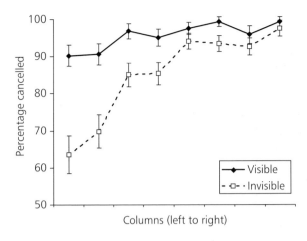

Figure 3 A group of neglect patients shows stronger neglect for cancellation with invisible marks than with highly visible thick red marks. The percentage of targets cancelled is shown for each of eight successive columns of elements (from the far left to far right) on an A3-size cancellation sheet. (Data from an unpublished study by Wojciulik et al.)

The results of this group study also show that our new version of the cancellation task, with invisible marks, may provide a more sensitive test for neglect than standard cancellation in a large number of patients. It may thus prove useful in assessment and diagnosis.

Conclusions

We have proposed that deficits in spatial working memory may contribute to visuospatial neglect. Specifically, we have suggested a role for a deficit in retaining which locations have already been examined, across saccades during search. When combined with some of the other deficits that undoubtedly characterize the sydrome (e.g. attentional biases which favor stimuli in more ipsilesional locations over their contralesional competitors), such a spatial working memory deficit could exacerbate neglect of contralesional locations by inducing recursive search through those locations already favored by the attentional bias. These locations would continue to be treated as potentially new locations to explore even after they have already been examined several times, thus exacerbating the attentional bias, with the result that search would rarely proceed to contralesional locations that have yet to be examined.

Initial support for this general idea was obtained from a detailed single-case study of a patient with enduring neglect after right inferior-parietal damage (Husain et al. 2001). He refixated ipsilesional items at an abnormal rate during search. Critically, when doing so he also judged that he was fixating these locations for the first time, at a highly abnormal rate, thus indicating a failure to retain which locations had already been searched. As the load on his deficient spatial working memory was increased, so his mistaken treatment of old locations as new discoveries increased, and his neglect became correspondingly more severe. An unpublished group study with the same basic search paradigm (i.e. eye-movement recording combined with explicit judgements of whether particular targets are being fixated for the very first time) provides some initial indication that this pattern can be found in many cases, but not all. We predict that, when present, spatial working memory deficits should exacerbate contralesional neglect (in effect by increasing the impact of the attentional bias towards the ipsilesional side), rather than simply being an additional deficit with no implications for neglect.

Consideration of how spatial working memory deficits might affect standard cancellation tests led us to develop, together with our collaborators, a new version of cancellation where marks are either invisible or highly visible (Wojciulik et al. 2001). Consistent with the predictions of our spatial working memory proposals, neglect can be more severe with invisible cancellation marks than with visible cancellation marks. An unpublished group study indicates that this may be a fairly general result, holding across a large group of patients overall. Cancellation with invisible marks may thus prove to be a more sensitive clinical measure than standard multitarget cancellation, which already provides the bedside test that correlates best with functional neglect in everyday life (Azouvi *et al.* 1996; Ferber and Karnath 2001).

Many questions about the possible role of spatial working memory in neglect remain. For example, the exact lesion sites responsible for the patterns we have described remain to be determined. Moreover, we have focused here on the role of retaining which locations have already been searched, across saccades, during search tasks. Future research may reveal whether the suggested deficits are specific to transaccadic updating of spatial information (as some related studies might suggest (Duhamel *et al.* 1992; Colby and Goldberg 1999)), or instead reflect more general difficulties in retaining spatial information regardless of whether saccades are involved. Other researchers have proposed that different aspects of spatial working memory may contribute to further aspects of neglect (e.g. to 'representational' aspects of neglect, as tapped by imagery tasks (Ellis *et al.* 1996; Beschin *et al.* 1997)).

It also remains to be determined whether the spatial working memory deficits we have emphasized, during search tasks, affect all display locations to the same extent or may be more pronounced for particular locations (consistent with some pioneering lesion studies in monkeys (Goldman-Rakic 1996). Note that the deficits uncovered in the search tasks described above can clearly apply to locations that have already been searched, which are typically those towards the ipsilesional side in most patients. Note also that other work on parietal patients in saccadic tasks (Duhamel *et al.* 1992; Heide *et al.* 1995) has suggested that such patients may be particularly impaired at retaining (or updating) *ipsilesional* locations after saccading away from them in the *contralesional* direction. Such saccades away from initially fixated ipsilesional locations will commonly arise in many search tasks before the patient returns recursively to the initial ipsilesional locations. Thus, transaccadic localization deficits might play a role in generating poor retention of which locations have already been searched. The possible role of pathologically disordered search strategies in generating poor retention could also be examined in the future.

Our existing research already suggests that impairments in retaining searched locations may be a fruitful avenue for further research on neglect. When combined with the attentional biases to the ipsilesional side which are conventionally suggested, such additional deficits may contribute substantially to one of the most characteristic features of the disorder. In both clinical tests and daily life, one of the most striking features of neglect is that patients recursively search ipsilesional locations, continuing to neglect contralesional locations even when given unlimited time. This behavior can appear highly paradoxical in patients who are demonstrably able to saccade towards contralesional locations when requested, and who can perceive stimuli there in isolation prior to any saccade. We suggest that their behavior may be less paradoxical given the combination of an ipsilesional attentional bias together with an impairment in retaining the locations that have already been examined, which exacerbates the effect of the attentional bias. Neglect patients may repeatedly look back towards their favored side in part because they do not realize that they have already looked there.

Acknowledgements

MH and JD are supported by the Wellcome Trust. JD was also supported by the McDonnell–Pew program in Cognitive Neuroscience. We thank the patients who participated in our studies, and our collaborators Karen Clarke, Tim Hodgson, Chris Kennard, Sabira Mannan, Dominic Mort, Chris Rorden, and Ewa Wojciulik. Thanks are also due to Angelo Maravita, Jason Mattingley, David Milner, and Patrik Vuilleumier for helpful comments, and to participants at the Como meeting for their robust response to this work.

References

Andersen, R. A., Snyder, L. H., Bradley, D. C., and Xing, J. (1997). Multimodal representation of space in the posterior parietal cortex and its use in planning movements. *Annual Review of Neuroscience*, **20**, 303–30.

Awh, E. and Jonides, J. (1990). Overlapping mechanisms of attention and spatial working memory. *Trends in Cognitive Science*, **5**, 119–26.

Azouvi, P., Marchal, F., Samuel, C., *et al.* (1996). Functional consequences and awareness of unilateral neglect: study of an evaluation scale. *Neuropsychological Rehabilitation*, **6**, 133–50.

Behrmann, M., Watt, S., Black, S. E., and Barton, J. J. S. (1997). Impaired visual search in patients with unilateral neglect: an oculographic analysis. *Neuropsychologia*, **35**, 1445–8.

Beschin, N., Cocchini, G., Della Sala, S., and Logie, R. H. (1997). What the eyes perceive, the brain ignores: a case of pure unilateral representational neglect. *Cortex*, **33**, 3–26.

Bisiach, E. and Vallar, G. (1988). Hemineglect in humans. In *Handbook of neuropsychology*, Vol. 1 (ed. F. Boller and J. Grafman,), pp. 195–222. Elsevier, Amsterdam.

Chedru, F., Leblanc, M., and Lhermitte, F. (1973). Visual searching in normal and brain-damaged subjects (contribution to the study of unilateral inattention). *Cortex*, **9**, 94–111.

Colby, C. L. and Goldberg, M. E. (1999). Space and attention in parietal cortex. *Annual Review of Neuroscience*, **22**, 319–49.

D'Esposito, M., Aguirre, G. K., Zarahn, E., Ballard, D., Shin, R. K., and Lease, J. (1998). Functional MRI studies of spatial and non-spatial working memory. *Cognitive Brain Research*, **7**, 1–13.

Driver, J. and Vuilleumier, P. (2001). Perceptual awareness and its loss in unilateral neglect and extinction. *Cognition*, **79**, 39–88.

Duhamel, J.-R., Goldberg, M. E., Fitzgibbon, E. J., Sirigu, A., and Grafman, J. (1992). Saccadic dysmetria in a patient with a right frontoparietal lesion: the importance of corollary discharge for accurate spatial behaviour. *Brain*, **115**, 1387–1402.

Eglin, M., Robertson, L. C., and Knight, R. T. (1989). Visual search performance in the neglect syndrome. *Journal of Cognitive Neuroscience*, **1**, 372–85.

Ellis, A. X., Della Sala, S., and Logie, R. H. (1996). The bailiwick of visuo-spatial working memory: evidence from unilateral spatial neglect. *Cognitive Brain Research*, **3**, 71–8.

Ferber, S. and Karnath, H.-O. (2001). How to assess spatial neglect—line bisection or cancellation tasks? *Journal of Clinical and Experimental Neuropsychology*, **23**, 599–607.

Goldman-Rakic, P. S. (1996). The prefrontal landscape: implications of functional architecture for understanding human mentation and the central executive. *Philosophical Transactions of the Royal Society of London. Series B, Biological Sciences*, **351**, 1445–53.

Halligan, P. W. and Marshall, J. C. (1992). Left visual neglect: a meaningless entity? *Cortex*, **8**, 525–35.

Heide, W., Blankenburg, M., Zimmermann, E., and Kömpf, D. (1995). Cortical control of double-step saccades: implications for spatial orientation. *Annals of Neurology*, **38**, 739–48.

Heide, W., Bikofski, F., Seitz, R. J., *et al.* (2001). Activation of frontoparietal cortices during memorized triple-step sequences. *European Journal of Neuroscience*, **13**, 1177–89.

Heilman, K. M., Bowers, D., Coslett, H. B., Whelan, H., and Watson, R. T. (1985a). Directional hypokinesia: prolonged reaction times for leftward movements in patients with right hemisphere lesions and neglect. *Neurology*, **35**, 855–9.

Heilman, K. M., Watson, R. T., and Valenstein, E. (1985b). Neglect and related disorders. In *Clinical neuropsychology* (ed. K. M. Heilman, R. T. Watson, and E. Valenstein), pp. 279–336. Oxford University Press.

Horowitz, T. S. and Wolfe. J. M. (1998). Visual search has no memory. *Nature*, **394**, 575–77.

Husain, M., Mattingley, J. B., Rorden, R., Kennard, C., and Driver, J. (2000). Separating perceptual and motor components in parietal and frontal neglect. *Brain*, **123**, 1643–59.

Husain, M., Mannan, S., Hodgson, T., Wojciulik, E., Driver, J., and Kennard, C. (2001). Impaired spatial working memory across saccades contributes to abnormal search in parietal neglect. *Brain*, **124**, 941–52.

Jonides, J., Smith, E. E., Koeppe, R. A., Awh, E., Minoshima, S., and Mintun, M. A. (1993). Spatial working memory inhumans as revealed by PET. *Nature*, **363**, 623–5.

Karnath, H.-O. and Fetter, M. (1995). Ocular space exploration in the dark and its relation to subjective and objective body orientation in neglect patients with parietal lesions. *Neuropsychologia*, **33**, 371–7.

Kinsbourne, M. (1987). Mechanisms of unilateral neglect. In *Neurophysiological and neuropsychological aspects of spatial neglect* (ed. M Jeannerod), pp. 69–86. Elsevier, Amsterdam.

Klein, R. M. (2000). Inhibition of return. *Trends in Cognitive Sciences*, **4**, 138–47.

Kristjansson, A. (2000). In search of remembrance: Evidence for memory in visual search. *Psychological Science*, **11**, 328–32.

Mark, V. W., Kooistra, C. A., and Heilman, K. M. (1988). Hemispatial neglect affected by non-neglected stimuli. *Neurology*, **38**, 1207–11.

Mazzoni, P., Bracewell, R. M., Barash, S., and Andersen, R. A. (1996). Spatially tuned auditory responses in area LIP of macaques performing delayed memory saccades to acoustic targets. *Journal of Neurophysiology*, **75**, 1233–41.

Mattingley, J., Husain, M., Rorden, C., Kennard, C., and Driver, J. (1998). Motor role for human inferior parietal lobule revealed in spatial neglect patients. *Nature*, **392**, 179–82.

Mesulam, M.-M. (1999). Spatial attention and neglect. *Philosophical Transactions of the Royal Society of London. Series B, Biological Sciences*, **354**, 1325–46.

Na, D. L., Adair, J. C., Kang, Y., Chung, C. S., Lee, K. H., and Heilman, K. M. (1999). Motor perseveration behavior on a line cancellation task. *Neurology*, **52**, 1569–76.

Niemeier, M. and Karnath, H.-O. (2000). Exploratory saccades show no direction specific deficit in neglect. *Neurology*, **54**, 515–18.

Owen, A. M., Downes, J. J., Sahakian, B. J., Polkey, C. E., and Robbins, T. W. (1990). Planning and spatial working memory following frontal lobe lesions in man. *Neuropsychologia*, **28**, 1021–34.

Petrides, M. and Milner, B. (1982). Deficits on subject-ordered tasks after frontal- and temporal-lobe lesions in man. *Neuropsychologia*, **20**, 249–62.

Posner, M. I., Walker, J. A., Friedrich, F. J., and Rafal, R. (1984). Effects of parietal injury on covert orienting of attention. *Journal of Neuroscience*, **4**, 1863–1874.

Rizzolatti, G., Fogassi, L., and Gallese, V. (1997). Parietal cortex: from sight to action. *Current Opinion in Neurobiology*, **7**, 562–7.

Robertson, I. and Marshall, J. C. (ed.) (1993). *Unilateral neglect: clinical and experimental studies*. Lawrence Erlbaum, Hove.

Rusconi, M. L., Maravita, A., Bottini, G., and Vallar, G. Is the intact side really intact? Perseverative responses in patients with unilateral neglect: a productive manifestation. (In press.)

Snyder, L. H. (2000). Coordinate transformations for eye and arm movements in the brain. *Current Opinion in Neurobiology*, **10**, 747–54.

Tobler, P. N., Felblinger, J., Burki, M., Nirkko, A. C., Ozdoba, C., and Muri, R. M. (2001). Functional organisation of the saccadic reference system processing extraretinal signals in humans. *Vision Research*, **41**, 1351–8.

Vallar, G. (1998). Spatial hemineglect in humans. *Trends in Cognitive Sciences*, **2**, 87–97.

Vallar, G. and Perani, D. (1986). The anatomy of unilateral neglect after right hemisphere stroke lesions: a clinical CT correlation study in man. *Neuropsychologia*, **24**, 609–22.

Wojciulik, E., Husain, M., Clarke, K., and Driver, J. (2001). Spatial working memory deficit in unilateral neglect. *Neuropsychologia*, **39**, 390–6.

Section 7 Rehabilitation of patients with neglect

7.1 Cognitive routes to the rehabilitation of unilateral neglect

Ian H. Robertson and Tom Manly

Cognitive neuroscience has long held out the promise of yielding tangible benefits to the development of effective cognitive rehabilitation of brain damage. In this chapter we will argue that in the field of unilateral neglect, this goal has been partly achieved. Furthermore, cognitive rehabilitation research in unilateral neglect has also contributed to theoretical developments in cognitive neuroscience, yielding a unique symbiosis which we hope will serve as an example for other domains of cognitive function and dysfunction.

For the purposes of this chapter, we will define cognitive rehabilitation as 'the systematic use of instruction and structured experience to manipulate the functioning of cognitive systems such as to improve the quality and/or quantity of cognitive processing in a particular domain' (Robertson 1999).

This definition has been influenced by the research literature of the last decade which has seen, for instance, the dramatic disconfirmation of a long-held central assumption about the brain—that new cell bodies cannot emerge in adulthood. Recent data for both humans and animals have shown that new cells can indeed be produced in the hippocampus (Eriksson *et al.* 1998). What is more, this process is partly experience dependent—animals kept in enriched compared with impoverished environments show more cell genesis in the hippocampus (Gould *et al.* 1999). This finding follows close on the heels of another revolutionary discovery of the last decade—the demonstration that the adult brain can show large experience-dependent changes in neural circuits, including dendritic and axonal sprouting (Recanzone *et al.* 1993).

There is every reason to believe that parallel plastic changes also occur in the damaged brain (Seitz *et al.* 1995), and that such changes mediate in part recovery of function after brain damage. Therefore rehabilitation can now turn its attention to the ambitious goal of directly altering neural circuitry through appropriately planned experience. Such direct effects on neural circuits have already been demonstrated in primates (Nudo *et al.* 1996). While some pioneering researchers on rehabilitation have argued that rehabilitation may under certain circumstances have direct neural effects (Bach-y-Rita 1989), the prevailing view has been that rehabilitation following brain damage had its effects by fostering what Luria (1963) termed 'functional reorganization'— the compensatory reorganization of surviving undamaged brain circuits in order to achieve the impaired behavioral goals in a different way—and such mechanisms do indeed underpin much behavioral recovery (Robertson and Murre 1999). A third way in which recovery from brain damage can take place is through the lifting of inhibition over damaged networks by healthy competitor circuits (Robertson and Murre 1999). This can take place either by damping down the inhibitory competition, or by boosting the activation in circuits in the lesioned network.

It is likely that many, if not all, of these mechanisms are important in recovery from brain damage—whether that recovery be spontaneous or guided by the planned experience we call rehabilitation. But precisely what kind of experience to provide in order to facilitate recovery is problematic; nonspecific stimulation may inadvertently strengthen nondamaged competitor circuits, for instance (Robertson and Murre 1999), or it may simply fail to provide the type of precisely shaped and timed input that may be needed to foster changes in a particular lesioned network. Cognitive neuroscience can make a significant contribution toward the development of a scientific basis for the practice of brain rehabilitation through elucidating the brain's functional architecture, because only on the basis of an adequate understanding of the inhibitory and facilitatory relationships between different modular systems in the brain can one establish the optimal routes for stimulation that will result in the various types of experience-dependent plasticity. The systematic application of cognitive neuroscience models to rehabilitation can not only foster better more theoretically grounded rehabilitation, but the models themselves can be tested and modified by the data generated by rehabilitation-oriented research. Nowhere has this been more true than in research on unilateral neglect.

'Spontaneous' recovery in unilateral neglect

The majority of patients with unilateral neglect in the acute post-lesion stage show apparently spontaneous recovery from the frank spatial biases of the disorder (Stone *et al.* 1992). In working with the minority of patients who are less fortunate, considering how these improvements take place—or why they do not—is an important starting point for targeted rehabilitation. Of particular interest is whether such changes better reflect recovery in the neural systems supporting spatial representation or the development of corrective compensatory strategies.

Goodale *et al.* (1990) studied a group of nine subjects at a mean of 21 weeks after a unilateral lesion of the right hemisphere. Although many of these patients had previously shown signs of unilateral neglect, clinically significant manifestations of spatial bias were largely absent by the time of testing. The experiment consisted of two tasks, one involving reaching out to touch lighted targets presented on a vertical screen, and the other requiring the participants to judge the midpoint in space between two of the targets. While the patients did not differ from healthy controls in the ultimate accuracy of their reaches, kinematic video analysis revealed significant rightward deviations in their movement trajectories that were only corrected in the final pre-target stage. In addition, the bisections (where there is no clear target to point to) continued to show significant deviations toward the right of the objective center. These and similar results (Mattingley *et al.* 1994) show that underlying distortions in spatial or attentional representations may be prevalent in apparently 'recovered' neglect patients. So how do patients minimize the effect of these persistent deficits on everyday activities?

There is evidence that a frontal-based system for the voluntary orienting of attention can functionally compensate for damage to more posterior systems (Làdavas *et al.* 1994*a*). Although the distinction between 'automatic' and 'controlled' processes can be somewhat arbitrary, one marker of the more volitional system is its vulnerability to interference from concurrent activity that makes common demands on limited resources. Therefore, if volitional orienting is a feature in functional recovery from neglect, we could predict a re-emergence of the deficit under challenging dual-task conditions. This seems to be the case. Robertson and Frasca (1992), for example, found exacerbations of neglect under dual-task conditions. Another study (Bartolomeo 2000) found that dual-task interference with a spatial task was relatively greater for 'recovered' neglect patients than for patients still showing clinical evidence of the disorder (who, by inference, were not yet using a compensatory strategy).

Thus, the lack of spontaneous improvement shown by some patients may stem from impairments in the more general resources necessary to maintain corrective 'top-down' control. One way to minimize the demands is to attempt to train such strategies to a point where they become more habitual.

Scanning training

Carefully evaluated attempts to train neglect patients in making leftward visual scans began in New York in the 1970s and has been continued, particularly in Rome, throughout the 1980s and 1990s. Early findings, using techniques such as training patients to find the left side of a line of text before attempting to read it or tracking moving lights across a board, revealed generally positive effects. Unfortunately, these seemed somewhat transient and rather specific to the trained context (Weinberg *et al.* 1977; Gouvier *et al.* 1987). Such specificity does not, in itself, preclude a useful rehabilitation effect, but does suggest that training would need to be carried out in a wide variety of settings relevant to a patient's day-to-day goals. Highlighting this, and the sometimes rather brief nature of the interventions, researchers in Italy have revisited scanning training using a wide variety of tasks and a much longer training periods. Over 40 sessions, significant improvements which generalized to nontrained tasks and semistructured everyday-life situations were observed in a radomized controlled study (Antonucci *et al.* 1995; Paolucci *et al.* 1996). An additional, and possibly crucial, feature of this training was the use of optokinetic stimulation (see below).

Further optimistic findings on the potential of scanning training have come from France. Wiart *et al.* (1997) trained patients to scan a large screen using a trunk-mounted pointer. The consequence of this technique was that, in order to orient to the left, patients would need to move their entire body midline into left space. Two months after the termination of training the experimental group showed significantly greater gains in everyday activities than the untreated controls—a finding that has recently been replicated (Seze *et al.* 2001). Làdavas and her colleagues have further demonstrated that training leftward orienting of covert attention (i.e. without eye or body movements) is possible, although the effects of such training on everyday function has yet to be assessed (Làdavas *et al.* 1994*b*).

Inducing corrective distortion to spatial representation

Scanning training encourages patients to use conscious volitional resources to overcome the effects of a persistent bias in the representation of space—resources that can be, for some patients, a rather scarce commodity. However, a number of interventions are known to induce distortions in the perception of (egocentric) space with healthy individuals regardless of their intentions. These have been harnessed to provide corrective input to neglect patients.

If healthy individuals watch a unidirectional moving background display, for example, optokinetic nystagmus and a subjective displacement of body midline occur. If neglect patients are exposed to such displays during the performance of a spatial task, bias can be magnified or minimized according to the direction of movement (Pizzamiglio *et al.* 1990). Similar temporary distortions can be induced via the vestibular system by irrigation of the contralesional ear with cold water and/or the ipsilesional ear with warm water (Cappa *et al.* 1987; Rubens 1985; Vallar *et al.* 1993), by vibration of the posterior neck muscle on the contralesional side (Karnath *et al.* 1993), or by wearing prism spectacles that bring the contralesional periphery into central vision (Rossi *et al.* 1990). Although these interventions have been theoretically useful in calibrating the spatial biases of neglect, the generally short-lived effects and requirement for less-than-portable apparatus have led to pessimism about their role in rehabilitation. However, the fact that they may not form a long-term solution does not exclude a useful role in training. Animal and human studies described earlier show the importance of experience in functional or plastic neural reorganization, and such interventions may foster plastic changes that make subsequent endogenously generated correction easier. For example, it is possible that some of the positive results of the scanning training developed by Pizzamiglio and coworkers (Pizzamiglio *et al.* 1992; Antonucci *et al.* 1995; Paolucci *et al.* 1996), compared with previous attempts, resulted from the additional use of optokinetic stimulation.

Activation of the right hemisphere

So far we have broadly discussed scanning training and the use of corrective distortions as interventions that functionally compensate for enduring biases in attention and the representation of space. However, it is possible that such techniques serve a more direct, if temporary, role in 'rescuing' or supporting neural representations of left space.

With many brain systems activated by visual input, it is likely that processing is competitive, with increased response to one object being associated with decreased response to another. The 'integrated competition model' (Duncan 1999), for example, suggests that unilateral neglect may be an extreme example of such competition, where the damaged visual attentional networks in the right hemisphere consistently lose out in the competition for selection, leading to phenomena such as extinction. Furthermore, as the competition is integrated between components of the sensorimotor network, as one object gains dominance in one system, responses to the same object are supported elsewhere.

This view provides one route whereby different manipulations, in that they enhance activity within the right hemisphere or inhibit activity within the left, may lead to the transient amelioration of neglect. For example Bottini *et al.* (2001) describe how both vestibular stimulation and neck vibration to the left induce increased right-hemisphere activation, including somatosensory and tempero-parietal cortex, and produced deactivation in left fusiform gyrus. A further area in which induced activation of the right hemisphere might play a role in reducing neglect comes from the study of contralesional movements.

Halligan and Marshall (1989) reported that use of the left hand to perform a spatial task resulted in a significantly less biased performance than use of the right. Robertson and colleagues (Robertson and North 1992, 1993, 1994; Robertson *et al.* 1992) systematically examined these effects by asking patients to describe spatial arrays whilst making hand movements under the table. In this manner the inevitable visual cue of a moving hand used to perform the task was avoided. The results showed an interaction between hand movements and the location of those movements. The greatest reduction in neglect emerged when the left hand was moved in isolation within left space (relative to the body midline). Movement of the right hand within left space, or of the left hand within right space, produced much less dramatic results. Simultaneous movement of both hands (the left hand in left space and the right hand to the right) abolished any benefits of left-hand movement.

These effects have been exploited for rehabilitation which has produced generalized and durable improvements in performance of everyday activities (Samuel *et al.* 2000; Wilson *et al.* 2000). In a full randomized controlled trial, patients with neglect receiving limb-activation training (LAT) showed significantly less neglect, improved body image, shorter hospital stay, and a lower requirement for physiotherapy input than a control group (Kalra *et al.* 1997). More recently, in a single-blind randomized controlled trial of home-based LAT 39 patients with left unilateral neglect were randomly allocated to perceptual training plus LAT or to perceptual training alone. Both groups received training of 12–45-minute sessions over a 12-week period. LAT treatment was associated with significantly reduced unilateral neglect at 3 months post-treatment, and with significantly improved left-sided motor function (measured by the motricity index) at 3, 6, and 18–24 months (Robertson *et al.*, in press).

The reason why movement of the left hand ameliorates a visual bias in attention remains somewhat unclear. It is possible that, in line with 'premotor' theories that view visual attention as intimately connected with preparation for action (Rizzolatti and Camarda 1987), the intention to move on the left enhances attentional representation of objects on the left. In a simple form, however, this would lead us to predict that directed action of the right arm toward left space would produce similar benefits to movement of the left hand, which has not been the case. An alternative possibility is, as discussed, that movement of the left hand produces a more general right-hemisphere 'activation' effect, enhancing its capacity to compete with the intact left hemisphere, and that this effect is modulated by the location of the action. A final view, in which the improvements are not directly linked to motor activity *per se*, would be that the difficulty in attending to or moving the left hand (due to the neglect), as with any difficult task, might heighten general phasic arousal levels, an intervention that can also lead to reductions in neglect (see below). This account is, however, difficult to square with the lack of an effect under bi-manual movement conditions.

Spatially nonselective attention

A key role for nonspatially selective attention deficits in unilateral neglect is another example of how multiple cognitive processes may underpin the set of phenomena associated with neglect. Heilman and his group have been at the forefront of research exploring this relationship. In a review of the behavioral and neural mechanisms of attention, they argue that '... the right hemisphere may have a special role in mediating the arousal response as well as in selective attention' (Heilman *et al.* 1987, p. 475). They argue that the greater incidence and severity of neglect from right-hemisphere lesions in humans is due to the asymmetry of the receptive fields for novel or significant stimuli. They propose that the temporal–parietal cortex in the right hemisphere may have receptive fields for novel stimuli for both left and right hemispace, whereas the equivalent area in the left hemisphere has receptive fields for novel or significant stimuli only in right hemispace. By this argument, left-hemisphere damage can relatively easily be compensated by a right hemisphere capable of responding to novel and significant stimuli in both hemispaces. Heilman and colleagues therefore make a distinction between hypoarousal associated with right temporal parietal damage on the one hand, and spatial selective attention on the other. While a clear formulation of the precise relationship between these two systems remains elusive, it is clear that the temporoparietal junction does play both a spatial-independent role (Fink *et al.* 1996) and a spatially specific role (Fink *et al.* 2000).

We examined the performance of a large number of right-hemisphere stroke patients on a nonspatial sustained attention measure (Robertson *et al.* 1997). Despite reasonable equity between groups on indices of functional severity, such as motor function, right-hemisphere patients who showed neglect were significantly more likely to have problems with this task than those who had no obvious neglect. Indeed, the discriminative power of this sustained attention measure, which consists simply of maintaining a count of tones, was greater than a conventional measure of visual neglect, namely line bisection. Samuelsson *et al.* (1997) similarly found that nonlateralized attentional deficits, such as in maintaining alertness during the interval between a temporal cue and the presentation of a target, are strong predictors of persisting unilateral neglect within a right-hemisphere group. Other studies that have examined the allocation of attention over time rather than space have reached similar conclusions. For example, Husain *et al.* (1997) demonstrated that neglect patients required a significantly longer period after processing one target before resources were available to process a subsequent target (an 'attentional blink'). Cusack *et al.* (2001) found that when neglect patients were asked to discriminate two tones within a single auditory event, their performance did not differ from that of healthy age-matched controls. However, when an interval was introduced between the tones, a significant impairment was apparent. Taken together with results showing reduced spatial capacity in the 'good' as well as the neglected hemifield (Duncan *et al.* 1999), these results suggest prevalent attentional deficits stressed by both time and space associated with unilateral neglect. Therefore it is possible that these more generalized deficits form the setting conditions under which the spatial biases of the disorder are perpetuated.[1,2]

We put these correlational links between arousal and neglect to experimental test (Robertson *et al.* 1998). The prediction was that phasically increasing the patients' alertness should transiently ameliorate the spatial bias in perceptual awareness, and indeed the results provided the first direct confirmation of this proposal. The task required right-hemisphere neglect patients to judge whether a left visual event preceded a comparable right event or vice versa. Neglect patients became aware of left events half a second slower than right events, on average. This dramatic spatial imbalance in the time course of visual awareness could be reversed if a warning sound alerted the patients phasically. Even a sound on the right dramatically accelerated the perception of left visual events in this way. Thus a nonspatial alerting intervention can overcome disabling spatial biases in perceptual awareness after brain injury.

In a clinical experimental corollary of the above study, we attempted direct rehabilitation of sustained attention in a group of patients with unilateral left neglect following right hemisphere lesions. These patients were trained while doing a variety of tasks with no lateralized scanning component; periodically the patients had their attention drawn to a routine task (e.g. a sorting task by combining a loud noise with an instruction to attend. Patients were then gradually taught to 'take over' this alerting procedure using a self-generated verbal cue so that eventually it became a self-alerting procedure. Among this group of eight patients, not only were there improvements in sustained attention, but there were also very significant improvements in spatial neglect over and above those expected by natural recovery (Robertson *et al.* 1995*b*).

In conclusion, the links between theoretical models of cognitive neuroscience and cognitive rehabilitation techniques have been particularly fruitful in the field of unilateral neglect. Most patients who show unilateral neglect in the immediate post-stroke phase recover quite rapidly from the frank spatial biases of the disorder. For many patients, however, this apparent recovery may reflect the use of compensatory strategies (volitional or otherwise) that mask a persistent distortion in the perception of space.

A number of early attempts to induce such compensation by training visual scans into left space found rather transitory improvements that were highly specific to the trained context. A number of reasons may account for the more successful outcome of recent scanning training research, including the use of a much wider set of training conditions, increased duration of training, and the use of techniques such as optokinetic stimulation. Techniques that lead to a distortion in the perception of egocentric space in healthy individuals have been used to temporarily correct the pathological biases of neglect. These techniques (caloric vestibular stimulation, neck muscle vibration, optokinetic stimulation, and the use of prism-lens spectacles), although largely impractical as long-term rehabilitation or compensatory aids, may form a useful adjunct to training.

---

[1] There is emerging evidence for a role of these attentional functions in mediating many aspects of recovery. We (Robertson *et al.* 1997) recently found that nonspatial sustained attention assessed 2 months after stroke was a significant predictor of functional (left-hand) dexterity when measured at a 2-year follow-up, an effect that was independent of stroke severity (see also Ben-Yishay *et al.* (1968)).

[2] The detection of neglect-like spatial biases in children defined by poor attention and lowered arousal (attention-deficit hyperactivity disorder) is consistent with this view (Manly *et al.* 1997; Nigg *et al.* 1997; Sheppard *et al.* 1999; Dobler *et al.* 2001).

In particular, their role in inducing processing of left-sided stimuli that does not rely on the expenditure of limited-capacity resources requires further examination.

Persuasive accounts of how the brain handles multiple simultaneous inputs view it as a competitive process whereby one object or event will dominate awareness and response preparation. In the case of neglect, damage to the right hemisphere leads to a dominance by the intact left hemisphere. Therefore a number of interventions, including training in leftward scanning, may serve a more direct role in rescuing representations of left space by increasing activation within the right hemisphere. Limb-activation effects, whereby movement of the patient's left hand within left space leads to a significant reduction in spatial bias, appear to be a striking example of this process. The cognitive deficits of neglect patients are rarely restricted to a spatial bias. In particular, patients seem disproportionately vulnerable to nonspatial attention deficits in maintaining an alert ready-to-respond state. In line with the view that such deficits may contribute to the setting conditions in which a spatial bias may be perpetuated, experimental evidence shows a direct modulatory role on external alerting procedures on neglect. This view has been used to develop tractable and somewhat paradoxical clinical interventions for the disorder that emphasizes encouraging patients to develop and maintain general alertness rather than to search for items on the left.

Thus, if the close and two-way theory–practice links of unilateral neglect research can be reproduced in other areas of cognitive function and dysfunction, we can be optimistic about the future development of both cognitive neuroscience and neuropsychological rehabilitation in a range of other areas of cognitive function and dysfunction.

References

Antonucci, G., Guariglia, C., Judica, A., *et al*. (1995). Effectiveness of neglect rehabilitation in a randomized group study. *Journal of Clinical and Experimental Neuropsychology*, **17**, 383–9.

Bach-y-Rita, P. (1989). Theory-based neurorehabilitation. *Archives of Physical Medicine and Rehabilitaton*, **70**, 162.

Bartolomeo, P. (2000). Inhibitory processes and spatial bias after right hemisphere damage. *Neuropsychological Rehabilitation*, **10**, 511–26.

Ben-Yishay, Y., Diller, L., Gerstman, L., and Haas, A. (1968). The relationship between impersistence, intellectual function and outcome of rehabilitation in patients with left hemiplegia. *Neurology*, **18**, 852–61.

Bottini, G., Karnath, H.-O., Vallar, G., *et al*. (2001). Cerebral representations for egocentric space— Functional-anatomical evidence from caloric vestibular stimulation and neck vibration. *Brain*, **124**, 1182–96.

Buccino, G., Binkofski, F., Fink, G. R., *et al*. (2001). Action observation activates premotor and parietal areas in a somatotopic manner: an fMRI study. *European Journal of Neuroscience*, **13**, 400–4.

Cappa, S. F., Sterzi, R., Vallar, G., and Bisiach, E. (1987). Remission of hemineglect and anosognosia during vestibular stimulation. *Neuropsychologia*, **25**, 775–82.

Cusack, R., Carlyon, R. P., and Robertson, I. H. (2001). Neglect between but not within auditory objects. *Journal of Cognitive Neuroscience*, **12**, 1056–65.

Dobler, V., Manly, T., Robertson, I. H., Polichroniadis, M., Verity, C., Goodyer, I., and Wilson, B. A. (2001). Modulation of hemispatial attention in a case of developmental unilateral neglect. *Neurocase*, **7**, 185.

Duncan, J. (1999). Converging levels of analysis in the cognitive neuroscience of visual attention. In *Attention, space, and action* (ed. G. W. Humphreys, J. Duncan, and A. Treisman), pp. 112–29. Oxford University Press.

Duncan, J., Bundesen, C., Olson, A., Humphreys, G., Chavda, S., and Shibuya, H. (1999). Systematic analysis of deficits in visual attention. *Journal of Experimental Psychology: General*, **128**, 450–78.

Eriksson, P. S., Perfilieva, E., Bjork-Eriksson, T., *et al*. (1998). Neurogenesis in the adult human hippocampus. *Nature Medicine*, **4**, 1313–17.

Fadiga, L., Fogassi, L., Gallese, V., and Rizzolatti, G. (2000). Visuomotor neurons: ambiguity of the discharge or 'motor' perception? *International Journal of Psychophysiology*, **35**, 165–77.

Fink, G. R., Halligan, P. W., Marshall, J. C., Frith, C. D., Frackowiak, R. S. J., and Dolan, R. J. (1996). Where in the brain does visual attention select the forest and the trees? *Nature*, **382**, 626–8.

Fink, G. R., Marshall, J. C., Weiss, P. H., *et al.* (2000). 'Where' depends on 'what': A differential functional anatomy for position discrimination in one versus two dimensions. *Neuropsychologia*, **38**, 1741–8.

Gallese, V., Fadiga, L., Fogassi, L., and Rizzolatti, G. (1996). Action recogniton in the premotor cortex. *Brain*, **119**, 593.

Goodale, M. A., Milner, A. D., Jakobson, L. S., and Carey, D. P. (1990). Kinematic analysis of limb movements in neuropsychological research: subtle deficits and recovery of function. *Canadian Journal of Psychology*, **44**, 180–95.

Gould, E., Beylin, A., Tanapat, P., Reeves, A., and Shores, T. J. (1999). Learning enhances adult neurogenesis in the hippocampal formation. *Nature Neuroscience*, **2**, 260–5.

Gouvier, W., Bua, B., Blanton, P., and Urey, J. (1987). Behavioural changes following visual scanning training: observation of five cases. *International Journal of Clinical Neuropsychology*, **9**, 74–80.

Halligan, P. W. and Marshall, J. C. (1989). Laterality of motor response in visuo-spatial neglect: a case study. *Neuropsychologia*, **27**, 1301–7.

Heilman, K. M., Watson, R. T., Valenstein, E., and Goldberg, M. E. (1987). Attention: behavioral and neural mechanisms. In *Handbook of physiology. Section 1: The nervous system* (ed. F. Plum), Vol. 5, pp. 461–81. American Physiological Society, Bethesda, MD.

Husain, M., Shapiro, K., Martin, J., and Kennard, C. (1997). Abnormal temporal dynamics of visual attention in spatial neglect patients. *Nature*, **385**, 154–6.

Kalra, L., Perez, I., Gupta, S., and Wittink, M. (1997). The influence of visual neglect on stroke rehabilitation. *STROKE*, **28**, 1386–91.

Karnath, H.-O., Christ, K., and Hartje, W. (1993). Decrease of contralateral neglect by neck muscle vibration and spatial orientation of trunk midline. *Brain*, **116**, 383–96.

Làdavas, E., Carletti, M., and Gori, G. (1994*a*). Automatic and voluntary orienting of attention in patients with visual neglect: horizontal and vertical dimensions. *Neuropsychologia*, **32**, 1195–1208.

Làdavas, E., Menghini, G., and Umilta, C. (1994*b*). A rehabilitation study of hemispatial neglect. *Cognitive Neuropsychology*, **11**, 75–95.

Luria, A. R. (1963). *Restoration of function after brain injury*. Pergamon Press, Oxford.

Manly, T., Robertson, I. H., and Verity, C. (1997). Development unilateral neglect: A single case study. *Neurocase*, **3**, 19–29.

Mattingley, J. B., Bradshaw, J. L., Bradshaw, J. A., and Nettleton, N. C. (1994). Residual right attentional bias after apparent recovery from right hemisphere damage: implications for a multicomponent model of neglect. *Journal of Neurology, Neurosurgery, and Psychiatry*, **57**, 597–604.

Nigg, J. T., Swanson, J. M., and Hindshaw, S. P. (1997). Covert visual spatial attention in boys with attention deficit hyperactive disorder: Lateral effects, methylphenidate response and results for parents. *Neuropsychologia*, **35**, 165–76.

Nudo, R. J., Wise, B. M., SiFuentes, F., and Milliken, G. W. (1996). Neural substrates for the effects of rehabilitative training on motor recovery after ischemic infarct. *Science*, **272**, 1791–4.

Paolucci, A., Antonucci, G., Guariglia, C., Magnotti, L., Pizzamiglio, L., and Zoccolotti, P. (1996). Facilitatory effect of neglect rehabilitation on the recovery of left hemiplegic stroke patients: A crossover study. *Journal of Neurology*, **243**, 308–14.

Pizzamiglio, L., Frasca, R., Guariglia, C., Incoccia, C., and Antonucci, G. (1990). Effect of optokinetic stimulation in patients with visual neglect. *Cortex*, **26**, 535–40.

Pizzamiglio, L., Antonucci, G., Judica, A., Montenero, P., Razzano, C., and Zoccolotti, P. (1992). Cognitive rehabilitation of the hemineglect disorder in chronic patients with unilateral right brain damage. *Journal of Clinical and Experimental Neuropsychology*, **14**, 901–23.

Recanzone, G. H., Schreiner, C. E., and Merzenich, M. M. (1993). Plasticity in the frequency representation of primary auditory cortex. *Journal of Neuroscience*, **13**, 87–103.

Rizzolatti, G., and Camarda, R. (1987). Neural circuits for spatial attention and unilateral neglect. In *Neurophysiological and neuropsychological aspects of neglect* (ed. M. Jeannerod) pp. 289–313. North Holland Press, Amsterdam.

Robertson, I. H. (1999). Setting goals in cognitive rehabilitation. *Current Opinion in Neurology*, **12**, 703–8.

Robertson, I. H. and Frasca, R. (1992). Attentional load and visual neglect. *International Journal of Neuroscience*, **62**, 45–56.

Robertson, I. H. and Murre, J. M. J. (1999). Rehabilitation of brain damage: brain plasticity and principles of guided recovery. *Psychological Bulletin*, **125**, 544–75.

Robertson, I. H. and North, N. (1992). Spatio-motor cueing in unilateral neglect: the role of hemispace, hand and motor activation. *Neuropsychologia*, **30**, 553–63.

Robertson, I. H. and North, N. (1993). Active and passive activation of left limbs: influence on visual and sensory neglect. *Neuropsychologia*, **31**, 293–300.

Robertson, I. H. and North, N. (1994). One hand is better than two: motor extinction of left hand advantage in unilateral neglect. *Neuropsychologia*, **32**, 1–11.

Robertson, I. H., North, N., and Geggie, C. (1992). Spatio-motor cueing in unilateral neglect: Three single case studies of its therapeutic effectiveness. *Journal of Neurology, Neurosurgery, and Psychiatry*, **55**, 799–805.

Robertson, I. H., McMillan, T. M., MacLeod, E., and Brock, D. (in press). Rehabilitation by Limb Activation Training (LAT) reduces impairment in unilateral neglect patients: a single-blind randomized control trial. *Neuropsychological Rehabilitation*.

Robertson, I. H., Manly, T., Beschin, N., *et al.* (1997). Auditory sustained attention is a marker of unilateral spatial neglect. *Neuropsychologia*, **35**, 1527–32.

Robertson, I. H., Mattingley, J. B., Rorden, C., and Driver, J. (1998). Phasic alerting of neglect patients overcomes their spatial deficit in visual awareness. *Nature*, **395**, 169–72.

Robertson, I. H., Tegner, R., Tham, K., Lo, A., and Nimmo-Smith, I. (1995). Sustained attention training for unilateral neglect: theoretical and rehabilitation implications. *Journal of Clinical and Experimental Neuropsychology*, **17**, 416–30.

Rossi, P. W., Kheyfets, S., and Reding, M. J. (1990). Fresnel prisms improve visual perception in stroke patients with homonymous hemianopia or unilateral visual neglect. *Neurology*, **40**, 1597–9.

Rubens, A. B. (1985). Caloric stimulation and unilateral visual neglect. *Neurology*, **35**, 1019–24.

Samuel, C., Loui-Dreyfus, A., Kaschel, R., Makiela, E., Troubat, M., Aselmi, N., Cannizzo, V., and Azouvi, P. (2000). Rehabilitation of very severe unilateral neglect by visuo-spatial cueing: two single case studies. *Neuropsychological Rehabilitation*, **10**, 385–99.

Samuelsson, H., Jensen, C., Ekholm, S., Naver, H., and Blomstrand, C. (1997). Anatomical and neurological correlates of acute and chronic visuospatial neglect following right hemisphere stroke. *Cortex*, **33**, 271–85.

Seitz, R. J., Huang, Y., Knorr, U., Tellmann, L., Herzog, H., and Freund, H. J. (1995). Large-scale plasticity of the human motor cortex. *NeuroReport*, **6**, 742–4.

Seze, M. D., Wiart, L., and Bon-Saint-Come, A. (2001). Rehabilitation of postural disturbances of hemiplegic patients by using trunk control retraining during exploratory exercises. *Archives of Physical Medicine and Rehabilitation*, **82**, 793–800.

Sheppard, D. M., Bradshaw, J. L., Mattingley, J. B., and Lee, P. (1999). Effects of stimulant medication on the lateralisation of line bisection judgements of children with attention deficit hyperactivity disorder. *Journal of Neurology, Neurosurgery and Psychiatry*, **66**, 57–63.

Stone, S. P., Patel, P., Greenwood, R. J., and Halligan, P. W. (1992). Measuring visual neglect in acute stroke and predicting its recovery: the visual neglect recovery index. *Journal of Neurology, Neurosurgery and Psychiatry*, **55**, 431–6.

Vallar, G., Bottini, G., Rusconi, M. L., and Sterzi, R. (1993). Exploring somatosensory neglect by vestibular stimulation. *Brain*, **116**, 71–86.

Weinberg, J., Diller, L., Gordon, W., *et al.* (1977). Visual scanning training effect on reading-related tasks in acquired right brain damage. *Archives of Physical Medicine and Rehabilitation*, **58**, 479–86.

Wiart, L., Bon-Saint-Come, A., Debelleix, X., Petit, H., Joseph, P. A., and Mazaux, J. M. (1997). Unilateral neglect syndrome rehabilitation by trunk rotation and scanning training. *Archives of Physical Medicine and Rehabilitation*, **78**, 424–9.

Wilson, F. C., Manly, T., Coyle, D., and Robertson, I. H. (2000). The effect of contralesional limb activation training and sustained attention for self-care programmes in unilateral spatial neglect. *Restorative Neurology and Neuroscience*, **16**, 1–4.

7.2 Reducing spatial neglect by visual and other sensory manipulations: noncognitive (physiological) routes to the rehabilitation of a cognitive disorder

Yves Rossetti and Gilles Rode

A large proportion of right-hemisphere stroke patients show unilateral neglect—a neurological deficit of perception, attention, representation, and/or performing actions within their left-sided space (Heilman *et al.* 1985), which induces many functionally debilitating effects on everyday life and is responsible for poor functional recovery and ability to benefit from treatment (Denes *et al.* 1982; Fullerton *et al.* 1986; Halligan and Marshall 1989). The history of neglect modulation by a specifically designed intervention started with Diller and Weinberg (1977) 25 years ago. It was the study by Rubens (1985) that renewed interest in rehabilitation methods for hemispatial neglect and a renewal of both theoretical questions and experimental approaches. The experimental neuropsychology approach to hemispatial neglect brought in clearer constraints for the precise quantification of the patients' performance and stimulated interest in the focal or partial aspects of this syndrome. At this stage local interventions with the patients were shown to alleviate most of the symptoms of hemispatial neglect (Vallar *et al.* 1997a). More recently, the idea that specific learning could produce improvements in patients has been revived and has incorporated the physiological aspects of sensory stimulation (Kerkhoff 2000). In addition, the need for public health systems to evaluate quantified but functional outcomes of rehabilitation procedures has motivated the use of a more global and ecological evaluation of patient recovery.

The various manifestations of unilateral neglect share one major feature: patients remain unaware of the deficit they exhibit or at least fail to attend to these deficits fully consciously. This deficit in awareness is dramatically expressed in anosognosia and hemiasomatognosia (Bisiach *et al.* 1986). Therefore it is surprising that the first methods proposed for the rehabilitation of neglect were mainly based on a voluntary orientation of attention to the left. This apparent contradiction was emphasized by Diller and Weinberg themselves: 'The first step in the treatment of hemi-inattention is to make the patient aware of the problem. This is particularly difficult in hemi-inattention since this failure in awareness appears to be at the heart of the patient's difficulty' (Diller and Weinberg 1977, p. 67). It may indeed appear paradoxical to base a rehabilitation procedure on awareness and intention in patients with a deficit in consciousness. How can a sustained overt orienting to the left be obtained from individuals whose pathology is precisely to remain unable to attend to the left? These techniques have produced significant results but clearly have several limitations. For example, rehabilitated patients may typically produce almost perfect performance on classical tests performed during a testing session and then walk into the door when leaving the room, i.e. their voluntary monitoring of attention is restricted to a specific context and does not apply as soon as more automatic control is required. Harvey and Milner (1999) have also shown that the training of visual scanning in hemispatial neglect may improve line bisection, which requires a sustained voluntary orienting of attention, but not other tasks. To act on higher-level cognition in such a way as to bypass the impaired conscious awareness and intention, one should, at least in principle, find another entry route to space representation systems. In their theory, Jeannerod and Biguer (1987) proposed that the transformation of the sensory input into the motor output is impaired in hemispatial neglect. This idea is compatible with current knowledge about the crucial role of the parietal cortex in coordinate transformation (Jeannerod and Rossetti 1993; Andersen 1995; Milner and Goodale 1995; Pisella and Rossetti 2000; Rossetti and Pisella 2002). Jeannerod and Biguer predicted that unilateral lesions 'produce an illusory "rotation" of the egocentric reference, somewhat as if the subject felt being constantly rotated toward the lesion side'. This idea has been recently revisited by Karnath (1997) and Vallar *et al.* (1997*b*) who proposed that the coordinate transformation system was biased by an internal constant error. Apparent experimental support for this hypothesis was provided by Rubens (1985), who stimulated the left ear of neglect patients with cold water in order to stimulate the vestibular input to the right hemisphere and found that they immediately improved.

The methods proposed to modulate neglect have evolved rather slowly from these initial results and framework. We will present here three main groups of physiological approaches to neglect modulation: passive physiological stimulation, active stimulation, and stimulation of sensorimotor plasticity. The main questions to be addressed concern the specificity of these methods with regard to the physiopathology of hemispatial neglect, and their possible outcome in terms of rehabilitation.

Passive physiological stimulation

Different manifestations of neglect may be alleviated by sensory stimulation. The first improvement of visual neglect was reported by Silberpfennig (1941) after a caloric vestibular stimulation applied to two patients with cerebral tumors. The stimulation led to a reduction of head and eye deviation and of neglect dyslexia. These preliminary results were confirmed later by Rubens (1985) who showed in 18 right-brain-damaged patients with neglect that a left cold caloric stimulation might improve left visual neglect, although a right stimulation might worsen the deficit. These exciting results had shown that a cognitive deficit related to damage of the right hemisphere might be positively influenced by a physiological stimulation (for a review of the effects of vestibular stimulation, see Rode *et al.* (1998*d*)). These investigations were followed by numerous studies assessing the effects of other kinds of stimulation and the nature of the improved symptoms. Following the work of Rubens (1985) and the striking results obtained with caloric stimulation, many studies have replicated this result and extended its conclusions. Several other types of sensory stimulation were proposed and tested in patients. Many manifestations of neglect have been shown to be alleviated by sensory stimulation (vestibular, optokinetic, transcutaneous electrical, transcutaneous mechanical vibration, auditory) (Vallar *et al.* 1997*b*; Kerkhoff 2000). The improvement has been mainly reported for extrapersonal neglect (classical neuropsychological testing), but many other aspects have been investigated including personal neglect and sensory and motor deficits of left hemibody associated with neglect or extinction. Even productive manifestations of hemispatial neglect, such as anosognosia or somatoparaphrenia, may be also reduced by sensory stimulation (Rode *et al.* 1992). Positive effects on postural instability in right-brain-damaged patients with neglect have also been reported. Table 1 summarizes the various techniques that have been tested with patients and the parameters investigated.

The second characteristic of effects reported through stimulation is their abrupt onset. In all studies the improvement was observed during or immediately following the stimulation. Unfortunately, a single application of these techniques produces positive effects lasting for only up to about 10 to 15 minutes, and then they vanish within minutes. These characteristics were reported in the early study by Rubens (1985) and have been reviewed in detail by Vallar *et al.* (1997*b*) and Kerkhoff (2000). The multiplicity of the effects and the transient characteristics of the improvement have raised questions about the specificity of sensory stimulation. The reduction of neglect symptoms might be simply due to an increased arousal level by a nonspecific action. Alternatively, they may be attributable to a reduction of attentional bias or spatial representation asymmetry by a selective action on physiopathological mechanisms involved in spatial cognition. Patients with extensive damage to the right cerebral hemisphere exhibit hemispatial neglect of the left side of space, but also a nonspatial deficit in alertness (ability to maintain arousal) (see Chapter 7.1). A short nonlateralized auditory stimulation (a 300-ms tone-burst) may increase the patient's alertness and ameliorate the spatial bias in awareness, suggesting that the spatial and non-spatial deficits may be linked (Robertson *et al.* 1998*a*). Although an effect of the various sensory stimulations on the patient's alertness is possible, several results have suggested that it may not be sufficient to explain the selective effects on cognitive deficits or the hemispheric asymmetry of the effects on somatosensory and motor deficits. First, a vestibular caloric stimulation with iced water in the left ear (Rode and Perenin 1994) or transcutaneous electrical nervous stimulation (TENS) of the left side of the neck (Guariglia *et al.* 1998) produced significant improvement of performance *only on the left side* of mental representations of mental images of space (description of the map of France and of Italian piazzas respectively).

Second, the effects of vestibular stimulation, optokinetic stimulation (OKS), and TENS on somatosensory and motor deficits are not symmetrical. Vallar *et al.* (1993*a*) have shown that ves-tibular stimulation improved left hemianesthesia in 15 out of 17 right-brain-damaged patients but in only two out of 11 left-brain-damaged patients (these two cases also had right visuospatial hemineglect). Similar asymmetric results on somatosensory deficits in right- and left-brain-damaged patients were reported by the same authors after TENS. A stimulation of the side of the neck contralateral to the side of the lesion reduced the somatosensory deficit in right-brain-damaged patients, whereas the ipsilateral stimulation did not modify it, and even worsened it in one case (Vallar *et al.* 1996). Interestingly, the same asymmetry was reported for motor deficit after vestibular stimulation in nine right-brain-damaged patients with neglect (Rode *et al.* 1998). Also for motor deficit, Vallar *et al.* (1997*a*) reported that two right-brain-damaged patients were improved whereas two left-brain-damaged patients were not when OKS was applied with a left-ward motion. As for somatosensory deficit (Vallar *et al.* 1993), the only left-brain-damaged patient who was improved after this stimulation was ambidextrous and had shown transient signs of right neglect. Therefore these physiological stimulations seem to modulate, through afferent sensory pathways, higher-order spatial representations of the body that are pathologically distorted toward the side of the lesion. They may affect the operation of specific neural systems, which are more frequently disrupted by lesions in the right hemisphere (Vallar *et al.* 1997*a*).

Third, the hypothesis of selective effect of stimulation on neglect is also supported by two case studies. Vallar *et al.* (1995*a*) assessed the effects of vestibular stimulation in a patient who had a lesion in the left parieto-occipital paraventricular white matter and suffered from both right visuospatial hemineglect and fluent dysphasia. Vestibular stimulation improved the right hemineglect, but did not affect the speech disorder. Moreover, Rode *et al.* (2002) studied a patient with a florid left visual neglect for whom a cold irrigation in the left ear improved the spatial deficit whereas an irrigation in the right ear worsened it. Despite the obvious prediction that a bilateral

Table 1 Effects of sensory stimulations on neglect

Reference	Symptoms of neglect							
	Extrapersonal neglect	Personal neglect	Imaginal neglect	Anosognosia Somatoparaphrenia	Sensory deficit	Motor deficit	Postural instability	Subjective Straight-ahead
Vestibular stimulation								
Silberpfennig (1941)	×							
Marshall and Maynard (1983)	×							
Rubens (1985)	×							
Cappa et al. (1987)	×	×						
Vallar et al. (1990)	×			×				
Bisiach et al. (1991)				×	×			
Rode et al. (1992)				×				
Geminiani and Bottini (1992)	×	×						
Vallar et al. (1993a)			×		×			
Rode and Perenin (1994)			×					
Karnath (1994)*	×							×
Vallar et al. (1995a)	×							
Ramachandran et al. (1995)				×				
Karnath et al. (1996)*	Ocular exploration							
Rode et al. (1998a)		×				×	×	
Rode et al. (1998b)				×				
Rorsman et al. (1999) (galvanic)	×							
Rode et al. (2002)	×							
Optokinetic stimulation (OKS)								
Pizzamiglio et al. (1990)	×							
Vallar et al. (1993b)					Position sense			
Vallar et al. (1995b)					Position sense			
Karnath (1996)								×
Vallar et al. (1997)						×		
Kerkhoff et al. (1999)	×							
Kerkhoff (2000)	×							

Table 1 (continued)

Reference	Symptoms of neglect							
	Extrapersonal neglect	Personal neglect	Imaginal neglect	Anosognosia Somatoparaphrenia	Sensory deficit	Motor deficit	Postural instability	Subjective Straight-ahead
Transcutaneous electrical nervous stimulation (TENS)								
Vallar et al. (1995c) (neck/hand)	×							
Karnath (1995)*	×							×
Vallar et al. (1996) (neck)					×			
Guariglia et al. (1998) (neck)			×					
Perennnou et al. (2001) (neck)							×	
Guariglia et al. (2000) (neck)	Spatial orientation							
Richard et al. (2001) (plantar)*								×
Transcutaneous mechanical vibration (TMV)								
Karnath et al. (1993) neck	×							
Karnath (1994) (neck)*								×
Karnath (1995)*	×							×
Karnath et al. (1996) (neck)*	Ocular exploration							
Richard et al. (2001) (plantar)*								×
Auditory stimulation (AS)								
Hommel et al. (1990) (auditory)	×							
Robertson et al. (1998) (auditory)	×							

*Studies assessing two stimulations made separately or together.

Vestibular stimulation was applied by cold water irrigation of the left external auditory canal with 30–60 ml of ice water for 1 min.

OKS was evoked by a constant linear moving pattern of randomly distributed white dots with a direction of the horizontal movement of the luminous dots contralateral to the side of the lesion.

TENS was administered by a stimulator with superficial electrodes used to stimulate the posterior neck (below the occiput, just lateral to the spine), the hand , or the sole of the foot contralateral to the side of the lesion.

TMV was applied by vibration of the left posterior neck muscles with an experimental vibrator (frequency, 80 Hz; amplitude, 0.4 mm).

stimulation would provide the maximal arousal stimulation, a bilateral irrigation produced no effect. Thus sensory stimulation seems to bring about a specific reorganization of lateralized spatial processes, which involves the whole representation of space and the body.

The reversibility of various symptoms of hemispatial neglect syndrome through physiological stimulation also calls into question the physiopathology of this condition. The spontaneous variability of the deficit strongly contrasts with the strength of primary motor or sensory deficits or with other cognitive deficit affecting language, memory, or executive functions on which these various stimulations exert no effect. This suggests that a specific functional component is associated with the lesion. This may be explained by the fact that neglect is a deficit consequent to damage to multimodal areas related to the orientation of spatial behavior and not to a specialized cortical area such as the primary motor or sensory areas. These associative areas can be activated by peripheral stimulation (visual, vestibular, somatosensory, optokinetic) (Bottini *et al.* 1994, 2001), and may be organized in parallel with other central nervous system structures which receive convergent inputs from several sensory systems. Following cerebral damage, undamaged cerebral structures may be activated by passive stimulation and contribute to a modulation of the functional deficit. However, this action remains highly transient despite its selectivity.

The common feature of all these techniques is that the sensory inputs that are manipulated are strongly linked to automatic levels of orientation behavior. Various submodules of the sensorimotor system can be more or less directly implicated, ranging from sensorimotor adjustments (tendon vibration), to orienting behavior (neck muscle vibration, vestibular or optokinetic nystagmus) or to whole-body posture (vestibular stimulation, plantar vibration) (Table 1). With the notable exception of the alertness reaction (Robertson *et al.* 1998a), these physiological responses are lateralized. The automatic nature of the orientation reactions stimulated by these stimulations is such that the patient is passively fed with a sensory input and that the sensorimotor reaction takes place without the patient being actively involved in the stimulus processing or in the response preparation or execution (e.g. optokinetic nystagmus (Mattingley *et al.* 1994)). Therefore the response to the stimulation is no longer activated when the stimulation is interrupted, and no residue is left in the nervous system once the phasic response has vanished. This feature is likely to explain the short duration of the effects generated by these techniques. In contrast, active stimulations may be expected to produce longer-lasting effects (Rode *et al.* 2001a).

Active training

Rather than just passively feeding sensory systems of neglect patients, several techniques have proposed the use of simple actions from the patients in normal or specific sensorimotor contexts. Two interesting characteristics can be distinguished within this category: the task effect, which can be observed at the level of a single trial, and the modulation effect which can be transferred to other tasks after completing a training session (Table 2).

The first clinical method of rehabilitation specifically designed to improve hemispatial neglect was proposed by Diller and Weinberg (1977). Based on clinical experience, it was proposed to focus on the awareness of the deficit exhibited by neglect patients and to repeat the orienting 'procedure so that it becomes automatic'. Following training periods of 1 h each day for a 1-month period, the treated groups improved more than controls receiving only traditional occupational therapy for eye–hand skills (Weinberg *et al.* 1977, 1979). Improvement in performance was assessed by tasks of reading, copying, written arithmetic, spatial localization, and spatial relationships. Following this first wave of training studies, a more recent wave incorporated more physiological parameters in the training procedures, i.e. exploration or orientation reactions. When compared with nonspecific cognitive training, the active training of efficient scanning has

Table 1 Active stimulation

Trial level	Less impaired	More impaired
Joanette et al. (1986)	Left-hand response	Right-hand response
Robertson (1991)	Left-hand response	Right-hand response
Milner and Harvey (1995)	Motor bisection	Perceptual bisection
Harvey and Milner (1999)	Motor action	Motor matching
Robertson et al. (1995)	Motor action	Motor designation

Training level	Training task	Training duration	Testing	Duration of improvement
Weinberg et al. (1977)	Scanning training	1 month (daily)	Classical tests	6 weeks
Antonucci et al. (1995)	Scanning training	2 months	Classical tests +functional	2 months
Wiart et al. (1997)	Scanning training +trunk rotation	2 months	Classical tests +functional (F.I.M.)	2 months
Kerkhoff (1998)	Visual scanning	6+4 weeks	Classical tests +visuospatial tests	Not tested
Schindler et al. (2002)	Visuospatial training Visual scanning +neck vibration	6 weeks	Classical tests +tactile exploration	2 months

The upper section of this table describes experimental studies showing that performance on a generic task can be strongly modulated by the type of effector used by the patients. For example, responding with the left versus the right hand (Joanette et al. 1986) or producing a manual (action) versus a verbal (perceptual) bisection reveal different levels of performance. The lower section of the table describes studies where active training of the patients was achieved by various techniques. The early training techniques focused on awareness training while the later studies emphasized more automatic orienting responses.

been shown to improve performance on related tasks (Antonucci et al. 1995). Wiart et al. (1997) have compared the efficiency of rehabilitation by both trunk rotation toward the neglect side and scanning training in two groups of neglect patients. The experimental group showed a significant improvement of neglect, assessed by cancellation and bisection tasks, and of incapacity, assessed by an 'activities of daily living' test at days 30 and 60.

Another approach in this domain was derived from the observation that tasks can be differentially affected by hemispatial neglect. For example, the intensity of visual hemineglect assessed by a cancellation task may be influenced by the hand used for the response. An improvement is observed when the patient performs the task with the hand contralateral to the lesion, suggesting a functional interaction between the hand and the side of space (Joanette et al. 1986). Performing an action with the left arm (corporeal space) in left extra-corporeal space improved the spatial disorder. Robertson et al. (1992) proposed spatiomotor cueing as a method of rehabilitation and a functional outcome assessment of this method was recently reported by Samuel et al. (1998).

A further interesting observation was that perceptual and motor versions of the same task were differentially affected by hemispatial neglect. Milner and colleagues (Milner and Harvey 1995; Milner et al. 1998) investigated the perception of size in hemispatial neglect. They presented the patients with two rectangles of different or identical size, one in each hemifield. In most of the trials the two rectangles were identical, but the neglect patients judged the left-sided object to be smaller than the right-sided one. Based on the famous anatomical and functional dissociation between the dorsal and the ventral pathways, two visual streams devoted to action control and to perceptual identification respectively (Milner and Goodale 1995; Rossetti 1998; Rossetti and Pisella 2002), a very interesting observation was then made on the manual responses to the rectangle size when a directed grasping response was compared with a size-matching task performed with the same hand (Pritchard et al. 1997). The action response (object grasping) was more accurate than the perceptual (matching) response, which was similar to the former perceptual response. Along the same lines, recovery from hemispatial neglect was observed to affect primarily manual bisection, whereas its perceptual equivalent (the Landmark test) remained impaired in a more chronic fashion (Harvey and Milner 1999). This finding was interpreted as the consequence of possible strategic learning of the manual bisection task which would not affect the perceptual version of the same task. It has also been reported that the manual prehension of a horizontal bar was performed closer to its center than the response obtained when patients were asked to point at its center (Robertson *et al*. 1995).

Kerkhoff (1998) also proposed training neglect patients on a visual orientation discrimination task (visuospatial training). Verbal feedback was provided to the patients during the learning phase. An improvement was observed for spatially related tasks but not for tests related to visual exploration (including visual search and reading). The reverse was observed when patients were trained for visual search; there was no improvement for visuospatial tasks such as orientation judgment or clock reading. This suggests that training with an explicit processing of error feedback may have only limited capacity for generalization.

To conclude, a patient's actions can be used in such a way as to provide error feedback to cognitive levels of spatial processing. These actions not only produce short-term effects but may also generate prolonged effects following repetitive training, although they do not generalize to many other task domains, as is the case for physiological stimulation (e.g. vestibular stimulation).

Stimulating sensorimotor plasticity

One interesting aspect of sensorimotor relationships is that they are highly susceptible to adaptive processes. The attractive feature of this plasticity is that it should produce prolonged effects on patients. Simple reaching behavior can be adapted to dramatic changes of the relationship between the body and its environment. For example, people can adapt to left–right or up–down reversal of the visual field within a few days (Sekiyama *et al*. 2000), or to the altered gravitational forces produced by weightlessness or a simple rotating chair (Coello *et al*. 1996). It may be useful to some neglect patients to reverse their visual field along the left–right axis and perform adaptation exercises. However, this technique implies a severe visual field cut, can be responsible for falls, and produces very uncomfortable effects for several days. A simpler technique, used extensively for about a century to investigate the plasticity of sensorimotor correspondences, consists of simply shifting the visual field to one side of space by means of prisms (review: Redding and Wallace 1997). This visual shift produces dramatic consequences on the reaching behavior of the subject exposed to the prisms, but adaptation to this condition can be obtained much faster than for the more complex visual manipulations mentioned above.

One very interesting correspondence between prism adaptation and spatial neglect is that prism adaptation can produce a shift in manual straight-ahead pointing in a direction opposite to the visual shift, just as has been described in some patients with spatial neglect (review: Jeannerod and Rossetti 1993). If a normal individual is exposed to right-deviating prisms, he or she will exhibit a leftward deviation of straight-ahead pointing, and the opposite is true for left-deviating prisms. One may therefore wonder whether the egocentric reference of patients with spatial neglect could be altered by prism adaptation, and whether a hypothetical shift could be accompanied by an improvement in other neglect symptoms. Initially based on the theory that neglect was attributable to a shift of the egocentric reference frame that is demonstrable by manual straight-ahead pointing, we have investigated the effect of prism adaptation in neglect patients. The rational for running this first study was that adaptation to wedge prisms can easily alter the manual straight-ahead pointing of normal subjects in a direction opposite to the visual shift. An identical procedure was actually used for many years to evaluate the patient's egocentric reference and the after-effects of prism adaptation in normal subjects. Since neglect patients had been reported to exhibit a shift of the egocentric reference to the right (which was thought to explain the left-side neglect) (Chokron and Imbert 1995), we selected right-deviating prisms in this study. The amount of visual displacement was set at 10°, chosen as being the best compromise between a significant shift, required to generate adaptation, and visual comfort (stronger displacement causes curvature distortion and color fringes). The procedure used to generate the adaptation was simply to require the patients to perform 60 pointing movements to visual targets presented in front of them. Attention was paid to keeping the head straight throughout the testing and the adaptation procedure, and to prevent any view of the hand at its starting position (Rossetti et al. 1998a,b). Patients were then always tested without the prismatic goggles. The results of the first experiment performed on five patients with left sided neglect clearly demonstrated that they adapted to the visual displacement. Not only did they show an improvement in their manual straight-ahead pointing, but the amount of the prism after-effect was about twice that of normal subjects (Fig. 1(a)).

Of course the main question was whether the adaptation would alter the performance of the patients in other tests. Line bisection (Schenkenberg et al. 1980), copy drawing (Gainotti et al. 1972), line cancellation, daisy drawing, and text reading were compared in two groups of five patients who were exposed to a similar pointing procedure. The test group wore prismatic goggles while the control group wore neutral goggles. All patients were tested prior to the adaptation, immediately upon goggle removal, and again 2 h later. A multiple analysis of variance showed that the prism group was significantly improved with respect to the control group and, to our own surprise, the improvement was sustained for at least the 2-h follow-up period, i.e. much longer than in healthy subjects. On average, all patients were improved and all tests exhibited better values after adaptation (e.g. Fig. 1(b)). Interestingly, aspects of object-based and space-based neglect were equally improved by the adaptation procedure (Rossetti et al. 1998a: Fig. 3).

This result raises a number of important theoretical and practical questions which can be clustered in three groups.

1.	What parameters of neglect can be improved by prism adaptation?
2.	What are the mechanisms of neglect improvement by prism adaptation?
3.	Could prism adaptation become a tool for the rehabilitation of hemispatial neglect?

We shall now describe some experiments performed to attempt to answer these questions.

It would seem logical that the effects of prism adaptation should be restricted to, or be best for, visuomotor tasks because they have more features in common with the visuomanual adaptation procedure. In the original study, the best improvement was observed for the Schenkenberg bisection test (all six patients markedly improved), whereas the least improvement was obtained for text reading (two out of six patients markedly improved). Therefore other tests of neglect were investigated (Table 3). Rode et al. (1998, 2001) explored the effect of prism adaptation on visual imagery and found a clear-cut improvement in two patients who could initially not evoke cities on the western half of an internally generated map of France. This result strongly suggested that the after-effects of visuomanual adaptation can no longer be considered to be restricted to visual and motor parameters (Rossetti et al. 1999). Farnè et al. (2001) compared visuomotor tasks (including line and bell cancellation tests, and two subtests taken from the Behavioural Inattention Test (BIT) battery, namely letter cancellation and line bisection.) with visuo-verbal tasks (the visual scanning test, also taken from the BIT, requiring a verbal description of the objects depicted on a colored picture, an object-naming task with 30 Snodgrass pictures of familiar objects intermingled with geometric shapes as distractors, and word and nonword reading) in six patients. They found that the two groups of tasks followed a strictly parallel improvement, which lasted for at least 24 h. Table 3 summarizes the various tasks used with patients. The fact that other sensory modalities can be improved (haptic circle centering (McIntosh et al. 2001), dichotic listening (Courtois-Jacquin

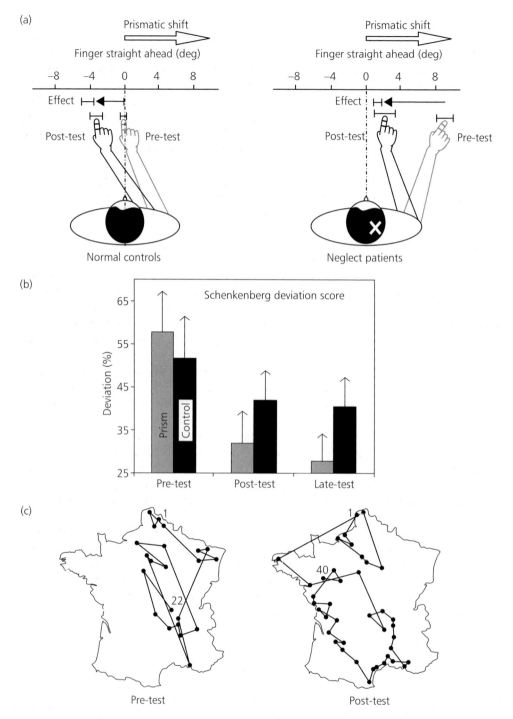

Figure 1 Some effects of prism adaptation. (a) Straight-ahead pointing by patients and healthy subjects before and after prism adaptation. Blindfolded subjects were required to point straight ahead while keeping their heads aligned with the body's sagittal axis. Ten pointing trials were run in the pre-test (without goggles) and in the post-test (immediately upon removal of the 10° prism (white arrow)). As expected, the midline demonstrations made by the neglect group were initially shifted to the right, whereas control subjects pointed straight ahead. Patients were more

et al. 2001), and haptic object recognition (Toutounji *et al.* (2001)) and that several nonmanual tasks (postural control, wheel-chair driving, imagery, verbal reports) were also improved suggests that the effects of prism adaptation are not restricted to visuomanual parameters as is known to be the case in normal subjects. Recent investigations have explored the effects of prism adaptation in both non-manual and non-spatial tasks (at least not explicitly spatial). Pisella and Mattingley (2001) have investigated the temporal order judgment task also used by Robertson *et al.* (1998*a*) and Jacquin-Courtois *et al.* (2002) have used the mental number bisection task described by Zorzi *et al.* (2002). In both studies a clear improvement was found following prism adaptation. These results strongly suggest that adaptation to wedge prisms somehow affects the very core of hemispatial neglect.

If prism adaptation can improve numerous aspects of neglect, then the possible mechanisms of this improvement are worth investigating because they could help us to develop a comprehensive description of neglect physiopathology and hence facilitate the development of more refined methods of rehabilitation. One obvious candidate would be the effect of prisms on the patient's egocentric reference, as it provided the rationale for initiating this series of experiments. However, Pisella *et al.* (2002*b*) showed that there was no significant correlation between the effect of prisms on manual straight-ahead pointing and on line bisection performance. Furthermore, they reported that these two parameters could be affected in contrasting ways by prism adaptation, such that a dynamic double dissociation could be observed between them. This result not only confirmed the dissociability between the egocentric reference frame and other aspects of neglect (Farnè *et al.* 1998; Bartolomeo et Chokron 1999), but also excluded a possible causal role of the sensorimotor after-effects of prisms on the general spatial deficit exhibited by the patients.

Another explanation for the effects of adaptation on the patients' deficits would be the existence of possible cross-talk or synergy between the short-term plasticity mechanisms involved in the adaptation and the longer-term plasticity mechanisms involved in recovery. This hypothesis was explored by Luauté *et al.* (2000) who compared the effects of left- versus right-deviating prisms. Because the sensorimotor after-effects produced by these two types of wedge prisms are symmetric in normal subjects, one might predict that they should generate a similar amount of plasticity and thus affect hemispatial neglect in the same way. However, adaptation to left-sided visual displacement did not improve a group of five patients (see Rossetti *et al.* 1998*a*). As for specificity, this result also demonstrated that nonlateralized parameters such as arousal could not account for the effect of adaptation.

The last candidate mechanism is obviously associated with the attentional theory of neglect (see Section 5 of this volume). Pisella (1999) showed that the strong left–right attentional gradient observed in neglect patients (see Chapter 5.4) could be reduced following prism adaptation. However, further investigations are required to confirm whether prism adaptation mechanisms alter the brain mechanisms for the spatial distribution of attention, as there is no suggestion of such a link in the classical prism adaptation literature.

Figure 1 *Contd*   affected by the adaptation than controls (black arrows), and the magnitude of this effect was less variable in patients (arrow's whiskers). (b) Schenkenberg test line bisection performed by a patient group exposed to prism adaptation and a control group. The mean percentage deviation (±SEM) is initially shifted to the right in both groups, and patients tend to omit lines on the left side (values close to 100 per cent). Following goggle exposure, this initial deviation was significantly shifted to the left in the prism group. No significant difference was observed between post-test and late test. (c) The effect of prism adaptation on mental imagery. Maps of France plotted from the mental evocation of the patient prior to a prism exposure (pre-test) and immediately after removing the goggles (post-test). The dots indicate the geographical loci of the different responses and the bold number indicates the total number of responses. ((a) and (b) adapted with permission from Rossetti *et al.*, *Nature*, **395**, 166–9 (1998); (c) adapted with permission from Rode *et al.*, *Behavioural Neurology*, **11**, 251–8 (1998)).

Table 2 Stimulation of sensorimotor plasticity

Reference	Symptoms of neglect								Duration of the improvement
	Extrapersonal Neglect	Personal neglect	Imaginal neglect	Wheelchair driving	Reading	Postural instability	Subjective straight ahead	Other	
Rossetti et al. (1998a)	x				Text: +			Classical tests	≥2 h
Jacquin et al. (1998)	x			x			x		96 h ??
Rode et al. (1998)	x		x					Daisy	<24 h
Tilikete et al. (2001)						x			Immediate
Pisella et al. (2001)	x						x	Bisection	≥96 h
Farnè et al. (2001)	x				Words: +			Visuoverbal	≥24 h
Rode et al. (2001b)	x		x				x		Immediate
McIntosh et al. (2002)	x				Text: −			Haptic centering	1 week
Courtois-Jacquin (2001)	x							Dichotic listening	>2 h
Toutounji (2001)	x							Haptic matching	

Several studies have explored various aspects of hemispatial neglect before and after a short wedge prism adaptation session. Surprisingly, many aspects of neglect can be improved by this technique. However, more functional assessments are still needed and long-term effects remain to be explored.

One of the side-effects of questions about basic mechanisms is that they should help us to answer the intriguing question of why the effects of prism adaptation last for so long in the patients, whereas the after-effects observed in normal subjects in the same conditions resolve within a few minutes.

The main interest of prism adaptation is that the effects produced by a single 5-min session of adaptation last for much longer than for any other method. Two group studies showed fully sustained effects after 2 h (Rossetti et al. 1998a,b) and 1 day (Farnè et al. 2002). Case studies have reported even more prolonged improvements, lasting for about 4 days (Pisella et al. 2001; Jacquin et al. 1998; quoted by Rossetti et al. 1999a). Although a recent group study found no improvement in neglect 1 week after the adaptation session (Farnè et al. 2001), it is possible that some patients are improved for a longer period than others (McIntosh et al. 2002). However, the best prospect for rehabilitation purposes is to repeat adaptation sessions. We have investigated the effects of a daily session of adaptation and found no further improvement in the days following the initial exposure to prisms.[1] Thus a controlled clinical trial has been initiated with a weekly exposure to prisms. So far only a few measures of the functional outcome for the patients have been provided (e.g. wheel chair driving or postural control) and the outcome will need to be investigated carefully.

One of the crucial questions raised by the observation of a strong and sustained improvement of hemispatial neglect by a single short adaptation session is whether this plastic effect is restricted to the acute phase of the deficit. In our original study patients were tested between 3 weeks and 14 months post-stroke (Rossetti et al. 1998a). We have now collected data on a group of patients who were exposed to the adaptation procedure between 5 and 12 years post-stroke and surprisingly found the same amount of improvement. Figure 2 shows the example of a patient who benefited from prism adaptation 6 years after her stroke.

One of the most striking aspects of prism exposure in neglect patients is that, in strong contrast with healthy subjects, they exhibit a reduced awareness of the optical effects of the prisms. Most patients performed accurate pointing movements with the prisms on, which implies that their initially misdirected pointing trajectories are corrected during the course of the movement. However, they do not report that the goggles are responsible for any visual distortion, even when specifically questioned. In a way, they show a kind of 'hypernosognosia', as if they had been so used to missing things on the left side that they over-attribute the prism-induced errors to themselves. This hypothesis would also explain why they develop more adaptation than healthy individuals in identical prism exposure conditions.

Taken as a whole, investigations of the effects of prism adaptation on unilateral neglect have been very frustrating in terms of the difficulty in providing plausible theoretical accounts for the strong positive effects produced. These effects can by no means be compared with the classical understanding of prism adaptation in healthy individuals, for which both the duration and the generalization of the adaptation after-effects are extremely restricted. However, two interesting perspectives have emerged from these studies. The theoretical perspective is that it seems possible to emulate hemispatial neglect in healthy individuals (Colent et al. 2000; N. Berberovic and J.B. Mattingley 2002, personal communication; Michel et al. 2002). The practical perspective is that the long duration of the improvement produced by prism adaptation should give rise to clinical studies proposing routine protocols for the rehabilitation of patients.

---

[1] The first study was published on this issue while this book was in press. It was observed that a group of patients performing a daily session of prism adaptation over two weeks presented a significant improvement of several neglect parameters (Frassinetti et al., Brain 2002, **125**, 608–23.)

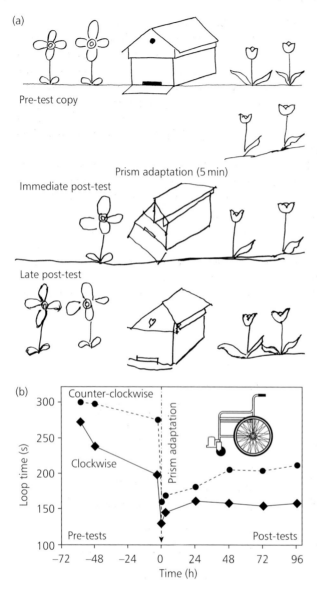

(a)

Pre-test copy

Prism adaptation (5 min)

Immediate post-test

Late post-test

(b)

Figure 2 Toward rehabilitation. (a) Prism adaptation in persistent neglect. Copy drawing was explored 5 years after the stroke in a case of persistent hemispatial neglect. The patient was a 72-year-old right-handed female who suffered from a severe left hemiplegia with left hemi-anesthesia, hemianopia, and neglect following a large hematoma of the right cerebral hemisphere. The patient had benefited from specific active training for neglect and caloric vestibular stimulation during the first year post-stroke. Before prism exposure (pre-test), she copied only the most rightward parts of the drawing, showing an associated object-centered neglect. In the immediate post-test, two items were added to the patient's drawing; in the late test (after 2 h), all items are drawn, the object-centered neglect was reduced (limited to the beehive), and the constructive apraxia had also improved. (b) The effect of prism adaptation on wheel-chair driving. A patient was repeatedly tested prior to and following a short prism adaptation session for his ability to make one tour of the medical unit (either clockwise or anticlockwise). An abrupt improvement was produced by prism adaptation and partly sustained over the 96 h follow-up (from Jacquin et al. 1998).

Toward rehabilitation of neglect

In most of the studies discussed above the improvement of neglect lasted for only a limited time. Even the prolonged improvement produced by a short prism adaptation session could not be used within the daily routine to cure neglect. However, there are several ways in which rehabilitation protocols could be based on physiological manipulations of neglect patients. First, several techniques could be combined to gain efficiency. Second, the single-application experiments that have been reported so far could be repeated in such a way as to increase the magnitude and/or the duration of the positive effects. Such approaches would open the way for devising effective rehabilitation procedures. Although these approaches are still in their infancy, a few recent trials have been conducted recently. One of the best examples of rigorous clinical research that has both combined techniques and used a daily application has been provided by Schindler *et al.* (2002). These authors have tested a rehabilitation paradigm where patients were subjected to neck muscle vibration for 6 weeks and then followed up for 8 weeks. Using a cross-over design, two groups of 10 patients were subjected to visual exploration training alone and then to visual exploration training plus neck muscle vibration (or the reverse). Each of the two types of treatment was applied daily for 3 weeks using simple tasks different from the pre- and post-probe tests. Not only the classical visual cancellation test and text reading were improved, but a tactile exploration task was also significantly ameliorated by the combined therapy. Only the horizontal size-matching task was not improved by either therapy.

For a functional approach, it is useful to distinguish which level of disease expression is altered by passive or active stimulation. Most studies reported improvement of symptoms of neglect corresponding to the clinical level of disease expression, according to the W.H.O. model (1973) (Fig. 3). Only a few studies have evaluated the effects of stimulations on incapacity, and none have evaluated the effect on handicap (Luauté, Halligan *et al.* 2001). One theoretical approach is to distinguish three types of procedures for cognitive neurovisual rehabilitation—restitution, compensation and substitution—according to their specific anatomical and physiological substrates (Kerkhoff 2000). One may also identify interest in a functional assessment of neglect rehabilitation. Wiart *et al.* (1997) reported a sustained improvement of disability and handicap due to neglect

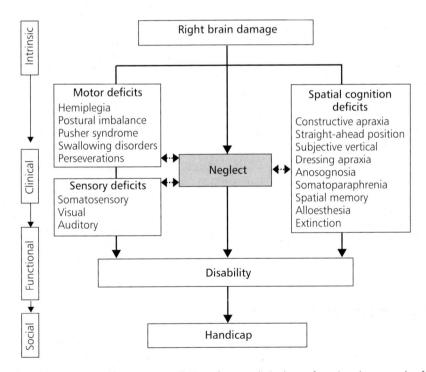

Figure 3 Levels of action of sensory stimulation: from a clinical to a functional approach of neglect rehabilitation. At a clinical level, a neglect syndrome is rarely pure. It is most frequently associated with other deficits according to the topography and size of the damage to the right hemisphere. These deficits may influence the manifestations of neglect and conversely neglect may worsen the severity of motor or sensory deficits (Vallar *et al.* 1997*b*). They may affect the locomotion, the posture, and activities of daily life. A precise identification of these deficits is necessary because they all contribute to the disability of the patient. Therefore it is difficult to identify the precise contribution of neglect *per se* to the disability.

produced by an original method combining voluntary trunk rotation (controlled by an orthosis) with scanning training. However, the hemispatial neglect syndrome is often associated with other disorders such as motor, sensory, or other spatial cognition deficits. These associated deficits are influenced by neglect; for example, motor or sensory deficits may be worsened by neglect and they then contribute to the handicap. It is indeed difficult, in a rehabilitation context, to distinguish clearly the components of disability that are specifically attributable to neglect from those due to motor, sensory, or other visuospatial disorders. A global improvement of the functional outcome and overall life quality of hemineglect patients is the ultimate goal of rehabilitation research.

As mentioned above, our preliminary observations suggested that a daily application of prism adaptation does not produce a cumulative gain. However, McIntosh et al. (2002) applied prism adaptation weekly for a 3-week period and observed a sustained improvement in one case.

So far, evaluation of functional parameters has rarely been reported in the literature, while classical neuropsychological testing has been used extensively. The effects of vestibular, somato-sensory, or proprioceptive stimulations on neglect constitute a powerful way of studying the integration of different sensory inputs in yielding reference frames based not on individual peripheral sensory codes, but on ego-centered and object- or environment-centered coordinates. On the other hand, the practical value for the rehabilitation of right-brain-damaged patients still appears to be rather limited. Previous studies reported the reduction of neglect symptomatology in sometimes very spectacular ways, but no accompanying general reduction of incapacity and disadvantage was reported. No functional improvement has been yet reported after the reduction of somatosensory and motor deficits through vestibular stimulation, TENS or OKS. The only functional improvement reported after sensory stimulation was the reduction of postural instability after vestibular stimulation (Rode et al. 1997), TENS (Perennou et al. 2001), or prism adaptation (Tilikete et al. 2001), but as for other symptoms this effect was transient after a single session. It is essential that such investigations are developed further in the near future (Fig. 3).

Conclusions

Two main points deserve discussion here: the question of the research strategy to develop an optimal technique for both the rehabilitation and the understanding of hemispatial neglect, and the question of brain structures participating in the recovery.

Two main aims have been followed by most of the techniques proposed for alleviating hemispatial neglect. A first pragmatic clinical approach is aimed at improving the perceptual and behavioral biases by acting on the patient's awareness of the deficit, i.e. on the highest cognitive levels. A second physiological approach is aimed at altering the balance of sensory inputs between the left and the right. Neglect is a deficit in spatial awareness which has been treated for years by *training* the patient to *intentionally* orient his or her attention to the left. The studies reviewed here suggest that an opposite view should be considered. Previous researchers have focused on *physiological* but *passive* maneuvers which allowed them to bypass the central awareness deficit. However, the passive processes at work in such cases do not produce long-lasting effects. These two strategies have now proved to be complementary. A combination of the learning aspects of the former methods with the physiological rational of the latter techniques seems to produce the best results so far. It is when a physiological level of learning (i.e. adaptation) is activated that the most prolonged positive effects are observed in the patients. Paradoxically, it thus seems that the lowest level of activation of the spatial functions of patients is associated with the strongest improvement of spatial neglect. It is interesting to note that even this approach has largely focused on the head level. Neck posture or tendon vibration could have been applied to other body segments, but it is only recently that tendon vibration has been applied to the sole of the foot (Richard et al. 2001), that TMS has been applied to the arm (Heldmann *et al.* 2000), and that a visual shift through wedge prisms has been coupled with an arm motor task (Rossett 1998*a*).

The optimal level of action that should be used clinically to treat hemispatial neglect still has to be precisely defined. Specifically, it does not appear to be sufficient that an action is involved in the rehabilitation procedure (Rode *et al.* 2001*a*). For example, the implicit low level of error processing involved in prism adaptation appears to produce longer-lasting effects (Farnè *et al.* 2001) than the more explicit high level of error processing involved in a bar-lifting task (see Chapter 7.2), even though an action is performed in the two cases. This is consistent with the idea that dorsal-like mechanisms (e.g. visuomotor, online feedback-based guidance) may be less impaired than perceptual judgments (e.g. offline error processing of the finger contact on the bar) in patients with hemispatial neglect. On the practical side, it may be that active training procedures would be most fruitfully employed after sensory stimulation has first produced an improvement of the patients' awareness of their deficit. The interaction of bottom-up and top-down mechanisms for neglect reduction may prove to be very efficient when appropriately coordinated.

These observations should further stimulate a reconsideration of the interpretations provided for the improvement of neglect through physiological manipulations. Specifically, the interpretations of the mechanisms of neglect improvement, and thus of the physiopathology of this condition, may have to be revised to lower levels. The recent observations that a minor form of hemispatial neglect can be emulated in healthy individuals by a simple visuomanual adaptation task using left-deviating wedge prisms (Colent *et al.* 2000; N. Berberovic and J.B. Mattingley 2002, personal communication; Michel *et al.* 2002) is particularly suggestive of such a close link between low-level sensory processing and higher-level spatial cognition (Rossetti *et al.* 1999).

It has often been stated that a hemispheric imbalance might be responsible for unilateral neglect and therefore that the weaker hemisphere should be stimulated in order to strengthen its weight in the balance. Thus most of the sensory stimulations used with hemispatial neglect have been aimed at activating the damaged hemisphere. However, these physiological maneuvers can be effective even in presence of large lesions of the right hemisphere, which suggests that other structures may be involved in the compensation of the deficit. It is obvious that most physiological maneuvers primarily stimulate subcortical structures, especially at the brainstem level. In the particular case of prism adaptation, a number of neuropsychological studies have shown that the only patients who are impaired in adapting to wedge prisms are patients with a lesion at the cerebellar level (review: Jeannerod and Rossetti 1993). Even patients with bilateral lesions of the posterior parietal cortex can adapt to prisms as well as normal subjects (Pisella *et al.* 2002*a*). Therefore one may suspect that the equilibrium between the two hemispheres can be counterbalanced by the equilibrium between symmetric subcortical structures such as the cerebellum, as was indicated by the famous cat lesion experiments reported by Sprague (1966). In support of this view it is interesting to note that a TMS-induced inhibition of the left parietal cortex and the adaptation to wedge prisms shifting vision to the left induce a similar bias in line bisection performed by normal individuals (Colent *et al.* 2000; Fierro *et al.* 2000). Although brain imaging studies are necessary for the precise elucidation of these neuroanatomical aspects, these observations may already lead to the paradigm shift of using low-level sensorimotor transformation for the systematic modulation of high-level spatial attentional processes.

In summary, the sensory stimulations used to alleviate the clinical and neuropsychological manifestations of unilateral neglect have failed so far to fulfil their main objectives. First, they have not been very instructive about the fundamental basis of unilateral neglect. However, recent new perspectives have been offered, for example via the association of several techniques during brain imaging (Bottini *et al.* 2001) or the simulation of neglect in healthy subjects (e.g. Colent *et al.* 2000), which should provide a tool for understanding the physiopathological basis of hemispatial neglect. Second, the functional outcome of exposure to these forms of stimulation has not been sufficiently investigated and therefore they have not yet given rise to practical rehabilitation routines. However, longer-term improvement of neglect symptoms is now available (Rossetti *et al.* 1998*a*; Farnè *et al.* 2001; Pisella *et al.* 2001) and studies of repetitive stimulation of single or combined techniques are now in progress (Schindler *et al.* 2002). Therefore the currently frustrating overview of the status of sensory manipulations in the understanding and rehabilitation of unilateral neglect should be positively moderated by several promising approaches.

Acknowledgements

This work was supported by INSERM (PROGRES), MENRT (French Ministry of Research, grant Cognitique). The authors wish to thank David Milner and Giuseppe Vallar for their constructive comments on an earlier version of this chapter, Dominique Boisson, Sophie Courtois-Jacquin, Peter Halligan, Jacques Luauté, Carine Michel, Laure Pisella, and Xavier Rochet for stimulating discussions, and Maurice Rossetti for his artistic touch.

References

Andersen, R. A. (1995) Encoding of intention and spatial location in the posterior parietal cortex. *Cerebral Cortex*, **5**, 457–69.

Antonucci, G., Guariglia, C., Judica, A., *et al.* (1995). Effectiveness of neglect rehabilitation in a randomized group study. *Journal of Clinical and Experimental Neuropsychology*, **17**, 383–9.

Bartolomeo, P. and Chokron, S. (1999). Egocentric frame of reference: its role in spatial bias after right hemisphere lesions. *Neuropsychologia*, **37**, 881–94.

Bisiach, E., Vallar, G., Perani, D., Papagno, C., and Berti, A. (1986). Unawareness of disease following lesions of the right hemisphere: anosognosia for hemiplegia and anosognosia for hemianopia. *Neuropsychologia*, **24**, 759–67.

Bisiach, E., Rusconi, M. L., and Vallar, G. (1991). Remission of somatoparaphrenic delusion through vestibular stimulation. *Neuropsychologia*, **29**, 1029–31.

Bottini, G., Sterzi, R., Paulesu, E., *et al.* (1994). Identification of the central vestibular projections in man: a positron emission tomography activation study. *Experimental Brain Research*, **99**, 164–9.

Bottini, G., Karnath, H.-O., Vallar, G., *et al.* (2001). Cerebral representations for egocentric space. Functional-anatomical evidence from caloric vestibular stimulation and neck vibration. *Brain*, **124**, 1182–96.

Cappa, S., Sterzi, R., Vallar, G., and Bisiach, E. (1987). Remission of hemineglect and anosognosia during vestibular stimulation. *Neuropsychologia*, **25**, 775–82.

Chokron, S. and Imbert, M. (1995). Variations of the egocentric reference among normal subjects and a patient with unilateral neglect. *Neuropsychologia*, **33**, 703–11.

Coello, Y., Orliaguet, J. P., and Prablanc, C. (1996). Pointing movement in an artificial perturbing inertial field: a prospective paradigm for motor control study. *Neuropsychologia*, **34**, 879–92.

Colent *et al.* (2000).

Courtois-Jacquin, S., Ota, H., Rode, G., Boisson, D., and Rossetti, Y. Visuo-manual adaptation to shifting wedge prisms improve mental number bisection. Unpublished manuscript.

Courtois-Jacquin, S., Rossetti, Y., Rode, G., *et al.* (2001). Effect of prism adaptation on auditory extinction: an attentional effect? Presented at International Symposium on Neural Control of space coding and action production, Lyon, 22–24 March 2001.

Denes G., Semenza, C., Stoppa, E., Lis, A. (1982). Unilateral spatial neglect and recovery from hemiplegia: a follow up study. *Brain*, **105** (Pt. 3), 543–52.

Diller, L. and Weinberg, J. (1997). Hemi-inattention in rehabilitation: the evolution of a rational remediation program. *Advances in Neurology*, **18**, 63–82.

Farnè, A., Ponti, F., and Làdavas, E. (1998). In search for biased egocentric reference frames in neglect. *Neuropsychologia*, **36**, 611–23.

Farnè, A., Rossetti, Y., Toniolo, S., and Làdavas, E. (2002). Ameliorating neglect with prism adaptation: visuo-manual vs. visuo-verbal measures. *Neuropsychologia*, **40, 7**, 1069–80.

Fierro, B., Brighina, F., Oliveri., M, *et al.* (2000). Contralateral neglect induced by right posterior parietal rTMS in healthy subjects. *NeuroReport*, **11**, 1519–21.

Fullerton, K. J., McSherry, D., and Stout, R. W. (1986). Albert's test: a neglected test of perpetual neglect. *Lancet*, **22**; 1(8478), 430–2.

Gainotti, G., Messerli, P., and Tissot, R. (1972).Qualitative analysis of unilateral spatial neglect in relation to laterality of cerebral lesions. *Journal of Neurology, Neurosurgery, and Psychiatry*, **35**, 545–50.

Geminiani, G. and Bottini, G. (1992). Mental representation and temporary recovery from unilateral neglect after vestibular stimulation. *Journal of Neurology, Neurosurgery, and Psychiatry*, **55**, 332–3.

Guariglia, C., Lippolis, G., and Pizzamiglio, L. (1998). Somatosensory stimulation improves imagery disorders in neglect. *Cortex*, **34**, 233–41.

Guariglia, C., Coriale, G., Cosentino, T., and Pizzamiglio, L. (2000). TENS modulates spatial reorientation in neglect patients. *NeuroReport*, **11**, 1945–8.

Harvey, M. and Milner, A. D. (1999). Residual perceptual distortion in 'recovered' hemispatial neglect. *Neuropsychologia*, **37**, 745–50.

Halligan, P. W., Marshall, J. C., and Wade, D. T. (1989). Visuospatial neglect: Underlying factors and test sensitivity. *Lancet*, **14**; 2(8668), 908–11.

Heilman, K. M., Watson, R. T., Valenstein, E. (1985). Neglect and related disorders. In *Clinical Neuropsychology*, (ed. K. M. Heilman and E. Valenstein). pp. 243–93. Oxford University Press, New York, 1985.

Heldmann, B., Kerkhoff, G., Struppler, A., Havel, P., and Jahn, T. (2000). Repetitive peripheral magnetic stimulation alleviates tactile extinction. *NeuroReport*, **11**, 3193–8.

Hommel, M., Peres, B., Pollak, P., *et al.* (1990). Effects of passive tactile and auditory stimuli on left visual neglect. *Archives of Neurology*, **47**, 573–5.

Jacquin, S., Luauté, J., Li, L., Rode, G., Rossetti, Y., and Boisson, D. (1998). Amélioration de la conduite en fauteuil roulant après adaptation prismatique chez le patient héminégligent. *Annales de Médecine Physique et de Réadaptation*, **41**, 320–1.

Jeannerod, M. and Biguer, B. (1987). The directional coding of reaching movements: a visuo-motor conception of spatial neglect. In *Neurophysiological and neuropsychological aspects of spatial neglect* (ed. M. Jeannerod), pp. 87–113. North-Holland, Amsterdam.

Jeannerod, M. and Rossetti, Y. (1993). Visuomotor coordination as a dissociable function : experimental and clinical evidence. In *Visual perceptual defects. Baillère's clinical neurology: international practice and research* (ed. C. Kennard), pp. 439–60. Baillière Tindall, London.

Joanette, Y., Brouchon, M., Gauthier, L., and Samson, M. (1986). Pointing with left vs right hand in left visual field neglect. *Neuropsychologia*, **24**, 391–6.

Karnath, H.-O. (1994). Subjective body orientation in neglect and the interactive contribution of neck muscle proprioception and vestibular stimulation. *Brain*, **117**, 1001–12.

Karnath, H.-O. (1995). Transcutaneous electrical stimulation and vibration of neck muscles in neglect. *Experimental Brain Research*, **105**, 321–4.

Karnath, H.-O. (1996). Optokinetic stimulation influences the disturbed perception of body orientation in spatial neglect. *Journal of Neurology, Neurosurgery, and Psychiatry*, **60**, 217–20.

Karnath, H.-O. (1997). Neural encoding of space in egocentric coordinates? Evidence for and limits of a hypothesis derived from patients with parietal lesions and neglect. In *Parietal lobe contribution to orientation in 3D space*, (ed. P. Thier and H. O. Karnath). pp. 497–520. Springer-Verlag, Berlin.

Karnath, H.-O., Christ, K., and Hartje, W. (1993). Decrease of contralateral neglect by neck muscle vibration and spatial orientation of trunk midline. *Brain*, **116**, 383–96.

Karnath, H.-O., Fetter, M., and Dichgans, J. (1996). Ocular exploration of space as a function of neck proprioceptive and vestibular input: observations in normal subjects and patients with spatial neglect after parietal lesions. *Experimental Brain Research*, **109**, 333–42.

Kerkhoff, G. (1998). Rehabilitation of visuospatial cognition and visual exploration in neglect: a cross-over study. *Restorative Neurology and Neuroscience*, **12**, 27–40.

Kerkhoff, G. (2000). Multiple perceptual distortions and their modulation in left sided visual neglect. *Neuropsychlogia*, **38**, 1073–86.

Kerkhoff, G., Schindler, I., Keller, I., and Marquardt, C. (1999). Visual background motion reduces size distortion in spatial neglect. *NeuroReport*, **10**, 319–23.

Luauté, J., Rode, G., Jacquin-Courtois, S., Pisella, L., Boisson, D., and Rossetti, Y. (2000). Improvement of left spatial neglect after prismatic adaptation: lateralized warning signal or cerebral plasticity? Presented at European Conference on Cognitive and Neural Bases of Spatial Neglect, Como, 14–17 September 2000.

Luauté, J. and Halligan, P. A. A systematic and critical review of attempts to remediate visuo-spatial neglect. Unpublished manuscript.

McIntosh, R. M., Rossetti, Y., and Milner, A. D. (2002). Prism adaptation improves chronic visual and haptic neglect. *Cortex*, in press.

Marshall, C. R. and Maynard, F. M. (1983). Vestibular stimulation for supranuclear gaze palsy: a case report. *Archives of Physical Medicine and Rehabilitation*, **64**, 134–6.

Mattingley, J. B., Bradshaw, J. L., and Bradshaw, J. A. (1994). Horizontal visual motion modulates focal attention in left unilateral spatial neglect. *Journal of Neurology, Neurosurgery, and Psychiatry*, **57**, 1228–35.

Michel, C., Pisella, L., Halligan, P., Rode, G., Luauté, J., Boisson, D., Rossetti, Y. (2002). Simulating unilateral neglect using prism adaptation: Implications for theory. *Neuropsychologia*, in press.

Milner, A. D. and Goodale, M. A. (1995). *The visual brain in action*. Oxford University Press.

Milner, A. D. and Harvey, M. (1995). Distortion of size perception in visuospatial neglect. *Current Biology*, **5**, 85–9.

Milner, A. D., Harvey, M., and Pritchard, C. L. (1998). Visual size processing in spatial neglect. *Experimental Brain Research*, **123**, 192–200.

Perennou, D. A., Leblond, C., Amblard, B., Micallef, J. P., Herisson, C., and Pelissier, J. Y. (2001). Transcutaneous electric nerve stimulation reduces neglect-related postural instability after stroke. *Archives of Physical Medicine and Rehabilitation*, **82**, 440–8.

Pisella, L. (1999). Multiples voies en interaction pour la perception et l'action: processus automatique et volontaire de guidage visuo-manuel et diversité des syndromes pariétaux. Ph.D. dissertation, Lyon University.

Pisella, L. and Mattingley, J. B. (2001). Prism adaptation improves temporal order judgement in unilateral neglect patients. Unpublished manuscript.

Pisella, L. and Rossetti, Y. (2000). Interaction between conscious identification and non-conscious sensori-motor processing: temporal constraints. In *Beyond dissociation: interaction between dissociated implicit and explicit processing* (ed. Y. Rossetti and A. Revonsuo), pp. 129–51. Benjamins, Amsterdam.

Pisella, L., Michel, C., and Rossetti, Y. (2002*a*). Prism adptation following a bilateral lesion of the posterior parietal cortex. Submitted for publication.

Pisella, L., Rode, G., Farnè, A., Boisson, D., and Rossetti, Y. (2002*b*). Dissociated long lasting improvements of straight-ahead pointing and line bisection tasks in two hemineglect patients. *Neuropsychologia*, **40, 3**, 327–324.

Pisella, L., Michel, C.,Tilikete, C., Vighetto, A., and Rosetti, Y. (2002*c*). Preserved prism adaptation following a bilateral lesion of the posterior parietal cortex. Submitted manuscript.

Pizzamiglio, L., Frasca, R., Guariglia, C., Incoccia, C., and Antonucci, G. (1990). Effect of optokinetic stimulation in patients with visual neglect. *Cortex*, **26**, 535–40.

Pritchard, C. L., Milner, A. D., Dijkerman, H. C., and MacWalter, R. S. (1997). Visuospatial neglect: veridical coding of size for graping but not for perception. *Neurocase*, **3**, 437–43.

Ramachandran, V. S. (1995). Anosognosia in parietal lobe syndrome. *Consciousness and Cognition*, **4**, 22–51.

Redding, G. M. and Wallace, B. (1997). *Adaptive spatial alignment*. Lawrence Erlbaum, Mahwah, NJ.

Richard, C., Rousseaux, M., and Honoré, J. (2001). Plantar stimulation can affect subjective straight-ahead in neglect patients. *Neuroscience Letters*, **301**, 64–8.

Robertson, I. H. (1991). Use of left versus right hand in responding to lateralized stimuli in unilateral neglect. *Neuropsychologia*, **29**, 1129–35.

Robertson, I. H. (1999). Cognitive rehabilitation: attention and neglect. *Trends in Cognitive Sciences*, **3**, 385–93.

Robertson, I. H., North, N., Geggie, C. (1992). Spatio-motor cueing in unilateral neglect: three single case studies of its therapeutic effects. *Journal of Neurology, Neurosurgery and Psychiatry*, **55**, 799–805.

Robertson, I. H., Nico, D., and Hood, B. M. (1995). The intention to act improves unilateral left neglect: two demonstrations. *NeuroReport*, **7**, 246–8.

Robertson, I. H., Mattingley, J. B., Rorden, C., and Driver, J. (1998*a*). Phasic alerting of neglect patients overcomes their spatial deficit in visual awareness. *Nature*, **395**, 169–72.

Robertson, I. H., Hogg, K. H., and MacMillan, T. M. (1998*b*). Rehabilitation of unilateral neglect: improving function by contralesional limb activation. *Neuropsychological Rehabilitation*, **8**, 19–29.

Rode, G. and Perenin, M. T. (1994). Tempory remission of representational hemineglect through vestibular stimulation. *NeuroReport*, **5**, 869–72.

Rode, G., Charles, N., Perenin, M. T., Vighetto, A., Trillet, M., and Aimard, G. (1992). Partial remission of hemiplegia and somatoparaphrenia through vestibular stimulation in a case of unilateral neglect. *Cortex*, **28**, 203–8.

Rode, G., Tiliket, C., and Boisson, D. (1997). Predominance of postural imbalance in left hemiparetic patients. *Scandinavian Journal of Rehabilitation Medicine*, **29**(1), 11–16.

Rode, G., Perenin, M. T., Honoré, J., and Boisson, D. (1998*a*). Improvement of the motor deficit of neglect patients through vestibular stimulation: evidence for a motor neglect component. *Cortex*, **3**, 253–6.

Rode, G., Tiliket, C., Honoré, J., and Boisson, D. (1998*b*). Postural asymmetry is reduced by caloric stimulation in left hemiparetic patients. *Scandinavian Journal of Rehabilitation Medicine*, **30**, 9–14.

Rode, G., Rossetti, Y., Li, L., and Boisson, D. (1998*c*). The effect of prism adaptation on neglect for visual imagery. *Behavioural Neurology*, **11**, 251–8.

Rode, G., Perenin, MT., Tiliket, C., and Boisson, D. (1998*d*). Apports des stimulations vestibulaires dans la négligence unilatérale. In *Les syndromes de négligence spatiale* (ed. D. Perennou, V. Brun, and J. Pélissier), pp. 278–84. Masson, Paris.

Rode, G., Rossetti, Y., Badan, M., and Boisson, D. (2001*a*). Role of action in the rehabilitation of hemineglect syndromes. (Rôle de l'action dans la rééducation du syndrome d'héminégligence). *Revue Neurologique*, **157**, 497–505.

Rode, G., Rossetti, Y., and Boisson, D. (2001*b*). Prism adaptation improves representational neglect. *Neuropsychologia*, **39**, 1250–4.

Rode, G., Tilikete, C., Luauté, J., Rossetti, Y., Vighetto, A., and Boisson, D. (2002). Bilateral stimulation does not improve visual hemineglect. *Neuropsychologia*, **39**, 11, 1250–4.

Rorsman, I., Magnusson, M., and Johansson B. B. (1999). Reduction of visuo-spatial neglect with vestibular galvanic stimulation. *Scandinavian Journal of Rehabilitation Medicine*, **31**, 117–24.

Rossetti, Y. (1998). Implicit short-lived motor representation of space in brain-damaged and healty subjects. *Consciousness and Cognition*, **7**, 520–58.

Rossetti, Y. and Pisella, L. (2002). Several 'vision for action' systems: A guide to dissociating and integrating dorsal and ventral functions. In *Attention and performance XIX: common mechnisms in perception and action* (ed. W. Prinz and B. Hommel). pp. 62–119. Oxford University Press.

Rossetti, Y., Rode, G., Pisella, L., Farnè, A., Li, L., and Boisson, D. (1998*a*). Prism adaptation to a rightward optical deviation rehabilitates left hemispatial neglect. *Nature*, **395**, 166–9.

Rossetti, Y., Rode, G., Cheikh-Rouhou, M., *et al.* (1998*b*). Amélioration durable des symptômes de la négligence par adaptation prismatique: quels arguments pour les théories référentielle, attentionnelle et intégrationnelle? In *Les syndromes de négligence spatiale* (ed. D. Perennou, V. Brun, and J. Pélissier), pp. 299–310. Masson, Paris.

Rossetti, Y., Rode, G., Pisella, L., Farnè, A., Ling, L., and Boisson, D. (1999*a*). Sensorimotor plasticity and cognition: prism adaptation can affect various levels of space representation. In *Studies in perception and action* (ed. M. Grealy and J. A. Thomson), pp. 265–9. Lawrence Erlbaum, Mahwah, NJ.

Rossetti, Y., Rode, G., Boisson, D., and Pélisson, D. (1999*b*). Tromper le cerveau pour le guérir. *La Recherche*, **324**, 31–4.

Rossetti, Y., Rode, G., and Boisson, D. (1999*c*). Sensori-motor plasticity and the rehabilitation of hemispatial neglect (Plasticité sensori-motrice et récupération fonctionnelle: les effets thérapeutiques de l'adaptation prismatique sur la négligence spatiale unilatérale). *Médecine/Sciences*, **15**, 239–45.

Rubens, A. B. (1985). Caloric stimulation and unilateral visual neglect. *Neurology*, **35**, 1019–24.

Samuel, C., Louis-Dreyfus, A., Kashel, R., *et al.* (1998). Apport de l'indiçage spatio-moteur dans la rééducation de l'héminégligence gauche. In *Les syndromes de négligence spatiale* (ed. D. Perennou, V. Brun, and J. Pélissier), pp. 244–53. Masson, Paris.

Schenkenberg, T., Bradford, D. C., and Ajax, E. T. (1980). Line bisection with neurologic impairment. *Neurology*, **30**, 509–17.

Schindler, I., Kerkhoff, G., Karnath, H.-O., Keller, I., and Goldenberg, G. (2002). Neck muscle vibration induces lasting recovery in spatial neglect. *Journal of Neurology, Neurosurgery, and Psychiatry*, in press.

Sekiyama, K, Miyauchi, S, Imaruoka, T, Egusa, H, and Tashiro, T. (2000). Body image as a visuomotor transformation device revealed in adaptation to reversed vision. *Nature*, **407**, 374–7.

Silberpfennig, J. (1941). Contributions to the problem of eye movements. III: Disturbances of ocular movements with pseudohemianopsia in frontal lobe tumors. *Confinia Neurologica*, **4**, 1–13.

Sprague, J. M. (1966). Interaction of cortex and superior colliculus in mediation of visually guided behaviour in the cat. *Science*, **153**, 1544–7.

Tilikete, C., Rode, G., Rossetti, Y., Li, L., Pichon, J., and Boisson, D. (2001). Prism adaptation to rightward optical deviation improves postural imbalance in left hemiparetic patients. *Current Biology*, **11**, 524–8.

Toutounji, N., Michel, C., Luauté, J., Rode, G., Boisson, D., and Rossetti, Y. (2001). *Prism adaptation improves haptic object recognition in hemispatial neglect*. Société de Neuropsychologie de Langue Française, Paris.

Vallar, G., Sterzi, R., Bottini, G., Cappa, S., and Rusconi, M. L. (1990). Temporary remission of left hemianesthesia after vestibular stimulation: a sensory neglect phenomenon. *Cortex*, **26**, 123–31.

Vallar, G., Antonucci, G., Guariglia, C., and Pizzamiglio, L. (1993a). Deficits of position sense, unilateral neglect and optokinetic stimulation. *Neuropsychologia*, **31**, 1191–1200.

Vallar, G., Bottini, G., Rusconi, M. L., and Sterzi, R. (1993b). Exploring somatosensory hemineglect by vestibular stimulation. *Brain*, **116**, 71–8.

Vallar, G., Papagno, C., Rusconi, M. L., and Bisiach, E. (1995a). Vestibular stimulation, spatial hemineglect and dysphasia. Selective effects? *Cortex*, **31**, 589–93.

Vallar, G., Guariglia, C., Magnotti, L., and Pizzamiglio, L. (1995b). Optokinetic stimulation affects both vertical and horizontal deficits of position sense in unilateral neglect. *Cortex*, **31**, 669–83.

Vallar, G., Rusconi, M. L., Barozzi, S. *et al.* (1995c). Improvement of left visuo-spatial hemi-neglect by left-sided transcutaneous electrical stimulation. *Neuropsychologia*, **33**, 73–82.

Vallar, G., Rusconi, M. L., and Bernardini, B. (1996). Modulation of neglect hemianestheisa by transcutaneous electrical stimulation. *Journal of the International Neuropsychological Society*, **2**, 452–9.

Vallar, G., Guariglia, C., Nico, D., and Pizzamiglio L. (1997a). Motor deficits and optokinetic stimulation in patients with left hemineglect. *Neurology*, **49**, 1364–70.

Vallar, G., Guariglia, C., and Rusconi, M. L. (1997b). Modulation of the neglect syndrome by sensory stimulation. In: *Parietal lobe contribution to orientation in 3D space* (ed. P. Thier and H.-O. Karnath), pp. 555–79. Springer Verlag, Heidelberg.

Wiart, L., Bon-Saint-Come, A., Debeilleix, X., *et al.* (1997). Unilateral neglect syndrome rehabilitation by trunk rotation and scanning training. *Archives of Physical Medicine and Rehabilitation*, **78**, 424–9.

Weinberg, J., Diller, L., Gordon, W. A., *et al.* (1977). Visual scanning training effect in reading related tasks in acquired right brain damage. *Archives of Physical Medicine and Rehabilitation*, **58**, 480–5.

Weinberg, J., Diller, L., Gordon, W. A., Gerstman, L. J., Lieberman, A., and Sawicki, J. (1979). Training sensory awareness ans spatial organization in people with right brain damage. *Archives of Physical Medicine and Rehabilitation*, **60**, 491–3.

W.H.O. (World Health Organisation). (1973). From the french translation: O.M.S. (Organisation Mondiale de la Santé) Classification internationale des handicaps: déficiences, incapacités et désavantages. Un manuel de classification des conséquences des maladies. Paris, CTNERRHI-INSERM, 1988, 202 pp.

Zorzi, M., Priftis, K., and Umilta, C. (2002). Neglect disrupts the mental number line. *Nature* **417**, 138–9.

Index